Lecture Notes: Emergency Medicine

To our parents, without whose help we would never have begun to learn about medicine

Contents

Preface to the Third Edition

Emergency medicine is changing. New developments, government targets, economic considerations and staffing problems have brought about rapid changes in traditional patterns of delivery of care. However, the injuries and illnesses, which cause patients to seek emergency assistance, are much less variable and thus their treatment forms a stable core for this book. We have tried to introduce change to clinical practice only when it is clearly an improvement. Although we have attempted to use the best available evidence, we have not been slaves to evidential doctrine when there were no clear or unequivocal recommendations to be found for commonly occurring problems. The format of this book is designed such that it is not only easy to use but also provides much more than just a simple set of lists and rules. We hope that it will guide and help the providers of emergency care, whoever they may be and wherever they may practise.

Chris Moulton and David Yates
Bolton, UK, 2006

Preface to the Second Edition

Emergency physicians work in an environment where measured interrogation is a luxury, where life-saving skills can be required urgently and where the art of rapid and effective communication is essential. Add to this list the expectation that the doctor will have an encyclopaedic knowledge of the emergency aspects of every medical condition – and not a few social crises – and it is not surprising that most medical students and young doctors approach the emergency department with an excitement that is tinged with anxiety.

This book is designed, in its approach, layout and content, to address these fears. Information is presented in an order that is relevant to the enquirer. It is demand led. Pathophysiology and relevant explanations follow. The reader learns how to deal with the emergency and then reads the background to the crisis and how, perhaps, it could have been avoided. This link with prevention is an increasingly emphasised part of emergency medicine, together with its concern to blur the boundaries between hospital and community care. Our primary aim has been to equip the reader with the knowledge to deal with crises, but we hope that we have shared, in these pages, our concern to ensure that doctors are also trained to try to avoid them.

Professor AD Redmond was the co-author of the first edition of this work, with Professor Yates. Although the book has been completely rewritten we have retained all the innovations that were so successfully introduced in *Lecture Notes on Accident and Emergency Medicine* in 1985. Professor Redmond has provided valuable advice on the development of this new edition and it is a pleasure to record our appreciation of this support and encouragement.

The authors are very grateful for the support of their families, whose accidents and emergencies were neglected during the writing of this book.

Chris Moulton and David Yates
Manchester, UK, 1999

Preface to the First Edition

Our aim has been to cover all aspects of the work of a doctor in a busy accident and emergency department. Much of the text should be of interest to medical students during their clinical studies, but we hope that the book will be of special value to doctors studying for postgraduate diplomas.

Clearly some restriction must be placed on our definition of accident and emergency work unless we are to be overwhelmed, both here as authors and in our departments as casualty officers. These lecture notes have not been conceived as comprehensive treatises on the management of the many topics discussed – for only some aspects of most diseases and injuries are germane to the accident and emergency department. But it is precisely these aspects that are often inadequately covered in the standard texts. This book is based on our daily experience of the plethora of conditions presenting to what is inevitably an unstructured environment.

Sections devoted to 'Urgent action' are designed to facilitate the book's use during emergencies. The remaining text continues this rather didactic format but is supported by background material, which attempts to justify our dogma. It is, however, not always enough to state that the advice given here has worked in practice (but it has!). Emergency medicine, like all other branches of medicine, must be based on sound scientific principles. A significant recent development has been the acceptance that emergencies are better treated by the experienced than used to gain experience. Future developments must ensure that the scientific method is woven into the fabric of the department.

The academic base for accident and emergency medicine in Manchester has been created by the foresight and hard work of three men. We wish to record our thanks to Professor M. H. Irving, Dr G. S. Laing and Professor H. B. Stoner who have given so much to the specialty in its early days and who have supported us during the preparation of this book. The doctors, nurses, clerical staff and patients of Salford and Stockport have also given us invaluable help. Their encouragement has been greatly appreciated. Jackie Fortin typed some of the preparatory work and Julie Rostron exercised great skill and patience in compiling the manuscript.

Veronica Yates responded to our vague requests for pictures with precise illustrations, and our publishers displayed remarkable tolerance during a long gestation.

D. W. Yates and A. D. Redmond,
August 1984

Chapter 1

The principles of emergency medicine

People from many different backgrounds, with an enormous variety of problems, present to an emergency department (ED) both by day and by night. Fortunately, certain basic principles are applicable to the care of them all.

Immediate (or primary) assessment and management of the patient

The priorities are as follows. In all cases, swift and accurate assessment must immediately lead to appropriate action.

For cardiac arrest protocols see page 156.
For further details of immediate assessment and management of children see Chapter 18, page 323.

A – Airway

The airway may be:
- patent, partially obstructed or completely obstructed (this results from physical obstruction or loss of muscle tone);
- adequately protected or at-risk (this depends on the protective reflexes of the airway).

Check for responsiveness
Is the patient alert and responsive to questions? A verbal reply confirms that there is:
- a maintained and protected airway;
- temporarily adequate breathing and circulation;
- cerebral functioning.

If responsive, then the patient will usually be able to elaborate on the cause of the sudden deterioration that has brought him or her to an ED.

Failure to respond indicates a significantly lowered level of consciousness and therefore an airway that may be obstructed and is definitely at risk. There may be a need for airway opening manoeuvres and action to protect the airway.

Look, listen and feel for breathing
The absence of breath sounds indicates the need to attempt airway opening manoeuvres (*see below*) and if unsuccessful to consider the possibility of a foreign body obstruction.

> Foreign body obstruction may initially present as a distressed, very agitated, cyanosed patient – 'choking'.

For choking protocols see page 205.
For respiratory arrest see page 208.
For cardiorespiratory arrest see Chapter 11, page 156.
If breathing is present then:

Look for the signs of partial upper airway obstruction
- *Snoring* – the familiar sound of obstruction caused by the soft tissues of the mouth and pharynx. Often it accompanies the reduced muscle tone of a lowered level of consciousness.
- *Rattling or gurgling* – the sound of fluids in the upper airway.
- *Stridor* – a harsh, 'crowing' noise, which is heard best in inspiration. It is thus different from

wheezing, which is usually loudest in expiration. Stridor suggests obstruction at the level of the larynx and upper trachea. General illness and temperature usually indicate an infection causing swelling. Obstruction by a foreign body is the other main cause.

> In cases of suspected supraglottic swelling, examination or instrumentation of the throat should not be carried out for fear of causing complete obstruction.

- *Drooling* – the inability to swallow saliva. It suggests blockage at the back of the throat.
- *Hoarseness* – gross voice change. This suggests obstruction at the level of the larynx.

> Cyanosis and reduced haemoglobin saturation readings on a pulse oximeter are very late signs of airway obstruction.

For clearance and protection of the airway *see below.*
For laryngotracheal obstruction see page 205.
For allergic reactions see page 295.
For surgical airways see page 23.

> Assess the need for cervical spine protection before any airway intervention.

Clearance and maintenance of the airway

A patent airway is a prerequisite for life; a blocked airway is a common harbinger of death in emergency situations. There are two main ways in which the airway becomes blocked.

1 The most common cause of airway obstruction is a depressed level of consciousness. The tone of the muscles controlling the patency of the mouth and the pharynx is under neural control in much the same way as is the activity of the other striated muscles of the body. When this control is lost the soft tissues around the airway prolapse and fail to maintain its patency (simplistically, the tongue falls back). This can be overcome by:

- tightening these tissues (chin lift manoeuvre);
- pushing the jaw and the hyoid bone and their attached soft tissues forward (jaw thrust manoeuvre);
- putting an artificial airway down the anatomical airway (oro- or naso-pharyngeal airways, endotracheal tubes, laryngeal masks, etc., *see Figure 1.1*).

2 The other way that the airway becomes blocked is by physical obstruction. Many things can do this (direct trauma, external or intramural mass, etc.) However, in emergency practice, there is usually

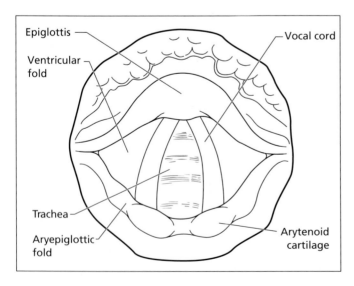

Epiglottis
Ventricular fold
Vocal cord
Trachea
Aryepiglottic fold
Arytenoid cartilage

Figure 1.1 Visualisation of the larynx.

either something in the airway (vomitus, blood or foreign body) or there is swelling in the wall of the airway (oedema, haematoma, etc.). This is overcome by:

- removing the cause of the obstruction (suction, manual removal or choking manoeuvres);
- passing an artificial airway (as detailed above) past the obstruction;
- reducing the swelling with vasoconstrictor drugs (adrenaline);
- bypassing the obstruction with a surgical airway.

Protection of the airway

The airway is normally kept clear of foreign matter by the gag, cough and laryngeal reflexes. These may be attenuated by specific palsies, the effects of drugs or a generalised depression of conscious level. They may also be impaired at the extremes of age and in states of general debilitation. Special vigilance is required in all such situations; the recovery position should be used whenever possible.

Paradoxically, these same reflexes may make advanced airway care extremely difficult in situations where they are not completely absent. At such times, the airway should be managed by a person skilled in both its assessment and the use of sedating and paralysing drugs.

> Over 10% of normal subjects have no gag reflex.

Laryngospasm, bleeding, vomiting and consequent hypoxia can result from ill-judged attempts at intubation. It should be noted that the absence of the gag reflex is not a good predictor of the need for (or the ease of) endotracheal intubation.

> In a patient with a reduced level of consciousness, the airway must be assumed to be at-risk until proved otherwise.

On-going protection of the airway requires continual vigilance. The following are also essential:
- The recovery position uses gravity, both to drain fluid matter away from the airway and to allow the soft tissues to be positioned in such a way that they do not cause obstruction. Once the airway is clear, this position can be used to both maintain and protect the airway.
- A high-flow suction catheter must always be near the patient's head.
- The patient's trolley must be capable of tilting "head down" so as to drain vomitus out of the airway.
- If endotracheal intubation is attempted, the airway must be protected by the manoeuvre known as cricoid pressure throughout the period of instrumentation. Pressure is applied to the front of the patient's cricoid cartilage by an assistant using the thumb and two fingers. This compresses the oesophagus against the cervical spine and thus prevents the passive regurgitation of gastric contents. The airway is vulnerable from the start of induced paralysis until the cuff is inflated on a correctly positioned endotracheal tube.

Protection of the cervical spine

If the patient has an injury to the cervical spine, there is a risk of damage to the spinal cord during the procedures needed to maintain the airway. Because of the terrible outcome of such damage, it is mandatory to protect the neck immediately in patients who are:

1 unresponsive with a history of trauma or no clear history;
2 suffering from multiple trauma;
3 difficult to assess;
4 showing any symptoms or signs that might be attributable to the cervical spine.

Adequate protection of the potentially unstable cervical spine consists of a rigid collar and either a purpose-made cervical immobiliser or sandbags and tape.

For exclusion of cervical spine injury see page 57.

B – Breathing

Breathing is the means by which oxygen is delivered to the alveoli and thus made available to the circulating red cells. At the same time carbon dioxide (CO_2) is eliminated.

Look for

- *Difficulty in talking.*
- *An abnormal respiratory rate* – usually fast, laboured breathing. Very slow respiratory rates may occur just before respiratory arrest or as a consequence of poisoning with narcotic drugs, for example, methadone.
- *Recession of the chest wall* – the indrawing of the elastic tissues of a child caused by increased respiratory effort.
- *Nasal flaring and use of the shoulder and neck muscles during breathing.*
- *Paradoxical respiration* – a see-sawing movement of the chest and abdomen, which indicates obstruction of either the upper or lower airways or fatigue of the diaphragm.

All the above suggest that the patient is struggling to achieve normal respiration. Failure to oxygenate the blood adequately and hence the tissues is shown by:

- *Tachycardia* – the nervous system has detected hypoxia and is stimulating the heart.
- *Pallor and sweating* – again caused by sympathetic stimulation.
- *Cyanosis* – a late sign.
- *Irritability, confusion or reduced responsiveness* – the brain is short of oxygen. This is an extremely worrying sign.
- *A low SaO$_2$ (<95%)* – pulse oximetry should be established as soon as possible.
- *Unequal, diminished or abnormal breath sounds.*
- *Hyper-resonance or dullness to percussion.*
- *Displacement of the trachea or apex beat.*
- *A flail segment.*

For oxygen therapy see below.

For decompression and drainage of the chest see page 77.

For severe allergic reactions see page 295.

For specific treatment of respiratory distress see page 205.

For injuries to the chest see page 75.

Oxygen therapy

The common denominator of all life-threatening illness, regardless of cause, is a failure to deliver adequate amounts of oxygen to the tissues. In normal circumstances, the oxygen content of atmospheric air (21%) is perfectly adequate but when the mechanisms for breathing are diseased or traumatised supplemental oxygen should be given. The physiological compensatory mechanisms for hypoxia and hypovolaemia all consume oxygen themselves; the immediate administration of supplemental oxygen may maintain these reflexes while more definitive measures are put in place.

There are really only two main types of oxygen therapy:

1 high-concentration oxygen (40–100%);

2 low-concentration oxygen (24–30%).

The dangers of high-concentration therapy are known to every medical student. The patient with a chronically raised blood CO_2 level may depend on a hypoxic drive to stimulate breathing – give him or her oxygen and the breathing slows, CO_2 levels rise even higher and the patient becomes comatose with CO_2 narcosis. In practice, these patients are a small group in whom the speed of onset of symptoms can be used to determine treatment – *see pages 215 and 208.*

Hypoxia is a swift killer and so patients in the resuscitation room invariably need a high concentration of oxygen. The use of a mask that has a reservoir bag will improve the effectiveness of oxygen delivery (to perhaps 60–80%) and should be standard. The reservoir bag is needed because a patient's inspiratory flow is always greater than the 15 L per min maximum flow from the oxygen supply.

Blood gases must be obtained at an early stage to monitor the effect of supplemental oxygen. If improvement is not satisfactory, then ventilation may be needed. Continuous positive airway pressure (CPAP) is another method of increasing oxygenation.

Mechanical ventilation

This should always be considered when:

- the patient cannot maintain a clear airway;
- oxygen enrichment of the inspired gases fails to prevent the signs of cerebral hypoxia;
- CO_2 narcosis is present;
- there has been a successful but prolonged resuscitation from cardiac arrest;

• the patient is multiply injured;

• the patient has a severe chest injury (particularly those with multiple rib fractures and/or flail segments);

• the patient is to be transferred and there is a risk of severe deterioration en route.

The emergency induction of anaesthesia for the purpose of intubation and ventilation in a hypoxic patient is a difficult and demanding task. It requires considerable anaesthetic skills.

> A pneumothorax is more likely to tension in a ventilated patient. Chest drains must be inserted prior to ventilating patients with chest injuries.

C – Circulation

Check for a central pulse (over 5 s).

The absence of a central pulse (or a rate of less than 60 beats per min in infants) indicates the need to follow procedures for cardiorespiratory arrest (*see page 156*).

The clinical significance of the different arrest rhythms – ventricular fibrillation (VF), asystole and electro-mechanical dissociation (EMD) – is discussed on *page 156*.

Look for

• *Pallor and coolness of the skin* – the body diverts blood away from the skin when there are circulatory problems and these signs are thus very useful indicators of shock.

• *Pallor and sweating* – signs of gross sympathetic disturbance.

• *Active bleeding or melaena.*

• *A fast or slow heart rate* – fast heart rates usually mean that either there is a cardiac arrhythmia or more commonly that the sympathetic nervous system has detected a problem with the body (such as hypoxia, hypoglycaemia, pain or fear) and is 'instructing' the heart to beat faster. A slow heart rate usually means that something is wrong with the heart itself. The worst cause of this is severe hypoxia (or hypovolaemia) and, in this case, it means terminal bradycardia and asystole are only seconds away.

• *Abnormal systolic blood pressure (BP).*

• *A raised capillary refill time* – it should be less than 2 s if the circulation is satisfactory. However, peripheral shutdown in a cold, wet patient can easily produce a prolonged refill time.

• *Absent or quiet heart sounds and raised jugular venous pulse (JVP)* – suggestive of tamponade if accompanied by hypotension and tachycardia; JVP will not be raised if there is hypovolaemia also.

• *A precordial wound.*

• *An abnormal electrocardiogram (ECG) trace on the monitor.*

• *Signs of left ventricular failure (dyspnoea, gallop rhythm and crepitations).*

• *Signs of abdominal, pelvic or occult bleeding (may need PR examination and a nasogastric tube or ultrasound scan).*

• *Signs of dehydration (especially in children).*

• *Purpura (meningococcal septicaemia).*

Inadequate circulation will reduce tissue oxygenation and thus may also cause:

• *a raised respiratory rate;*

• *altered mental status.*

> Bolus fluid therapy should be calculated at 20 mL per kg and repeated as necessary after further assessment. (Reduced to 10 mL per kg for patients with bleeding following trauma in hospital and no more than 5 mL per kg for patients with trauma in the prehospital setting – *see page 7*.)

For the types of shock and their treatment see page 242.
For blood transfusion see page 26.
For the renal effects of shock (acute tubular necrosis and acute cortical necrosis) see page 252.
For severe allergic reactions see page 295.
For decompression of a cardiac tamponade see page 82.
For emergency thoracotomy see page 83.
For intra-abdominal bleeding see page 84.
For bleeding from the pelvis see page 88.
For cardiac arrhythmias see page 170.
For anaphylaxis see page 233.
For LVF see page 217.

Cardiac function

The stroke volume is the amount of blood ejected from the heart with each beat. It is determined by the left-ventricular filling pressure, myocardial contractility and the systemic vascular resistance.

The product of heart rate and stroke volume is the cardiac output – the most important parameter of cardiac function. (Cardiac index is cardiac output divided by body surface area.) An increase in heart rate will directly increase the cardiac output and is the earliest cardiac response to hypoxia. However, the faster the heart beats the less time there is for it to fill and, eventually, a rise in heart rate will no longer be matched by a rise in cardiac output.

> Myocardial function is compromised at high pulse rates because coronary blood flow occurs chiefly in diastole. When the heart rate rises above about 130 bpm in an adult, the filling time is so reduced that cardiac output will actually fall.

Pulse and blood pressure

The autonomic response to hypovolaemia is complex. Rapid blood loss produces a reflex bradycardia, but when associated with tissue damage, it produces the more familiar tachycardia. Systolic blood pressure is the product of the cardiac output and the systemic vascular resistance. A high catecholamine response to hypoxia and hypovolaemia will produce a high systemic vascular resistance. This will maintain a 'normal' blood pressure in the presence of a falling cardiac output.

> Knowledge of the systemic blood pressure provides only very limited information about cardiac function and is a very late indicator of haemodynamic instability.

Blood pressure when measured by a cuff depends upon the production of Korotkoff sounds by turbulent flow in the artery. When systemic vascular resistance is high and flow through the artery is relatively low (e.g. in the immediate aftermath of cardiac arrest) these sounds may not easily be heard, even when the mean arterial pressure is good. Great care must be taken when deciding if such patients are beyond salvage or in electromechanical dissociation (PEA).

Maintenance of systemic vascular resistance is a vital response to hypovolaemia and hypoxia. (Skin pallor reflects this early on but is an imprecise clinical sign.) Like other compensatory mechanisms to hypoxia, this vasomotor response consumes oxygen and will eventually fail.

Measurements of pulse and blood pressure are very poor indicators of haemodynamic function in critically ill patients. Central venous pressure may not reflect the functioning of the left side of the heart and is thus of limited use in the assessment of overall cardiac performance. Indwelling pulmonary artery flotation and systemic arterial catheters will provide much more useful information and allow measurement of the cardiac output. Critically ill patients should be moved to an intensive care unit where such monitoring facilities are available as soon as possible. Direct ultrasound measurement of cardiac output may soon become routine in emergency departments, but this facility must not delay consultation with intensivists.

Fluid replacement

Left-ventricular filling pressure (and hence cardiac output) is a function of the circulating blood volume. Increases in heart rate, systemic vascular resistance and myocardial contractility can maintain cardiac output and blood pressure in the early stages of hypovolaemia. However, this will be at the expense of increased oxygen demands by the cardiovascular system and reduced tissue perfusion in many other areas. The rapid restoration of circulating volume will prevent a sudden failure of these mechanisms and an often irreversible fall in cardiac output.

> Early restoration of blood pressure by transfusion does not necessarily indicate correction of the circulatory deficit.

The delivery of oxygen to the tissues depends not only on the pumping mechanism of the heart but also on the red cells in the circulating blood. A modest fall in haematocrit can reduce viscosity and increase blood flow while maintaining oxygen delivery but will still require an increase in cardiac output to be effective. Maintenance of haemoglobin levels by blood transfusion reduces the impact of hypoxia by increasing the effectiveness of each cardiac cycle and reducing the need for an increase in cardiac output. Transfused blood will also maintain the oncotic pressure of the circulating fluid, thereby increasing the filling pressure. However, adequate levels of 2,3-diphosphoglycerate

(2,3-DPG) are also necessary for satisfactory oxygen delivery – *see page 26*.

Maintenance of adequate tissue perfusion is not synonymous with the return of a normal blood pressure. Indeed, the latter may be contraindicated in the ED in an actively bleeding patient (e.g. with an aortic aneurysm). Resuscitation can be achieved while keeping the blood pressure relatively low. This has been shown to improve survival until definitive surgery can be undertaken. A similar approach is recommended in the prehospital management of injured adults and older children with presumed blood loss. Intravenous (IV) fluids should not be administered if a radial pulse can be felt (or, in the case of penetrating torso injuries, if a central pulse can be felt). In the absence of these pulses, IV crystalloids should be administered, en route to hospital, in boluses of no more than 250 mL until the relevant pulse becomes palpable. The same advice is probably applicable for young children and infants also, in which case boluses of 5 mL per kg should be used. When rapid fluid replacement is required, warmed IV fluids (40°C) should be be used. A ratio of crystalloids to colloids of at least 50 : 50 has been shown to be safe. Many doctors believe that Hartmann's solution is preferable to normal saline if large volumes are to be given. The role of hypertonic saline in resuscitation looks promising but has yet to be fully established.

D – Disability

After A, B and C (airway, breathing and circulation) have been attended to, it is necessary to look at the state of the brain. The term disability is now widely used to describe a brief assessment of neurological functioning.

Look for

1 A reduced level of consciousness – this is the most important sign of any problem affecting the brain. AVPU scoring is useful initially.

   A Alert.

   V Voice elicits a response.

   P Pain elicits a response. [Attending relatives are usually in a highly distressed state so be careful

how you elicit this sign. Pressure on a finger nail (with a pencil) is probably the most subtle way.]

   U Unresponsive.

Later, the Glasgow Coma Scale (GCS) should be used (*see page 36 for GCS in adults and page 327 for children*).

> Always consider hypoglycaemia as a cause for a reduced level of consciousness.

2 Abnormal pupils – look for size, equalness and reactivity. These features can be affected by both drugs and brain disease.

3 Abnormal posture and limb movements.

Severe intracerebral problems may also cause:

- airway obstruction;
- respiratory depression (respiration, unlike the heart beat, requires an intact brainstem);
- bradycardia and hypertension (Cushing's response);
- neurogenic pulmonary oedema (caused by massive sympathetic vasoconstriction).

For hypoglycaemia see page 9.

For poisoning see Chapter 15 on page 267.

For head injury see Chapter 3 on page 34.

For intracranial pathology see Chapter 14 on page 226.

For brainstem death see page 381.

Depression of consciousness

A decreased level of consciousness indicates that something is wrong with the brain or its fuel supply – *see Box 1.1*. There is a continuum of consciousness that ranges from an alert and orientated patient to one with brainstem death.

Box 1.1 Causes of Impaired Consciousness

Hypoxia, hypovolaemia or cerebral ischaemia
Hypoglycaemia
Hypothermia
Poisoning or gross metabolic disturbance (including CO_2 narcosis)
Injury to the brain
Intracranial pathology (bleeding, thrombosis, embolism, infection, swelling, tumour, fits, etc.)

If prolonged, many of the above problems (including hypoxia, ischaemia, hypoglycaemia and status epilepticus) will lead to a remarkably similar outcome – selective neuronal necrosis and permanent brain damage.

> Coma is defined as a Glasgow Coma Score of 8 or less.

Unconsciousness is an imprecise term usually describing a condition of an unaware patient with whom verbal communication is not possible; unresponsive is thus a better description. Such patients will usually be amnesic for the duration of the unresponsiveness.

The ability to maintain the airway decreases as the coma score falls and finally the ability to protect the airway is also lost. Breathing indicates a functioning brainstem; in an arrested patient it often returns quickly after cerebral circulation is restored. Sudden cerebral trauma may cause transitory apnoea and all of the causes of impaired consciousness listed in Box 1.1 may lead to terminal apnoea. The heart beat is less immediately dependent on an intact brain but asystole is inevitable within hours of brainstem death.

E – Environment and exposure

Control of the body temperature is increasingly recognised as important to a successful outcome in resuscitation. Wet clothes should be removed and consideration given to the use of warm IV fluids. In cases of trauma, collapse and depressed conscious level, the whole body must be exposed so that nothing important is missed. Even at this early stage care must be taken to avoid extrinsic factors that may harm the patient.

Look for
- Cold extremities.
- Shivering.
- Wet clothing.
- Pyrexia and clamminess.
- The position in which the patient is most comfortable.
- Uncomfortable splints (including collars and spinal boards).
- Loss of the protective reflexes of the eyes.
- Areas where pressure sores might form (*see page 229*).
- The proximity of the next of kin.

Attention to these details early on can radically change the well being (and demeanour) of a patient.

> If a patient cannot blink, then the eyes should be covered to protect them.

For hypothermia see page 248.
For hyperpyrexia and hyperthermia see pages 250 and 270.

F – Fits

It is very difficult to assess adequately or manage a patient with convulsions. Hence termination of the convulsion must be an immediate aim and often precedes satisfactory care of the airway or breathing.

Look for
- Frank tonic or clonic activity.
- Spasmodic twitching.
- Post-ictal drowsiness.
- Gurgling, rattling or other signs of post-ictal airway obstruction.
- Cyanosis. There is increased demand for oxygen and also respiratory distress.
- Signs of head injury.
- Signs of other injury caused by a convulsion (e.g. a bitten tongue and intra-oral bleeding).
- Reasons to consider hypoglycaemia.
- Pyrexia or other signs of infection (especially in children).

Convulsions must be terminated before any further action can be effective. Meanwhile, the patient must be prevented from harming himself or herself.

For hypoglycaemia see pages 246 and 327.
For treatment of convulsions see page 237.
For treatment of convulsions in childhood see page 339.

Fitting indicates that something is wrong with the brain or its fuel supply. The list of possibilities is almost the same as that for causes of reduced consciousness – *see Box 1.2*. Convulsive activity causes a dramatic increase in cerebral and muscle oxygen demand; a post-ictal acidosis is inevitable. The uncoordinated muscle action that occurs during the tonic or clonic stages of a fit makes control of the airway extremely difficult; some regurgitation may also occur. Ventilation of the lungs is usually reduced for the same reason. Alveolar oxygenation is thus poor at a time of high oxygen

> **Box 1.2 Causes of Fits**
>
> Hypoxia or shock
> Hypoglycaemia
> Poisoning or gross metabolic disturbance
> Injury to the brain
> Intracranial pathology (bleeding, thrombosis, embolism, infection, swelling, tumour, epilepsy, etc.)

demand. This combination probably explains why prolonged fitting is associated with permanent neurological damage.

G – Glucose

The human body can be compared to an engine that needs an oxygen supply (airway and breathing) delivered in the blood stream (circulation). However, we should not forget that the oxygen is required to burn fuel (glucose). Fat and protein are, of course, also important but the brain uses glucose almost exclusively.

Look for

- Restlessness, agitation or other mental change ('jitteriness' in a neonate).
- Inappropriate lack of cooperation or aggression.
- A reduced level of consciousness.
- Convulsions.
- Signs of insulin usage.
- A low blood sugar level on testing with a reagent strip.

A reagent-strip measurement of blood glucose should be performed in all patients who have depression of consciousness. If hypoglycaemia is found it should be immediately treated with IV glucose solution (50 mL of 50% glucose for a normal adult; 0.2 g per kg for a child). If no venous access can be found, then glucagon 1 mg by IM injection is a useful standby.

For hypoglycaemia see also pages 246 and 327.

> Hypoglycaemia is always waiting to catch you out. A comatose patient with profuse sweating should always make you think of a low blood sugar.

H – History

At this juncture a brief history becomes a necessity and brief is AMPLE:

A Allergies.
M Medication.
P Past and present illnesses of significance.
L Last food and drink.
E Events leading up to the patient's presentation.

The people who accompany the patient to the department are a vital source of this information; hence the need to collect facts before the paramedical staff leave the ED.

> Patients who are undergoing prolonged treatment with steroids (i.e. for more than 3 weeks) may develop adrenocortical suppression. This can also occur for up to a year after stopping long-term steroid therapy. During a medical crisis, such patients should be given supplementary corticosteroids (e.g. hydrocortisone 200 mg IV in the ED).

I – Immediate analgesia and investigations

> This is the point (if you have not already done it) to call for help. There should be no hesitation in seeking another pair of hands or a more experienced opinion.

In many patients who are not in extremis, the above will only take a matter of seconds. Once life-threatening problems have been identified and treated, it is necessary to perform the tasks that are at the very heart of emergency medicine – the immediate relief of suffering. This will include:

- administration of analgesia *(for the assessment of pain see Box 1.3)*;
- provision of splintage and support for injuries;
- further relief of dyspnoea;
- reassurance.

This is not just a matter of humanity. The trust of the patient (and their relatives and friends) is

> **Box 1.3 Assessment of Pain**
>
> Pain is a subjective experience. Clinical assessment of a patient's level of pain depends upon:
> - the patient's description of the pain;
> - the patient's behaviour;
> - the known injuries or condition;
> - any observed signs of pain (sweating, etc.);
> - the use of visual pain scales – analogue or image type (pain ladders and faces, etc.).

more easily gained by staff who are seen to 'do something'. This trust leads to the provision of more information and better compliance with treatment. Conversely, nothing agitates relatives more than the sight of a doctor or nurse asking endless questions while the patient continues to suffer. It is always better to overestimate pain rather than to underestimate it.

Major radiographs can now be requested. In patients who have suffered multiple trauma, these are views of the chest, lateral cervical spine and pelvis. In other instances a chest X-ray is usually sufficient. Twelve-lead ECG and blood gas analysis are also helpful early on.

Box 1.4 Summary of Immediate Assessment and Management

Airway
  Establish and maintain a clear airway.
  Ensure airway protection.
  Consider the need for cervical protection.
Breathing
  Give high-concentration oxygen.
  Ensure adequate ventilation of the lungs.
  Decompress pneumothoraces.
  Begin to correct severe respiratory problems.
Circulation
  Restore the circulating blood volume.
  Ensure adequate cardiac function.
  Commence monitoring.
Disability
  Assess cerebral functioning.
  Consider causes of depression of consciousness.
Environment/exposure of the whole body
  Check the body temperature and positioning.
  Ensure protection from further harm.
  Expose the whole body for examination.
Fits
  Control convulsive activity.
Glucose
  Correct hypoglycaemia.
History
  Take brief but AMPLE details.
Immediate analgesia and investigations
  Provide analgesia and splintage.
  Relieve remaining dyspnoea.
  Give reassurance.
  Request major investigations.

Analgesia

The administration of analgesia does not mask significant clinical signs. Conscious level is not greatly depressed by the judicious administration of small doses of IV opioids and abdominal signs also remain unchanged. Tenderness can still be located and guarding is an involuntary mechanism, which is unaffected. The biggest change will be in the ease of examining a trusting, cooperative patient who was previously distressed and agitated.

> The immediate relief of suffering, in all its forms, is the most important function of an ED.

For a summary of this section on immediate assessment and management of emergency patients see Box 1.4.

Further (or secondary) assessment and management of the patient

The needs of the relatives and friends

The needs of the carers cannot be ignored. These may vary from simple reassurance to medical treatment. As soon as practicable, the relatives must be informed of the patient's current situation and what is going to happen next.

History and examination

History-taking in emergencies should be guided by the presenting complaint. The familial medical history will rarely be relevant in a patient with a dog bite; it might be vital in a haemophiliac with a swollen joint. The art of adjusting the acquisition of information is a difficult one. Most new ED staff take an over-long history for the first few days; they then record less than a bare minimum for the next few months. Mechanism of injury is particularly important in trauma; events leading to presentation are essential in medical cases.

The examination must also be tailored to the patient. At times it can be limited; often it must be thorough. Experience teaches the relative uselessness of some physical signs and the enormous value of others. The examination in trauma patients is usually performed from top to toe rather than in systems and is called the secondary survey. The back of the patient and the perineum are the parts that are often missed.

Investigations

Investigations should only be requested if the results could have an impact on immediate care or disposal. Specific tests have been described above. Other tests should be performed for precise indications rather than as a general screen. The exception to this is in elderly patients who present with non-specific events such as collapse. They can be very difficult to evaluate clinically. Consequently, before considering sending them home, it is best to carry out a brief screen including Chest X-ray, ECG, haemoglobin, white cell count and blood urea level.

Definitive care

This may involve:
- accurate liaison with other specialists in the hospital or the community;
- safe transport to another facility;
- careful follow-up arrangements;
- rehabilitation.

For observation wards see page 15.
For review clinics see page 15.

The patient and his problem

For ED attendance figures in the United Kingdom see Box 1.5.

Box 1.5 Patients Attending EDs in the United Kingdom

Over 15 million patients attended EDs in the United Kingdom in 2004. Of these patients, around:
- 25% were children;
- 20% arrived by emergency ambulance;
- 20% were admitted to hospital.

Attendance figures are increasing by 6% per annum (2005).

The sorting of patients (triage)

The word triage originally referred to the sorting of coffee beans. Later the term was used to describe the way in which an army divided the mass casualties of war into three categories, depending on their likelihood of returning to the front line. In normal civilian practice, triage means the prioritising of patients such that those with the most urgent or life-threatening conditions are seen and treated first; immediate assessment is a more easily understood description of this process.

Different departments use varying terms and labels for their assessment categories but there is increasing acceptance of the definitions in *Box 1.6*.

Box 1.6 Categorisation of Patients

Category	Label colour	Condition
Category 1	Red	Immediate resuscitation required
Category 2	Orange	Very urgent, major illness or injury
Category 3	Yellow	Urgent, serious problem but apparently stable
Category 4	Green	Standard, routine case without immediate danger or distress
Category 5	Blue	Non-urgent problem, which may be redirected to a more appropriate facility

---

Patients with pain should be placed in a category that reflects their need for analgesia. This may be higher than that dictated by the apparent severity of their injury. Category blue is often best determined in retrospect (*see inappropriate attenders on page 12*).

The process of immediate assessment is usually undertaken by experienced nursing staff and should logically take place before registration and documentation. The provision of immediate therapies such as analgesia, splintage and ice-packs increases the usefulness of this early clinical contact with the patient.

Management rather than diagnosis

Accurate diagnosis is a skill that every doctor strives to acquire but we can only diagnose conditions that we know exist. Outside of these, a whole gamut of uncertainty remains to be explored. In the meantime, the patient still needs help. This requires flexibility of mind and a good knowledge of basic principles.

Management of a condition is possible without a firm diagnosis: you may not know what the underlying cause of the problem is, but you must know what to do about it. This approach is life-saving in the primary phase of resuscitation. As each problem presents, immediate action is taken to resolve it – long before the whole clinical picture becomes apparent.

Inappropriate attenders and minor problems

The label inappropriate attender is often given to patients whose problems are thought to be trivial or that are more suitably managed in general practice. However, the perception of trained health providers may not be shared by the lay public. This is because it takes a considerable amount of knowledge to differentiate confidently between major and minor conditions. Moreover, small injuries can be disproportionately distressing and help can seem difficult to find in the complex healthcare systems of today. Whatever your view of the apparent inappropriateness of the patient's attendance, it is best to examine first and criticise later.

Social problems

It is the nature of the work of an ED to take all-comers. Most of these patients will fall into standard medical and surgical categories. However, many people are unaware that suffering must be classified before they can gain relief. For ED staff to complain that many of the problems that they see are vague, ill-defined or social is on a par with a geriatrician complaining that most of his or her patients are elderly.

Homelessness

> The standardised mortality rate for homeless people is three times higher than that of the United Kingdom population as a whole.

Many patients who come to an ED have nowhere to sleep or to shelter. People suffering from psychiatric disease often become homeless and there are many other illnesses (such as tuberculosis and alcohol abuse), which are associated with homelessness.

> The average life expectancy for someone on the streets is just 47 years.

Efforts should always be made to find temporary accommodation for these patients. The most likely sources of help are:

- the social services;
- the Salvation Army;
- Shelter Nightline (in London).

> Health inequalities in the United Kingdom are increasing. The differences in life expectancy between rich and poor areas of the country are at their greatest since the Victorian era.

Placebo therapy

Do not be afraid to acknowledge this very important aspect of medical practice. Human health is inextricably linked with mental functioning and fear and worry play a large part in many consultations. Improvement rates of up to 40% may be obtained with placebo therapy. The doctor's reassurance is the greatest placebo and his or her apparent casual dismissal of a problem has the reverse effect.

Communication

Good communication is the hallmark of the good doctor, the good nurse and the good ED. In addition to the obvious patience and direct verbal skills required, this may encompass:

- information cards to take out;
- telephone advice help-lines;
- translation facilities;
- good quality records and letters.

It is not just the patient who is concerned with communication. Special care is also needed with:

- relatives;
- other health professionals in the hospital;
- paramedics;

- GPs, health visitors and district nurses;
- police officers.

Dealing with complaints properly is a further example of good communication – *see page 382*.

National alert systems. MedicAlert® is a UK-registered charity that provides an identification system for individuals with hidden medical conditions and allergies. This takes the form of bracelets or necklets (known as 'Emblems') that are engraved with the wearer's main medical condition(s) or vital details, a personal ID number and a 24-h emergency telephone number. Medical and emergency personnel can telephone the alert service and, by quoting the patient's ID number (and after clearing security checks), they can receive details of the person's name, address, general practitioner, current medication, next of kin and other medical information.

Record-keeping and letters in an ED

Medical records must be concise and relevant but at the same time sufficiently comprehensive and legible to allow other doctors to understand what happened during the consultation. With increasing litigation (and emergency medicine is a high-risk area for claims), the notes have taken on a new importance as the major source of information for medical defence. Moreover, police statements and other legal reports are impossible to prepare from illegible, inadequate notes. The records should be in a problem-orientated form but must also contain:

- the name of the practitioner (in capitals) and the date and time;
- an adequate history (including mechanism of injury or events leading to presentation);
- a relevant examination (with drawings and measurements as required);
- a list of investigations and the results of them;
- a treatment plan;
- details of any follow-up and instructions given; any factors complicating discharge must be given written consideration.

For medicolegal aspects of record-keeping see page 365.

General practitioners should receive a notification of their patient's attendance at the ED which, as a minimum, tells them:

- who the patient is (the name and address as a minimum);
- on what date he or she attended the ED;
- the diagnosis;
- the results of any investigations;
- treatment and medications given;
- details of any follow-up arranged or required.

Health promotion

The ED is an ideal situation for giving information and advice about health. Patients in the department are in a receptive state and form a captive audience while in the waiting areas. Health information may address:

- accident prevention, home and road safety;
- the importance of routine immunisations;
- healthy eating and lifestyles (*see Box 1.7*);
- domestic and other violence;
- the problems of alcohol, drug and substance abuse;
- hygiene and dental care;
- venereal disease;
- access to local facilities;
- other areas of perceived local and national importance.

Leaflets, films and advice may all have a part to play. There should be a liaison with the local agencies for health education and with the local area child accident prevention group. Some departments will be involved with campaigns in neighbourhood schools.

Box 1.7 Common Health Problems in the United Kingdom in 2005

66% of men and 50% of women are overweight.
25% of children are overweight; 14% are obese.
70% of men and 80% of women take insufficient exercise.
31% of men and 28% of women smoke.
28% of men and 11% of women drink more than the UK recommended limit.

Detection of osteoporosis

Fractures occurring in patients who are over 45–50 years old may be related to bone fragility caused by osteoporosis. This is not visible on plain radiographs until the disease is well advanced. Those patients with fractures that have resulted from relatively minor trauma, should be referred to their GP for further investigation. Treatment may include exercise, diet, hormone replacement therapy and specific drugs.

> More than 1 in 3 women and 1 in 12 men are at risk from osteoporosis. It causes 200,000 fractures every year in the United Kingdom.

The staff and their surroundings

Learning and teaching

A good department of emergency medicine is a forum for ideas and discussion, which should help with personal and professional advancement as well as benefiting the department. Research is just one aspect of this progression. All staff should participate in learning and teaching.

Clothing, appearance and cleanliness

Unlike the GP or ward-based staff, the emergency practitioner has only a few minutes in which to form a relationship with the patient and his or her relatives. This means that first impressions are extremely important. Some factors can be predicted to create a caring but professional image:
• a smart, clean and appropriate appearance (greatly enhanced by a white coat or a uniform and a name badge);
• pleasant body and breath odours;
• courtesy;
• a concerned and attentive attitude.

The reaction of the patient to other factors (such as the sex, age and race of the doctor) is less predictable; some patients may also have a preconceived view of a doctor's attitudes. Personal and intimate problems may sometimes justify a request for a doctor of another sex and it is certainly true

that age is often assumed to be synonymous with wisdom. Racial prejudice, however, is always totally unacceptable. If it occurs it must not be tolerated. Senior staff must be informed without delay.

Clean hands. Healthcare-associated infection leads to the deaths of many patients every year in the United Kingdom and costs the NHS millions of pounds. Studies have shown that infection rates can be reduced by 10–50% if hospital staff clean their hands regularly. Unfortunately, hand-washing is often performed infrequently and inadequately. The ED is an ideal place to learn and practise good habits in all aspects of cleanliness.

For the prevention of the spread of infectious pathogens see SARS on page 222.

For the prevention of nosocomial respiratory infections see hospital-acquired pneumonia on page 219.

Health and safety at work

Health and safety legislation. The Health and Safety at Work Act 1974 places a legal duty on employers to provide for the health and safety of their employees. NHS trusts have been subject to the full requirements of this legislation since 1991. These obligations were extended further under the Management of Health and Safety at Work Regulations 1992, which require employers to assess risks to their employees and implement a comprehensive system of safety management. There are several additional UK regulations and three EU Council Directives that are relevant to the health and safety of workers.

Departmental facilities. A suitable working environment is a prerequisite for good practice in emergency medicine. Some of the less subtle aspects of this are:
• adequate and well-maintained equipment (this is the responsibility of all staff, not just a few);
• good support from departmental and other hospital staff;
• reasonable working rotas for all members of the team;

- streamlined and clear procedures for most eventualities;
- measures to ensure the health and safety of staff (e.g. security procedures and hepatitis B immunisation).

Prevention of blood-borne infections. There are more than 20 dangerous transmittable blood-borne diseases. The three main infections are hepatitis B, hepatitis C and HIV/AIDS, of which hepatitis B is by far the greatest danger. However, other blood-borne pathogens include:

- Human T lymphotrophic retroviruses (HTLV I and II).
- Hepatitis D and hepatitis G viruses (HDV and GBV-C).
- Cytomegalovirus (CMV).
- Epstein Barr virus (EBV).
- Parvovirus B19.
- Transfusion-transmitted virus (TTV).
- West Nile virus (WNV).
- Malarial parasites and prion agents.

These organisms may be transmitted through contact with blood or any other body fluid from an infected person. This can be via a 'needlestick' injury, a human bite, a splash into the eyes or directly into an open wound or cut.

> The high-risk patient cannot be confidently detected and so precautions must be taken to avoid transmission of infection at all times.

Every effort should be made to avoid exposure to blood and body fluids through safe systems of practice. The principle of following standard ('Universal') precautions means never assuming that there is no risk. The same precautions to prevent transmission of infection should be used for every single procedure:

1 Cuts and grazes should always be covered with a waterproof dressing.
2 Gloves should be worn when dealing with blood or other body fluids. (Although a needle or other sharp instrument can easily penetrate latex, it is said that a surgical glove will remove 80% of the blood on the offending instrument before it reaches the underlying hand.)

3 Eye protection should be worn when there is a high risk of splashing of body fluids.
4 Needles should not be re-sheathed.
5 Needles and other sharp objects should be disposed of carefully into an appropriate bin in the room where they are used and not carried around.

For the identification of high-risk patients see Box 21.7 on page 398.

For the management of blood and body-fluid exposure incidents see page 397.

Observation wards

The College of Emergency Medicine recommends that there is one ED-managed 'short stay' or observation bed per 5000 new emergency patients. The exact case-mix of the patients admitted to this ward will vary between departments but might include those with:

- head injuries;
- chest injuries;
- soft-tissue injuries;
- soft-tissue infections;
- acute alcohol intoxication;
- some other poisonings;
- alcohol withdrawal;
- social problems.

The acceptable level of severity of some of the above conditions will depend on unit policy, as will maximum length of stay on the ward. To make the best use of the available bed space, ward rounds are required at least twice a day with interventions and investigations as necessary.

Review clinics

Some patients (but certainly less than 10%) may be best managed by follow-up in a review clinic, which is run under the auspices of the ED. This clinic can provide:

- specialised dressings and other wound care;
- reassessment of burns and certain other wounds;
- review of cellulitis and other infections;
- reassessment of soft-tissue injuries where complete resolution is not inevitable (e.g. some joint sprains);

15

- follow-up of particular conditions (e.g. scaphoid injuries, chest injuries, some head injuries, minor fractures).

> Neither the review clinic nor the short stay ward should be used as a substitute for proper examination, investigation and treatment at first presentation.

Organisation – the team approach

To carry out the rapid assessment of patients with almost simultaneous treatment of life-threatening conditions requires a team effort. The team must have an acknowledged leader and a clear line of command. The team should be identified beforehand and should practise and prepare for an emergency. Horizontal integration with concurrent actions that are undertaken by team members who are allocated to specific tasks is the most effective system. The ED staff will form the nucleus. Other specialists called to the department must know beforehand that they will be required to function as part of this team under the supervision of the team leader. Training according to the tenets of Advanced Life Support for trauma, cardiac and paediatric emergencies is recommended.

Prehospital care

Outside of the hospital situation, there is a clear organisational hierarchy.
- The police are in overall control of the scene.
- The fire service is in charge of rescue and extrication, and scene safety for the other personnel.
- The ambulance service is responsible for the evacuation of casualties.
- The medical team is present at the request of the ambulance service.

Entrapment of casualties is now the most common reason for paramedics to request the assistance of a hospital team – either prolonged entrapment (more than 20 min) or situations where release requires analgesia.

An on-site medical team must be formed from experienced, regularly trained staff who have:

- high-visibility protective clothing;
- adequate equipment;
- insurance cover for this type of work.

Furthermore, the parent department must be left adequately staffed.

The only measures which have been shown conclusively to save lives in the prehospital situation are ABC:

Airway	Clearance, maintenance and protection
Breathing	Oxygen and ventilation
Circulation	Chest compression and defibrillation

> In cardiac arrest, the time taken to initiate the above interventions is crucial to survival – *see page 157.*

Extensive clinical examination and the establishment of IV infusions are of no proven benefit. Nevertheless, other prehospital treatments may contribute greatly to the relief of pain and suffering.

> Time at the scene must not be extended by anything other than essential treatment. The priority is to get the patient to hospital as soon as possible.

The basic principles of prehospital care are the same as those for in-hospital care. Specific resuscitation courses are now available where the applied skills may be mastered.

Major incidents

A discussion of the management of major incidents is outside the scope of this book. However, all departments should have a written policy for dealing with events that have the potential to overwhelm the standard facilities of the hospital. Action cards for all personnel should be available together with a special supply of equipment and drugs. Regular practice sessions are a necessity. (NB. This is a legal obligation under the Civil Contingencies Act 2004. The Act is divided into two parts – Civil Protection (Part I) and Emergency Powers (Part II). For the purposes of Civil Protection, local responders are divided into two categories. The Category 1 responders (which include hospitals, primary care trusts and ambulance services) have a duty to make and execute effective plans for major incidents. Category 2 organisations (such as utility and transport companies) are obliged to co-operate with other responders.)

For contamination and irradiation see page 297.

The administration of sedation or general anaesthesia in the ED

The unique circumstances of the ED lead to special problems with the safe administration of sedative drugs. However, a unit that treats comatose patients as part of its daily workload must inevitably have the personnel and facilities available for the care of sedated patients.

The techniques used for assessment and monitoring of pathological coma are also applicable to depression of consciousness during sedation. The safety of the patient is paramount; emergency situations do not obviate the need for standard precautions. Consideration must be given to the medical preparedness and fasting state of all patients. If in doubt, senior staff should be consulted.

Special problems associated with sedation in an ED

Most ED patients are self-referred and many will return to their homes or workplaces within a matter of hours. Moreover, the very nature of accidents and emergencies is that they are unplanned. This combination of circumstances leads to special problems with the safe administration of sedative drugs.

- Most patients are not fasted; in addition, painful conditions delay gastric emptying.
- Many patients will have ingested alcohol in the preceding few hours.
- There is no opportunity for preplanned assessment of fitness or review of case notes.

- The need for sedation is invariably immediate.
- The fitness of patients for discharge and the circumstances to which they depart require very careful consideration.

Preparation for sedation and selection of patients

The immediacy of the situation does not obviate the need for a concise but adequate work-up of the patient. Most patients will not require investigations to assess their fitness for the procedure; those that do are generally not suitable for sedation in the ED. Pulse oximetry (while breathing air) is a useful screening test – a fit patient will invariably have an SaO_2 of above 94%.

Some patients will be found to be unsuitable for sedation in the department. They include those who:

- are severely intoxicated;
- have a full stomach;
- have had previous problems with sedation;
- have chronic illnesses, which may complicate sedation or aftercare;
- have other severe injuries;
- have a co-existent significant head injury;
- are at the extremes of age;
- have inadequate circumstances for discharge.

Patients who are deemed unsuitable for sedation but whose condition does not allow delay (e.g. vascular compromise distal to a dislocation) must be discussed with a senior colleague immediately.

The urgency of most of the conditions that present to an ED, does not allow for the conventional period of preoperative fasting. However, in all but the most pressing circumstances, a period of 2 h should separate sedation from the last ingestion of food or drink to allow for gastric emptying. No further food or drink must be allowed from the moment of entering the department.

Painful conditions, such as dislocations, must be alleviated with parenteral analgesia (before X-ray) and the subsequent doses of sedative drugs then adjusted accordingly.

> Sedation is not the same as analgesia.

17

Facilities for the administration of sedation or general anaesthesia

The minimum requirements include:
- medical and nursing staff trained in the management of patients with a depressed level of consciousness;
- areas suitable for high-dependency observation;
- a full range of resuscitation and monitoring equipment;
- all necessary drugs for resuscitation, including the specific benzodiazepine antagonist flumazenil and the opioid antagonist naloxone.

> When a doctor is performing a procedure on a sedated patient, a separate member of staff must be responsible for the overall care of that patient. The operator should never try to monitor the patient at the same time.

Conditions during the period of sedation

During sedation, and until recovery is complete, all patients should:
- be accompanied by a responsible member of staff;
- be on a trolley with side rails, which can be tipped head-down;
- have an IV cannula *in situ*;
- be given a high concentration of oxygen by mask;
- be monitored by pulse oximetry as a minimum standard (respiratory rate, ECG and BP recording are also highly desirable);
- have a high-volume suction catheter in place under their pillow.

The protective reflexes of the airway are depressed by all sedative and narcotic drugs to an unpredictable degree. Even at a high GCS there may be enough impairment of airway protection to allow aspiration of gastric contents. Therefore, all sedated patients must be placed in the recovery position as soon as is practically possible.

Effective sedation is greatly facilitated by pleasant, quiet surroundings and the presence of attentive, reassuring and obviously competent staff.

Assessment of the level of sedation

> The scores for measuring coma (AVPU and GCS) are understood and practised by all staff in an ED. They are thus ideal for use in assessing the level of sedation.

General anaesthesia and sedation are both induced states of depression of consciousness. Sedation is characterised by the fact that verbal contact should be maintained with the patient throughout – V on the AVPU scale. (This does not mean that the patient either speaks sensibly or remembers the conversation afterwards.) In the language of an ED, sedation is equivalent to a GCS of 10 or above and is certainly not the same as a GCS of 8 (coma). Full general anaesthesia is characterised by a GCS of 3. Gentle stroking of the upper eyelashes usually causes blinking (the eyelash reflex) and the loss of this reflex (at a GCS of around 8) is a good guide as to the imminent onset of general anaesthesia.

Drugs for sedation in the ED

All drugs that are used for sedation are capable of inducing general anaesthesia and vice versa. The main difference between the two groups of agents is the speed of onset of action and thus the ability to control the level of consciousness. (Thiopental acts in 20 seconds whereas diazepam takes several minutes to work.)

Sedation should always be accompanied by adequate analgesia, both before, during and after the procedure. Anti-emetics may be given as required but there is little evidence that their routine use reduces the risk of aspiration.

For sedation and analgesia for children see page 347.
For sedation of the disturbed patient see Chapter 19 on page 352.

Intravenous benzodiazepines

Intravenous benzodiazepines such as midazolam or diazepam emulsion are the standard drugs for ED sedation.
- Initial adult dose of IV midazolam = 1–2 mg.
- Initial adult dose of IV diazepam = 2.5–5 mg.

The correct initial dose can be estimated from the age, weight and general health of the patient. The elderly may need only very small amounts. Subsequent doses, given after a delay of a few minutes, should be titrated against apparent effect. The muscle relaxation that is a feature of sedation with benzodiazepines makes these drugs ideal for use in the reduction of dislocations.

Short-acting opioids

Short-acting opioids such as fentanyl can provide an excellent combination of sedation and analgesia:
- IV dose of fentanyl = 1–3 μg per kg.

This should be titrated slowly at a rate of no more than 1 μg per kg per min up to a maximum dose of 5 μg per kg in 1 h. The onset of action is within 3 min and the effects of a single dose wear off in less than 1 h. Opioids may cause some muscular rigidity.

Low-dose inhaled nitrous oxide

Low-dose inhaled nitrous oxide is useful as a supplement to other drugs or to give background sedation. It is often administered, for the purpose of analgesia rather than sedation, in a fixed concentration (50%) from a cylinder premixed with oxygen (e.g. Entonox) via a demand valve. Such valves require a negative pressure to open them (which varies greatly with the make of the demand apparatus). The generation of this pressure may be beyond the ability of younger children and some adults.

Proper sedation with nitrous oxide requires a constant flow of gas and this is best achieved with a purpose-built system such as the Quantiflex machine. Using this apparatus, nitrous oxide may be administered in sub-anaesthetic concentrations of 30–70% via a non-rebreathing circuit with a guaranteed minimum of 30% oxygen.

Ketamine

Ketamine is a derivative of phencyclidine and is often recommended as an anaesthetic for prehospital use. This is because it has both sedative and analgesic effects and does not compromise the airway or the circulation as much as other comparable drugs. In a lower range of doses, it is also an excellent and safe sedative for use in the ED:
- IV dose of ketamine for sedation = 0.5–1 mg per kg. The sedation starts within less than 60 s and lasts for 5–10 min.
- IM dose of ketamine for sedation = 2–4 mg per kg. When 2 mg per kg is given IM (as recommended by the authors), the onset of sedation is around 5 min with an effective duration of up to 35 min. A top-up dose of a further 1 mg per kg can be given if either the first dose proves to be inadequate or there is a requirement to prolong the duration of the sedation. The effects of ketamine are surprisingly predictable and reliable when it is administered by the IM route.

In these low doses, dysphoria is uncommon and excess salivation is not a problem. Consequently, emergence from sedation is usually uneventful and prior administration of atropine is unnecessary.

Discharge of patients who have received sedative drugs in the ED

The patient who is fit for discharge after sedation must fulfil all of the following criteria:
- alert and orientated;
- able to walk steadily and unaided;
- able to drink liquids;
- not suffering from any disabling condition such as vomiting, dizziness, shortness of breath or severe pain;
- accompanied by a responsible adult;
- suitable for available transport; and
- returning to adequate home circumstances.

For aftercare advice to be given to a patient who has received sedative or narcotic drugs in the ED see page 385.

Chapter 2

Major trauma and multiple injuries

There is a pandemic of trauma throughout the world. In the developed countries, trauma is the leading cause of death in the first three decades of life and is surpassed only by cancer and atherosclerosis throughout life. Moreover, because it affects young people, trauma wastes more years of life than any other cause; it is responsible for 8.3% of all 'life-years' lost in people under the age of 75 years in the United Kingdom. In addition, for every death from trauma, there are more than two permanent disabilities.

In the United Kingdom, accidents cause nearly 1 in 50 (2%) of all deaths in all age groups and account for 7% of the total NHS expenditure.

The absolute number of accidental deaths is greatest in people aged 65 years and over. In this age group, more than half of all fatal trauma results from falls. However, for the majority of the population, road traffic is the greatest danger, being responsible for about 40% of trauma deaths in the United Kingdom. Falls from a height and motor vehicle accidents commonly lead to multiple injuries (sometimes called polytrauma).

People from deprived backgrounds are more likely to be injured than those from higher social classes.

Alcohol is a significant factor in about one in seven of all fatal car crashes and in over 40% of deaths from falls. (For other details about the enormous part alcohol plays in injury see page 370). The other major ingredient in road traffic accidents is high speed. When pedestrians are struck by moving cars:

- at 20 mph, 5% are killed;
- at 30 mph, 45% are killed;
- at 50 mph, 85% are killed.

Deaths from trauma are often said to occur in a triphasic distribution:

1 Immediate death within seconds to minutes of injury (damage to the brain, brainstem, proximal spinal cord, heart, aorta or other large vessels).
2 Delayed deaths within minutes to hours after injury (intracranial bleeding or blood loss into the chest, abdomen or pelvis).
3 Late deaths occurring days or weeks after the initial injury (sepsis and organ failure).

However, in the United Kingdom, the majority of fatalities (around 80%) actually occur at the site of the injury. Prevention is thus the most important factor in the reduction of deaths from trauma.

The Advanced Trauma Life Support (ATLS) system, developed by the American College of Surgeons in the late 1970s, has become the standard method for initial assessment and management of trauma victims. There are three main phases:

1 primary survey and resuscitation;
2 secondary survey;
3 definitive care.

> This chapter adopts the ATLS approach but is no replacement for attendance on the 3-day course. The practical skills and team approach to trauma care cannot be learned from a book.

Preparation for reception of trauma victims

If warned of the imminent arrival of patients who are multiply injured:
- assemble a team in the resuscitation area;
- warn appropriate in-patient specialties;
- allocate tasks: doctor/nurse to airway and breathing, doctor/nurse to circulation, nurse to record findings and interventions, nurse to support relatives, senior doctor as team leader;
- check equipment and don protective clothing;
- meet the ambulance with doctor/nurse to ensure continuous care of the airway;
- detain the ambulance crew for a subsequent report on the biomechanics of impact (*see Box 2.1*), initial clinical state and prehospital care.

The primary survey and resuscitation phase (initial assessment and management)

See also Chapter 1.
- Assess and secure the airway while guarding the neck. Manual in-line stabilisation may be needed.
- Give high flow 100% oxygen.
- Protect the neck with a rigid cervical collar and a head holder (or sandbags and tape).
- Assess the breathing; exclude/treat tension pneumothorax and other critical chest injuries. Cover 'sucking' chest wounds with a flap dressing.

> **Box 2.1 Factors Associated with Severe Injury**
>
> Fall from a height of 5 m or more or a road traffic accident involving:
> - impact at high speed;
> - fatality of other passenger(s);
> - ejection from vehicle;
> - pedestrian struck by vehicle;
> - motorcyclist with no crash helmet;
> - steering wheel or windscreen damage;
> - significant intrusion into passenger compartment.

- Stop external bleeding by direct pressure and establish venous access at two sites – large cannulae in large veins.
- Take 20 mL of blood for cross-matching, a coagulation screen and baseline glucose, electrolytes and haemoglobin.
- Commence infusions of normal saline and then colloid (a 50 : 50 ratio of the two is probably a good start).
- Take and record the pulse, BP and respiratory rate. Attach the patient to a pulse oximeter and a cardiac monitor.
- Determine the level of consciousness (*AVPU – see page 7*) and the size and reactivity of the pupils.
- Assess limb movements to confirm spinal cord integrity.
- Remove remaining clothing and expose the patient to allow further assessment.
- Measure the blood glucose with a reagent stick in all unresponsive patients.
- Obtain brief details of the patient and the trauma that he or she has suffered (*AMPLE – see page 9*).

> An understanding of the biomechanics of the trauma will suggest the likely extent of the injuries – many of which may not be obvious at this stage.

- Consider early analgesia.
- Request the three major radiographs of trauma: chest, lateral cervical spine and pelvis.

The secondary survey (further assessment)

- Begin a head-to-toe examination. This assumes that resuscitation is underway and successful. If any features in the primary survey are still giving cause for concern, return to the assessment of oxygenation and circulation.
- When the front of the trunk and the limbs have been assessed, call for help to log-roll the patient. Four people are required, one controlling the head alone and taking charge of the timing of the turn.
- When rolled, examine the thoracolumbar spine, listen to lung fields, examine the perineum and do a rectal examination. The latter will reveal the anal tone, the presence of perineal injuries, the position of the prostate and any blood.

- Document the injuries discovered.
- Consider the priorities for investigation and treatment. Discuss the patient with doctors from other specialties who should, by now, have arrived in the resuscitation room.
- Maintain contemporary notes and repeat the ABCs and baseline observations frequently.

The chain of care

> Patients appear deceptively stable even after significant injury – particularly blunt trauma. Inadequate assessment and treatment is commonplace, yet the consequences are not immediately evident. Complications on the intensive care unit (ICU) may be a result of inadequate resuscitation in the emergency department (ED) and deterioration in an ED may be caused by inadequate treatment at scene.

In urban areas, with short transfer times and no delay involved in releasing the injured patient, a 'scoop and run' prehospital policy (pausing only to secure the airway and protect the neck) is best. In other situations (e.g. entrapment or prolonged transfer time) field resuscitation may be helpful (*see Box 2.2*). These procedures must not delay transfer to a definitive care centre; treatment in transit may be possible. Prolonged and inappropriate attempts at resuscitation in the field are harmful.

> **Box 2.2 Prehospital Management**
> - Secure the airway – jaw thrust, oropharyngeal or nasopharyngeal airway. Consider intubation.
> - Protect the cervical spine – collar and head holder.
> - Ensure adequate ventilation and oxygenation. (This may necessitate decompression of the chest.)
> - Cover open chest wounds.
> - Control external haemorrhage by direct pressure.
> - Commence IV infusions only if this does not delay transfer.
> - Protect thoracic and lumbar spine – backboard or 'scoop' stretcher.
> - Provide analgesia.
> - Record initial assessment of cardiorespiratory and neurological status.
> - Communicate with the hospital – assessment, management and expected time of arrival.

> In the prehospital management of injured adults and older children with presumed blood loss, it is now recommended that IV fluids should not be administered if a radial pulse can be felt (or, in the case of penetrating torso injuries, if a central pulse can be felt). In the absence of these pulses, IV crystalloids should be administered, en route to hospital, in boluses of no more than 250 mL until the relevant pulse becomes palpable. The same advice is probably applicable for young children and infants also, in which case boluses of 5 mL per kg should be used.

Primary concern in the ED is:

1 adequate oxygen delivery to vital tissues;
2 treatment of critical problems as soon as they are identified,
3 prevention of further deterioration.

This can be achieved by a well-rehearsed team working to agreed protocols and integrated into a comprehensive trauma care system.

Primary survey and resuscitation

This must be carried out in a strict order of priority. Problems are corrected as they are identified. The ATLS formula for the primary survey is:

A Airway.
B Breathing.
C Circulation.
D Disability.
E Exposure.

Airway

Check for responsiveness.

> In an unresponsive patient the airway is always at risk.

Then look for:
- no movement of air (complete airway obstruction or apnoea);
- noises from the upper airway (partial airway obstruction). There may be snoring, rattles, stridor or other sounds.

For causes of upper airway obstruction in trauma see Box 2.3. Any injury severe enough to compromise the airway may also have damaged the cervical spine.

Box 2.3 Causes of Upper Airway Obstruction in Trauma

Oropharyngeal – tongue, teeth, dental plates, foreign bodies, blood and vomit.
Facial – fractures of the maxilla or mandible.
Cervical – laryngeal injury.
Intracerebral – altered level of consciousness after head injury, alcohol or drugs.

Tx

All severely injured patients require a high inspired oxygen concentration. The airway must be:
- *cleared* of foreign material with suction, Magill's forceps and fingers, if necessary;
- *maintained* using a jaw thrust manoeuvre, a Guedel oropharyngeal airway, a nasopharyngeal airway or by endotracheal intubation (the nasopharyngeal airway is safe and well tolerated in the conscious patient and is much less likely to stimulate gagging than the Guedel airway); and
- *protected* by vigilance, suctioning and positioning.

When traumatic disruption of the facial or laryngeal structures prevents intubation, surgical access to the airway must be obtained. Emergency tracheostomy is difficult and dangerous and has been superseded by the technique of cricothyroidotomy. Needle puncture of the cricothyroid membrane is preferable in children under 12 years old. *For artificial airways in trauma see Box 2.4.*

The cervical spine

Neck injury must be assumed to have occurred in all patients who have sustained polytrauma until clinical examination and good quality radiographs prove otherwise. Patients at particular risk include those who have sustained:
- any injury above the clavicle;
- head injury associated with depressed consciousness;
- a high speed injury;
- a fall from a height.

A normal neurological examination does not exclude cervical spine injury. Moreover, conscious patients with other painful injuries may not always complain of neck discomfort.

Box 2.4 Artificial Airways in Trauma

Standard orotracheal intubation. This is the route of choice in the apnoeic patient or where cervical spine injury has been excluded by good quality radiographs.

Nasotracheal intubation. Nasotracheal intubation may be useful in cases in which cervical spine injury has not been excluded as it involves less extension of the neck. It is also a valuable technique in some special situations, such as for the non-paralysed patient. It should not be performed in the presence of a possible fracture of the base of the skull. The traditionally advocated method of 'blind' nasal intubation requires considerable skill (to say the least!) and thus should not be attempted by the inexperienced.

Surgical cricothyroidotomy. This is the method of choice in adults. It is contraindicated in children under 12 years of age because of the importance of the cricoid cartilage in tracheal support and the long-term problems that result if it is damaged – *see Box 2.5.*

Needle cricothyroidotomy. This procedure is performed using a large cannula. Bag and mask ventilation is ineffective via such a small opening. The patient must be ventilated with high-flow oxygen from either a flow meter or the wall supply (at 50 psi or 4000 cm H_2O pressure). Intermittent flow is achieved using a Y-piece, a three-way tap or a hole in the side of the tubing. Exhalation takes place through the upper airway and not through the cannula. CO_2 retention occurs and thus this technique should not be used for more than 20 min if a more effective airway can be obtained – *see Box 2.6.*

Box 2.5 Cricothyroidotomy

- Extend the patient's neck while controlling the head.
- Mark the skin over the centre of the cricothyroid membrane (which lies between the thyroid and cricoid cartilages, *see Figure 2.1*).
- Support the larynx and tighten the overlying skin with the non-dominant hand.
- Make a small transverse incision through the skin and spread the edges outwards.
- Make a transverse incision through the cricothyroid membrane and open the wound with the handle of the scalpel.
- Insert an appropriate size of endotracheal or tracheostomy tube.
- Start ventilation and check for air entry.
- Secure the tube.

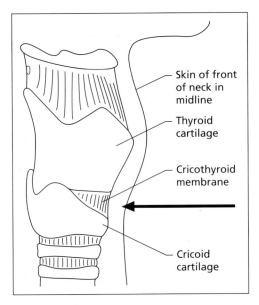

Figure 2.1 The site for cricothyroidotomy.

Box 2.6 Needle Cricothyroid Puncture

- Extend the patient's neck while controlling the head.
- Mark the skin over the centre of the cricothyroid membrane (which lies between the thyroid and cricoid cartilages *see Figure 2.1*).
- Attach a cannula and needle of an appropriate size (at least 12 G for an adult) to a small syringe.
- Support the larynx and tighten the overlying skin with the non-dominant hand.
- Puncture the skin and cricothyroid membrane with the needle, aiming for the small of the back, aspirating as the needle is advanced.
- When air is easily aspirated, advance the cannula and withdraw the needle.
- Recheck the ease of aspiration of air. (It is surprisingly easy to miss the trachea with a needle, especially in children.)
- Attach the cannula to either the wall or the flow meter oxygen supply via an in-line Y-connector. In a child, start with a flow meter set at a delivery rate in litres equal to the child's age in years.
- Adjust the flow rate and inspiratory time until adequate chest movement is achieved. Expiration may take several seconds.
- Secure the cannula.

Tx

The neck must be splinted to prevent damage to the cord from the movement of an unstable injured spine. This should be achieved with a well-fitting hard collar and a purpose-built head holder. However, if the patient is struggling violently, attempts to control the head may inadvertently lead to further injury. In these circumstances, it is best to use a collar alone. The cause of the agitation should be sought. It is often hypoxia, pain or both. In a patient with a depressed level of consciousness, a full bladder may be responsible.

Breathing

Look for
- External signs of injury.
- Abnormal respiratory rate or pattern.
- Unequal chest movement.
- Tracheal shift and displacement of the apex beat.
- Decreased breath sounds.
- Increased or decreased resonance.
- Low SaO_2.
- Signs of hypoxia (tachycardia, agitation or confusion and cyanosis).

There are five major chest injuries that require immediate recognition and treatment during the primary survey. They are:

1 tension pneumothorax;
2 open pneumothorax (sucking chest wound);
3 massive haemothorax;
4 flail segment of the chest;
5 cardiac tamponade.

Other injuries, which may cause dyspnoea or shock, may become apparent in the secondary survey:

- pulmonary contusion;
- myocardial contusion;
- aortic disruption;
- traumatic diaphragmatic hernia;
- tracheobronchial disruption;
- oesophageal disruption.

Tx

For the diagnosis and treatment of major chest injuries see Chapter 6.

Upper airway patency does not ensure adequate ventilation. Assisted breathing using a bag, mask and airway or tracheal intubation may be required. Prior to attempted intubation, the patient must be pre-oxygenated using a bag, mask and airway technique, and intubation should be performed quickly by an experienced operator. Prolonged, unsuccessful attempts at intubation must be avoided.

> Attempted intubation in a patient who is not paralysed may cause a dramatic rise in intracranial pressure.

Therefore, even the apparently 'flat' apnoeic patient should ideally be assessed by an anaesthetist before intubation. (These cases are not analogous to the cardiac arrest patient, where intubation without paralysis is acceptable.)

A small, uncomplicated, and possibly undiagnosed, simple pneumothorax may rapidly develop into a life-threatening tension pneumothorax if the patient is mechanically ventilated, either in theatre or ICU. Prophylactic chest drains should be considered in any patient with chest injury requiring ventilation.

Circulation

In the primary survey the state of the circulation is quickly assessed by observation of:
- skin colour and temperature;
- pulse rate and volume;
- capillary refill time at a finger pulp or nail bed (this is usually < 2 seconds);
- BP;
- jugular venous pressure (JVP) and heart sounds (for tamponade);
- level of consciousness (in the patient who has not sustained a brain injury).

> Hypotension with a raised JVP and absent heart sounds suggests the presence of a cardiac tamponade.

The assessment of hypovolaemia in the trauma patient is notoriously difficult for the following reasons.
- The interaction of autonomic reflexes, head injury, pain, drugs and blood loss is complex and still not fully elucidated.

- Compensatory mechanisms may prevent a fall in systolic blood pressure until 30% of the blood volume has been lost.
- Rapid blood loss may produce a reflex bradycardia.
- In the elderly, tachycardia may not be present as a result of a limited cardiac response to catecholamines or treatment with beta-blockers.
- Haematocrit is an unreliable index of shock; a nearly normal value does not rule out significant blood loss.

> All abnormalities of colour, pulse, BP and consciousness should be regarded with suspicion.

For signs of shock see Box 2.7. For methods of assessing organ perfusion see Box 2.8. The blood loss potential of evident injuries should be considered (*see Box 2.9*); the mechanism of injury may suggest occult blood loss. Hypovolaemia is seldom caused by head injury alone, except occasionally in infants. Open fractures will cause greater blood loss than similar closed injuries.

Box 2.7 Signs of Shock

- Altered mental state.
- Delayed capillary refill (> 2 s).
- Tachycardia.
- Pale, cool skin.

Box 2.8 Guides to Organ Perfusion

- Mental state.
- Urinary output.
  Adequate volume replacement will produce a urine output in the adult of about 50 mL per h.
- Arterial blood gases.
  Metabolic acidosis implies inadequate tissue oxygenation requiring increased oxygen and fluids (not bicarbonate).
- Shock index.
  Shock index is calculated by dividing the pulse rate in beats per minute by the systolic BP in mmHg. The normal range is 0.5–0.7. Values in excess of 0.9 are suggestive of significant haemorrhage.
- Core/periphery temperature gradient.
- Aortic flow (measured by Doppler ultrasound probe).
- Serum lactate.
  High lactate is increasingly recognised as a good indicator of tissue hypoxia and a poor prognostic sign.
- ICU determination of oxygen demand and supply.

Box 2.9 Estimation of Traumatic Blood Loss in an Adult (closed injuries)

Site	Volume (L)
Pelvis	0.5–3
Shaft of femur	1–2
Tibia	0.5–1
Chest	>2
Abdomen	>2
Arm	0.5–1
Forearm	0.5–1

Tx

• Control external blood loss by direct pressure at the bleeding site.

• Insert at least two large-calibre (14 G) cannulas into large veins. If percutaneous venous access is difficult, cut down to the antecubital veins, the long saphenous vein or the femoral vein. Central veins should not be used as routes for fluid replacement in the initial stages of resuscitation, but should be preserved for use in the ICU. In small children, if venous access is not achieved within a few minutes, the intra-osseous route is the most suitable (*see page 326*); femoral venous access is an alternative.

• Take a sample of blood (20 mL in an adult) for grouping and cross-matching and coagulation screen.

• Commence rapid fluid replacement with a bolus of 10 mL per kg. After reassessment of the patient, this can be repeated. (In the prehospital management of patients with presumed blood loss, it is now recommended that IV fluids should not be administered if a radial pulse can be felt or, in the case of penetrating torso injuries, if a central pulse can be felt. In the absence of these pulses, IV crystalloids should be administered, en route to hospital, in boluses of not more than 250 mL (5 mL per kg for infants and young children) until the relevant pulse becomes palpable.) Whenever rapid fluid replacement is required, warmed IV fluids (40°C) should be be used. A ratio of crystalloids to colloids of at least 50 : 50 has been shown to be

safe. Many doctors believe that Hartmann's solution is preferable to normal saline if large volumes are to be given. The role of hypertonic saline in resuscitation looks promising but has yet to be fully established.

• Consider the possibility of intra-abdominal bleeding and the need for surgical advice.

• Consider the possibility of blood loss from a major pelvic fracture. This is difficult to identify surgically and is best treated with an external fixation device. A pelvic fixator can be applied rapidly in the ED by the orthopaedic team. This should be thought of as a resuscitation manoeuvre to help control the circulation in the primary survey.

Military anti-shock trousers (MAST) or pneumatic anti-shock garments (PASG) are no longer recommended. Controlled trials have not shown them to be of benefit and their sudden removal causes significant volume loss into the lower limbs.

The return of a normal BP after the infusion of, for example, 1000 mL does not mean that only a litre has been lost – the true amount is likely to be much higher. Normotension, which can only be maintained by continuing infusion, is a sign of impending collapse; the cause of the hidden loss must be sought. Failure to respond to fluids is usually a result of the administration of inadequate aliquots or to other (unrecognised) fluid losses. However, it may also be caused by:

• tension pneumothorax – *see page 77*;
• cardiac tamponade – *see page 81*;
• myocardial infarction;
• acute gastric distension; or
• neurogenic shock – *see page 52*.

Blood transfusion

Modest haemodilution and a fall in haematocrit to 30% improve erythrocyte passage through the microcirculation. This allows optimal oxygen delivery to the tissues – until the haematocrit falls below 25%. However, when estimated blood loss exceeds 1.5 L in an adult, blood should be transfused to maintain the haematocrit above 25%.

SAG-M blood (which consists of plasma-poor red blood cells in saline, adenine, glucose and mannitol) is frequently supplied by the National Blood Service in the United Kingdom. (The adenine maintains 2,3-DPG activity in stored blood to allow more normal uncoupling of oxygen from oxyhaemoglobin and thus improved tissue oxygenation.) This red cell concentrate is presented in units of 300 mL, each with a packed cell volume (haematocrit) of 0.55–0.65.

If a blood sample is taken when the initial intravenous lines are established, grouped blood (type-specific) should be available within 20 min. Cross-matched blood (whether by urgent or full cross-match) is seldom available within 1 h and is therefore not normally appropriate for unstable hypovolaemic patients. These patients should receive blood that is matched only for the recipient's ABO and rhesus group. This will, of course, increase the incidence of transfusion reactions.

In situations of such urgency that delay – even for grouped blood – is unacceptable, O negative (universal donor) blood should be given. However, the risks of a transfusion reaction must be outweighed by the benefits of immediate blood replacement; such occasions are rare.

Rapid blood transfusion may produce:
- *coagulopathy* – requiring platelets and/or fresh frozen plasma;
- *hypocalcaemia* – as a result of calcium binding by anticoagulants in stored blood (at infusion rates of less than 50 mL per min this should not be a problem and most authorities do not now recommend giving additional calcium);
- *hypothermia* (which may itself cause a significant reduction in coagulation).

Thus, if a large volume of blood is transfused rapidly, it should be filtered and warmed.

For the indications for transfusion of different blood components see Box 14.25 on page 262.

Control of severe bleeding

Severe bleeding from damaged tissue, blood vessels or even organs may sometimes be controlled by the application of haemostatic substances. The most effective of these is MPH (microporous polysaccharide hemospheres), a patented powder synthesised from raw materials derived from potatoes! The MPH particles dehydrate the blood and concentrate blood solids on their surfaces, thus creating a high concentration of gelled, compacted clotting material.

With intractable bleeding, deficiency of clotting factors should be considered and haematological advice sought. In particular, in the absence of any known disease, acquired haemophilia may be a possibility – *see page 263*.

Emergency thoracotomy

Emergency thoracotomy may be life saving for some patients with penetrating injuries to the chest (*see page 83*). A left anterolateral thoracotomy in the fourth intercostal space allows cardiac tamponade to be relieved; cross-clamping of the thoracic aorta optimises cerebral circulation during the critical period. Thoracotomy is of no value if the patient is already lifeless on arrival at the department or has sustained blunt trauma.

Disability

A rapid assessment of the patient's neurological status completes the primary survey:
- level of consciousness;
- pupil size and reaction;
- posture and spontaneous movements.

A simple classification of level of consciousness is the AVPU system:

A Alert.
V Responds to voice.
P Responds to pain.
U Unresponsive.

Alternatively, if time allows, the Glasgow Coma Scale can be used.

Exposure

All parts of the patient should be exposed and examined. The spine must be well controlled when clothing is disturbed. Some clothes can only be safely removed during log-rolling. The areas most often missed are the back and the perineum.

> Beware of hypothermia.

Further care of the trauma patient

At the end of the primary survey, attention must be given to the following:

• *Glucose* – check for hypoglycaemia with a reagent stick. Some degree of hyperglycaemia is inevitable in most trauma patients; hypoglycaemia can precipitate trauma – *see pages 246 and 327*.
• *History* – the AMPLE format (*see page 9*).
• *Immediate analgesia* – small aliquots of IV morphine are carefully titrated against response.
• *Investigations* – the three initial X-rays of multiple trauma (chest, lateral cervical spine and pelvis).

> Do not forget to communicate as frequently as possible with the patient's relatives (*see pages 10 and 330*).

The secondary survey

On completion of the primary survey – when resuscitation is well underway and appropriate inpatient team members have been called – remove all of the patient's remaining clothing while controlling the entire spine. The detailed secondary survey can now begin. It should be carried out in a top-to-toe rather than in a systems-orientated order.

> Much of the information of the secondary (and primary) surveys is best recorded on a purpose-designed trauma form.

The following features must be included in the examination:

Head and neck
• Glasgow Coma Score.
• Pupillary size and reactions.
• Posture, movement and cranial nerve function – lateralising signs.
• Scalp – haematomata, lacerations, depressed fractures. Insert a gloved finger into the lacerations to detect fractures.
• Ears and nose for cerebrospinal fluid and/or bleeding. Look with an auroscope for haemotympani.
• Facial skeleton.

• Mouth and teeth.
• Neck – swelling, wounds and tenderness.

Chest
• Respiratory rate, pattern and depth. Watch and feel for the abnormal movement of a flail segment.
• Clothing imprints or bruising.
• Wounds – especially small penetrating injuries.
• Surgical emphysema.
• Rib tenderness.
• Tracheal displacement.
• Air entry, percussion note and breath sounds.
• Heart sounds and position of the apex beat.
• Trends in SaO_2.
• Arterial blood gases.
• ECG.

Abdomen
• Clothing imprints or bruising – which usually indicate severe compression.
• Wounds.
• Localised or generalised tenderness and guarding.
• Bowel sounds – an unreliable guide to injury.
• Buttocks, anus, genitalia and perineum.
• Consider rectal and vaginal examination (*see page 301*).

Back (will need log-roll)
• Bruising, swelling and wounds.
• Gaps and swellings in the line of the spinous processes.
• Tenderness – especially ribs, spine and loins.
• Perineum and anus (*see page 88*).

Limbs
• Swelling and bruising.
• Tenderness.
• Wounds.
• Deformity and compound fractures.
• Circulation, nerve and tendon function distal to injuries.
• General peripheral neurological function.

At the end of the secondary survey, re-examine the ABCs.

Tx

• Summon further appropriate specialist help.
• Reduce any fracture or dislocation, which is threatening distal circulation or overlying skin.

A mixture of IV morphine and inhaled nitrous oxide will be the minimum analgesia required for this in a conscious patient – *see page 17*.
- Splint other fractures.
- Clean and dress wounds.
- Catheterise the bladder and measure the urine output.
- Obtain further information from the patient, paramedics, bystanders, relatives or the GP.
- Consider the need for further investigations (*see later*).

Prophylactic antibiotics. Prophylactic antibiotics are indicated for:
- severe contaminated wounds with tissue destruction;
- compound limb fractures;
- penetrating intestinal injuries.

> Antibiotics are not indicated for simple contaminated wounds but thorough surgical toilet is always required. Delayed primary suture may be appropriate.

Tetanus prophylaxis. Tetanus immune status should be confirmed as soon as possible and antitetanus toxoid and immunoglobulin given as appropriate (*see page 390*). If no history is available, the patient should be treated as unimmunised.

Investigations in trauma

Blood tests

Blood should be taken for full blood count, blood grouping and cross-matching, coagulation screen and biochemistry (including glucose). In some cases – where the cause of coma is in doubt – a plasma osmolality can be useful (*see page 228*). Arterial blood gases should be checked as soon as possible.

Radiological priorities

In the severely injured patient, the radiological priorities are the chest, lateral cervical spine and pelvis. Radiographs should be obtained using portable or overhead machines, so that the patient does not have to be moved out of the resuscitation area. Further radiographs of the skull, dorsal and lumbar spine or extremities may be delayed until resuscitation is underway and the patient is stable. *For assessment of chest injury see page 75.*
For assessment of injury to the cervical spine see page 51.
For assessment of pelvic injury see page 88.

Trauma radiograph of the chest

The ideal view of the chest is the erect posteroanterior (PA) film, which will demonstrate:
- pneumothorax;
- haemothorax;
- mediastinal widening;
- subphrenic air;
- rib fractures.

However, positioning the patient upright is potentially hazardous if spinal injury has not been excluded or if the patient is unresponsive. Diagnosis of intrathoracic injury on an anteroposterior (AP) (supine) film is difficult. A lateral decubitus film, ie., taken with a patient lying on his or her side (literally 'elbow down') may be helpful in diagnosing pneumothorax, free intraperitoneal air or fluid levels but to achieve the correct position requires careful in-line log-rolling.

Trauma radiograph of the cervical spine

A good cross-table lateral view of the cervical spine will exclude many significant injuries. Often, the body of C7 and the C7/T1 junction are not adequately visualised on the initial film and a coned view of this area with gentle shoulder traction is needed.

If the lateral radiograph of the neck is normal and the patient is fully conscious without significant neck pain, then the cervical collar may be removed to allow clinical assessment of the cervical spine. In the patient with depressed consciousness, the cervical spine must remain immobilised while awaiting AP and odontoid peg views, discussion with an orthopaedic surgeon and, if necessary, a CT scan. *For clearance of the cervical spine see page 57.*

Trauma radiograph of the pelvis

Clinical assessment of pelvic injury by pressure on the anterior superior iliac spines is unreliable. Furthermore, any movement elicited may restart or exacerbate pelvic bleeding. An AP radiograph of the pelvis is taken to assess the potential for blood loss rather than to obtain detailed information about the nature of any fractures.

CT scan

This provides excellent assessment of intracranial injuries and their sequelae. Sequential cuts of the cervical spine, chest and abdomen may also be obtained. Do not ask for 'CT trunk' as a replacement for clinical assessment – widely based cuts can overlook spinal injuries, are time consuming and involve a large amount of radiation exposure. Reasonable requests for a CT scan (other than brain) in a trauma patient might be for:
- clearance of the lower cervical spine;
- further assessment of spinal injuries seen on plain films;
- examination of the mediastinum;
- assessment of abdominal injuries;
- assessment of pelvic fractures.

Requests for CT scanning should be discussed with a senior radiologist who will be able to advise as to the appropriateness of the intended investigation.

Ultrasound scan

In experienced hands, ultrasound can be a highly sensitive diagnostic technique. It is particularly useful for the detection of free fluid and the identification of solid organ injury. It is less valuable in the assessment of bowel damage.

Further assessment of the abdomen in multiple trauma

Abdominal injuries have special significance because of the following:

1 They can cause profound haemorrhage.

2 They can be difficult to diagnose clinically – especially in unresponsive patients. Signs may be poorly localised or equivocal.

Exclusion of intra-abdominal damage is particularly important in any patient who:
- is shocked or unstable;
- has signs attributable to the abdomen;
- has a reduced level of consciousness or is otherwise difficult to assess clinically;
- is about to be anaesthetised or transferred to another department for the management of other injuries.

Methods of abdominal assessment include:
- immediate laparotomy;
- diagnostic peritoneal lavage;
- ultrasound examination;
- CT scanning.

For a full discussion of the assessment of abdominal injuries see Chapter 6 on page 75.

Definitive care of the trauma patient

Every effort should be made to get the trauma patient to the area of definitive care as soon as possible. This may be a theatre, a specialised surgical unit, an ICU or a bed in a ward. Rapid disposal of a properly assessed and stabilised patient is associated with a decreased risk of complications and is (obviously) a reassurance for both patients and relatives.

> Do not forget the continuing need for analgesia.

See also the appropriate chapters on specific areas of injury.

Special situations

For major burns see page 146.
For electrocution see page 154.
For irradiation see page 298.
For choking see page 205.

Drowning

Drowning is suffocation resulting from submersion or immersion in a liquid and as such causes injury by the effects of fluid in the airway and lungs and by generalised hypoxia. There may also be coexisting:
- hypothermia;
- injury (from a fall or dive into water – especially involving the cervical spine);

- illness (which precipitated the drowning – such as myocardial infarction, hypoglycaemia or a fit);
- alcohol or drug intoxication.

Toddlers and teenagers are the most common victims of drowning and drowning is the leading cause of accidental death in children worldwide.

The difference between the effects of sea water (hypertonic) and fresh water (hypotonic) drowning is probably less important than once believed. In many cases, there is immediate laryngospasm and thus little inhalation into the lungs (dry drowning). The patient is likely to be unresponsive and hypotensive with signs of cerebral hypoxia and perhaps also pulmonary oedema.

Tx

For cardiac arrest see page 156.
In other patients carry out the following:

- Clear the airway of debris and then secure it. Consider the need for cervical spine protection.
- Give high-flow oxygen with a continuous positive airway pressure (CPAP) circuit if possible. Patients in whom breathing is inadequate should be ventilated immediately – with the help of an anaesthetist if possible. These patients will usually need decompression of the stomach with a wide-bore tube.
- Establish IV access and fluid infusion.
- Monitor SaO_2, respiratory rate, pulse, BP, ECG and core temperature.
- Send blood for FBC, blood chemistry, glucose and blood gases.
- Obtain a 12-lead ECG and Chest X-ray.
- Treat hypotension, wheezing or pulmonary oedema. Severe acidosis can be corrected with bicarbonate.
- Treat hypothermia (*see page 248*).

All patients must be admitted – most to the ICU. Delayed exacerbations may occur up to 24 h after injury. Patients with signs of cerebral hypoxia (usually unresponsive) should be ventilated even in the presence of satisfactory oxygenation as they are likely to have cerebral oedema.

Suffocation and asphyxiation

Suffocation is a state where there is inadequate availability of air for inhalation – usually as a result of external obstruction of the mouth and nose. Asphyxiation describes oxygen deficit from a wider range of causes such as gassing and strangulation. The signs of both are those of prolonged hypoxia and developing cerebral oedema. The treatment is similar to that detailed above for drowning.

Paediatric trauma

The principles of the management of trauma are the same for both adults and children. Differences in anatomy, physiological parameters and equipment are dealt with in *Chapter 18*. The most important aspects of a child when compared to an adult in trauma care are as follows:

- The airway is narrower, floppier and more difficult to maintain.
- The lungs have a very limited oxygen reserve but the body has a higher metabolic rate.
- The circulation may suddenly decompensate and thus shock appears with very little warning.
- The vertebrae are relatively elastic and so there may be spinal cord injury without radiological abnormality (abbreviated to the acronym SCIWORA).
- The ribs are also elastic and so may not protect the underlying viscera from trauma.
- A child becomes hypoglycaemic and hypothermic very easily.

> A child's lungs, liver and spleen are like fresh eggs in an AMBU bag. Hit the bag with a hammer and the eggs are smashed but the bag (the ribs) returns to its former shape. An adult's organs are like hard-boiled eggs in a tin can. Hit the can and it is damaged (there are rib fractures) but the eggs may survive intact.

Trauma in pregnancy

The anatomical and physiological changes of pregnancy must be considered during assessment.

- The tidal volume is increased, respiratory rate is stable and so $PaCO_2$ is slightly reduced.
- The BP is normally slightly reduced and the pulse is increased.
- Compression of the inferior vena cava in the supine patient in the last trimester of pregnancy is

very significant and reduces cardiac output. The risk of sudden collapse is reduced by turning the patient partially onto the left side.

• Gastric emptying is delayed.

Systemic (maternal) hypovolaemia results in a selective reduction in placental blood flow. The foetus is very vulnerable to hypoxia but the maternal circulation is partially protected by a physiological hypervolaemia. Deterioration in oxygen supply to the foetus can occur very rapidly after a period of apparent normality.

XR

Consider early ultrasound scan of the abdomen, uterus and foetus.

For other methods of foetal assessment see below.

TX

Management of a pregnant patient with injuries involves the care of two patients:

1 *The mother*. For the most part, the care of a pregnant woman is identical to that of a nonpregnant patient. Important additions are the following:

• Hypoxia and hypovolaemia must be treated particularly quickly and vigorously.

• Patients who are in the last trimester of pregnancy should be nursed wedged on to the left side. This is to prevent compression of the inferior vena cava by the pregnant uterus with consequent reduction in cardiac filling and circulatory collapse.

• All pregnant patients suffering from trauma are at risk of aspiration pneumonia (Mendelson's syndrome), especially if they have a reduced level of consciousness or may need sedation or anaesthesia. Prophylaxis is aimed at reducing the acidity of the gastric contents as quickly as possible and thus IV therapy with ranitidine (50 mg diluted to 20 mL and given over 2 min) or omeprazole (40 mg diluted to 100 mL and given over 20 min) is indicated for all such patients.

• Rhesus-D-negative women with abdominal injury are at risk of developing antibodies against a rhesus-positive foetus. Consequently, any pregnant woman who may have suffered from abdominal trauma should be blood grouped and, if found to be Rhesus-D- negative, given anti-D immunoglobulin.

2 *The foetus*. The well-being of the foetus depends almost entirely on the state of the mother.

> The initial management of the foetus is the support of the maternal airway, breathing and circulation.

Once the mother is stabilised, then obstetric advice should be sought. Methods of assessing the foetus include:

• auscultation with a Pinnard's stethoscope or Doppler foetoscope;

• foetocardiotocography (FCTG);

• abdominal ultrasound.

In some cases, in late pregnancy, caesarean section will be required for the health of both parties. Postmortem caesarean section may occasionally save the life of the baby when the mother is recently deceased. For this purpose, the modern operation of lower uterine segment caesarean section is too slow. A 'classical' section is usually performed through the muscle of the upper uterine segment leading to a rapid delivery.

For other aspects of abdominal trauma in pregnancy, see page 87.

Other aspects of trauma care

Bereaved relatives

As with cardiac arrest, a fatality from trauma will leave relatives in a state of sudden and unexpected bereavement. The care of these people is part of the complete spectrum of trauma management.

For an outline of bereavement care, see page 169.

Trauma scores

Trauma scoring systems are useful for audit, research and planning purposes but should not be used to determine in-hospital care. They have a limited use in prehospital triage. There are four main types:

1 Scores used at the site of an incident, which are based on direct observation of evident abnormalities (e.g. the Circulation, Respiration, Abdomen, Movement and Speech Score or CRAMS).

2 Scores that are based – retrospectively – on the anatomical injuries (e.g. the Injury Severity Score or ISS).

3 Scores that are calculated from the observed physiology of the patient at the time of presentation (e.g. the Revised Trauma Score or RTS).

4 More complex scores – usually derived on ICU – which take account of both the current status and the pre-existing health of the victim (e.g. the Acute Physiology and Chronic Health Evaluation or APACHE score).

Chapter 3

Head injuries

In the United Kingdom, about 1.4 million people come to departments of emergency medicine every year after a head injury – approximately 10% of all new patients; half are children.

> Over 5000 people die from traumatic brain injuries in England and Wales every year. In addition, it is estimated that over 1500 patients survive with severe brain damage. Most will have a severely reduced employment potential and many will require long-term nursing care. The majority are men, with a mean age of 30 years.

Primary damage to the brain occurs at the time of injury. Secondary damage is the result of extracranial factors such as hypoxia or hypovolaemia, which lead to impaired cerebral oxygen delivery. Reperfusion of damaged brain (with the release of oxygen free radicals and lipid peroxidation) is now recognised as an additional secondary factor that can complicate recovery from traumatic brain injury. The problems that cause secondary damage can be minimised by systemic resuscitation. In the future, intracranial factors may be amenable to pharmacological interventions.

A decreased level of consciousness indicates that something is wrong with the brain or its fuel supply. It may be:
- hypoxia or shock;
- hypoglycaemia;
- hypothermia;
- poisoning or gross metabolic disturbance (including CO_2 narcosis);
- injury;
- intracranial pathology (bleeding, thrombosis, embolism, infection, swelling, tumour, fitting).

> Over half of all patients who are in a traumatic coma for more than 6 h will die; only one-fifth will recover without significant disability.

Biomechanics and brain injury

Direct trauma may cause:
1 Focal scalp injury
2 Depressed vault fracture
3 Extradural haemorrhage
4 Focal brain injury
5 Contra-coup injury
6 Brain laceration and intracerebral haemorrhage
7 Subdural haemorrhage
1–5 may not be associated with loss of consciousness.

Sudden acceleration/deceleration causes shearing injury to the brain and diffuse axonal injury (DAI). This is associated with loss of consciousness but external evidence of head injury may be lacking.

DAI is more common with the longer deceleration time characteristic of restrained passengers in traffic crashes. Extradural haemorrhage is more common in falls.

Cervical spine injury is more likely if the mobile head hits a fixed object (deceleration/acceleration), than if a mobile object hits the fixed head (assault).

The patient with a markedly depressed level of consciousness

This section deals with the management of those patients who when first seen have a Glasgow Coma Score (GCS) of 13 or less. Serious brain injury must be suspected. The principal objective of emergency management is to limit the effects of this primary insult by preventing deleterious secondary events, which could impair cerebral oxygen supply. A detailed neurological examination to determine the extent of the primary injury must be deferred until treatable secondary events have been controlled.

Immediate assessment and management

The ABC approach is vital.
• Clear and maintain the airway and give high-concentration oxygen. Have suction available.
• Ensure that the cervical spine is protected.
• Obtain anaesthetic assistance as soon as possible. Emergency induction of anaesthesia, intubation and ventilation is likely to be required.

> Ensure that cardiorespiratory resuscitation is initiated and the neck is protected before assessing brain injury.

• Obtain IV access.
• Monitor and record pulse, BP, SaO$_2$, respiratory rate and ECG.
• Assess neurological status by AVPU criteria:
  A Alert
  V Responds to voice
  P Responds to pain
  U Unresponsive
and assess the pupils for size, equality and reaction.
• Check the blood glucose with a reagent strip.

• Treat reversible conditions (and reassess after therapy):
Hypoglycaemia: Take blood for glucose estimation prior to giving IV dextrose (0.2–0.5 mg per kg); avoid hyperglycaemia.
Fits: Give lorazepam 4 mg (0.1 mg per kg) or diazepam 10 mg (0.25 mg per kg) slowly IV.
Narcosis: Give naloxone IV 0.4 mg.
Aggression and restlessness: Give 100% oxygen. Check the airway and the SaO$_2$. Catheterise the bladder. Sedation should only be given after consideration of the causes.

• Ask witnesses/paramedics if the level of consciousness has changed since the impact. Did the patient briefly recover and speak and then deteriorate? Obtain a brief history (*AMPLE see Chapter 1*). Try to establish the mechanism of the injury.
• Obtain radiographs of the cervical spine. Measure the blood gases.

> The administration of steroids has been shown to be of no benefit in the treatment of head injuries.

Further assessment and management

• Carry out a detailed secondary survey.
• Seek surgical/neurosurgical advice.
• Catheterise the bladder.
The secondary survey should look for other injuries and elaborate the neurological status of the patient. This must include examination of:
• the scalp;
• the auditory canals and tympanic membranes (with caution – *see page 45*);
• the pupils and limbs;
• the face;
• the neck.

Neurological assessment

There are three groups of observations.
1 Level of consciousness. This is the main indicator of global brain function. It should be assessed

using the GCS (*see Box 3.1*). This score is a sensitive and reproducible indication of early neurological deterioration.

2 Focal neurological signs. For example, variation in muscle tone, asymmetrical limb movement and reflexes, disconjugate eye movements.

3 Pulse (down), BP (up), pupil size (up) and pupillary response (down). These parameters are easily measured but are late indicators of high intracranial pressure. The combination is known as Cushing's response.

These observations should be repeated at appropriate intervals and plotted on a chart.

GCS maximum score = 15 (not necessarily equivalent to alert and orientated)
GCS minimum score = 3 (even if dead!)
GCS of 8 or less = coma

For the children's coma score see page 327.

Other injuries

About 50% of patients with major brain injury have serious injuries elsewhere. The more injuries there are, the greater the risk of missing some of them.

For multiple injuries see Chapter 2 on page 20.

Imaging

As soon as the patient is stabilised, a CT scan of the brain should be obtained. The majority of patients will be intubated and ventilated prior to scanning. *For the indications for CT imaging of the brain in patients with head injuries see Box 3.2.*

Skull X-rays do not contribute to initial management. Therapy is directed towards the brain injury rather than any bony injury, and this is initially detected by the neurological signs. A lateral cervical spine view is more valuable. It must show the C7/T1 junction (*for advice on interpretation see page 55*). Special neck views in flexion and extension and basal skull radiographs are dangerous and contraindicated at this early stage of assessment.

For the indications for imaging of the cervical spine in patients with head injuries see Box 3.3.

For safety, logistical and resource reasons, MR imaging is not currently indicated as a primary investigation in patients with head injuries. Moreover, it is contraindicated in both head and cervical investigations unless there is absolute certainty that the patient is not harbouring an incompatible device, implant or metallic foreign body.

Box 3.1 The Glasgow Coma Scale (GCS)

Response elicited	Score
Response of eyes	
Open spontaneously	4
Open to speech	3
Open to pain	2
No response	1
Best motor response	
Obeys commands	6
Localises pain	5 (supraorbital ridge pressure)
Withdraws from pain	4 (normal flexion)
Abnormal flexion	3 (decorticate response)
Extension to pain	2 (decerebrate response)
None	1
Best verbal response	
Oriented	5
Confused	4
Inappropriate words	3
Incomprehensible sounds	2
None	1

Management of specific problems

Airway and breathing

Inadequate respiration leads to hypoxia, hypercarbia and acidosis. This results in cerebral vasodilatation and a rise in intracranial pressure. Although simple manoeuvres to clear and maintain the airway may be initially successful, intubation and ventilation is required for most patients with impaired respiration.

For the indications for immediate intubation and ventilation after a head injury see Box 3.4.

Box 3.2 Indications for CT Imaging of the Brain in Patients with Head Injuries

(The content of this box is adapted from the UK National Institute for Clinical Excellence's head injury guideline)

1 *The threshold for CT examination should be lowered if there are other life-threatening injuries, particularly if these will require operation under GA.*

2 *It is recommended that the CT scan of the head should extend down to the second cervical vertebra with 3 mm cuts from the level of the foramen magnum to C2. If the lower cervical spine has not been well-visualised on plain radiographs, then this should also be scanned.*

3 *Patients who return to the emergency department after discharge with persistent complaints that could be attributed to their head injury should be discussed with a senior clinician and considered for CT imaging.*

Immediate CT scan = *imaging performed and results analysed within 1 h of the request*

GCS less than 13 at any time since the injury.

GCS still less than 15 at 2 h or more post-injury.

Suspected open or depressed skull fracture.

Penetrating injury.

Any signs of basal skull fracture (*see page 44*).

Focal neurological signs.

Deteriorating neurological signs.

Post-traumatic seizure.

More than one episode of vomiting (Clinical judgement should be used regarding the cause of vomiting in children aged 12 or less and whether imaging is necessary).

Age 65 years or more with a history of loss of consciousness or amnesia.

Coagulopathy with a history of loss of consciousness or amnesia (history of bleeding or clotting disorder or current anticoagulant treatment).

Delayed CT scan = *imaging performed and results analysed within 8 h of the time of injury*

Dangerous mechanism of injury with a history of loss of consciousness or amnesia (e.g. pedestrian hit by motor vehicle, occupant ejected from a motor vehicle or fall from a height of greater than 1 m or more than five stairs. Lower heights are applicable for infants and young children).

Amnesia for greater than 30 min for events before the impact (Almost impossible to assess in children under the age of 5 years).

Persistent severe headache (not included by the National Institute for Clinical Excellence).

Linear fracture of the skull on plain radiographs (not included by the National Institute for Clinical Excellence).

Box 3.3 Indications for Plain X-ray Imaging of the Cervical Spine in Patients with Head Injuries

(The content of this box is adapted from the UK National Institute for Clinical Excellence's head injury guideline)

Patients with any one of the following features after head injury require urgent imaging of the cervical spine:

GCS less than 15 when assessed.

Focal neurological signs.

Parasthesia in the extremities.

Neck pain or tenderness and aged 65 years or above.

Neck pain or tenderness following dangerous mechanism of injury (fall from height of more than 1 m or 5 stairs; axial load to head such as diving injury, high speed RTA, rollover motor accident, ejection from a motor vehicle, accident involving motorised recreational vehicles, bicycle collision. A lower threshold for height of falls should be used for infants and children under the age of 5 years).

Failure to actively rotate the neck by 45° to left and right.

Clinical reasons for not wanting to move and examine the neck. *(For patients with neck pain who can be safely examined see Box 4.4 on page 57).*

Box 3.4 Indications for Immediate Intubation and Ventilation After Head Injuries

Aiming for PaO$_2$ greater than 100 mmHg (13 kPa) and PaCO$_2$ of 35–38 mmHg (4.5–5 kPa)

Coma or deteriorating conscious level.

Apparent loss of protective airway reflexes.

Ventilatory insufficiency as judged by oximetry/blood gas measurement:
- PaO$_2$ of < 75 mmHg (10 kPa) on air or < 100 mmHg (13 kPa) on oxygen;
- PaCO$_2$ of > 45 mmHg (6 kPa).

Spontaneous hyperventilation causing a PaCO$_2$ of < 25 mmHg (3.5 kPa).

Irregular respiration.

Multiple fits.

Significant facial injuries.

Bleeding into the airway.

Extreme agitation.

Intubation should not be attempted without sedation, analgesia and muscle paralysis (even in apparently 'flat' head-injured patients) as this would cause a sudden rise in intracranial pressure.

In ventilated patients with a head injury, aim for a PaO_2 of >100 mmHg (13.3 kPa) and a $PaCO_2$ of 35–38 mmHg (4.5–5.0 kPa).

Even patients with no apparent respiratory disturbance may benefit from controlled ventilation. *For reasons for intubating and ventilating patients with brain injuries see Box 3.5.* Hyperventilation to a $PaCO_2$ of below 40 mmHg (5.3 kPa) causes cerebral vasoconstriction and a consequent fall in intracranial pressure. Excessive hyperventilation, however, can be dangerous. Only the undamaged brain responds to changes in blood gas tension and vasoconstriction in normal areas may result in redistribution of blood flow to the injured tissue. This increases the penumbra around the damaged area. Brain ischaemia leads to lactic acidosis and reflex vasodilatation.

Box 3.5 Reasons for Intubating and Ventilating Patients with Brain Injuries

1 To clear, maintain and protect the airway.
2 To maintain adequate gas exchange.
3 To reduce intracranial pressure (ICP) and $PaCO_2$.
4 To facilitate CT scanning.
5 To allow safe patient transport.

Circulation

Changes in arterial BP between 80 and 200 mmHg do not influence normal cerebral blood flow. Brain injury impairs this autoregulatory function and hence cerebral blood supply in damaged areas is less well protected from changes in the systemic circulation.

Hypotension is only very rarely caused by brain injury. Trauma to the trunk and neck must be considered together with the biomechanics of the impact.

Cushing's response (bradycardia and hypertension) is a late sign and indicates rising intracranial pressure.

Neurogenic pulmonary oedema is occasionally seen. It is thought to be caused by vasoconstriction resulting from sympathetic overactivity (an alpha effect). It should be treated aggressively with standard drugs and always necessitates ventilation (*see page 217*).

Raised intracranial pressure

Hyperglycaemia increases brain swelling and must be avoided. Mannitol (1 g per kg IV) is used as a short-term agent to reduce brain swelling before clot evacuation; furosemide (frusemide) (0.5 mg per kg IV) is an alternative. Mannitol actually causes a transient intracranial pressure rise and leaks into the extracellular space, exerting an osmotic effect. Furosemide does not have these deleterious effects and causes a reduction in cerebrospinal fluid production. Neither drug should be used for long-term management of cerebral oedema.

Fits

Both intracranial pressure and metabolic demand for oxygen rise dramatically during a fit and this may increase the extent of the brain damage. Intravenous lorazepam or diazepam is usually effective, but be aware of the possibility of respiratory arrest.

Suspected alcohol intoxication

Drunkenness increases the risk of sustaining a head injury and of that injury causing brain damage. Nevertheless, changes in conscious level must not be attributed to alcohol or other drugs except by exclusion and in retrospect. The plasma osmolality may be a useful investigation in this circumstance (*see page 228*) if direct measurement of plasma alcohol is unavailable.

Patients with alcohol intoxication who have not regained full consciousness within 6–8 h of arrival should have a CT scan of the brain.

Urine output

Catheterisation of the bladder is mandatory in an unresponsive, brain-injured patient. A full bladder leads to increasing restlessness. In addition, the urine output is a good indicator of adequate tissue perfusion – it should be at least 1 mL per kg per h.

Pain

Analgesia may be needed if the patient is not deeply unconscious and has other painful injuries. Initially, it can be achieved by fracture splintage. Once baseline observations are established, give small doses of opiates intravenously.

Bleeding from the scalp

Examination of the scalp must be meticulous and so the hair must be shaved off to a distance of at least 1 cm from around the wound edges. Lacerations should be palpated with a gloved finger to detect fracture lines and foreign bodies. Severe bleeding can be controlled with a single layer of deep sutures, using 2–0 silk on a hand-held needle. A pressure dressing should then be applied. The application of Raney clips to the wound edges can be a useful holding measure.

Deterioration

Early, rapid, neurological deterioration is very rarely caused by a remedial intracranial lesion but more often is due to:

- severe primary brain injury;
- hypoxaemia;
- hypovolaemia.

Guidelines for neurosurgical consultation

> Do not attempt neurosurgical intervention in the ED, no matter how experienced you are or how ill the patient seems to be. Burr-hole exploration – even by neurosurgeons with good facilities – frequently fails to reveal a haematoma.

Seek neurosurgical/neuro-intensive care advice in any of the following instances:

- positive findings on CT scan including cerebral oedema;
- penetrating injury;
- depressed skull fracture;
- basal skull fracture;
- skull fracture with any depression of consciousness, repeated fits, severe headache, persistent vomiting or acute focal neurology;
- GCS = or < 13 after resuscitation;
- confusion or other neurological disturbance persisting after 8 h;
- deterioration of conscious level or of neurological signs.

> Before telephoning a neurosurgeon, ensure that resuscitation has been initiated.

The ambulant patient with a head injury

These patients will mostly have a GCS of 15. This score does not necessarily imply normal mental functioning as the GCS is not sensitive to changes in alertness or higher intellectual function. Some ambulant patients may be confused (GCS = 14).

The diagnosis of a minor head injury can only be made in retrospect. The following points should help to distinguish between those with no significant brain injury and those at risk of serious complications.

The history

The history of the incident is important as it often influences management. When the history is unknown or unreliable the patient must be considered for admission to hospital.

- Establish the speed of impact and the nature of the object struck by the head. The part of the head involved and the area of contact are also important (e.g. occiput hitting a carpeted floor is less serious than temple hitting the corner of a radiator).
- Establish the pattern of subsequent behaviour and ask about any period of unconsciousness, confusion, amnesia or fitting. Ask about the occurrence of headache and vomiting. Changes to hearing and vision, including diplopia, must also be noted.

Post-traumatic amnesia

The duration of post-traumatic amnesia (PTA) correlates fairly well with the degree of primary brain injury. Under 1 h usually denotes mild injury, whereas over 24 h is associated with severe injury. PTA is often underestimated. It should be measured up to the time when memory of consecutive events returns. This usually corresponds with the duration of spatial disorientation and is much longer than the period during which the patient did not speak.

PTA is often longer than initially estimated.

Retrograde amnesia

Retrograde amnesia (for events before the accident) is very unreliable and extremely variable. It may be grossly prolonged in patients who have been drinking alcohol.

Drugs and alcohol

These are often implicated in the aetiology of head injury, but deterioration in a patient should not be attributed to their effects. Very high blood alcohol levels (> 6000 mg per L) have been recorded in ambulant patients. Put alcohol at the bottom of the list of causes of altered consciousness.

Medical history

A medical history is usually obtained from relatives, neighbours, a phone call to the GP or by searching clothing. It is valuable in two respects:

1 factors relevant to present management (e.g. diabetes, steroid treatment);
2 factors relevant to the prevention of a further incident (e.g. transient ischaemic attack, alcohol abuse).

Always enquire about any bleeding diathesis or anticoagulant therapy.

Assessment of an ambulant patient with a head injury

- Assess the patient's behaviour. It is common for a patient to appear normal on casual assessment whereas enquiry a few days later reveals no recollection of the first interview.
- Assess the patient's higher cortical function. This is essential. Pupil changes and the other classical signs of raised intracranial pressure are very late indicators of deterioration. Eighty per cent of the rise in pressure required to cause brainstem coning occurs without any change in clinically detectable brain function.
- Examine the pupils.
- Watch the patient move, looking especially for loss of coordination and ataxia. Examine the limb movements, sensation and reflexes if there is any reason to think that the patient's gross movements are abnormal or if there are any other neurological signs.
- Calculate the GCS (*see Box 3.1*).
- Examine the head, noting any wounds, swellings or depressions. This requires palpation as well as inspection. Interpretation of imaging is facilitated by being able to link common areas of radiological and clinical abnormality.
- Examine the neck and exclude injuries elsewhere.
- Record the BP, pulse, respiratory rate, SaO_2 and temperature.

Imaging of the skull and brain

CT scanning allows visualisation of the brain and almost all pathology that may require operative treatment. Fractures of the base and vault of the skull may also be seen on 'bony windows'. Depressed fractures may be identified and the depth of depressions calculated. Most hospitals without a resident neurosurgeon have the facility to send CT scans to a neurosurgical centre by electronic transfer. *For the indications for CT imaging of the brain in patients with head injuries see Box 3.2.*

Skull X-rays have been largely replaced by CT scanning and observation on short-stay wards. However, they still have a place in the management of physical child abuse and the assessment of some complicated patients. Moreover, 24 h CT scanning is not readily available in all countries (and in some parts of the United Kingdom). *For radiology of the skull see page 47.*

Patients at risk of developing complications after a head injury

Patients with one or more of the following features have a significant risk of developing intracranial complications:

• impaired level of consciousness at time of presentation (including those who are showing GCS = 15 but not fully alert);

• post-traumatic amnesia of over 15 min duration;

• abnormal neurological signs;

• fits;

• symptoms of raised intracranial pressure (severe headache, persistent vomiting);

• vault fracture on X-ray (*see Boxes 3.6 and 3.7*);

• clinical evidence of basal skull fracture (*see page 44*).

For the indications for observation in hospital following a head injury see Box 3.8.

Box 3.6 Risk of Intracranial Haematoma in Adults with Head Injuries

	No skull fracture	Skull fracture
Fully conscious	1 in 8 000	1 in 45
Impaired consciousness	1 in 180	1 in 5
Comatose	1 in 27	1 in 4

Box 3.7 Risk of Intracranial Haematoma in Children with Head Injuries

	No skull fracture	Skull fracture
Fully conscious	1 in 13 000	1 in 157
Impaired consciousness	1 in 580	1 in 25
Comatose	1 in 65	1 in 12

Box 3.8 Indications for Observation in Hospital Following Head Injuries

(The content of this box is adapted from the UK National Institute for Clinical Excellence's head injury guideline)

Patients with head injuries who have any of the following features should be admitted to hospital for observation:

New abnormalities on imaging

Failure to return to GCS of 15 regardless of any imaging results

Fulfils the criteria for CT imaging (*see Box 3.2*) but cannot be scanned because of patient state or equipment failure

Continuing symptoms or signs for concern (e.g. persistent vomiting, severe headache)

Other co-existing problems (e.g. drug or alcohol intoxication, other injuries, CSF fluid leak, suspected non-accidental injury).

In patients who are fully alert on examination, a history of an altered level of consciousness before arrival at hospital increases the risk of intracranial haematoma by a factor of 4.

XR

Computed tomography is of great value in this group of patients.

TX

All patients with a significant risk of developing complications must be admitted and observed carefully by nurses who understand the GCS and are trained in the early detection of changes in neurological status. The following observations should be made, initially at half-hourly intervals, and then hourly if the patient is stable:

• best eye-opening response;

• best motor response (noting lateralising signs);

• best verbal response;

• pupil size and reaction to light;

• respiratory rate;

• pulse and BP;

• temperature.

For changes requiring urgent review in patients admitted to hospital with head injuries see Box 3.9.

Box 3.9 Changes Requiring Urgent Review in Patients Admitted to Hospital with Head Injuries

(The content of this box is adapted from the UK National Institute for Clinical Excellence's head injury guideline)

Patients under observation in hospital after head injury should be reviewed urgently if any of the following features occur:

Development of agitation or abnormal behaviour.

Drop of one point in GCS for 30 min or more (especially in the motor score).

Drop of two of points or more in GCS.

Development of persistent severe headache.

Development of persistent vomiting.

Development of new or evolving focal neurological symptoms or signs (e.g. pupil inequality or asymmetry of limb or facial movements).

Box 3.10 Discharge Criteria for Patients with Head Injuries

Patients who fulfill all of the following criteria may be discharged home to a caring relative or friend:

Fully conscious on presentation.

No abnormal neurological signs.

Loss of consciousness or post-traumatic amnesia of less than 5 min.

No severe headache or vomiting.

No suspicion of skull fracture.

No bleeding disorder.

Good home conditions.

Reliable relative or friend available to take patient home from the ED (in appropriate transport).

Ambulant patients with head injuries who are not obviously at risk

There is a remote possibility that intracranial complications will occur after the most trivial head injury. A counsel of perfection might suggest that all patients should be admitted. This would result in a vast number of people being admitted to make an uneventful recovery. Quite apart from economic and social implications, this would be counterproductive. Staff would have an increased threshold for the recognition of abnormalities when their everyday experience was of large numbers of relatively well patients. Thus only those patients who have histories, symptoms or signs that put them at risk (see before) should be detained. However, if the home conditions appear inadequate or the relatives are unhappy about looking after the patient, admission is essential.

For the discharge criteria for patients with head injuries see Box 3.10.

Advice to discharged patients (head injury instructions)

1 Insist on the presence of a relative or a friend and never discharge a head-injured patient unless a third party is aware of the injury and will accompany the patient home.

2 Ensure that there is a telephone in or near the patient's home and encourage the relatives to phone the hospital if they have any anxieties.

3 Provide verbal and written advice. The following points should be made:

- Nausea and mild headache are common but the ED should be contacted if these symptoms persist or increase. Any vomiting must be taken seriously.

- Alterations in the level of consciousness are an important early sign of the development of complications and necessitate urgent referral back to hospital. Changes should not be attributed to drugs or alcohol.

- Any other unusual change in vision, hearing or movement should prompt a discussion with the hospital.

- Recovery from a mild traumatic brain injury often takes much longer than commonly expected. A period of rest and time off work is usually appropriate. Alcohol may delay recovery.

Head injuries in children

In a school-age child the most common cause of death is a brain injury from a road traffic accident. Minor head injuries are also important, even if they do not produce immediate major complications, as repeated minor head trauma in children has been linked to lowered IQ. Young children are less likely to lose consciousness than adults.

Significant brain injury may thus occur without a history of unconsciousness.

Assessment can be difficult. The children's coma scale (a modified GCS) should be used for children aged below 5 years (*see page 327*). In the evening, children may be sleepy but, nevertheless, a normal child is easily woken. Parents are in the best position to judge minor alterations in their children's level of consciousness.

Children are more prone to head injury when fractious, feverish or in the prodromal stage of an acute illness. A cause for unsteadiness should always be sought and the temperature recorded.

Child abuse

Unexplained or atypical head injuries may be a result of non-accidental injury, especially if bilateral. Severe intracranial haemorrhage, usually without skull fracture, may occur in an infant who has been violently shaken. Such babies may present as generally unwell with drowsiness and poor feeding or may have fits and apnoeic attacks. Retinal haemorrhage is a characteristic sign of this injury. Skull X-rays have a valuable part to play in the assessment of children under the age of 12 years with suspected abusive injuries.

For radiology of the skull in both adults and children see page 47.

For a full discussion of child abuse see page 348.

Xʀ

Early cerebral oedema may not be visible on the CT scan of a child's brain.

Separation of the suture lines of the skull (diastasis) may sometimes be seen after injury. This can fail to close, resulting in a growing fracture.

Most serious head injuries in the first year of life result from abuse. There may be multiple, branching fractures that involve more than one skull bone. Occipital fracture is characteristic and underlying brain injury is relatively common.

Tx

Most aspects of the management of a child's head injury are identical to that in the adult. Children are unique in invariably having a carer with them. This means that most can go home with their parents and a set of head injury instructions. They often sleep after trauma and should not be kept awake. Instead, they should be examined by their parents two or three times during the night. All that is required is for the parents to be confident that their child has a normal response to a mild stimulation (verbal or tactile). It is not necessary to wake the child completely or to examine the pupils. Parents are much better judges of their children's night-time behaviour than hospital doctors or nurses.

Some injuries, especially those to the occiput, may cause severe and prolonged vomiting. Children in this situation require observation in hospital and a CT scan is usually indicated – *see Box 3.2*.

Delayed presentations

Occasionally, young children are brought to the ED by their parents with a large fluctuant swelling over the parietal area (cephalohaematoma). There is a history of an injury a few days before but the child is otherwise well. CT scan (or skull X-ray) usually shows a long, linear fracture that may extend over most of the side of the skull. It is normal for the swelling to be delayed and for a relatively late presentation. Although unlikely, child abuse must still be considered and excluded. Most of these children will need observation over a period of 24 h and assessment by paediatricians.

Specific injuries

Fracture of the vault of the skull

Fracture of the skull vault most commonly results from a fall on to a hard surface. The lateral parts of the skull are the most vulnerable and intoxication is a predisposing factor. The indications for skull X-ray in the absence of a CT scan (*see Box 3.11*) lists details of the associated features such as swelling of the scalp and vomiting.

> Child abuse is the most common cause of a skull fracture in an infant – *see page 348*.

XR

A CT scan of the cranium will detect most fractures of the vault of the skull.
For radiology of the skull see page 47.

TX

All patients with a new skull fracture should be admitted for observation. In the same way that a broken egg box may contain smashed eggs, a skull fracture (a broken head box) may contain traumatised brain. Expressed more scientifically, the presence of a skull fracture greatly increases the risk of a patient developing an intracranial haematoma – *see Boxes 3.6 and 3.7.*

Around 70% of intracranial haematomata occur in the presence of a skull fracture.

Compound fracture of the skull

Antibiotics are not routinely indicated for compound linear fractures of the skull. Lacerations over fractures that are not depressed can be closed in the normal way and the injury then treated in the same way as a simple vault fracture.

Depressed fracture of the skull

Depressed fractures are often missed. The history is the key to the diagnosis – direct force will have been applied over a small area of the head, for example, a blow from a hammer or a golf club. The injury is usually compound. Cerebral irritation may manifest itself as fitting.

XR

A CT scan is required when there is a suspicion of a depressed skull fracture – *see Box 3.2.* Fractures can be easily overlooked on plain skull films. It appears as an area of whiteness rather than as a black line. This is because of the increased density of the compressed and overlapping bone. The fracture may be stellate in appearance. In the absence of a CT scan, a plain film tangential view can be used to assess the amount of the depression but will give no indication as to the extent of any underlying damage.

TX

Signs of brain injury should be treated as described in the relevant section. All depressed fractures should be discussed with a neurosurgeon. Surgical elevation of the fragments is usually indicated.

Fracture of the base of the skull

This is usually the result of indirect violence. It often occurs in a drunken patient and may follow uncontrolled 'rag doll'-type falls.

The patient may sometimes feel unwell and vomit. A complaint of reduced hearing in one ear points to a haemotympanum. There will be one or more signs:

• bleeding from the ear canal;
• haemotympanum (causes reduced hearing);
• bleeding from the nose in the absence of direct injury;
• nasopharyngeal bleeding (this may be torrential and even severe enough to compromise the airway);
• cerebrospinal fluid leakage from the nose or ear;
• subconjunctival haemorrhage without a posterior edge;
• retro-orbital haematoma (*for emergency treatment see page 68*);
• bilateral periorbital haematomata ('raccoon or panda eyes');
• bruising around the mastoid area (Battle's sign) (occurs late).

Blood in the external auditory meatus after trauma is usually caused by basal fracture but is occasionally secondary to temperomandibular joint injury.

> Deep auroscopic examination of the canal should be avoided as it may introduce infection via torn meninges.

Xʀ

A CT scan of the cranium will detect most fractures of the base of the skull. High-resolution sections may be required.

There are usually no plain radiographic signs of a basal skull fracture. However, there may be:

1 blood in the sphenoid sinus (look for a fluid level); and
2 a fracture line that appears to continue towards the base of the skull.

Tx

• Admission for observation for 48 h or until any discharge has ceased for at least 24 h.
• Discussion with a neurosurgeon, ophthalmologist or ENT surgeon as appropriate.

Antibiotics (e.g. penicillin V or ampicillin) are not of proven value.

Aerocoele

A fracture involving a bony sinus may result in intracranial air. The presence of this aerocoele is suggested by periorbital surgical emphysema.

Xʀ

An aerocoele is usually an incidental finding on a CT scan of the brain or a plain skull X-ray. On a brow-up lateral film it will lie anteriorly.

Tx

The aerocoele may expand if the pressure in the sinuses is increased and so the patient should be warned not to blow his or her nose. The patient must be discussed with a neurosurgeon as early decompression is sometimes necessary.

Extradural haematoma

A blood clot in the extradural space results from direct trauma and, in adults, is usually associated with a skull fracture (of the squamous temporal bone). A lucid interval between initial trauma and the onset or return of depressed consciousness is said to be characteristic but is by no means inevitable.

The signs are those of increasing intracranial pressure. An impaired level of consciousness is the first feature. The classical unilateral, fixed, dilated pupil is a very late sign; it occurs as the result of an ipsilateral third nerve palsy that is caused by cerebral herniation. Limb weakness, from direct pressure on the motor cortex, is usually found on the contralateral side. Lateralising signs may be preterminal.

Xʀ

CT scanning will detect almost all extradural bleeds. In the very early stages, the blood may have the same density as the brain tissue and thus be difficult to identify. Extradural collections usually appear biconvex on CT scan, whereas subdural collections have inner concave borders.

On plain skull X-rays, a fracture that overlies the vascular markings of the middle meningeal artery may be associated with an extradural bleed.

Tx

Resuscitation and stabilisation of the patient as detailed on *page 35* should precede transfer to a neurosurgical centre. Major coincidental extra-cranial injuries must always be identified before transport is initiated.

> Outcome in a patient with an extradural haematoma is compromised if the time to decompression is more than 2 h from the point of deterioration.

Acute subdural haematoma

Bleeding from the veins that traverse the subdural space results in a more insidious clinical picture than extradural haemorrhage. Alteration in conscious level is the cardinal feature; lateralising signs may be absent or minimal. A unilateral increase in limb tone is sometimes apparent.

Subdural haematomas are most commonly seen in the cases below:

1 Patients who are intoxicated with alcohol. There may be no apparent injury. The first sign may be a failure to wake-up after an episode of heavy drinking. CT scan is thus indicated in all patients who are intoxicated but fail to reach a GCS of 15 within 6–8 h.
2 Those who are on anticoagulant therapy. The trauma may be minimal.
3 Patients who have coexisting extensive brain injury from major trauma (lacerations and contusions).

XR

CT scan is diagnostic, showing a collection with an inner concave border (cf. extradural).

Tx

Patients with subdural haematomas must be discussed with a neurosurgeon immediately.

> Outcome in a patient with an acute subdural haematoma is compromised if the time to decompression is more than 4 h from the accident.

Sub-arachnoid haemorrhage

Sub-arachnoid haemorrhage (SAH) may some-times occur after trauma. In a conscious patient there may be severe headache, neck stiffness and photophobia (*see page 231*). Diagnosis is con-firmed by CT scan and then neurosurgical advice must be sought. IV nimodipine is no longer indi-cated in the treatment of traumatic SAH.

Cerebral contusions

Bruising to the brain may result in a similar clini-cal picture to subdural haematoma, with a delayed recovery from trauma or alcohol intoxication. Frontal contusions cause disinhibition.

XR

CT scan is diagnostic.

Tx

All patients with contusions should be discussed with a neurosurgeon. Spontaneous resolution may take several weeks.

Cortical blindness

Sudden visual loss following a head injury is uncommon but very frightening for the patient. The loss of vision can be confirmed by testing for the absence of the blink reflex (i.e. an object rapidly approaching the eye will not cause blinking).

XR

A CT scan of the brain should be requested.

Tx

The patient should be admitted and examined by an ophthalmologist. Vision usually returns spontaneously within a few hours.

Abducens palsy

Unilateral sixth nerve palsy is occasionally seen after an otherwise uncomplicated minor head injury. CT scan should be obtained to exclude significant intracranial pathology. The condition resolves spontaneously.

Chronic subdural haematoma

This is usually seen in elderly patients with a history of a trivial head injury, or no injury at all. The symptoms and signs develop after a latent period of days or months and characteristically fluctuate in severity as a result of alternating bleeding and resorption of clot. There is headache, memory loss, confusion and drowsiness. Localising signs are rare.

CT scan should be performed if the diagnosis is suspected. Neurosurgical intervention has a good outcome.

Prolonged symptoms after apparently minor traumatic brain injury

Many patients with a minor traumatic brain injury who do not have demonstrable intracranial lesions or abnormal signs will have persisting symptoms for a surprisingly long period of time. These complaints include:
- minor lapses in concentration and memory;
- inability to undertake complex tasks;
- fatigue;
- occipito-frontal headache.

Symptoms may progress to a more chronic post-concussional stress disorder. It is probable that some patients will have structural brain damage – a minor form of diffuse axonal injury – although this may not be evident on CT scan.

XR

CT scan may be undertaken (as a delayed procedure) to exclude treatable causes and to give a more reliable prognosis.

TX

The patient should be reassured that recovery will occur but may take several weeks. Advise against alcohol and propose a gradual resumption of normal activities. Follow-up by the GP or specific care by a psychologist or neurologist may be valuable.

Radiology of the Skull*

Skull X-rays must be taken with suitable equipment (not portable) and should include an AP, a Towne's and a lateral view. Basal views should not be requested as they require extreme extension of the cervical spine. Occipito-mental and special tangential views may be required after the first set of films has been viewed. *For the indications for skull X-rays in the absence of CT imaging see Box 3.11 on page 44.*

Interpretation of skull X-rays

- Insist on good-quality films.
- Look at them carefully on a good viewing box with a rear spotlight.
- Use specific films for specific purposes.
  1 AP view for frontal bone, orbits and upper occiput. The calcified pineal gland – which is identified on the lateral film above the shadow of the ear lobe – should appear in the midline on the AP view.
  2 Towne's view for occipital injury.
  3 Left lateral (plate next to the left side of the head) shows lesions on the left clearly but those on the right will be slightly out of focus (*see Figure 3.1*).
  4 Laterals taken from both sides, together with a careful examination of the head for bruising and haematoma, will help to indicate the significance of linear markings in the temporal regions.

---

* This section is included in the recognition that in many countries (and in parts of the United Kingdom) CT scanning is not readily available.

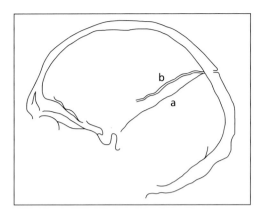

Figure 3.1 Characteristics of an extensive linear vault fracture. This shows as a crisp thin line (a) on the side of the skull adjacent to the X-ray film, but as a wide hazy line (b) on the opposite side of the skull.

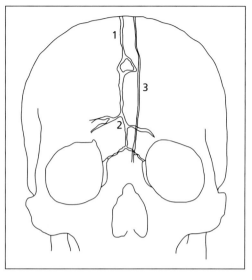

Figure 3.3 AP view of child's skull. Note the persisting metopic suture in the frontal bone. This does not overlie the sagittal suture because the radiograph has not been correctly centered. The division of the sagittal suture into the two lambdoid sutures, at the lambda, is an imprecise feature in this particular skull. 1, sagittal suture; 2, lambdoid suture; 3, metopic suture.

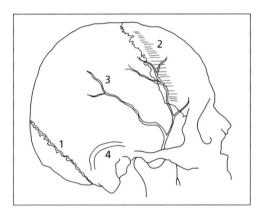

Figure 3.2 Lateral view of adult's skull. The coronal and lambdoid sutures are fused but persist as wide irregular structures in contrast to the curvilinear branching radiolucencies produced by the meningeal vessels. Note the superoposterior radiation of the vessels. Darker lines at right angles in the region of the pterion (just in front of and above the pinna) usually represent undisplaced vault fractures. 1, lambdoid suture; 2, coronal suture; 3, meningeal vessels; 4, pinna.

It is essential to be aware of the characteristics of the normal suture lines and vascular markings of the skull in both adults and children – see *Figures 3.2–3.4*. The common anatomical variants should also be recognised – see *Figures 3.5–3.7 and the accompanying legend in Box 3.12*.

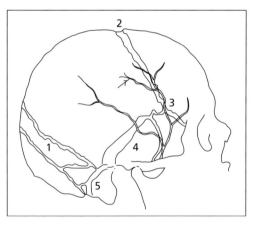

Figure 3.4 Lateral view of child's skull. Note that sutures on both sides of the skull are seen on this projection. Whilst the bregma is often very thin, the lambda is thick and irregular. 1, lambdoid suture; 2, bregma (position of anterior fontanelle in infant); 3, coronal suture; 4, squamosal suture; 5, pinna.

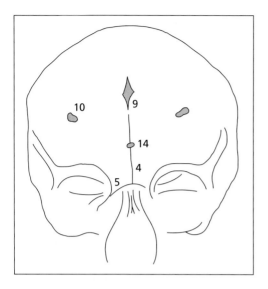

Figure 3.5 Normal anatomical variants – AP view (*see Box 3.12*).

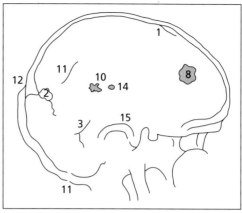

Figure 3.7 Normal anatomical variants – lateral view (*see Box 3.12*).

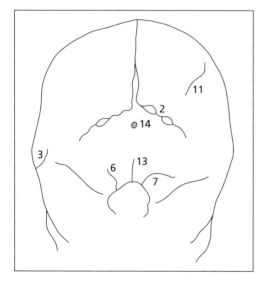

Figure 3.6 Normal anatomical variants – Townes' view (*see Box 3.12*).

- A fracture classically produces a finite, crisp, linear mark (*see Figure 3.1*). Fractures of the skull may persist on X-ray for many years. However, if there is any doubt about the age of a fracture, it should be presumed to be new.

- A vascular marking is usually of indefinite length, wide and curvilinear. Vessels in the temporal region tend to radiate upwards from the base of the skull, predominantly posteriorly. Any markings at right angles to these should be considered to represent fractures.

- A shift of the calcified pineal gland from the midline is evidence of movement of the falx, usually by an expanding haematoma. If only the choroid plexi are calcified, they cannot be used reliably to indicate brain shift because of their variable positions in the normal brain.

- The small linear fracture, which is classically overlooked and overlies an extradural haematoma, is often near the soft-tissue marking of the pinna as seen on the lateral film.

Skull X-rays in children

The normal suture lines and vascular markings on a child's skull X-rays are shown in *Figures 3.3 and 3.4*. Separation of the suture lines (diastasis) may sometimes be seen after injury. This can fail to close, resulting in a growing fracture.

Box 3.12 Normal Anatomical Variants (Numbers Correspond with Those in Figures 3.5–3.7)

Neonate
Vault disproportionately larger in neonate than in adult (vault: face ratio in neonate 4:1 but in adult 3:2).
Overlapping sutures may be seen in neonate secondary to moulding occurring during labour.
Scalp folds may mimic fracture line (e.g. wrinkle in occiput).

Child
Suture spreading is very common between the ages of 4 and 8 years.
1 Anterior fontanelle. Fusion may mimic depressed fracture on lateral projection but is clearly outlined on Townes view.
2 Wormian (accessory) bones. Normal variant in both children and adults.
3 Posterior part of squamosal suture. May simulate a fracture.
4 Metopic suture. May persist throughout life.
5 Prominent nasofrontal suture. May persist into adult life.
6 Persistent membranous fissure. May simulate a fracture. Most common in infancy but may persist into adult life.
7 Normal synchrondrosis between two parts of occipital bone in infant.

Adult
8 Localised focal dural calcification.
9 Focal calcification of falx cerebri.
10 Calcification in the glomus of the choroid plexus of the lateral ventricle.
11 Subsagittal suture of parietal bone.
12 Overlapping of occipital bone (bathrocephaly). May be confused with a fracture.
13 Midline occipital suture. Also a common site for a fracture!
14 Calcified pineal. Visible on lateral view in 50% of adults. Less frequently seen on AP view.

All ages
15 Upper part of the pinna. Often seen on the lateral projection.
Matted hair, lacerations, clothing, hair buns and pillows may all simulate a fracture. However, the line may be seen to extend out past the bone into the soft tissue shadow.

Simple frontal trauma is very common in small children who have fallen. There is usually a swelling on the forehead. These children do not often meet the criteria for skull X-rays (*see Box 3.11*). However, all children who are not yet walking (i.e. less than 11–13 months) require skull X-rays after a head injury for the following reasons:

• The mechanism of injury must be significant. The infant will have been dropped or have fallen from a height.

• Most serious head injuries in the first year of life result from abuse. There may be multiple, branching fractures that involve more than one skull bone. Occipital fracture is characteristic and underlying brain injury is relatively common.

Chapter 4

The neck and the back

Potentially serious injuries of the spine

The possibility of spinal injury should always be considered in:
- major trauma;
- multiple injuries;
- high-speed injuries;
- falls;
- sports injuries (especially in diving, trampolining, riding and rugby accidents);
- head injuries;
- all unresponsive patients.

Immediate assessment and management

- Ensure an adequate airway and give high-concentration oxygen. The jaw-thrust manoeuvre is safer than the chin-lift technique in this situation. The neck must be protected by manual in-line stabilisation if more extensive airway intervention is needed. As soon as possible, immobilise the neck with a hard collar fitted with a chin piece and prevent head movement with a purpose-made head-holder (or sandbags and tape).
- Assess respiratory function and rate and measure oxygen saturation with a pulse oximeter.
- Set up an IV infusion and monitor BP and pulse.
- Record the GCS. Check if the patient can move and feel his or her fingers and toes. *For spinal cord injury see later.*

- Protect the thoracolumbar spine with a long spinal board wherever the signs or mechanism of injury suggest thoracolumbar injury or when there are evident injuries both above and below the spine.
- Log-rolling will be necessary to examine the back of the patient. Look for bruising, swelling, tenderness and palpable steps in the vertebral column.
- Pay special attention to pressure points (sores develop rapidly) and core temperature (the patient may be thermolabile).
- Consider the need for early analgesia.
- Complete the primary survey and continue resuscitation.
- Call for senior advice and then start the secondary survey.

For radiographs in spinal trauma see page 55.

> Whenever spinal protection is removed to aid examination, the neck and spine must be held still by one staff member who has no other responsibilities.

Injury to the spinal cord

In the fully conscious adult, the presence of paralysis and anaesthesia after trauma immediately points to spinal cord injury. However, in the obtunded patient the diagnosis may be difficult. Similarly, incomplete cord damage is often misdiagnosed – *for cord syndromes see page 54.*

Initial management of spinal cord injury

- *See section Initial Assessment and Management on page 51.*
- Keep the patient calm, warm, splinted and immobile.
- Request orthopaedic advice.
- Record respiration and SaO_2. The onset of respiratory failure may be insidious.
- Monitor pulse, BP and ECG. Watch carefully for peripheral vasodilatation and the onset of neurogenic shock. Copious IV fluids may be required, but there is a potential for volume overload if too much is given.
- Catheterise the patient.

Anaesthetic help will be required for both respiratory failure and neurogenic shock – *see later*.

> Paralysis may mask multiple injuries. Pain may be absent as may the signs of intra-abdominal trauma.

Steroid therapy

High-dose steroid therapy in patients with spinal cord injuries remains controversial. However, in the light of the recent evidence of the negative effects of steroids in acute head injury, it would seem inadvisable to give steroids routinely to patients with spinal cord damage.

Special problems that may accompany injury to the spinal cord

Respiratory failure

Intercostal muscle paralysis occurs with most cervical cord lesions. High lesions transect the phrenic nerve nucleus (C3/4/5) and are usually fatal. Even when the diaphragm is spared, vital capacity is greatly reduced and a compensatory tachypnoea occurs. The tidal volume and vital capacity should be measured if possible.

Paradoxical respiration is an important sign. As the diaphragm descends during inspiration to create a negative intrathoracic pressure, intercostal muscle paralysis allows rib retraction rather than the normal expansion. Deteriorating respiratory function (rate > 35 breaths per min) is an indication for senior anaesthetic advice to consider the need for ventilation.

Neurogenic shock

Impairment of descending sympathetic pathways in the spinal cord leads to relative hypovolaemia and bradycardia. Other injuries may have been sustained and can cause true hypovolaemia and either a bradycardia or a tachycardia. Any reduction of blood supply to the damaged cord will further impair its function. Hypotension from loss of sympathetic tone is one of the very few indications for therapy with vasopressor agents (e.g. ephedrine). The bradycardia usually responds to atropine.

Retention of urine

Bladder tone is lost immediately after spinal transection. Distension leads to ureteric reflux and renal damage. Intermittent catheterisation may be the treatment of choice in the spinal unit, but it is preferable to insert and retain a fairly thin catheter during the initial period of resuscitation and inter-hospital transfer. Catheterisation must be performed by an experienced member of staff using an aseptic technique.

Impaired thermoregulation

The patient is unable to sweat and thereby lose heat at high ambient temperatures. More commonly, too much heat is lost at low temperatures because of a failure of cutaneous vasoconstriction. The environmental temperature should be near to normal body temperature if the patient has to be exposed for long periods (e.g. for the diagnosis and treatment of other injuries). At other times, insulation is used to prevent heat loss to a cooler environment. Core temperature must be measured regularly.

Associated injuries

The signs of abdominal, pelvic and major limb injury may be masked by the motor and sensory loss. Peritoneal lavage or ultrasound examination should be performed if there are external signs of abdominal trauma or if the patient is haemody-namically unstable. Abdominal swelling may occur with a full bladder. Severe swelling from any cause may splint the diaphragm.

Localisation of spinal cord damage

Twisting forces are most likely to cause fractures at the junction of mobile and fixed parts of the column, that is, at C7/T1 and T12/L1. Upper thoracic spine injury may be associated with sternal fractures; massive forces attempting to buckle the thoracic cage. Direct blows are commonly associated with injuries elsewhere.

Partial transection of the cord may be inflicted by a knife or a bullet but complete separation is unusual. A twisting or bending movement resulting from indirect blunt violence is more common. This causes a combination of crushing and tearing which produces a mixed picture of neuronal damage. There is often total loss of neural continuity with complete distal motor and sensory loss.

Distal reflex activity may not be clearly related to the extent of cord section in the immediate post-injury phase. Complete section usually causes immediate flaccid paralysis with later return of reflex activity. Rarely, some reflexes are preserved throughout.

The level of cord injury may be difficult to determine because of the following:
1 Most muscles receive efferent fibres from more than one level.
2 Dermatomes have imprecise boundaries.
3 Closed cord lesions usually extend over several centimetres, involving more than one level.
It is important to detect change in neurological status over time. Identify and document the lowest functional muscle groups and the extent of skin anaesthesia (see Box 4.1 and Figure 4.1).

Delayed improvement or deterioration after spinal cord injury

Spinal shock

This is rare. After a cord injury, spinal concussion causes a generalised flaccidity below the level of

Box 4.1 Nerve Roots Supplying Tendon and Superficial Reflexes			
Tendon reflexes		**Superficial reflexes**	
Biceps	C5	Abdominal	T8–T12
Supinator	C5/6	Cremasteric	L1/2
Triceps	C7	Plantar	S1
Knee	L3/4	Anal	S3/4
Ankle	S1/2		

the lesion. Reflex activity may initially be present but later disappears. Neurological signs begin to improve spontaneously within 8 h and the effects of the concussion are variably reversed within 48 h.

This diagnosis can only be made in retrospect. An initial finding of proximal paralysis with sparing of distal neurological function (e.g. sphincter tone) is likely to be associated with cord concussion and carries a more favourable prognosis. Concussion and permanent cord damage may coexist.

Late-onset paralysis

Secondary deterioration can occur after spinal injuries in a similar way to the much commoner complications of brain injury. Paralysis that develops hours after the incident is rare and is usually a result of cord ischaemia or oedema (causing infarction or vascular occlusion, respectively). An extradural haemorrhage may cause cord compression. Delayed signs are very unlikely to result from direct injury. Gentle handling, as described above, will not further damage a spine that has been subjected to forces sufficient to render it unstable. The doctor would be expected to be less violent than the injuring agent.

Cord syndromes

Incomplete cord damage produces a number of discrete syndromes. Some degree of recovery is more likely than in complete lesions where there

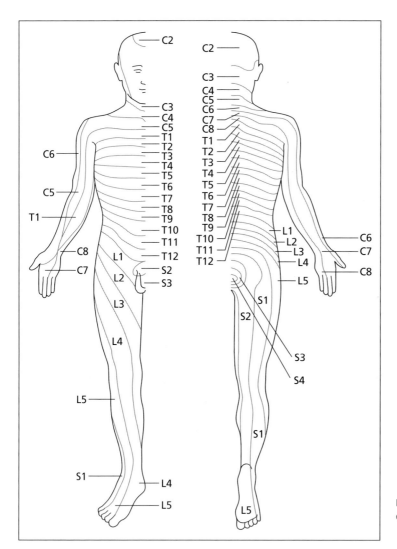

Figure 4.1 Sensory dermatomes of the body.

is no sign of any spinal cord function below the level of the injury. The mixed nature of the signs leads to misdiagnosis.

Central cord syndrome

This usually occurs in older patients with spondylitic spines following a relatively minor hyperextension injury. The spinal cord is compressed between the osteophytic vertebral body anteriorly and the stiff ligamentum flavum posteriorly. The more centrally situated parts of the corticospinal and spinothalamic tracts are the worst injured. These fibres supply the arms where the damage results in a flaccid (lower motor neuron) paresis. The legs are less affected with a spastic (upper motor neuron) type of weakness. The sacral fibres are often spared and so perineal sensation and bladder and bowel function may be normal.

Central cord syndrome should be suspected in the elderly patient with a forehead injury who can walk but complains of altered function in the upper limbs. These symptoms are often mistakenly diagnosed as hysterical.

Anterior cord syndrome

The anterior part of the spinal cord is usually injured by a mixture of bony encroachment and ischaemia. Typically, a flexion–rotation force causes a dislocation or a compression fracture of the vertebral body with accompanying anterior spinal artery compression. There is loss of power as well as reduced pain and temperature sensation below the lesion.

Traumatic herniation of a cervical vertebral disc

This may occur during an acute flexion injury and cause extensive injury to the anterior part of the spinal cord. There is impaired motor function with reduced pain and temperature sensation. The posterior horns and posterior columns are usually undamaged so that touch and proprioception remain intact. *See also page 60.*

Posterior cord syndrome

Hyperextension injuries with fractures of the posterior elements of the vertebrae may injure the posterior columns. Loss of proprioception may cause profound ataxia in the presence of normal power and pain and temperature sensation.

Brown–Séquard's syndrome

This lateral cord syndrome can only be precisely produced by a knife or gun, although closed injuries (lateral mass fractures) may also give rise to some of its classical features. These are the signs of a hemisection of the cord. On the injured side there is reduced power, but relatively normal pain and temperature sensation because the spinothalamic tract crosses over to the opposite side. The uninjured side has normal power, but reduced sensation for pain and temperature.

Imaging of the spine in trauma

Radiographs taken to confirm a clinically proven injury to the spine are less important initially than those requested for patients who are asymptomatic but at risk. Splints should be radiolucent and retained during radiography.
For the use of CT and MR imaging in spinal trauma see Box 4.2.

Box 4.2 Indications for CT and MR Imaging in Spinal Trauma

CT scan:
- Areas of the spine poorly visualised on plain films
- Fracture not excluded by plain films
- Significant or possibly significant fracture on plain films (requiring further visualisation)
- Unexplained neurology following trauma

MR scan:
- Fracture on plain films or CT scan with unknown associated soft tissue injuries
- Suspected ligament or disc injury
- Neurological symptoms and signs referable to the spine
- Suspicion of vascular injury to the spinal cord

Radiographs of the cervical spine

These should be obtained for all patients with:
- multiple injuries;
- injuries caused by the mobile head striking a fixed object.

For clearance of the spine see page 57.

There are three standard views of the cervical spine in UK practice:
1 lateral view;
2 upper AP ('open-mouth' or 'peg') view;
3 lower AP view.

Supplemental oblique views are used to visualise the apophyseal joints, looking for facet joint dislocation. Radiographs in flexion and extension are used to reveal instability. They should only be taken in the presence of a senior clinician.

Lateral view

Adequacy
This is the view that causes the most trouble. The first film is adequate (C7/T1 disc space shown) in only about two-thirds of cases. Often, only the

first five vertebrae are demonstrated. *For a suggested sequence to be followed, if the lateral radiograph of the cervical spine is inadequate, see Box 4.3.*

The lateral view of the cervical spine must include the C7/T1 junction.

Alignment

Confirm the continuity of the curve along the following 4 lines:
1 anterior borders of the vertebral bodies;
2 posterior borders of the vertebral bodies (the anterior edge of the vertebral canal);
3 posterior edge of the vertebral canal;
4 tips of the spinous processes.
Look for steps. Normal slight lordosis is lost when there is painful muscle spasm.

C2 may appear to be subluxed forward on C3 in young children; the same appearance is less frequently seen of C3 on C4. These are normal variants that occur in up to 10% of children under 7 years of age and disappear on extension of the neck.

Bones

Compare the height and shape of each vertebral body, looking for wedging and fractures.

Examine each apophyseal joint and spinous process for malalignment and fractures.

Look at the integrity of the odontoid peg and for increased space between the peg and the anterior arch of C1. Look for fracture of the posterior arch of C1 and for "hangman's fracture" of the pedicles of C2.

Cartilages

Examine each intervertebral joint looking for osteophytes and narrow disc spaces.

Soft tissue

The soft-tissue shadow, anterior to the vertebral bodies, is increased if there is a fracture, haematoma or anterior ligament injury. Air is trapped in this area if there is damage to the posterior pharyngeal wall. Above the larynx, the width of the prevertebral soft tissue space should be less than one-third of the diameter of the vertebral body. Below this level, the space is accepted as normal if it is no wider than a whole vertebral body.

Look for widening of the space between the spinous processes (torn interspinous ligaments).

Upper AP (odontoid peg) view

Adequacy

The upper AP view is adequate in only about two-thirds of first films. The odontoid peg may be superimposed on the base of the skull or on the upper incisors. Simple repositioning is usually sufficient.

Alignment

Look at the lateral masses of C1, on either side of the odontoid peg. They should line up with the equivalent parts of C2. Spread suggests a burst (Jefferson's) fracture.

Bones

Look at the integrity of the odontoid peg.

Anteroposterior view

Adequacy

The first attempt at this view is invariably adequate.

Alignment

Look for symmetry of the apophyseal joints.

Bones

Examine the transverse processes for fracture, buttressing of C7 or cervical rib. Thyroid cartilage wings are often misinterpreted as calcified vertebral arteries.

Cartilages

Confirm that the disc spaces are equal. Spaces above and below the centre of the X-ray beam appear narrower but should be bilaterally symmetrical.

Soft tissue

Confirm the central shadow of tracheal air.

> A CT or MR scan may be necessary for absolute clearance of the cervical spine.

Radiographs of the thoracolumbar spine

These are indicated when:
• the history suggests violent impact;
• there are significant injuries above and below the diaphragm; or
• there are positive clinical findings on log-rolling (such as bony tenderness, swelling or a palpable step).

Thoracolumbar films must include good views of the T12/L1 junction. Transverse process fractures, although not associated with spinal cord damage, are often overlooked and are important indicators of retroperitoneal injury. They may also cause severe pain.

Clearance of the spine

Patients with circumstantial evidence of multiple injuries – for example, those involved in high-speed incidents or falls – are assumed to have neck injuries until proven otherwise. Appropriate splintage will have been applied by the resuscitation team or paramedics. To remove this cervical protection, the examiner must be satisfied of the following points:
1 The patient is able to cooperate fully with the assessment, that is:
  • is fully conscious, cooperative and mentally normal;
  • is an adult or older child;
  • is free from severe pain in other regions of the body.
2 The patient has no neck pain.
3 The patient has no neurological deficit (normal peripheral movements and no paraesthesia).

Also, when the splintage is gently removed:
4 The patient has no bony tenderness of the cervical spine.
5 The patient has a good range of movements without pain or paraesthesia (specifically lateral rotation to 45° bilaterally).

Patients who fulfil the above criteria will not generally need radiographs of the cervical spine unless the mechanism of injury indicates the possibility of significant forces applied to the neck (*see page 51*).

Clearance of the cervical spine with the aid of radiographs is more difficult.
• A single, plain, lateral film will reveal about 80% of the fractures.
• The addition of the two standard AP views will increase the detection rate to about 90% of fractures.
• A CT scan of the neck will pick up about 98% of bony injuries.

The removal of splintage from the thoracolumbar spine should follow the same principles.

> Patients who have sustained injuries more than 48 h ago (and have been mobile since) should not have immediate splintage applied in the emergency department.

Cervical injury and neck pain

For patients with neck pain who can be safely moved and examined see Box 4.4.

> **Box 4.4 Patients with Neck Pain who can be Safely Moved and Examined**
>
> Even in the presence of neck pain, a patient who is fully conscious with no parasthesia or neurological deficit and no significant midline cervical tenderness can be safely moved and examined if any of the following apply:
> • no history of trauma;
> • simple rear-end motor vehicle collision (excludes rollover, hit by bus or large truck or high-speed vehicle, or pushed into oncoming traffic);
> • ambulatory at any time since the injury;
> • sitting position when seen;
> • delayed onset of neck pain.

Cervical spine fractures and dislocations

Bony injury is suggested by:
- a likely mechanism of injury (*see page 51*);
- severe pain of immediate onset;
- marked paraesthesia;
- other neurological signs.

XR

For interpretation of plain cervical films see page 55. Fractures may be difficult to see. The most common cause of a step on the lateral view is a unilateral facet joint dislocation with or without an accompanying fracture.

TX

For immediate assessment and management of potentially serious spinal injuries see page 51. The patient must be kept splinted and immobile. Orthopaedic advice must be sought immediately.

> The atlantoaxial joint of the cervical spine in a patient with Down's syndrome can be unstable. Subluxation and subsequent cord compression may occur after comparatively minimal force or even vigorous exercise. Similar problems are sometimes seen in rheumatoid arthritis.

Whiplash injury

This is caused by sudden hyperextension and flexion of the cervical spine, usually in a road traffic accident. The circumstances of the incident will help assessment of the forces applied to the neck and so aid prognosis. The most common story is of a stationary vehicle being hit from behind. Whiplash-type injuries are often the cause for legal claims and so notes should, as usual, be of a high standard.

Mobility may be good initially, with little pain and then symptoms typically increase over the first 24 h. There may be an associated headache, and pain may radiate to the shoulders. Sometimes there is slight paraesthesia in one or both hands, but there are no long tract signs. Occasionally, the patient complains of difficulty in swallowing as a result of inflammation of adjacent muscles.

> The patient may arrive in the ED wearing a cervical collar. *For advice on safe removal of splintage see clearance of the cervical spine on page 57.*

On examination, there is usually tenderness of the paravertebral areas. Movements are restricted, particularly lateral flexion (in the direction of tenderness) and flexion and extension of the lower cervical spine. Movement at the atlanto-occipital joint is normal and will allow the head to flex forwards without movement of the rest of the cervical spine. Rotation is variably restricted; forward flexion against resistance is always painful.

XR

Radiographs of the cervical spine should only be taken if any of the following apply:
- The patient is over 50 years old.
- The mechanism of injury suggests a violent application of force (e.g. the vehicle rolled over or the patient's head hit the windscreen).
- The pain occured immediately after the accident or is unusually severe.
- There is bony tenderness.
- There are abnormal physical signs additional to those described above (including severe paraesthesia).

Radiographic findings include the following.
- *Evident recent bony injury.* A cervical collar should be applied and no further radiographs taken without orthopaedic advice.
- *Loss of the normal lordosis with no bony injury.* This is caused by muscle spasm and usually indicates a more severe injury. Recovery may take longer than average but treatment remains as described below.
- *Pre-existing osteoarthritis.* The patient may have been asymptomatic previously. Some clinicians believe that spondylosis is associated with prolonged symptoms.
- *No radiographic abnormality.* This is the most common finding but does not equate to nothing wrong. There is a problem and it will get worse over the next 24 h.

> The prognosis is difficult to determine on initial presentation to the ED. Symptoms are usually worse and more protracted than most clinicians anticipate.

Tx

- Reassure the patient that symptoms will gradually settle over the next few weeks but warn him or her that they may increase over the first 24 h.
- Prescribe an oral NSAID (exclude peptic ulcer and asthma). Consider a parenteral NSAID for patients in severe pain.
- Do not prescribe a soft cervical collar. The use of these devices has been shown to prolong symptoms without short-term benefit.
- Consider physiotherapy (heat lamp and massage at home may suffice). Early treatment probably reduces the incidence of chronic symptoms.

Clay shoveller's shoulder

The muscular effort associated with strenuous digging – classically in clay – may avulse the spinous process of C7. There is localised pain over this vertebra prominens, which worsens on attempted flexion and extension.

XR

Lateral radiographs clearly demonstrate the lesion.

Tx

Fracture clinic referral is indicated for all spinous process fractures, although they heal spontaneously with conservative treatment.

Torticollis

Pain and spasm of one of the sternomastoid muscles may occur spontaneously (wry neck) or reflect local or generalised pathology. Most commonly, the symptoms occur on waking or following a sudden neck movement. The head is turned to the opposite side and cannot be rotated, but slight flexion and extension are usually possible. The muscle may be locally tender.

Local causes include throat infection, direct trauma, overuse or strain of neck muscles and spinal pathology. In small children, a submandibular abscess may cause painful torticollis. Athetoid movements as a result of extrapyramidal excitation may present as atypical torticollis (*see acute dystonias on page 296*).

XR

When there are no other positive findings and there is no history of trauma, radiographs are unnecessary.

Tx

Idiopathic torticollis may be extremely painful but usually responds to reassurance, oral analgesia and the local application of NSAID cream. The neck should be manipulated gently with slight longitudinal traction into the neutral position and a soft collar applied. Consider referral for physiotherapy. If symptoms persist for more than two or three days, review with radiographs is indicated.

Atlanto-axial rotary subluxation is one of the commonest structural neck injuries of childhood. It may present with torticollis after trauma and is very difficult to identify on plain radiographs. If suspected, CT scan of the neck is indicated.

Cervical spondylosis

Degenerative disease of the cervical spine is very common and often asymptomatic. The condition is usually diagnosed incidentally in the ED, on radiographs taken to exclude bony injury after trauma. Neurological function should be assessed and recorded.

If symptoms are longstanding and attributable to the cervical spondylosis, referral to the orthopaedic department or the patient's GP is appropriate.

Diffuse neck pain

The history is important:
- mode of onset;
- site and character of pain and any radiation;
- associated headache and systemic symptoms.

The temperature must be taken and the mouth, ears and neck examined. A brief neurological examination should also be performed. Consider:
- meningeal irritation (meningitis or subarachnoid haemorrhage);
- spinal disease (infection, degenerative disease or rheumatoid arthritis);
- intervertebral disc herniation;
- herpes zoster;
- pathology in the chest (e.g. myocardial infarction or pneumomediastinum – *see page 203*).

Standard cervical spine radiographs should be taken in most cases. The direction of further investigation and treatment is dictated by the clinical findings.

Cervical nerve root pain

This usually arises in the C7 distribution and causes pain and parasthesia in the upper arm, dorsal forearm and the dorsum of the hand, extending to the index and middle fingers. There may be weakness of the triceps and the extensors of the wrist and fingers. The triceps reflex may be absent.

Xʀ

A plain cervical radiograph may show degenerative changes.

Tx

This is difficult. Initial analgesia may be followed by physiotherapy and cervical traction. Specialist review may be indicated for patients whose symptoms or signs fail to settle rapidly.

Prolapse of a cervical intervertebral disc

This may arise in a young adult after a sudden twisting movement. There is acute pain and spasm of the neck muscles with pain and parathesia radiating down the arm. In severe cases, there is anaesthesia, weakness and loss of reflexes in the arm. Treatment consists of a soft collar, analgesia and physiotherapy. Patients with prolonged symptoms (more than three weeks) or neurological signs require specialist referral. *See also page 55.*

Back injury and back pain

Fractures of the thoracolumbar spine

> Injuries to the thoracolumbar spine are easily overlooked in patients with polytrauma.

Knowledge of the mechanism of the injury will help in the assessment of the forces involved. The spine should be assumed to be unstable until cleared by X-ray and a senior clinician.
- Log-roll the patient carefully. Look for swelling, bruising, tenderness and steps in the vertebral column. Examine the bony spines, paravertebral structures and perineum.
- Perform a neurological examination. This should include the anus (tone) and the rectum (blood and swelling).
- Consider the possibility of renal injury; test the urine for blood.

Chest injuries may coexist and include:
- aortic rupture;
- haemopneumothorax;
- fractures of the sternum and ribs.

Xʀ

Obtain radiographs of the thoracic and/or lumbar spine – *see page 57.* Visualisation of the thoracolumbar junction is important as there is a high incidence of fractures at this site. Look carefully for separation of the transverse processes.

Tx

For immediate assessment and management of potentially serious spinal injuries see page 51.

The patient must be kept splinted and immobile. Orthopaedic advice should be sought immediately. Urinary catheterisation is required.

For suspected renal injury see page 87.

Severe soft tissue injury to the back

Patients with severe bruising to the back are often unable to walk. Many such patients require admission for analgesia and mobilisation. The possibility of renal injury must always be considered; the urine should be tested for blood.

Fractures of the transverse processes

These fractures, which are often multiple, are caused by either direct trauma – usually a fall from a height – or by psoas muscle avulsion. Significant force is required and so other concomitant injuries are common. The retroperitoneal structures are particularly vulnerable; the urine must always be tested for the presence of blood. Over 10% of patients with a fractured transverse process also have a further lumbar spine fracture.

XR

The bisected transverse process is often missed on a plain AP radiograph. A CT scan is usually indicated to detect both retroperitoneal and more severe spinal injuries.

TX

Admission is required for observation, bed rest and especially for analgesia.
For suspected renal injury see page 87.

Acute back pain

Back pain of sudden onset is a common presentation in young or middle-aged patients. It usually occurs while lifting. The clinician should enquire about:
- onset of the pain/relation to lifting or injury;
- site and character of the pain;
- aggravating and relieving factors;
- radiation and referral of the pain, especially sciatica;
- neurological symptoms, including bladder and bowel function;
- previous episodes;

- coexisting diseases and drug therapy (especially steroids).

The clinician should then:
- Observe the patient's degree of mobility.
- Examine the spine and paravertebral areas for tenderness.
- Check the mobility of the lumbar spine with the patient erect and supine.
- Determine the extent of sciatic nerve sheath tethering by measuring straight-leg raising bilaterally.
- Record subjective or objective sensory loss in the lower limbs.
- Look for muscle weakness (commonly at ankle or toe) and reflex loss.
- In severe cases, examine the perineum for sensory loss and sphincter laxity.

Atypical (and thus worrying) features in a patient with back pain of sudden onset are listed in *Box 4.5*.

> Mechanical low back pain is usually exacerbated by movement in specific directions. Global pain (with all movements) is either more sinister or associated with psychological overlay.

XR

Urgent plain radiography is unhelpful in most younger patients – *see Box 4.6*. Older men (> 55 years) and postmenopausal women should have radiography to exclude osteoporotic collapse of the vertebrae or other diseases. The differentiation between new and old collapse of the bone can be very difficult on plain films.

Box 4.5 Atypical ('Red Flag') Features in a Patient with Back Pain

- Age less than 20 years or over 55 years
- Recent onset of pain without trauma or lifting
- Severe pain at rest or progressively worsening pain
- Bilateral sciatic pain
- Thoracic pain
- Obvious structural deformity
- Urinary or bowel symptoms
- Malaise or weight loss
- History of carcinoma, HIV infection, drug abuse or recent steroid therapy

---

Box 4.6 Indications for Radiography of the Lumbar Spine in Patients with Back Pain

- History of significant trauma – *see page 51*
- History suggestive of non-mechanical back pain (i.e. The pain is constant, progressive, worse at night and unrelated to activity)
- History of coexisting condition that may give rise to non-mechanical back pain (i.e. malignancy or inflammation)
- Patient at risk of spontaneous vertebral collapse (on steroids, elderly)
- Neurological signs
- Pain persisting for more than 4–6 weeks

Tx

Negative neurological findings in the presence of low back pain suggest minor ligamentous injury in the young or degeneration in the older patient. Most patients will be helped by:

- an immediate injection of an NSAID (e.g. Tenoxicam 20 mg IM);
- analgesia to take home (to be taken on a regular basis). The muscle relaxant baclofen may occasionally be helpful, especially where muscle spasm is a prominent feature;
- written instructions on the care of the injured back;
- review by the GP after this time if there is no improvement. A letter should accompany the patient.

Physiotherapy should also be considered. Regular exercise is important and patients should be advised to return to work as soon as possible. Some patients may be confined to bed as a consequence of their pain but this should be limited to two days as a maximum and should not be considered as a primary treatment.

Over 95% of patients with simple mechanical low back pain will recover spontaneously within 6 weeks. However, there is an 85% chance of recurrence with around 8% of affected patients becoming chronically disabled. Psychosocial factors are the only known predictors of long-term problems.

Collapsed vertebral bodies are an indication for an orthopaedic opinion. Nursing care and analgesia is usually required prior to mobilisation. Female patients with osteoporotic collapse who are referred back to their GP should be considered for hormone replacement therapy (*see page 14*).

Bladder, bowel and perineal symptoms and signs suggest central prolapse of an intervertebral disc. Immediate orthopaedic referral is essential. Positive findings in the limbs suggest lateral intervertebral disc protrusion (*see page 63*).

Atypical back pain

No one would be satisfied with a diagnosis of front pain so why accept back pain? A more specific diagnosis should be sought.

If back pain is not related to direct trauma and did not come on while the patient was lifting or twisting, the insidious onset of a more sinister disease should be considered. (*For atypical or warning features also see Box 4.5.*) This could include:

- secondary deposit (breast, bronchus, prostate, thyroid, kidney);
- myeloma;
- pelvic neoplasm or infection;
- aortic aneurysm;
- renal or pancreatic disease or peptic ulceration;
- ankylosing spondylitis;
- Paget's disease;
- herpes zoster.

Leaking aortic aneurysm commonly presents with pain experienced in the back and myocardial infarction may cause isolated back pain.

The examination should be tailored to the history but may need to include:

- abdominal palpation and rectal examination;
- urinalysis;
- breast examination;
- a search for causes of weight loss.

FBC, blood chemistry and ESR may be helpful as screening tests.

Xr

To obtain radiographs of the lumbar spine requires the highest doses of radiation of any plain films and thus these views should only be requested in specific circumstances – *see Box 4.6*. CT and MR scans are often of more diagnostic value than plain films. The advice of a radiologist should be sought.

Tx

Assess the patient and ask for advice. Older people with backache tend to be under-investigated.

Sciatica

Pain in the distribution of the sciatic nerve is most commonly caused by the lateral prolapse of an intervertebral disc (PID). The pain, which may be severe, radiates across the buttock, down the back of the thigh and along the medial aspect of the leg to the foot. Backache may be absent, especially when the sciatic pain is of more gradual onset. Bilateral buttock and thigh pain, which does not cross the knee joint, is not usually associated with PID.

The examination should be the same as that detailed above for low back pain. Consider alternative, particularly vascular, causes of the pain.

Xr

Plain films are not helpful.

Tx

The initial management of sciatica is similar to that for back pain. In severe cases, strong analgesics may be needed. A short course of prednisolone can sometimes speed resolution but should generally be avoided. The patient should be warned that sciatica can be slow to settle. Fortunately, the majority of sufferers will be better in 6 weeks and many of the remainder will have resolved before 6 months have elapsed.

Cauda equina syndrome

Central prolapse of the L4/L5 or L5/S1 intervertebral disc may cause compression of the terminal branches of the spinal cord. In the absence of prompt treatment, this cauda equina syndrome results in severe and permanent neurological damage. Consequently, the presenting symptoms and signs must not be missed:

• acute low back pain (which may be superimposed upon a chronic history of recurrent pain);
• radiation of pain to the legs – usually but not always bilateral;
• weakness or sensory disturbance in the legs – often present but not invariable. This may cause an abnormal gait;
• alteration of perineal sensation ('saddle anaesthesia') – usually but not exclusively bilateral;
• sphincter dysfunction presenting as urgency, frequency or incontinence;
• alteration of bladder and bowel habit (leading to retention and constipation).

Tx

Immediate admission and referral for urgent decompression is essential. Surgery undertaken more than 48 h after presentation is rarely successful.

Injury to the coccyx and coccygodynia

The coccyx may be injured by a fall on to the buttocks. There is local pain and extreme tenderness. Dyschezia (pain on defaecation) may also occur. A haematoma can sometimes be felt between the coccyx and the rectum, but pain usually prevents a rectal examination. Prolonged symptoms are inevitable; sitting is likely to be uncomfortable for months.

Pain in this region (coccygodynia) can also be caused by prolapse of an intervertebral disc, pelvic inflammatory disease and tumours of the spine and sacrum.

Xr

Films of the sacrum and coccyx are often of poor quality, especially in obese patients. Moreover, management is rarely changed by an initial X-ray. If imaged, a fractured coccyx is often seen to be anteverted or displaced. Anterior subluxation of the entire coccyx can also occur, with or without an accompanying fracture of the distal sacrum.

Tx

Analgesia is the mainstay of treatment and the patient should be advised to sit on an inflatable rubber ring cushion. A swimming ring is a cheap and easily available alternative. Constipation must be avoided. The patient should be warned that pain will persist for several months. Physiotherapy (ultrasound treatment) can sometimes be helpful. For severe, prolonged coccygodynia, excision of the coccyx may be necessary.

Wounds to the neck and the back

Major wounds to the neck

A major neck wound is defined as any injury in which the platysma muscle is thought to be divided. Look for further wounds if the patient has been stabbed. Neck wounds are often deeper than a casual examination might suggest and wounds near the base of the skull and the root of the neck are particularly dangerous.

• Major vascular injury may remain occult for many hours or even days. A normal carotid pulse does not exclude arterial damage.
• Air embolisation may follow venous injury.
• Surgical emphysema will follow division of the trachea or oesophagus.
• Hoarseness and stridor are associated with laryngeal trauma.

Xr

A lateral soft tissue view of the neck may show surgical emphysema or air tracks.

Tx

Position the patient with a slight head-down tilt to lessen the risk of air embolism. Gain venous access and ensure anti-tetanus cover.

Major neck wounds should not be explored under local anaesthesia in the ED. Patients with such wounds must be referred for specialist assessment, observation and surgical exploration.

Stab wounds to the back

Stab wounds to the back are common.

Xr

A chest X-ray should be taken to exclude pneumothorax.

Tx

The wound should be cleaned, dressed and anti-tetanus cover given. Suturing usually creates a large haematoma under the stitches. The injury will need to be inspected and the dressing changed on the following day.

Leakage of cerebrospinal fluid

Midline wounds to the back may occasionally puncture the dura and cause leakage of cerebrospinal fluid. Wet dressings are often the first clue. Patients with a suspected cerebrospinal fluid leak need admission for bed rest and antibiotics (e.g. oral penicillin V and flucloxacillin). The inevitable 'spinal' headache will be slow to settle and need prolonged analgesia.

For injuries to the trunk see also Chapter 6 on page 75.

Chapter 5

Facial injuries

Facial injuries are commonly seen following assaults in adults and falls in children. They need special consideration because of the following reasons:

- The possibility of interference with the airway is always present.
- The important areas of the eye, nose, mouth and ears need special care.
- The unique relationship between facial skin and the underlying tissue demands special techniques of wound care and may make adequate local anaesthesia difficult to achieve.
- Deep tissue injuries may be masked, and delay in their treatment can lead to major disability.
- A good cosmetic result is clearly essential.

Fractures of the facial bones

Management in the ED is confined to the following:

- airway care (may be difficult);
- control of profuse bleeding;
- pain relief;
- initial clinical and radiographic assessment;
- administration of antibiotics for compound fractures;
- tetanus prophylaxis;
- consideration of other injuries.

The airway

Airway patency may be threatened by profuse bleeding and distortion of the skeleton and soft tissues. The airway may be maintainable in a fully conscious patient, but in the unresponsive patient endotracheal intubation becomes essential. Rarely, very extensive facial injuries may make this technically difficult or impossible and warrant urgent cricothyroidotomy or tracheostomy – *see pages 23 and 24*.

Neck injuries

These must be considered when facial injury is sustained by the moving head striking a fixed object (e.g. in a car). Although neck damage is less likely if the immobile head is struck by a mobile object (e.g. in an assault) it is essential to examine the cervical spine of all patients with facial injuries.

An elderly patient with a bruise on the forehead and weak arms should be assumed to have sustained a central cord injury – *see page 54*.

The facial skeleton is designed to withstand the vertical forces associated with mastication, but it collapses readily when struck from the front. Injuries can be divided into lower third (mandible), middle third and upper third (frontal). The last type is considered in *Chapter 3*.

Facial fractures are not always obvious. Examination begins with an assessment of facial contours – often best achieved by looking at the face from above and behind. Bony tenderness may be difficult to detect if soft-tissue bruising and swelling is already present. However, pressure for a few seconds over bony points (e.g. the infraorbital margin) will usually displace sufficient interstitial fluid to allow assessment of bony contours and orbital contents.

Facial radiography

The head position required to obtain basal skull and occipitomental views can be dangerous in the presence of cervical spine injuries. The latter can never be excluded immediately in the severely injured patient and so it is unwise to request these views in such patients. The usual brow-up, lateral view has two advantages: (a) minimal patient movement and (b) easier demonstration of paranasal sinuses. A CT scan overcomes these problems but should not be undertaken at the expense of treating more immediately important injuries.

Antibiotics for compound fractures

Flucloxacillin is appropriate prophylaxis for fractures associated with skin wounds. When there is a fracture into a sinus, then penicillin V or equivalent is probably a better choice.

Special features associated with facial fractures

Surgical emphysema of the face

This indicates the presence of a fracture into an air-containing sinus. Antibiotics and follow-up are required.

Facial sensory loss

Anaesthesia in the area of distribution of the infraorbital nerve (terminal branches of Vb) is often present with:
- fractures of the malar complex;
- fractures of the floor of the orbit;
- Le Fort II and III fractures;
- severe soft-tissue injuries to the cheek.

The area of numbness may include the ipsilateral upper lip and also the anterior gums and teeth (anterior superior alveolar nerve). Oedema in the infraorbital canal is the usual cause. This is where the dental nerve separates off, leaving the terminal part of the maxillary nerve to exit from the infraorbital foramen as the infraorbital nerve. Oral surgical follow-up is indicated.

Intra-oral damage

Examination inside the mouth is very important. Malocclusion of teeth, or displacement of dentures in the absence of primary dental damage, is always associated with injury to bone or to the temperomandibular joint. Palatal irregularities suggest a Le Fort fracture. Inability to open the mouth fully should provoke a careful look at the mandible.

Injuries affecting the eye

Assessment of visual acuity, conjunctival sac, cornea, anterior chamber and fundus is an essential part of facial assessment. Displacement of the eye, inwards or downwards, is associated with injury to the infraorbital plate. Extraocular muscle damage or distortion may complicate any damage to the bony wall of the orbit and is clearly demonstrated on testing the full range of eye movements. The presence of a subconjunctival haemorrhage without evidence of direct trauma to the eye is a strong indication of the presence of a facial fracture, usually in the infraorbital region.
For other causes of subconjunctival haemorrhage see pages 45 and 408.

Wounds associated with major fractures

Closure of major wounds associated with displaced facial fractures must await reduction of the fractures. The wounds may offer surgical access to bone and facilitate reduction. Until this has been carried out it may not be possible to achieve cosmetically acceptable reconstruction of the soft tissues.

Mandibular fractures

The most common mandibular fracture, through the extracapsular part of the neck of the condyle, is usually sustained by a blow on the chin. It can be unilateral or bilateral. Examination reveals dental malocclusion, often a lateral cross-bite and absence of forward movement of the condylar head on opening the mouth. The force may have been sufficient to drive the head of the condyle backwards and cause a fracture of the squamous temporal bone. This produces bleeding and a cerebrospinal fluid leak into the external auditory meatus.

Fractures of the ramus, angle and body will be revealed by local tenderness of the cheek and difficulty in opening the mouth. There may be surprisingly little swelling. The presence of mucosal lacerations and irregular dentition helps confirmation. Displacement is determined by the configuration of the fracture line in relation to the pull of the masticatory muscles. Mental anaesthesia may reflect damage to the inferior dental nerve.

> The ability to open the mouth fully and to clench the teeth normally makes the presence of a fracture of the jaw very unlikely.

XR

The best radiographs are lateral obliques, PA and Towne's views (for the condyles). Orthopantomogram (OPT or OPG), a rotational tomogram that gives a circumferential view of the face, is especially helpful and easy to interpret.

TX

No immediate treatment is required in the ED for any of these fractures *per se*. Unstable and painful fractures will require early repair; the remainder – the majority – can be referred for specialist management later. Some displaced condylar fractures can be managed conservatively with good functional results, but there is an increasing trend towards internal fixation. All patients will need analgesia and a light diet.

> Mumps is often unilateral in its early stages and all unwell children are more likely to fall. Swelling at the angle of the jaw may reflect parotid engorgement and not a mandibular fracture. Take the temperature.

Temporomandibular joint dislocation

This may occur spontaneously as when the patient is unable to close his or her mouth after yawning, or may result from a blow to the open mouth. It is often recurrent and is particularly common in the elderly.

XR

Exclude fracture by radiography (*see before*).

TX

Reduction can usually be achieved without general anaesthetic, but must be carried out by an experienced clinician using appropriate analgesia or sedation. The jaw is held by putting both thumbs inside the mouth along the line of the lower teeth on each side while the forefingers grasp the bone from outside. Pressure is then applied downwards and backwards by the intra-oral thumbs pressing bilaterally against the angle of the jaw. Post-reduction radiographs are taken to confirm relocation although the patient is usually in no doubt. Specialist follow-up on an outpatient basis is appropriate.

Malar fractures

The malar complex provides the bony prominence on the cheek and is commonly fractured in isolation by a blow to that area. The strong central part of the bone usually remains intact, the force being transmitted to the three buttresses. These bones then fracture or dislocate either individually or, more frequently, simultaneously (a 'tripod fracture'):

1 *Infraorbital fracture*. Fracture in the infraorbital region usually causes neuropraxia of the infraorbital nerve. Subconjunctival haemorrhage may also be seen.

> Sensory loss following a facial injury merits specialist follow-up. It may involve the upper lip, the gum and the front teeth on the affected side (*see page 66*).

2 Displacement of the zygomaticofrontal suture. This may be associated with injury to the suspensory ligament of the eye.

3 Fracture of the zygomatic arch (zygoma). This may be sufficiently displaced to impinge on the coronoid process of the mandible and prevent normal jaw movement. Even if this does not occur at the time of injury, exuberant callus formation may cause problems later.

Examination will reveal tenderness over one, or all three, malar processes. Bony irregularity is sought for by intra-oral examination behind and above the upper molars and by careful palpation along the inferior and lateral borders of the orbit and along the line of the zygomatic arch. Diplopia may occur because of injury to the suspensory ligament or displacement and damage to the extraocular muscles. The latter is usually transient.

> Surgical emphysema in the area of a malar injury indicates a (compound) fracture into an air sinus. Antibiotics and follow-up are indicated.

XR

Facial views, which vary in their exact inclination from hospital to hospital, confirm the diagnosis. The two most common views supplied are occipitomental projections at 10° and 30°.

TX

Once the diagnosis has been made, the patient should be referred for specialist care. If reduction and elevation of the displaced malar are required, this can be achieved relatively simply, under a short general anaesthetic on a day-case basis within the following week.

Retrobulbar haemorrhage

This may occasionally occur following a fracture of the zygomatic complex. It causes:

- retrobulbar pain;
- very marked proptosis;
- diminished vision (which may quickly become permanent);
- massive facial swelling.

> Severe retrobulbar bleeding with orbital displacement is a surgical emergency. The area must be decompressed by lateral canthotomy. This entails division of the lateral check ligament, which extends between the edge of the globe and the lateral bony margin of the orbit. Seek urgent ophthalmic advice.

Middle third fractures

When the face is struck directly from the front, the delicate bony skeleton formed by the maxilla, palatine, nasal and ethmoid bones may be crushed and forced backwards and downwards. The nasal bones may be broken in isolation (*see page 69*) but the other bones tend to collapse *en masse*. Le Fort first described the three fracture complexes that are commonly seen – *see Box 5.1*.

Examination may reveal a dished-in face if the middle third has moved backwards and downwards. The nose appears flattened and widened. This appearance is best confirmed from the side and from above. Swelling and bruising are usually marked. Holding the vault of the skull with one hand and the maxilla complex with the other (between gloved index finger on the hard palate and thumb over the upper incisors), instability may be elicited with surprising ease – and without too much pain.

There may be diplopia on upward gaze and damage to the lacrimal system. Damage to the cribriform plate may produce anosmia, but this can be difficult to confirm in the ED as blood is usually present in the nasal cavity and will seriously impair the sense of smell even in the absence of damage to the olfactory apparatus. Any minor occlusion deformity is readily appreciated by the patient and is a reliable indicator of bony injury. The backwards displacement of the middle

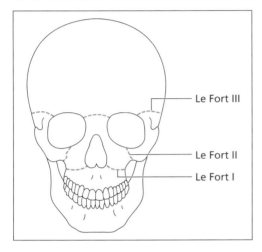

Figure 5.1 Le Fort classification of fractures of the middle third of the face.

third of the face will produce a reverse overbite (upper incisors behind lower incisors). The associated tilting results in an anterior open bite.

XR

Le Fort fractures can be difficult to spot on facial views, but once the fracture line is pointed out it usually becomes obvious.

TX

Immediate specialist inpatient care is required. Significant bleeding and airway compromise may occur, and in this case an anaesthetist should be called.

Nasal fractures

The nasal bones may be dislocated from their normal relationship with the maxilla or may be fractured. The nasal cartilages usually deform to accommodate violence and do not break. The nasal septum may be deformed, deviated laterally and fractured.

> Trauma to the nose may produce a large septal haematoma that can obstruct the nostril and damage the nutrient vessels to the septum. This can result in avascular necrosis of the bone and septal collapse.

The nose has a good blood supply and all these injuries are associated with epistaxis.

Examination should first exclude more serious facial injuries. Local tenderness over the nasal bones will be present but the appearance of swelling may be delayed. The tip of the nose may be upturned. Lateral deviation may not be obvious to the examiner. The patient should be given a mirror and asked to compare present and previous facial appearance. An obvious deformity may relate to a previous injury.

More extensive fractures involving the ethmoids are associated with widening of the intracanthal distance, a transverse cleft across the glabella and cerebrospinal fluid rhinorrhoea. Intranasal examination should be carried out with a speculum and a good light; it is essential to exclude a septal haematoma.

XR

Radiological confirmation of nasal fractures is of no immediate value. Indeed, an undisplaced fracture may be difficult to distinguish from a vascular marking.

TX

Bleeding usually settles with alar pressure – *see page 414*. Septal haematoma or uncontrolled bleeding are indications for immediate referral. Patients with clearly deformed noses should be seen at the next ENT clinic. However, there is a large group of patients who have marked swellings but an uncertain amount of deformity. They should be told to let the swelling settle over 5–7 days and then return to the ED for reassessment if they are unhappy with their appearance.

Facial wounds

See also Chapter 21.

Facial skin is unusual. It is an integral part of the deep structures, bound to them by the facial muscles that arise from and insert into the subcutaneous tissues. Consequently, it is difficult to undermine and close quite small defects without causing deformity. Wounds near the circular muscle around the eyes or mouth may influence their function.

Ask about
- Mechanism of injury and wounding agent (especially glass).
- Contamination.
- Delay to presentation.

Look for
- Function, before anaesthetising the wound.
- Involvement of specialised areas.

Record details of wound site, size and configuration. A drawing on a rubber-stamped facial outline is best. Many such injuries are the result of assaults and you may be called to describe the wound in court.

> Wounds to the chin may be associated with fractures of the condyles of the jaw.

Certain conditions are required before repair in the ED should be undertaken:
- patience (and time);
- good operating conditions;
- adequate anaesthesia;
- an immobile patient;
- a knowledge of facial anatomy;
- a knowledge of the general principles of plastic surgery;
- technical skill.

Standard suture sets, provided in EDs, often contain large and unreliable instruments. A special set of fine, good-quality instruments for face and hand use should be available.

Anaesthesia

This is essential to permit adequate exploration and cleaning. In children, a general anaesthetic may be required for a relatively small wound.

> Do not use local anaesthetics containing adrenaline near the extremities of the nose and ears.

Exploration

Deep wounds may damage the facial or infraorbital nerves or the parotid, submandibular or tear ducts. The suspicion of damage to any of these structures requires expert assessment by the appropriate specialist. Early referral is essential.

Cleaning

This must be very thorough. Dirt and foreign bodies such as windscreen glass may be driven deep into facial wounds. An appreciation of the direction and force of the injuring agent will facilitate exploration. Remove dirt from grazes as soon as possible, otherwise some of it is taken up by inflammatory cells, producing a tattoo effect. It may be necessary to use a scrubbing brush or toothbrush to remove ingrained dirt. A second operation to retrieve a foreign body is always more difficult and produces a more pronounced scar.

Special areas

Wounds involving the eyelid margins should always be referred to an ophthalmic surgeon. Incorrect apposition of the various layers may produce entropion or ectropion. Extreme care is also required when repairing wounds that involve the red margin of the mouth and nose. A slight malalignment will produce a major cosmetic defect.

Similarly, the line of the eyebrows must be carefully preserved. Adequate local anaesthesia can be difficult to achieve around the nose and ears.

Tissue loss

Undermining facial wound edges is technically difficult and can increase rather than decrease the deformity associated with tissue loss. Large defects are best closed by swinging whole flaps of facial tissue. An experienced plastic surgeon should be involved in the management of such wounds from the outset. The excellent blood supply of the face allows even the most tenuous flap to survive. Trimming of wound edges should be left to a senior doctor with plastic surgery experience.

Closure with sutures

Two layers are usually adequate. Troublesome bleeding may require the occasional ligature, but haemostasis is usually achieved on wound closure. Haematoma formation is rarely a problem. Subcutaneous closure with interrupted, plain catgut (about 4–0) is advisable in larger wounds. The skin is then apposed with interrupted sutures. Tension must be avoided. Correct alignment is best achieved by initial insertion of a few sutures at intervals along the wound.

Fine diameter sutures are generally recommended for use on the face but the contused wounds often seen in an ED do not lend themselves to very fine sutures. Placing adhesive tapes (e.g. steristrips) on top of a sutured wound may reduce the tension on the sutures and improve the final result.

Suture removal

Facial wounds heal rapidly. Those not subject to undue stress (e.g. on the forehead or the cheek) will be sufficiently strong to allow suture removal at 4–5 days. Wounds over convex surfaces may open up at this stage and can be protected by adhesive tapes. The early replacement of sutures by tapes has the advantages of reducing scarring around the needle puncture marks. This is not recommended under the chin and other areas where saliva or excessive movement may impair their adhesion.

Closure with adhesive tapes

Some facial wounds can be closed with adhesive tapes. Cleaning prior to the application of these tapes must be just as thorough as cleaning prior to the insertion of sutures. This often requires local anaesthesia. Wounds on convex surfaces will tend to open up in the early stages of healing, as a result of a combination of reduced tissue strength and oedema. Tapes should not be used if the wounds cannot be kept dry and immobile (e.g. the chin or eyebrows of children), but are ideal for small wounds of the forehead and cheek.

Closure with tissue glue

This can also be considered for some small wounds. The same precautions apply as for adhesive tapes.

Bites

This type of wound is considered in detail on *page 394*. The general principle of leaving bites open, to heal by secondary intention, does not apply to the face. Primary closure usually gives good cosmetic results. The wounds must be cleaned meticulously and then a broad-spectrum antibiotic (e.g. co-amoxiclav) prescribed. Follow-up in the ED is advisable.

Injuries inside the mouth

> Wounds associated with dental damage should be explored for tooth fragments which may lead to a severe infection if not removed. The possibility of aspiration should also be considered.

Injuries to the tongue

Isolated lacerations rarely require any specific treatment. Healing is rapid and the cosmetic result good, despite initial deformity caused by the pull of the intrinsic muscles. An antiseptic, analgesic, oral rinse (e.g. benzydamine HCl 0.15% solution) may be valuable. This is particularly important in patients who are reluctant to drink and in whom a dry mouth may predispose to secondary infection.

Injuries to the buccal mucosa and gingiva

Simple lacerations are treated in the same way as injuries to the tongue; if more extensive then look for a fracture.

> The patient (or the parents) should be warned that a yellow exudate will form over the wound. This is caused by the normal commensal bacteria of the mouth. It will last a few days and may give rise to slight halitosis.

Injuries to the permanent teeth

Teeth may be chipped, displaced or avulsed. The site of injury should be described using the dental formula shown in *Box 5.2*.

Tx

For conditions that require immediate dental advice see Box 5.3.

- A chip confined to enamel or dentine (*see Figure 5.2*) will be very sensitive but does not pose any immediate threat to the viability of the tooth. Varnish may be applied to reduce thermal pain and the patient referred to his or her own dentist the next day.
- If the pulp is exposed (see *Figure 5.2*) there is a risk of infection and immediate dental referral is necessary. The pulp is recognised by its red colour.
- Incisor teeth may be displaced (subluxed) but otherwise be apparently undamaged. Immediate specialist advice should be obtained in the case of permanent teeth as there is only a 4 h window of opportunity for easy repositioning. Manipulation of the tooth in the ED may loosen it further, with subsequent risk of inhalation.

> **Box 5.2 Dental Formula**
>
> 1) Determine the quadrant (as if you are looking into the mouth):
>   - upper right ⌋   upper left ⌊
>   - lower right ⌐   lower left ⌐
> 2) Count out from the midline:
>   - 1,2 incisors   3 canine
>   - 4,5 premolars   6,7,8 molars
>
> e.g. outer upper right incisor 2⌋
>
> lower left canine |3̄

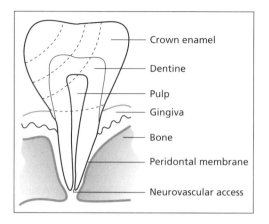

Figure 5.2 Types of dental injury in relation to the dental anatomy.

Labels: Crown enamel, Dentine, Pulp, Gingiva, Bone, Peridontal membrane, Neurovascular access

> **Box 5.3 Dental Injuries for which Immediate Specialist Advice is Needed**
>
> Exposed pulp of any tooth
> Avulsed permanent tooth
> Subluxed permanent tooth
> Mobile segment of alveolar bone
> Severe soft-tissue injury with dental damage

- Sometimes, several incisor teeth are loosened together with a segment of the underlying alveolar bone (alveolar plate fracture). Again, this needs immediate specialist treatment including splintage and antibiotics.
- Avulsed (permanent) teeth should be:
1 washed very gently with saline;
2 kept in saline;
3 handled as little as possible;
4 reimplanted and splinted in place by a dental surgeon.

Reimplantation is often successful but the chances of a good outcome are directly related to the speed of reimplantation – within 30 min is ideal. If definitive care is delayed, the socket can be cleaned with saline, local anaesthetic gel instilled and the tooth replaced. Temporary stabilisation is obtained by the patient biting on damp gauze. Aftercare includes tetanus prophylaxis and antibiotics.

Damage to deciduous (milk) teeth

For the purposes of treatment, it is important to differentiate the permanent dentition from the deciduous teeth. Permanent teeth are bigger and have a different shape from milk teeth. They usually appear after 6 years of age in the lower jaw and after 7 years of age in the upper jaw. The 32 permanent teeth replace 20 deciduous teeth. The first milk tooth erupts at about 6 months of age and thereafter one or more appears every month. They are all shed by the age of 13. For children, the dental formula is written in the usual way (*see Box 5.2*) but the letters A to E are used to designate the deciduous teeth.

Avulsed milk teeth are common and require no immediate treatment. However, there are two possible long-term effects on the permanent teeth.
1 The gap may affect their positioning.
2 The trauma may impair their development. This risk is increased by attempts at reimplantation.
The child should see his or her own dentist on the following day.

Deciduous teeth that are subluxed or intruded (pushed into the jaw) should also be seen by the dentist on the following day.

Very loose deciduous teeth should be removed but other loose milk teeth can be safely left to the patient's dentist. We all have 20 loose milk teeth at sometime in our lives and survive without aspiration.

Chipped deciduous teeth are dealt with in the same way as the permanent dentition – *see before*.

Injuries to the ear

Injuries involving the cartilage of the ear

The elastic cartilage of the ear receives its blood supply from the overlying skin. If exposed on both sides by skin avulsion or separated from the skin by haematoma it will necrose and collapse resulting in a 'cauliflower' ear.

Tx

Most lacerations of the pinna involving cartilage require specialist care. Small pieces of cartilage exposed at the edge of the pinna may be trimmed, prior to skin closure, without causing significant cosmetic problems.

Bites to the ear

Bites to the ear may result in extensive mixed flora infection and cartilage destruction. They are usually caused by humans.

Tx

Most such injuries should not be closed. Clean the area thoroughly, give antibiotics (e.g. co-amoxiclav) and ensure protection against tetanus. The advice of an ENT or plastic surgeon will usually be required.

Injuries around the eye

For assessment of the eye see page 405.
For corneal and other ocular injuries see page 406.

Blow-out fractures of the orbit

These injuries result because the eyeball is stronger than the floor of the orbit. A direct blow on the eye by a fairly large object (e.g. a squash ball) may cause little damage to the eye – acuity may not be impaired – but only push it backwards and downward through the infraorbital plate. Surprisingly, the condition may go unrecognised. Suspicion is aroused by the mechanism of injury and sometimes by restriction of the extraocular muscles resulting in double vision.

Xr

There may be a fluid level in the maxillary antrum on the AP radiograph and sometimes a 'tear-drop' soft-tissue shadow at the top of the antrum. An associated fracture of the malar may occur but the infraorbital plate fracture is often difficult to identify. CT scan shows the 'tear-drop' to be orbital contents herniating into the antrum through the fracture.

Tx

Elevation and reconstruction of the orbital floor may be necessary – early referral is essential.

Eyelid lacerations

These require expert assessment and repair and so must be referred to an ophthalmic surgeon. Injuries below the medial canthus may involve the lacrimal apparatus and this damage is easily overlooked.

Chapter 6

Injuries to the trunk

Injuries to the trunk can be difficult to diagnose and are easily overlooked, especially when associated with:

- a depressed level of consciousness;
- painful skeletal injuries.

They may be immediately life-threatening but can also cause delayed deterioration. Primary survey and resuscitation are described on *page 3*; details specifically concerned with injury to the trunk are dealt with in this chapter. A careful and repeated systematic review of the chest, abdomen, pelvis and thoracolumbar spine should be undertaken in all patients who may have sustained multiple injuries.

> If blunt trauma results in injuries both above and below the trunk (e.g. to the head and femur), then the trunk itself is also likely to be injured.

Bruises, clothing imprints and friction burns, together with any history available from the patient or witnesses, can help to determine the direction and severity of the injuring agent.

> Stab wounds must be assumed to involve vital organs until proven otherwise.

Repeated physical examination is essential.

> Always examine the back and the perineum – they are often forgotten.

Chest injuries

Chest injuries may:
- disrupt the mechanism of respiration;
- impair gas exchange;
- produce hypovolaemia;
- cause cardiogenic shock.

Immediate assessment and management

- Attend to ABCs as described in *Chapter 1*.
- Give high-concentration oxygen.
- Consider tension pneumothorax (*see page 77*).
- Cover open (sucking) wounds of the chest wall with firm, waterproof dressings. NB This may allow a tension pneumothorax to develop.
- Obtain IV access. *For a discussion of the rate and type of fluid infusion see page 6 and page 326.*
- Connect the patient to appropriate monitors (SaO$_2$, ECG and BP) and measure the respiratory rate.
- Request an urgent chest X-ray.
- Obtain an urgent 12-lead ECG.
- Consider early analgesia.
- Consider blood gas analysis.

Further assessment and management

Ask about
- site and character of pain;
- dyspnoea;

- mechanism of injury;
- past medical history.

Look for
- sweating, pallor and cyanosis;
- increased respiratory rate and work of breathing;
- uneven or abnormal chest movements;
- areas of tenderness, bruising, abrasions or crepitus;
- dullness or hyper–resonance on percussion;
- reduced air entry and abnormal breath sounds;
- abnormal position of apex beat or trachea;
- increased pulse rate or paradoxical pulse;
- inaudible heart sounds (tamponade);
- distended neck veins;
- abdominal tenderness;
- SaO$_2$, BP and ECG abnormalities.

> Remember the chest has a back as well as a front: log-roll the patient to examine it.

Radiographs of the chest

Ideally, the chest X-ray should be performed with the patient erect to permit fluid level detection (*see Figure 6.1*). With the patient supine, fluid present in the pleural cavity will lie behind the lung and produce a diffusely opaque lung field. A lateral decubitus film ('sick side down') may also reveal a fluid level, even in a supine patient.

> Radiography must not precede or prevent careful initial clinical assessment.

Injury to the chest wall and lungs

Wounds to the chest wall

Sucking wounds, although unusual, attract immediate attention. In contrast, small stab wounds may be underestimated. They must be assumed to penetrate the parietal pleura until proved otherwise. This entails confirmation of the mechanism of wounding, observation of progress (if necessary, with repeat chest radiographs) and occasionally careful examination of the anaesthetised wound by an experienced surgeon in an operating theatre. A long, incised wound at right angles to the line of the ribs is usually superficial.

X$_R$

All patients with stab wounds to the trunk should have a chest X-ray.

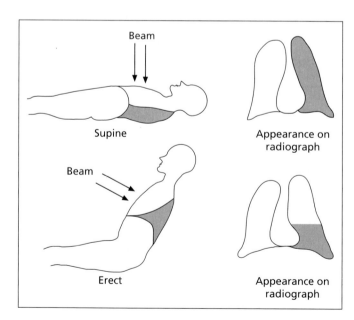

Figure 6.1 The appearance of fluid on erect and supine chest X-rays.

Beam

Supine

Appearance on radiograph

Beam

Erect

Appearance on radiograph

Tx

The presence of surgical emphysema, pneumothorax or haemothorax confirms pleural penetration. A chest drain will usually be required but should not be inserted through the wound (*see later*). Most cases settle without operative management; thoracotomy is only indicated if bleeding is severe or if a large air leak persists.

Anti-tetanus cover must be established and the wound covered with an antiseptic dressing. Be aware that an open wound may effectively prevent a tension pneumothorax. Stab wounds are best left unsutured to allow drainage of any intramuscular bleeding.

Pneumothorax and haemothorax

Traumatic pneumothorax may follow rib injury, stab wounds or barotrauma. The degree of pleuritic pain and dyspnoea is very variable. Clinical suspicion should be followed by radiographic confirmation except in the case of tension pneumothorax (*see later*).

> A simple pneumothorax may develop into a tension pneumothorax – particularly when the patient receives intermittent positive-pressure ventilation.

For management of spontaneous pneumothorax see page 201.

Haemothorax may also follow multiple rib fractures as a result of intercostal vessel damage. The bleeding is often brisk and continuous from the high systolic pressure of the intercostal arteries. In contrast, bleeding from the low-pressure pulmonary vessels usually stops with the collapse of the lung. A stab wound may cause profound bleeding from the internal thoracic artery or other intrathoracic structures. Symptoms and signs usually reflect the initial injury.

Xr

Look carefully for small pneumothoraces – especially apically, laterally and medially (close to the heart border). Haemothorax may appear as blunt-

ing of the costophrenic angles. A large quantity of blood lying parallel to the diaphragm is often missed (a sub-pulmonary haemothorax). If this area looks slightly abnormal consider requesting a lateral decubitus film (*see page 76*) that may reveal the problem.

Tx

- Give high-concentration oxygen by mask.
- Monitor SaO_2, BP and ECG.
- Consider early analgesia.
- Insert a chest drain (*see Box 6.1 and Figure 6.2*).

The 'open' technique is described but new equipment is now available on the market that makes 'closed' techniques much safer than was previously the case. In particular, small diameter wire-guided (Seldinger-type) catheters are quick and easy to insert and relatively comfortable for the patient.

Some small haemopneumothoraces can be managed conservatively if the patient is stable and there are no plans to institute IPPV. Such patients should be discussed with senior staff and must be observed closely for signs of deterioration. A repeat X-ray will be needed after 4 h to check for radiological enlargement of the pneumothorax.

> Do not use nitrous oxide mixtures for pain relief if there is a possibility of pneumothorax or pneumomediastinum. It may result in expansion of a gas-filled space.

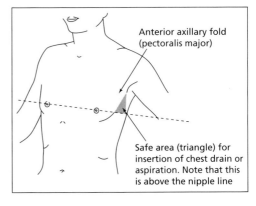

Anterior axillary fold (pectoralis major)

Safe area (triangle) for insertion of chest drain or aspiration. Note that this is above the nipple line

Figure 6.2 The triangle of safety for insertion of a chest drain.

Box 6.1 Insertion of a Chest Drain

In a dire emergency, the need for a chest drain should be determined clinically, without waiting for radiographic confirmation. However, this is the exception rather than the rule. Bilateral drains may sometimes be needed. The preferred site in emergency practice is the fifth intercostal space in the mid-axillary line – *for the correct area see Figure 6.2*. There are three equally important phases to the procedure.

Analgesia and preparation
- Position the patient in a semi-recumbent position with the affected side uppermost.
- Administer oxygen, attach a pulse oximeter and obtain venous access.
- Consider IV morphine if there is adequate respiratory effort. Sedation with a small dose of midazolam is also an option in some patients.
- Perform intercostal blocks posterior to the anticipated site of drain insertion. This is done by injecting 2 mL of 1% lidocaine around the neurovascular bundle (just below the inferior border of the rib). About three intercostal nerves should be blocked to include a space above and a space below.
- Infiltrate local anaesthetic down to the parietal pleura at the site of insertion. Aspiration of air bubbles into a syringe containing residual local anaesthetic is a useful confirmatory sign.

Insertion technique
- Clean the skin and use surgical gloves and drapes.
- Make a 2 cm incision down to parietal pleura. Aim for the upper border of the lower rib, to avoid the neurovascular bundle.
- Open the incision with forceps. Some blunt dissection over the superior border of the rib may be required with the tips of scissors.
- Consider inserting a gloved finger and sweeping the cavity to establish lung collapse.
- Insert a chest drain (up to 28 G in an adult) using either a pair of curved artery forceps or a blunt trocar. Better still, use a modern drainage tube that includes a flexible introducer within its lumen.
- Attach the drain to an underwater seal or a double Heimlich ('flutter') valve. In the case of the former, check for movements with respiration.
- Advance the drain up to 15–20 cm in an upwards, posterior direction.

Fixation of the tube
- Close the wound with large sutures on either side of the drain.
- Cover the site with a waterproof dressing.
- Cover the dressing completely with strips of tape.
- Secure the drain with a 'mesentery' of adhesive tape.
The position of the chest drain must be confirmed on chest X-ray.

Remember that the patient will have to live with the tube for several days and some other poor doctor will have to remove it!

Tension pneumothorax

This is a life-threatening emergency with the rapid increase in intrapleural pressure moving the mediastinum, compressing the opposite lung and impairing venous return. The patient has:
- dyspnoea;
- unilaterally reduced breath sounds;
- distended neck veins;
- tracheal deviation;
- impaired cardiac output;
- cyanosis (a late sign);

and may look and feel as if they are 'about to die'. (They are!)

The clinical picture may be mistaken for that of a cardiac tamponade (*see page 81*). However, tension pneumothorax:

- is more common;
- may be differentiated by the hyper-resonance to percussion over the affected side.

XR

This delays treatment and so is inappropriate in the case of a clinical tension. If taken, it would show a hyperexpanded lung field that is displacing the mediastinum, depressing the diaphragm and compressing the opposite lung.

Tx

Immediate needle decompression – *see Box 6.2*. This is part of the initial assessment or primary survey and resuscitation phase of management.

Box 6.2 Treatment of Tension Pneumothorax (Needle Thoracocentesis)

- On the affected side, identify the second intercostal space in the mid-clavicular line.
- Insert a cannula with a syringe attached just above the rib, until air is aspirated. (A cannula of at least 4.5 cm in length will be required.)
- Remove the syringe and needle. There should be a hissing decompression followed by an immediate clinical improvement.
- Tape the cannula in place.
- Proceed to chest tube drainage (*see Box 6.1 and Figure 6.2*).
- Once the chest drain is working, remove the cannula and dress the site.
- Obtain a chest X-ray.
NB A syringe with the plunger removed can be attached to the needle instead of a normal syringe. If it is filled with saline and the needle inserted with the patient supine, air bubbles will reveal the presence of a pneumothorax.

Insertion of a needle does not always decompress a tension pneumothorax as the underlying pleura and lung are 'sucked' into the needle and occlude it. If this happens, a second attempt should be made. Failure to achieve decompression at this point indicates the need to proceed immediately to rapid insertion of a chest drain.

Surgical emphysema

This may:
- complicate injury to gas-containing structures (usually lung or oesophagus – rib fracture is the most common cause);
- follow assault with a high-pressure hose;
- be a result of infection with gas-forming organisms.

Subcutaneous gas in the chest or neck can usually be felt as crepitus. Other symptoms and signs result from the original insult.

Surgical emphysema after blunt trauma is usually a direct result of damage to the lung, but clinical and radiological examination may not initially confirm this. Stab and gunshot wounds may injure the pharynx or oesophagus. Infection spreading from such wounds into the mediastinum is a major, life-threatening complication.

XR

Subcutaneous or mediastinal gas may easily be seen on a plain chest X-ray as streaking in the soft tissues.

Tx

Look for the injury that has caused the air leak. Observe in hospital.

For treatment of rib fractures see page 80.

For pneumothorax see page 77.

For pneumomediastinum and pneumopericardium see page 203.

In the case of suspected oesophageal or pharyngeal injury, prophylactic antibiotics should be started and surgical advice sought.

Rib fractures

Fractured ribs are common and result from direct blows or falls. There is pain on inspiration and coughing and also considerable difficulty with trunk movements. Local tenderness is inevitable. The patient must be asked about shortness of breath and previous cardiorespiratory problems. Careful observation should reveal any significant dyspnoea. The chest should be examined thoroughly to exclude underlying pneumohaemothorax and contusion.

Xr

A chest X-ray is mandatory in the presence of dyspnoea or past history of respiratory problems. There are usually more ribs fractured than you can easily see on the X-ray.

> Multiple old rib fractures on an adult's chest X-ray usually indicate past episodes of alcohol abuse; non-accidental injury should be considered in a child.

Tx

For simple pneumothorax/haemothorax see page 77.

Multiple rib fractures
- Give high-concentration oxygen by mask.
- Monitor SaO_2, BP and ECG and measure the respiratory rate.
- Consider early analgesia.
- Measure the blood gases.
- Request an urgent anaesthetic opinion; the patient often requires intensive care. The inevitable underlying contusion will cause severe hypoxaemia. Pain may require a thoracic epidural infusion.

Less than three fractured ribs
- Exclude underlying problems and respiratory difficulty.
- Assess mobility in the light of home circumstances.
- Assess the level of pain.

The patient may go home if the above considerations do not contraindicate it. Adequate analgesia and GP follow-up will be required. For patients with a past history of cardiorespiratory problems, also consider:
- prophylactic antibiotics;
- prophylactic steroids; and
- community physiotherapy.

The patient must take analgesics and cough rather than refuse to do both. Winding a scarf around the chest and pulling on the crossed-over ends while coughing provides a surprising amount of pain relief. Strapping of the ribs, however, is contraindicated.

Patients with clinical signs of chest injury who do not have fractures on X-ray should be treated in exactly the same way as those with radiographic signs.

Flail segment

This is best detected clinically but is often overlooked. A large area of crepitus is usually apparent. Respiratory movements are observed from the bottom of the trolley, looking for an area of the chest wall that moves out in expiration. Apparently minor degrees of this 'paradoxical respiration' cause significant hypoxaemia, as there is usually a large underlying pulmonary contusion.

Xr

Radiographs may initially look normal, as rib fractures and costochondral junction separation may not be visible; later, a pulmonary contusion becomes apparent. An erect chest film is helpful before intubation to exclude other major intrathoracic injuries.

Tx

- Give high-concentration oxygen by mask.
- Monitor SaO_2, BP and ECG.
- Consider early analgesia.
- Consider local direct pressure to stop gross flailing.
- Request an urgent anaesthetic opinion; intubation and ventilation is usually required.
- Measure the blood gases.

Tracheobronchial tree injuries

Larynx

There is localised pain, hoarseness, subcutaneous emphysema and local crepitus. An urgent ENT opinion is indicated and a surgical airway may be required – *see page 22*.

Trachea

The signs may be subtle and overlooked. If suspected, obtain anaesthetic and surgical advice. Plain radiographs may be followed by CT scan and bronchoscopy.

Bronchus

This is rare, difficult to detect and often fatal. A large air leak after thoracotomy is suspicious. Bronchoscopy is diagnostic. Ventilation of patients with tracheobronchial injuries may be difficult and indeed hazardous.

Fracture of the sternum

Sternal fractures are not usually associated with instability of the rib cage and may be overlooked in patients having multiple injuries. Local examination reveals tenderness and sometimes swelling. Respiratory movements may not be affected. Consider associated injury to the heart and great vessels. The ECG should be checked. There may also be associated crush injuries to the upper thoracic spine.

XR

Chest radiographs do not show sternal injuries clearly. Specific lateral views are required.

Tx

This consists of observation, exclusion of associated injuries and symptomatic pain relief. Reduction or internal fixation are not indicated, although fractures with a large amount of depression of the inner table should be discussed with a cardiothoracic surgeon.

Traumatic asphyxia syndrome

Diffuse crushing of the chest (e.g. by a trench collapse) will cause transient venous engorgement and petechial haemorrhages over the upper chest and face. There may also be subconjunctival haemorrhages. Maximal barotrauma occurs in the presence of airway obstruction.

The prognosis is good if the patient is rescued promptly. If crushing is not quickly relieved, hypoxia is severe with lung contusion and alveolar collapse. Some patients may initially appear deceptively well. Pulmonary oedema gradually develops and gas exchange is impaired – a form of adult respiratory distress syndrome.

Tx

Oxygen is given in high concentration and the patient admitted for intensive care. Steroids are of no benefit. If there is associated bronchospasm in the early stages nebulised salbutamol will be useful.

Injury to the heart and great vessels

Damage may be inflicted by a gunshot, stabbing or blunt decelerating forces. Contrary to popular belief, these injuries may not be instantly fatal and may remain undetected in the patient who is slowly dying from 'multiple injuries'. The paucity of specific signs may frustrate early and precise diagnosis.

Injury to the heart

Stab wounds anywhere between the mid-clavicular lines, from the lower one-third of the neck to the epigastrium, have the potential to involve mediastinal structures. Beware of small entry wounds, especially in the back.

Laceration of the thick left ventricular wall may not be as catastrophic as damage to less-muscular structures. Pump failure may occur because of valve damage, hypovolaemia or tamponade.

Haemopericardium may produce a life-threatening cardiac tamponade at any time, with high venous pressure, muffled heart sounds and falling BP (Beck's triad). There may be distended neck veins. Classically, the systolic BP is lower during inspiration (pulsus paradoxus). Tamponade may also cause a paradoxical rise in venous pressure during inspiration (Kussmaul's sign). Profound shock and IPPV may invalidate these signs.

Blunt injuries are more common. Most minor contusions probably resolve without detection. At the other extreme, fatal dysrhythmias may not be associated with structural damage at autopsy. A few patients, in between, present with symptoms and signs typical of myocardial ischaemia, including ECG changes.

Direct damage to coronary arteries is rare but septal rupture, damage to papillary muscle and chordae tendineae and tears of the atria or right ventricle do occur. Rupture of the sturdy left ventricle is rare.

It is useful to distinguish between cardiac contusion and concussion. The latter is defined as the occurrence of a dysrhythmia without ECG or biochemical evidence of muscle necrosis. Most of these dysrhythmias are transient, but sudden death has been reported after relatively minor blows to the sternum.

Tx

- Give high-concentration oxygen.
- Obtain IV access.
- Consider aspiration of the pericardium (*see Box 6.3 and Figure 6.3*).
- In dire cases of penetrating injury consider emergency thoracotomy (see later).
- Seek cardiothoracic advice.

Box 6.3 Needle Aspiration of the Pericardium (Pericardiocentesis)

The subxiphisternal approach is recommended (*see Figure 6.3*) although parasternal and apical approaches have also been described. Ideally, the procedure should be performed under ultrasonic (e.g. echocardiographic) guidance.

- Consider the need for sedation or general anaesthesia.
- Position the patient with a 30° head up tilt.
- Monitor the patient's SaO_2 and ECG.
- Clean and anaesthetise the subxiphoid area with 2% lidocaine, if time allows.
- Make a 5 mm long incision through the skin, just below a point midway between the tip of the xiphoid process and the left costal margin (*see Figure 6.3*).
- Attach a 20 mL syringe to a three-way tap and a long 16 G over-the-needle catheter (or use a central venous Seldinger-type set).
- Enter the skin through the small incision described above (*see Figure 6.3*), just below and to the left of the xiphochondral junction, at a 30–45° angle to the skin.
- Carefully advance the needle, aiming for the tip of the left scapula. Contact with the pericardium will occur at about 6–8 cm. Watch the ECG – ventricular ectopics suggest myocardial irritation while QRS or ST changes may indicate actual entry into the ventricular muscle. If these ECG changes are seen, the needle should be withdrawn and repositioned.
- Once fluid is reached (i.e. the needle has entered the pericardial sac), remove the needle and aspirate blood or straw-coloured fluid down the cannula. Removal of as little as 15 mL of blood may result in a dramatic clinical improvement. Large amounts of blood suggest that the ventricle has been entered.
- After aspiration remove the syringe, leaving the cannula *in situ* with a closed three-way tap attached.
- Secure the cannula to the skin. If the symptoms recur, aspiration can then be repeated.
- Obtain an ECG and chest X-ray and arrange definitive care.

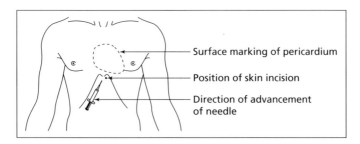

Surface marking of pericardium

Position of skin incision

Direction of advancement of needle

Figure 6.3 The site of entry for percutaneous pericardiocentesis.

In less urgent cases the problem is always the initial paucity of physical signs. Admit the patient to a high-dependency area and monitor carefully.

Emergency thoracotomy may be life-saving after stab wounds, but is rarely helpful after gunshot wounds, and never after blunt trauma. The criteria for this operation are defined in *Box 6.4* and the technique is described in *Box 6.5*; some possible intrathoracic procedures are listed in *Box 6.6*.

Box 6.4 Criteria for Thoracotomy in the Emergency Department

- History of penetrating trauma
- Signs of life in the field
- Short transport time to hospital (up to 15 min)
- Agonal vital signs or EMD (for less than 5 min)
- Cardiopulmonary resuscitation in progress if pulseless (for less than 5 min)

Patients with asystole or VF will not benefit from thoracotomy

---

Box 6.5 Technique of Thoracotomy in the Emergency Department

1 Intubate and ventilate the patient.
2 Start the incision in the fourth left intercostal space, 2 cm to the left of the sternum (to avoid the internal mammary artery, runs within 2 cm of the sternal border).
3 Extend the incision along the upper border of the rib as far as the anterior axillary or even the mid axillary line.
4 Incise the pleura and sweep the area with a gloved finger.
5 Insert a rib spreader and crank it open to allow visualisation of the thoracic cavity.
6 Open the pericardium transversely parallel to and above the phrenic nerve, without damaging surface vessels on the heart.

Injuries to the great vessels

Immediate survival depends on the formation of an acute false aneurysm. Stab wounds may inflict injury at any site, but the more common deceleration injury usually produces a lesion at the level of

---

Box 6.6 Procedures after Emergency Thoracotomy

- Pericardotomy to relieve tamponade
- Open cardiac massage
- Internal defibrillation (with up to 10 J energy)
- Cardiac haemostasis (An 18 FG Foley catheter may be inserted through a wound in the heart and the balloon inflated inside. Gentle traction on the distal catheter then achieves temporary haemostasis. If the catheter is connected to an IV infusion, fluids and drugs can be given by the intracardiac route.)
- Clamping of major lacerations of the lung
- Cross-clamping of the descending aorta to optimise cerebral circulation and to reduce major abdominal blood loss

---

the aortic isthmus. The intima and media rupture, but the adventitia and adjacent mediastinal structures may provide a sufficiently strong sheath to contain the arterial pressure for a few hours, or indeed many years.

The expanding haematoma may occlude the origin of one or more of the vessels arising from the aortic arch. Blood pressure and pulse may differ in the two arms. Pain radiating to the back is more common than precordial pain.

These injuries can be overlooked, even at thoracotomy. The history is important. Most are associated with injuries elsewhere after high-speed road traffic accidents or falls.

XR

A plain Chest X-ray may show haemorrhage into the mediastinum and other indirect signs of blood vessel injury:

- widened mediastinum (mediastinum/chest width > 25%) (may be obscured by lung injury and not present in 10% of cases);
- trachea (or nasogastric tube) displaced to the right;
- left mainstem bronchus depressed;
- aortic knuckle absent;
- left apical pleural cap (The left paraspinal line is displaced laterally and extends up and over the apex of the left lung.);
- broad right paratracheal stripe;

- separation of calcium deposits in the aortic wall;
- other signs of severe chest trauma (rib fractures, pulmonary contusion, haemopneumothorax, ruptured diaphragm).

On an AP (portable) film the mediastinum always appears to be widened. Other benign causes of a widened mediastinum are:

- supine as opposed to upright film;
- rotated positioning of the patient;
- X-ray beam directed cranially (lordotic view);
- short distance between the film and the X-ray source;
- poor inspiratory effort.

High resolution CT scan provides much more information, especially with CT angiograms. Transoesophageal ultrasonography and arch aortography may also be useful in some circumstances.

Tx

The role of the ED is to:
- have a high index of suspicion;
- begin fluid replacement (but beware of overload);
- refer urgently for specialist care.

Other injuries in the chest

For diaphragmatic injuries see page 86.

Oesophageal injury

This is usually caused by penetrating trauma. Blunt rupture may follow vomiting or a direct blow to the epigastrium; it may also complicate endoscopy. Consider oesophageal injury if there is:
- gas in the mediastinum on X-ray;
- inexplicable shock after trunk injury;
- left pneumothorax without rib fracture;
- gastric contents in a chest drain.

Mediastinitis develops insidiously and is usually fatal.

XR

There is mediastinal gas on the chest X-ray.

Tx

Early diagnosis, antibiotics and surgery are essential.

Abdominal injury

Immediate action

- Repeat ABCs as described in *Chapter 1*.
- Cover eviscerated gut with warm saline packs – do not try to push it back. Manipulating mesentery potentiates shock.
- Obtain IV access and commence an IV infusion.

> Fluid loss into the abdomen is usually underestimated.

- Examine the abdomen, noting areas of tenderness, guarding and lacerations; clothing imprints; and grazes. Listen for bowel sounds.
- Consider early analgesia.

> Intravenous analgesia is unlikely to mask significant signs in the abdomen. On the contrary, it usually makes the following procedures much easier to perform.

- Log-roll the patient and examine the back and perineum.
- Consider performing a rectal examination, noting injuries, sphincter tone, the presence of blood, the wall and contents and prostate.
- Obtain details of the incident, the past medical history, medication and time of last food and drink.
- Insert a urinary catheter if there is no urethral injury (*see page 88*).
- Consider passing a large-bore nasogastric tube if there is no basal skull fracture (*see page 44*).

> Closed abdominal injuries may be easily overlooked especially when they are less painful than injuries elsewhere and not immediately associated with signs of hypovolaemic shock.

- Give antibiotics if gut perforation is suspected.
- Obtain surgical advice early on. There are three possible courses of action:
1 immediate operation for obvious injury;
2 admission and observation of a stable patient; or
3 further assessment of a patient with equivocal signs or an impaired level of consciousness.

Techniques for assessment of intra-abdominal damage

Diagnostic peritoneal lavage

Diagnostic peritoneal lavage (DPL) is decreasingly used where sophisticated imaging is available. However, in its absence the technique may be useful and so it is described in *Box 6.7*. DPL is carried out in the resuscitation area of the ED but normally only after discussion with the admitting general surgeons. Iatrogenic damage to intraperitoneal structures and false positive taps are unusual (2% of cases) and may be reduced by

using the mini-laparotomy technique described. False negatives may also occur (again in 2% of cases) especially with diaphragmatic and pelvic injuries.

The other disadvantages of DPL are as follows:
1 It may change the clinical signs in the abdomen.
2 It introduces air into the peritoneum and thus prevents a subsequent CT scan.
3 It is unsuitable for young children.
4 It does not rule out hollow visceral perforation (bladder and bowel), diaphragmatic tears or retroperitoneal injuries (i.e. to pancreas or duodenum).
5 It is contraindicated in patients with bleeding diatheses, morbid obesity and advanced pregnancy.

Box 6.7 Peritoneal Lavage

- Catheterise the bladder to decompress it.
- Insert a nasogastric tube if the stomach is distended.
- Clean and drape the abdomen.
- Inject local anaesthetic in the midline, one-third of the distance from the umbilicus to the symphysis pubis. The use of lidocaine with adrenaline helps to limit bleeding from the wound into the abdomen.
- Make a small longitudinal skin incision.
- Identify and open the peritoneum under direct vision.
- Introduce a dialysis catheter, directing it towards the pelvis.
- Connect the catheter to a syringe and attempt to aspirate blood.

If gross blood is not obtained
- Flush in 500 mL (10 mL per kg) of warm isotonic saline. Gentle agitation of the abdomen with turning of the patient ensures distribution of the fluid throughout the peritoneal cavity.
- Leave the fluid in the peritoneum for 5–10 min, then lower the infusion bag to the floor to allow drainage.
- Send a sample of the lavage fluid to the laboratory.

A positive result is shown by
- Immediate aspiration of heavily blood-stained, non-clotting fluid.
- Lavage fluid containing more than 100,000 erythrocytes per mm^3.
- Lavage fluid containing more than 500 leucocytes per mm^3.
- Lavage fluid leaking from other sites (e.g. bladder catheter or chest drain).
- Lavage fluid containing bile, food, faecal matter or bacteria.

CT scanning or ultrasound examination of the abdomen are more appropriate for children than peritoneal lavage. There are equally good reasons for their superiority in adults.

Computed tomography

Computed tomography is increasingly available but the inherent delay may be dangerous. It should only be performed in stable patients with continuous monitoring. It is good for retroperitoneal examination but may miss gastrointestinal injury.

Ultrasonography

This is widely used in the ED. In experienced hands, it is good for solid organ assessment and detection of free fluid.

Stab wounds to the abdomen

Small lacerations should be assumed to be deep until proved otherwise. Injury to the intestine and mesentery may not be accompanied by the rapid clinical deterioration usually associated with stab wounds to the liver, spleen and major vessels.

X_R

An erect chest X-ray is the most important plain radiograph. Free gas is a strong, but not absolute, indication for laparotomy. Consider requesting an ultrasound scan (*see before*).

Tx

Obtain surgical advice. Laparotomy has an associated morbidity. This can be reduced if a selective approach is used.

Patients with immediate evidence of an intra-abdominal catastrophe must be taken straight to theatre. They will need resuscitation with oxygen and IV fluids in the ED and 4–8 units of blood should be cross-matched.

The remaining patients (the majority) can be treated by admission and careful observation. This must include serial examination of the abdomen (initially every 1–2 h) and frequent recordings of pulse and BP.

Early administration of antibiotics (e.g. metronidazole and cefotaxime) reduces the risk of intraperitoneal infection and septic shock. Patients with perineal injuries may develop gas gangrene and so should also receive benzylpenicillin.

The wound should be covered with an antiseptic dressing. Anti-tetanus prophylaxis is required. Stab wounds are best left unsutured when first seen, to allow drainage of any deep bleeding or infection.

Blunt abdominal trauma

Blunt abdominal injury should be considered if any of the following apply:
- There are localising symptoms or signs.
- There are marks on the abdominal wall.
- The mechanism of injury suggests trauma to the abdomen.
- There are injuries to areas both above and below the abdomen.
- There is unexplained hypovolaemia.
- The patient is abnormally pale following an injury.
- The patient has a reduced conscious level and is therefore difficult to assess.

In the conscious patient, the site and character of abdominal pain will help to determine the need for laparotomy. It may be possible to determine the direction and severity of the injuring agent from details of the incident, an examination of clothing and distribution of skin injuries and clothing imprints.

Most bleeding is caused by damage to the liver or the spleen. As in the case of stab wounds, damage in the absence of bleeding is much slower to present and more difficult to diagnose.

XR

An erect chest X-ray is likely to be difficult to obtain. *For techniques of assessment of intra-abdominal damage see page 85.*

Tx

Resuscitation should be started and blood should be cross-matched. Patients need close observation and laparotomy at the first indication of significant problems.

Abdominal pain may be caused by acute gastric dilatation or paralytic ileus associated with an injury elsewhere. Gastric dilatation is a well-recognised complication of head injury, particularly in children. Insertion of a nasogastric tube may resolve distension and pain. If the tube is wide-bore it will also remove partially digested food and thus reduce the risk of aspiration into the lungs.

Splenic injuries are common. They may occur with very little in the way of external signs. There is an increasing trend, especially in children, to preserve the spleen because of the risk of sudden, overwhelming sepsis that can occur at any time of life after splenectomy. Operation may be avoided or the spleen repaired. Very careful monitoring with repeat ultrasound or CT scan is essential.

Rupture of the diaphragm

This injury is often overlooked. It is commoner on the left side. Blunt injury usually causes a large defect in the diaphragm whereas stab wounds may cause a small defect with delayed presentation.

Xʀ

Rupture of the diaphragm may be missed on chest X-ray. If suspected, the insertion of a nasogastric tube will aid X-ray interpretation.

Tx

The stomach should be decompressed with a nasogastric tube and the patient kept sitting up if possible. Surgical repair will be necessary.

Retroperitoneal injuries

These are associated with back pain, significant blood loss, and paralytic ileus. Consider the involvement of:
• the paravertebral muscles with avulsion of lumbar transverse processes (*see page 61*);
• the kidneys and ureters; and
• the pancreas and duodenum.

Xʀ

A plain film may show associated bony damage as above. Confirmation of retroperitoneal injury may need CT scan. Investigate renal injury as below.

Tx

Resuscitation should be followed by surgical referral. Blood should be cross-matched. A raised serum amylase may point to pancreatic injury.

Renal injury

Injuries to the loins are common after falls and assaults. Many soft-tissue injuries in this area cause severe pain. The urine should always be tested for blood to identify renal involvement.

Xʀ

In a stable patient, with only microscopic haematuria, ultrasound scan can be performed during the next 24 h. CT scan (with contrast) or IVP is indicated for macroscopic haematuria and prior to exploratory laparotomy in an unstable patient.

Tx

All patients with suspected renal injury should be admitted for observation and analgesia.

Abdominal trauma in pregnancy

For general principles concerning the management of major trauma in pregnant women see page 31.
Signs of intra-abdominal bleeding tend to be reduced or modified in pregnancy. Gastric emptying is delayed.

Xʀ

Consider early ultrasound scan of the abdomen, uterus and fetus.

Tx

The treatment of an injured pregnant patient follows the usual ABCs, but in addition there should be the following:
• Maintenance of the patient in the left lateral position to avoid IVC compression.
• Extra vigilance in treating early hypovolaemia. Signs of shock are delayed because of maternal hyperaemia.
• Confirmation of the normal fetal heart beat (usually for maternal reassurance, as the fetus is well protected inside the amniotic sac). A Doppler ultrasound probe is better for this purpose than a fetal stethoscope. Consider early monitoring of the fetal heart rate by fetocardiotocograph (FCTG) in seriously injured patients – *see also page 32.*
• Prophylaxis against aspiration pneumonia with IV ranitidine – *see page 32.*
• Administration of anti-RhD immunoglobulin to rhesus-D-negative women.

Pelvic injury

Bony injury to the pelvis

There are two types of pelvic fracture:

1 After violent injury, the fracture is:
- unstable;
- crushed or displaced at more than one point;
- associated with major blood loss and visceral injury.

2 After a fall in an osteoporotic patient, the injury is:
- stable;
- anterior and minimally displaced;
- associated with pre-existing general medical problems.

Tenderness is usually apparent. Testing stability by attempting to move the iliac wings is unreliable. Straight-leg raising is usually reduced or impossible.

XR

An anteroposterior radiograph is essential initially. Oblique views and CT scan are useful later. A cone view of the pubic rami may sometimes be helpful.

Tx

Initial management of major pelvic fractures includes:
- fluid resuscitation;
- assessment of visceral injury;
- pain control;
- external fixation.

External fixation is now considered an emergency intervention in the management of an unstable pelvic fracture. Modern fixators are quick to apply and are suitable for use in the ED to control haemorrhage.

Single fractures of the pubic rami are rarely associated with visceral injury or significant blood loss. They are, however, painful and restrict the mobility of the elderly patients in whom they most commonly occur. Hospital admission is usually required for a few days prior to gentle mobilisation. No specific treatment is necessary in the ED. Look for the cause of the fall. Also consider fracture of the neck of the femur (*see page 93*). This presents itself in a similar way in the same group of patients.

Injury to the pelvic viscera

Injury within the pelvis may cause profound blood loss.

Tx

Transfuse and refer. External fixation may be helpful with pelvic instability (*see before*).

Urogenital injuries

Perineal injury is easily missed. Following trauma there may be:
- a painful desire to micturate;
- local swelling or bruising;
- blood at the external meatus;
- cranial migration of the prostate (the 'missing prostate' sign). This is associated with rupture of the membranous urethra and is diagnosed by rectal examination in the male.
- bogginess of the anterior vaginal wall on pelvic examination in the female.

Extravasation of urine into the perineal tissues is unusual immediately after injury, more commonly developing after 1 or 2 h. It suggests injury to the extraperitoneal part of the bladder or urethra. Intraperitoneal rupture of the bladder produces the earlier abdominal signs of pain and shock.

XR

Retrograde urethrography is easy to perform and must precede catheter placement. Alternatively, a suprapubic catheter may be inserted directly into the bladder.

Tx

The majority of urethral injuries are incomplete transections. The maintenance of urothelial continuity will reduce the severity of late stricture formation. It is therefore important that these injuries are diagnosed early and treated gently by an experienced surgeon.

Other perineal injuries

Lacerations of the perineal body or the anal or vaginal margins should be assumed to penetrate deeply until proven otherwise. This will entail careful and skilled examination under good operating conditions. If there is any suggestion of intraperitoneal extension, laparotomy will be required – possibly with faecal diversion. Early referral is essential. Antibiotics should be commenced in the ED.

Chapter 7

The lower limb

General approach to limb problems

This section should be read before turning to the relevant anatomical site.

For more details on the upper limb see page 117.

For more details on the hand see page 136.

For more details on the management of small wounds see page 386.

For more details on crush injuries and myoglobinuria see page 255.

> Four four-letter words describe a structured approach to examination of the limbs: LOOK, FEEL, MOVE, X-RAY.

Immediate assessment and management

- Start with the ABCs as discussed in *Chapter 1*.
- Apply direct pressure to stop any bleeding.
- Expose the affected part. Cut off clothes as necessary.
- Take a brief but comprehensive history.
- Confirm that the presenting problem is confined to the limb.

> Do not consider the limb in isolation as:
> - injuries around the shoulder and thigh may cause hypovolaemia;
> - painful limb injuries may be associated with life-threatening but less painful trunk trauma;
> - limb infection may have systemic effects; and
> - limb pain may be symptomatic of trunk pathology (e.g. cardiac pain, sciatica and herpes zoster infection).

- Confirm the presence of distal pulses and the integrity of the nerve supply.
- Splint fractures.
- Give analgesia early on. This may be systemic or local.
- Finally undertake a detailed local examination including a comparison with the opposite limb.

If there is a clear history of trauma, it is useful to reconstruct the incident to appreciate the forces applied and to consider the biomechanics of the injury:

- Healthy young bones will undergo considerable elastic deformation (e.g. the femoral shaft will bend over 10° before breaking). At breaking point, stored energy is released and the limb suddenly deforms further, inflicting secondary soft-tissue injury. Often, this is more important than the underlying fracture.
- Twisting tends to produce spiral fractures.
- Direct blows cause transverse fractures, which may be compound.
- Sheering forces raise contused skin flaps.
- Forces applied to the heel of the falling body and causing a fracture of the os calcis will be transmitted cranially and may produce a fracture of the lumbar spine or the base of the skull.
- An evident knee injury, sustained by a front-seat car passenger, may draw attention away from an occult hip dislocation.

Wounds

Wounds should not be explored at this stage. Sterile dressings or iodine soaks are the only necessary treatment. An instant photograph of the injury will prevent the need for frequent re-examination by attending doctors. Foreign bodies must be left alone, even if they are grossly protruding, until resuscitation has begun and the environment and staff are prepared for a careful, controlled assessment. Patients with grossly contaminated wounds and compound fractures should receive IV antibiotics (e.g. flucloxacillin) and antitetanus prophylaxis as soon as possible.

Pain

Splintage and reassurance are very important. Pain may be controlled by nitrous oxide while a splint is applied. Intravenous injection of opiates should be given as soon as contraindications have been excluded. In some situations a local anaesthetic block may be preferable.

Radiographs

Radiographs complement but do not replace a full clinical examination. Good radiographs demand good viewing facilities. The doctor should have viewing box, spotlight, magnifying glass and charts showing times of appearance and fusion of primary and secondary ossification centres.

> Do not attempt to interpret a colleague's radiographs without first examining the patient.

Vascular problems related to injury

For specific vascular problems see page 113.

> All urgent limb problems are related to blood supply.

Occlusion

Fractures around the elbow and the knee are commonly associated with vascular occlusion. Do not assume that distal ischaemia has been caused by transient vascular spasm. Urgent specialist referral is necessary. Limb viability is threatened if a major occlusion persists for 4 h or more.

> Healthy young limbs are more at risk from vascular occlusion of main vessels than are old ischaemic limbs because the latter have had time to develop a collateral circulation.

Bleeding

Elevation is an effective first-aid measure for major venous haemorrhage but is often impossible to achieve because of associated bony injury. Applying artery clips to spurting vessels in the ED will usually inflict further injury, especially as most major limb vessels run alongside peripheral nerves. Instead, local pressure should be applied. Bleeding into damaged muscle is a much more common problem.

Compartment syndrome

The closed fascial compartments of the limbs prevent contused muscles and haematomas from expanding indefinitely. Interstitial pressure rises causing pain and ischaemia – *see page 116.*

Plaster casts

Application of a cast is the most common way of immobilising an injured area of a limb, be it an injury to the bone or to the soft-tissue. It must be remembered, however, that acute injuries may swell up considerably in the first 48 h and severe ischaemia may then develop, caused by restriction of expansion by either the cast or a fascial compartment.

Splitting a cast (a single, longitudinal split is the best) or prescribing an incomplete slab-type plaster does not necessarily protect the limb from the underlying ischaemia. All ED plasters must be well padded, especially over bony protuberances, and the patient must have:
- instructions to elevate the limb and crutches or a sling if needed;
- advice on the care of the cast and a written list on the signs of ischaemia (plaster instructions);
- early review.

It is important that all staff who deal with patients in casts are aware of the need to look out for the signs of compartment syndrome (*see page 116*) as well as the more widely appreciated changes to the warmth, colour and capillary refill of the digits.

Physiotherapy

The help of the physiotherapist can be invaluable in treating a wide range of soft-tissue injuries and other conditions. Particular benefits are seen with early physiotherapy and include:
• reduction in pain, bruising and swelling;
• maintenance of muscle fibre length and range of movements; and
• early mobilisation and restoration of function.
The physiotherapist also offers:
• re-examination of the injury and the level of function;
• assessment for and training with walking aids;
• restoration of the patient's confidence;
• skilled follow-up.

Crutches

Crutches are required for emergency patients with a large variety of differing problems. They may be designed to enable a limb to be:
• non-weight-bearing (axillary crutches);
• partial weight-bearing (elbow crutches).
All patients given crutches must be instructed about their safe usage and should also be observed in action.

Local injection of steroids

The injection of a long-acting steroid-type drug into a joint, a tendon sheath, a bursa or other suitable area can bring long-lasting relief to a large number of inflammatory soft-tissue conditions. The steroid is often premixed with local anaesthetic to:
• minimise the discomfort of the injection;
• give some immediate relief of the underlying condition;
• act as a marker of successful localisation of an injection.

> The patient must be warned that symptoms may increase over the first 24 h prior to gradual resolution.

Complications of depot steroid injection include:
• local damage;
• introduction of infection;
• rupture of a tendon;
• fat necrosis and atrophy and disfigurement of overlying skin.
As such, it is a technique that requires knowledge of:
• the local anatomy;
• the best approaches to the target area;
• the correct drug dosage for each site (*see Box 7.1*).
Local injections of steroid should not be given by the inexperienced or in circumstances where there are no facilities for review of the patient.

Sports injuries

Soft tissue and bony injuries, secondary to trauma sustained during sport are common presentations. Many such injuries can also occur during non-sporting activities. The specific needs of the sportsman are:
1 a quick return to normal training and activity;
2 maintenance of muscle fibre length; and
3 protection from re-injury when the activity is resumed.

Box 7.1 Dose of Methylprednisolone for Local Injection

Large joint (knee, ankle, shoulder)	20–80 mg	(0.5–2 mL)
Medium joint (elbow, wrist)	10–40 mg	(0.25–1 mL)
Small joint (MCPJ, IPJ, ACJ)	4–10 mg	(0.1–0.25 mL)
Bursa	4–30 mg	(0.1–0.75 mL)
Periarticular (for epicondylitis)	4–30 mg	(0.1–0.75 mL)
Tendon sheath (never into a tendon)	4–30 mg	(0.1–0.75 mL)

Accurate diagnosis is essential. A good general recipe for treating sports injuries is:
- 3 days' complete rest (crutches/sling if required);
- appropriate analgesia; and
- early physiotherapy.

Ice, compression and elevation are useful in the early stages to reduce discomfort and swelling. There should be a return to about 50% training levels as soon as possible and then a gradual build-up to full activity.

See also the appropriate anatomical sections of this chapter and Chapters 8 and 9.

The hip

> The hip joint capsule is innervated from the L2/3/4 level. These dermatomes extend to the knee, hence the common complaint of hip pathology apparently arising in the knee. The hip must be examined whenever a patient complains of a knee problem.

Dislocation of the hip

This is caused by axial violence such as a force applied to the knee. The dislocation is usually posterior with a fracture of the acetabular rim. Sometimes the sciatic nerve is injured – most frequently that part destined to be the common peroneal nerve. Pain is usually severe and the hip is held partially flexed and adducted. Central dislocation into the pelvis is associated with major (concealed) blood loss. Dislocation of an arthroplasty of the hip is often seen after relatively minor trauma.

XR

When resuscitation has been established and analgesia given, X-rays are obtained. Later CT scan will aid identification of complex acetabular rim fractures.

Tx

Resuscitate and provide analgesia; support the limb but do not attempt reduction in the ED. The distal neurovascular function must be assessed and the secondary survey completed, looking for other injuries. The patient needs an urgent referral to the orthopaedic department.

Both types of traumatic dislocation can be difficult to reduce by closed manipulation. Posterior dislocation may be treated more appropriately by open reduction and internal fixation of the bone fragments.

Fracture of the neck of the femur

There are three circumstances in which this may occur:
1 at any age – associated with major violence and multiple injuries;
2 in the elderly – after a simple fall;
3 spontaneously – as a result of osteoporosis or bony secondary deposits.

> Fractures of the hips account for 90% of the enormous cost of osteoporosis to the NHS. The human cost is equally high – of the 68 000 patients with hip fractures in the United Kingdom each year, nearly a third die within 12 months of the injury.

A detailed history must be taken and other injuries excluded. Consider the reason for an unexplained fall (medication, domestic disorganisation) and assess general health. The following notes assume systemic examination has been undertaken and relate to the care of the typical elderly patient with an isolated injury.

The patient (usually female) presents as unable to weight-bear after a relatively minor fall. Some patients may be able to walk, albeit with a painful limp. There is pain in the hip, thigh or knee but usually no visible swelling, bruising or deformity. The affected leg may be shortened and externally rotated but this classical appearance is dependent on the grade of the fracture. A more valuable sign is pain on gentle passive rotation of the extended leg. If the fracture has impacted, other movements may be good with minimal pain including even straight leg raising. Tenderness is most marked posteriorly. Significant blood loss is unusual and associated vascular and tendon damage is rare.

Box 7.2 How to Examine the Hip Joint

• Assess gait and continue inspection of mobility and pain as clothes are removed and the patient gets onto the couch.
• Look for shortening or rotation of the leg. True shortening is caused by collapse or angulation of bone (distance between anterior superior iliac spine and medial joint line of knee – both legs in the same position). Apparent shortening is the difference between the two sides when the patient is lying supine (distance from umbilicus to medial malleoli). It is usually caused by pelvic tilt or fixed deformity at the hip joint.
• Look at the groin, perineum, buttock and lateral bony prominences and feel for tenderness in these areas. A sinus or old scar may point to established disease but there are usually no surface signs of acute inflammation or of joint effusion.
• Assess flexion, abduction, adduction and rotation in each leg (active before passive). Keep one hand under the lumbar spine when testing flexion and one hand on the opposite iliac crest when testing abduction and adduction. Rotation is most accurately measured with the knee at right angles (lower leg over the end of the couch or patient prone). With the patient lying on his or her side attempt to extend the hip joint backwards; 5–10° is often possible.
• Examine the relationship between hip movement and lumbar spine and pelvic movement. Fixed flexion of the hip can be camouflaged by excessive lumbar lordosis. Fixed adduction is usually compensated for by pelvic tilt. The easiest way to abolish the lordosis is to fully flex the leg that is not being measured. Any passive movement off the bed of the leg under assessment is fixed flexion. Similarly, setting the pelvis square may cause fixed adduction of one leg.
• Finally, ask the patient to stand on one leg. The pelvis should raise on the non-weight-bearing side. Failure to do this is a positive Trendelenburg's sign and indicates disease in the weight-bearing hip or its associated abductor muscles.

For a method of examining the hip joint see Box 7.2.

Xʀ

Radiological examination must include an anteroposterior view of the hips and pelvis and a lateral radiograph of the affected hip. In the anteroposterior view, look for a break in the normal apparent continuity of trabeculae across the joint.

Osteoarthrosis is associated with intertrochanteric rather than subcapital fractures, so it is very unlikely that an undisplaced subcapital fracture will be hidden in the disorganised radiological pattern around an arthritic joint.

The lateral view may be difficult to obtain and interpret but is nevertheless the best film on which to see a minimally displaced fracture.

Tx

A box splint may be used to control leg movements and analgesia should be given. Long waits on hard trolleys must be avoided as these patients acquire pressure sores very quickly. (*For risk factors for pressure sores see page 229.*) Internal fixation or hemiarthroplasty is usually performed within 24 h.

Fracture of the pubic rami

The anterior pelvis should be carefully examined in all cases. Fracture of the pubic rami occurs in the same group of patients as those with fracture of the hip and gives a very similar clinical picture. The pain may be felt in the buttock or groin but otherwise symptoms are localised to one leg and may divert attention away from the pelvis. Patients with this injury need initial bed rest and analgesia and then gradual mobilisation – *see also page 88.*

The elderly patient with failure to weight-bear after a fall

All such patients must be admitted for reassessment and mobilisation. A considerable number prove to have a fracture that was not evident on the initial X-ray. Other patients with soft-tissue injuries require prolonged rehabilitation before they are ready for discharge. Local policy dictates whether care for these patients is provided by the geriatric or the orthopaedic department.

Irritable hip

This is a common condition in children. The child, usually under the age of 5 years, presents with a limp that is unrelated to trauma. Occasionally, the sore hip gives way and creates the illusion of a traumatic injury. Pain in the hip region may not be immediately evident and passive movements are usually normal. Sometimes mild protective spasm may limit abduction. There may be a history of a prodromal upper respiratory infection.

The condition is thought to be caused by a transient synovitis, possibly of viral origin, and is invariably unilateral. It is important to exclude a septic arthritis.

For the management of a young child with a limp see Box 7.3.

Xᴿ

Radiographs of the affected limb from hip to ankle are usually required. The foot may need to be included if there is any tenderness in this area. The main differential diagnosis is a toddler's fracture or other tibial injury – *see page 105*.

Ultrasound examination can demonstrate an effusion in the hip joint but cannot differentiate between synovial fluid, blood and pus. A difference of more than 3 mm of effusion between the

---

Box 7.3 The Management of a Young Child who is Limping or Not Weight-Bearing

- Ask about duration and severity of limp.
- Ask about a history of trauma, viral infection or previous episodes.
- Take the temperature.
- Observe the gait.
- Ask the child to stand on alternate legs.
- Examine the whole limb, feeling carefully especially for tibial tenderness and hip spasm in abduction.
- Consider the need to obtain radiographs of the whole limb.
- If there are no specific clinical or radiological findings, reassure the parents and recommend rest and paracetamol elixir for the child. Arrange for review within 72 h.

---

normal and the affected hip is considered to be pathological. A positive ultrasound scan obviates the need for X-rays.

Tx

If there is an unexplained pyrexia and/or hip muscle spasm refer the child to the orthopaedic department for admission. A child who is apyrexial with no hip spasm and no evidence of bony injury can be discharged with analgesia and instructions to rest. Such a child must be reviewed in the clinic within 72 h.

The age of a limping child will help with diagnosis:
- *Irritable hip* – usually seen in children who are under 5 years.
- *Perthes' disease* – most common in children aged 5–10 years.
- *Slipped femoral epiphysis* – occurs at the age of 10–15 years.

Perthes' disease

Perthes' disease is an idiopathic avascular necrosis of the proximal femoral epiphysis. It is often called an 'osteochondritis' and belongs to a group of similar diseases of epiphyseal growth (*see page 345*). In the United Kingdom, it affects 1 in 10 000 children and is four times more common in boys than in girls. In 10% of cases it is bilateral. Children aged between 3 and 15 years may be affected, although it is most common in children between 5 and 8 years of age. It presents with a painful or painless limp or sometimes with hip or knee pain after exercise. Pain may be mild and is often of several months duration. There is restriction of hip movements with muscle spasm, especially internal rotation and abduction. Flexion is usually unaffected.

Xᴿ

Radiographs may be normal in very early disease. However, they often show remarkably advanced changes in contrast to the short clinical history. The femoral neck may be widened, bone density reduced, joint space increased and the femoral head fragmented (*see Figure 7.1*). Ultrasound scan reveals an effusion and bone scanning shows reduced uptake in the affected epiphysis. Blood tests are all normal.

Tx

The child should be referred to the orthopaedic department for admission. Bed rest until the muscle spasm has resolved is now the mainstay of treatment for this condition.

Slipped proximal femoral epiphysis

The capital epiphysis may slip suddenly or gradually in a child just before puberty, causing pain and limping. The onset may be linked to minor

trauma. Hip abduction is restricted but adduction is often increased.

XR

Radiographs may be difficult to interpret and should include anteroposterior and lateral views of both hips. Posterior movement of the epiphysis is usually the first radiographic sign and is best seen on the lateral view. Slight medial displacement of the epiphysis may sometimes be the initial change – *see Figure 7.2*.

Tx

Immediate referral to the orthopaedic department is essential. Operative reduction of an acute slip

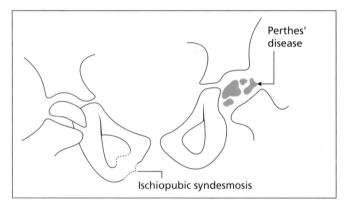

Figure 7.1 Perthes' disease, with incidental normal enlargement of the ischiopubic syndesmosis.

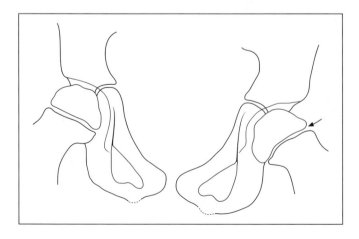

Figure 7.2 Slipped left proximal femoral epiphysis (arrowed) (anteroposterior view).

followed by prophylactic pinning is usually recommended.

Degenerative disease of the hip

The patient presents with pain and stiffness and may relate this to a recent injury. The hip joint has a restricted range of movement. Fixed flexion may be obscured by compensatory lumbar lordosis. Fixed adduction causes pelvic tilt and an apparently short leg. Pain is usually most marked at the extremes of the range and there is little muscle spasm. A general examination is always indicated to exclude systemic disease and injury.

XR

Radiographs show reduced joint space, irregular articular surface, osteophytes, sclerosis and bone cysts. Such changes, however, are common and may not be related to the patient's symptoms.

TX

In the absence of other pathology, symptomatic treatment with analgesia and a walking aid should be offered. The patient should be advised to consult his or her general practitioner. Physiotherapy may help with initial mobilisation.

Extra-articular problems around the hip

Spinal and abdominal lesions may present with hip symptoms.
• Infection of the lumbar spine may produce a psoas abscess, which points just below the inguinal ligament. This may be tuberculous or may be as a result of a variety of agents in drug addicts.
• A femoral hernia may be overlooked, especially in an obese, elderly lady.
• A high lumbar disc lesion may present with anterior thigh pain and limitation of hip extension (the femoral stretch test).
• Constriction of the lateral cutaneous nerve of the thigh as it passes through the inguinal ligament may cause persistent pain over the thigh (meralgia paraesthetica).
• A child with haemophilia may present with hip joint spasm caused by haemorrhage into the psoas muscle.

The thigh

Fracture of the femoral shaft

This is associated with extensive soft-tissue injury and internal bleeding but is not usually compound. The level of trauma required to fracture the femur should suggest the possibility of serious injuries elsewhere in the body.

XR

The diagnosis should be clinically evident without immediate resort to radiographs. X-rays are mainly used to exclude other injuries and to check the position of the bone after the application of a splint.

TX

Priorities are the following:
• Complete ABCs.
• Give effective analgesia, initially nitrous oxide mixture and then IV opiates – if not contraindicated – or a femoral nerve block (*see Box 7.4*).

Box 7.4 Femoral Nerve Block

Indications: Fractures at any level of the femur.
Contraindications: Hypersensitivity to local anaesthetics and neurovascular complications of the injury.
Method: Clean and drape the skin. Insert a short needle lateral to the femoral artery just below the inguinal ligament. Advance it perpendicularly to the skin. Feel for loss of resistance when the fascia is penetrated. Inject up to 10 mL of 0.5% bupivacaine. The patient may experience paraesthesia during the injection.
Onset: Within 15 min.
Duration: Variable, but often over 5 h.

- Apply a Thomas' or other traction splint (*see Box 7.5*).
- Check distal pulses. Vascular damage can occur with supracondylar fractures.
- Withdraw blood for baseline values and cross-match.
- Complete the secondary survey.
- Take X-rays as appropriate.
- Involve the orthopaedic team early in management.

Box 7.5 Splinting a Femoral Shaft Fracture

Traction splints and Thomas' splints are commonly available. Apply the splint before X-ray. It will give immediate pain relief and reduce blood loss.

- If a Thomas' splint is to be used, obtain the appropriate size and cover it with tubular bandage or webbing slings. If a traction splint is to be used much of the following can be omitted, but ensure you know how it works before trying to apply it.
- If skin traction is to be applied, shave both sides of the thigh and lower leg and apply tincture of benzoin.
- Apply the adhesive strapping from the skin traction kit to the leg. Adhesive strapping must not be used on elderly or fragile skin as its removal later may damage the skin. Instead, use a non-adhesive traction kit.
- Protect the malleoli by padding.
- Secure the strapping with crepe bandages.
- Ensure adequate analgesia. Intravenous analgesia can be supplemented with nitrous oxide while applying the splint.
- Grip the heel and forefoot of the injured leg and apply firm continuous traction. Muscle spasm will gradually disappear and angulation of the thigh will decrease. Transient increase in pain is usually reduced by continuous traction.
- Instruct an assistant to manoeuvre the splint over the foot and ankle.
- Maintain constant traction while the assistant pushes the splint towards pelvis.
- Protect the genitalia.
- Fasten the strapping by the ropes to the end of the splint.
- Tighten the traction by inserting a wooden spatula between the two ropes and twisting it until the required tension is achieved (Chinese windlass method).
- Check the foot pulses and toe movements.
- X-ray to check the position of the splint.

The knee

Assessment of the knee joint

The knee can be very difficult to assess acutely. A detailed history will help to distinguish between the many types of injury and symptoms, which may occur.

- Ask about the relationship between the onset of symptoms (especially pain and swelling) and the time of injury.
- Ask about and observe the ability to weight-bear.
- Look, feel and move the joint (*see Box 7.6*).
- Confirm the presence of distal pulses.
- Exclude referred pain, especially from the hip and spine.

Vascular problems are relatively common in fractures around the knee. They are of two types:
1 direct trauma to a major vessel by a bone fragment or by the interosseous ligament at the trifurcation of the popliteal artery;
2 raised interstitial pressure within a closed fascial compartment of the lower leg (*see page 116*).
Damage to the distal part of the popliteal artery is particularly serious in the young, because here it is an 'end' artery. Elderly patients may have developed a collateral circulation around the knee in response to the main vessel disease.

For a method of examining the knee joint see Box 7.6. For the indications for radiography of the knee following injury see Box 7.7.

Wounds around the knee

Even apparently trivial wounds around the knee may involve the joint capsule and synovium.

XR

Intra-articular air may be seen on the radiograph as a radiolucent area.

TX

Suspicion of joint involvement warrants orthopaedic referral, thorough assessment, (usually under general anaesthesia) and prophylactic antibiotics (flucloxacillin, started before surgery).

Box 7.6 A Method of Examining the Knee Joint

- Watch the patient climb on to the couch.
- Look for scars, sinuses, muscle wasting and joint swelling.
- Ask patient to point to the site of the pain.
- Test for the presence of an effusion or haemarthrosis (*see page 99*).
- Palpate bony landmarks for irregularities and tenderness.
- Confirm the ability of the quadriceps mechanism to extend the joint.
- Check for the ability to hyperextend the knee so that the heel lifts off the couch while the back of the knee remains in contact with it. This usually signifies that the joint is not severely injured.
- Determine the range of true extension and flexion and compare this with the normal side.
- At 90° flexion (or as near as the pain allows) rotate the tibia on the femur by twisting the foot. Pain at the joint line suggests meniscal injury. Repeat this test with the patient prone, applying compression along the tibia. This increases pain of meniscal origin and lessens the pain of a collateral ligament lesion.
- Keeping the joint at 90°, sit on the foot and attempt to pull and push the upper tibia on the femur to test the cruciate ligaments. The hamstrings must be flaccid; assess this by having the index fingers up against them while pulling forward. There is considerable variation in cruciate laxity between patients, but not between their two knees.
- Test collateral ligament integrity at 10° flexion. Stand facing the patient, put the foot in your axilla and hold the leg just below the knee in both hands. All muscles must be flaccid while you attempt to shake the knee sideways. Normally, there will be painless – if alarming – clunks at the limits of valgus and varus stressing. A 'rubbery', painful end point suggests collateral ligament injury. Complete rupture may be less painful than partial rupture.
- Move the patella sideways on the femur with the knee fully extended. If lateral pressure causes anxiety and pain, consider potential dislocation. If downward pressure is painful consider chondromalacia.

Box 7.7 Indications for Radiography of the Knee following Injury

Any of the following:
- history of fall, blunt trauma or penetrating injury;
- age under 12 years or over 55 years;
- obvious deformity;
- severe swelling of rapid onset;
- tenderness at the head of the fibula;
- isolated tenderness of the patella;
- inability to flex to 90°;
- inability to raise leg straight;
- inability to walk four weight-bearing steps unaided in the ED;
- atypical features;
- return visit with no improvement.

presentation. The patient generally has variable degrees of:
- pain;
- difficulty weight-bearing;
- swelling; and
- reduction of the range of movements. This is due to restriction by fluid, pain and sometimes by mechanical blocks.

Serious intra-articular problems are probable in the presence of any of the following:
- a large, rapidly developing effusion;
- complete inability to weight-bear; or
- demonstrable collateral or cruciate laxity.

> If the patient can lie with the joint fully extended so that the back of knee is on the couch while the heel is a few centimetres off it, and also squat down with the knee fully flexed, then serious injury is extremely unlikely.

Effusions in the knee joint

- Modest effusions can be detected by balloting the patella against the femur (patella tap).
- Large effusions will prevent bony contact, but are obvious.
- Small effusions are best detected by emptying the suprapatellar pouch with one hand and testing for lateral fluid shift with the other. The normal concavity on either side of the patella

Soft-tissue injuries to the knee

Ligamentous and meniscal injuries to the knee are often difficult to diagnose precisely on first is obliterated by quite small amounts of fluid. Pressure on one side of the patella will push fluid to the opposite side and increase the parapatella convexity there.

The speed of onset of an effusion is as important as the size:

• Rapid collection suggests the presence of blood and thus damage to vascular structures such as the bone or ligament. The most common cause of a haemarthrosis is a partial tear of the anterior cruciate ligament. Fractures of the lower femur and upper tibia may extend into the joint and produce a haemarthrosis.

• Onset of swelling over 24 h is typical of a synovial response, commonly associated with damage to the avascular menisci.

Injury to a meniscus

This is suggested by the ability to walk immediately after the incident followed by a gradual onset of swelling with increasing pain. Tenderness is maximal at the joint line. The knee may lock or give way days later.

Damage will have been inflicted by tibial rotation on the partially flexed joint and pain at the joint line can be reproduced by recreating these stresses. The medial meniscus is the more commonly injured of the two because it has more restricting peripheral attachments than the lateral meniscus and is therefore subjected to greater shearing forces.

Minor injury to a collateral ligament

This may result in a very similar picture to meniscal injury. There is pain on valgus/varus stressing but no significant laxity.

XR

Radiological examination is usually unrewarding, but must be carried out to exclude intra-articular fracture. There may be an avulsion injury at the site of attachment of collateral or cruciate ligaments.

Tx

For knee problems that require immediate referral see Box 7.8.

Early arthroscopy is increasingly used to aid diagnosis and to give appropriate treatment. Minor meniscal and collateral ligament injuries can be treated on an outpatient basis. A support bandage should be applied and crutches and analgesia given as necessary. Follow-up must be arranged and physiotherapy may be very helpful.

Withdrawal of fluid from the knee may relieve the pain caused by a tense swelling, facilitate examination and distinguish between blood and serous effusion. However, aspiration of an effusion should not be attempted in an unsuitable environment by an inexperienced doctor.

Box 7.8 Knee Problems which require Immediate Referral

Haemarthrosis.
Ligamentous instability.
Locked knee.
Complete failure to straight leg raise.
Fracture on X-ray.
Possibility of septic arthritis.
Penetration of the joint.

Fractures of the tibial condyles

Fractures of the upper tibia may occur after a forcible valgus or varus strain (e.g. knee hit by a car bumper). The patient is in pain, unable to walk and has an obvious haemarthrosis. However, the tibial plateau may be depressed to a lesser degree in elderly patients after relatively minor trauma, in which case the knee is not very swollen and the patient is able to walk.

There is:

• localised pain and tenderness at the joint line;
• a modest effusion;
• a reasonable amount of movement of the knee;
• pain on valgus/varus stressing.
(See Figure 7.3).

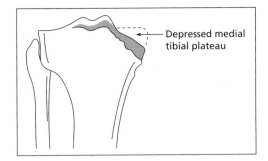

Figure 7.3 Fracture of the medial tibial plateau.

Xʀ

Minor degrees of depression of the tibial plateau are often overlooked on X-ray. The anteroposterior radiograph requires especially careful scrutiny. Osteoporotic bone is often present, as a causative factor. The radiological appearance of osteoarthrosis may obscure the fracture.

Tx

Patients with tibial condyle fractures generally require referral for operative fixation. Some minor crush fractures of the tibial plateau may be treated on an outpatient basis in a plaster cast, but most patients will need to be admitted.

Fracture of the neck of the fibula

This injury may be associated with damage to the common peroneal nerve (causing drop-foot, paralysis of ankle everters and loss of sensation over the lateral aspect of the lower leg). It may be an isolated injury or may accompany rotational injuries of the ankle (Maisonneuve's fracture).

Xʀ

Radiographs of this area are indicated when there is direct injury or tenderness accompanying an obvious ankle injury.

Tx

The uncomplicated injury may be treated with an elastic bandage, analgesia, crutches and fracture clinic follow-up. Other variants require immediate referral.

Diffuse inflammation of the knee

See also page 399 in Chapter 21.
Septic arthritis may be florid, with acute joint pain, fever and systemic illness or more insidious with only modest pain and some joint movement. Be alert to this possibility in elderly patients and those with rheumatoid disease. Also consider the diagnosis of gonorrhoea.

Crystal arthropathy may present with exquisite local pain and joint stiffness.

Deformity secondary to osteoarthrosis and bone destruction decreases locomotor efficiency. Muscle work is increased and the patient complains of fatigue as well as joint pain. The joint line is prominent and irregular as a result of osteophytes and there are usually a few degrees of fixed flexion. Collateral ligament instability follows tibial condyle collapse and instability predisposes to trauma. Osteoarthrosis extends recovery time after injury.

Xʀ

Radiographs may show calcified menisci or nonspecific changes.

Tx

Referral to an orthopaedic surgeon or rheumatologist should be decided by the most likely diagnosis. Diagnostic tap may be indicated but should not be performed in the ED.

Loose bodies in the knee joint

Intra-articular fragments may arise from an area of osteochondritis dissecans (*see Figure 7.4*), degenerate menisci, osteophytes or the synovium. The patient complains of intermittent locking of the knee, typically in a different position each time. There may be a small effusion.

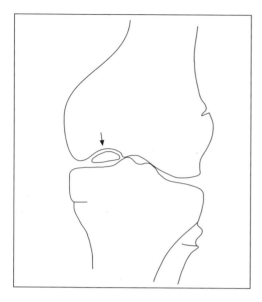

Figure 7.4 Osteochondritis dissecans (arrow).

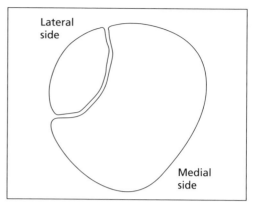

Figure 7.5 Bipartite patella.

The action of the quadriceps muscle should be assessed by active knee extension; failure to straight leg raise suggests a significant injury.

XR

Occasionally, the patella is bipartite. The upper lateral part is separated from the rest of the patella by a curved line mimicking a fracture (*see Figure 7.5*). This is a normal variant, but may not be present in both knees.

Tx

Refer for specialist care. Comminuted fractures are excised. Minimally displaced fractures may be wired together. Undisplaced fractures are treated in a plaster cylinder. Transverse fractures of the patella, which extend laterally to involve the quadriceps expansion, require surgical repair as do serious injuries of the quadriceps.

XR

The loose fragments are usually easily seen on an X-ray.

Tx

If the knee is locked, no attempt should be made to manipulate it but orthopaedic advice should be sought. In other cases, the patient is given a tubular support bandage and referred to the next orthopaedic clinic.

Fracture of the patella/quadriceps injury

The patella may be fractured by a direct blow or fall or by sudden quadriceps contraction. Indirect traction force can break the quadriceps mechanism at different levels. The older the patient the higher the lesion:

- *young* – patella tendon;
- *middle-aged* – across the patella;
- *older* – rectus femoris muscle.

Dislocation of the patella

The patella may dislocate laterally during active quadriceps action. Teenage girls are most often affected. All knee movements are painful and the deformity is obvious. If spontaneous reduction has occurred, the diagnosis can be confirmed by a positive patella apprehension test: pushing the patella laterally (usually in either knee) causes pain and a feeling of imminent dislocation.

XR

Radiographs should be taken to exclude bony injury.

Tx

Reduction under sedation may be undertaken in the ED. This entails a gentle straightening of the leg by the application of distal traction. A plaster cylinder or other suitable straight leg splint is then applied and the patient referred to the next fracture clinic, non-weight-bearing on crutches. Patients with a clear history of dislocation of the patella in whom spontaneous relocation has occurred should be treated in the same way.

Patellofemoral osteochondritis

Pain behind the patella is a common cause of knee pain in young women. Trivial direct trauma may be implicated. Symptoms are exacerbated by exercise, especially going down steps. Pain is reproduced by pressing on the patella. There may be a small effusion but the knee joint is otherwise normal.

XR

Radiographs are usually normal.

Tx

A support bandage and physiotherapy (to prevent wasting of the quadriceps muscles) are indicated. The condition is self-limiting and rarely requires surgical intervention. Initial referral to the patient's GP is usually appropriate.

Peripatellar bursitis

Both the prepatellar and infrapatellar bursae may become inflamed and then secondarily infected following repeated minor trauma. Colloquial names for these conditions viz housemaid's and clergyman's knee respectively, were derived from the most commonly affected professions and their differing kneeling positions. Nowadays, because of changing priorities in society, tradesmen are the people most prone to these conditions. The affected area is red, swollen and tender. Pain may limit full movements but there is no communication between the bursa and the knee joint.

Acute traumatic bursitis may follow a direct blow or fall. In this case, the prepatellar area is very tender and swollen. There often appears to be a fluid-filled area that could be aspirated but attempts to do this are usually unsuccessful.

XR

Following severe direct trauma, the knee should be radiographed to exclude an underlying fracture of the patella.

Tx

When there is no clinical evidence of infection (as indicated by body temperature), the patient can be treated with an elastic bandage, NSAIDS and follow-up. The condition usually resolves spontaneously but occasionally the bursa has to be removed. Any suspicion of knee joint involvement demands immediate orthopaedic referral. If there is an acute localised infection of the bursa alone, incision and drainage under a general anaesthetic should be carried out by the orthopaedic team.

Rupture of a Baker's cyst

Bursae in the popliteal fossa may be connected to the knee joint. An enlarged and isolated popliteal bursa (a Baker's cyst) is associated with rheumatoid involvement of the knee. If it ruptures, there is sudden pain in the upper calf as the synovial fluid is squeezed between the calf muscles. The condition is often misdiagnosed as either a tear of the calf muscles or a deep vein thrombosis (*see pages 106 and 114*).

Exclude a popliteal aneurysm before considering other extra-articular swellings.

Xʀ

Arthrography is diagnostic.

Tx

Advice should be sought from the orthopaedic or rheumatology departments.

Osgood–Schlatter's disease

Adolescents may experience pain around the insertion of the patella tendon after exercise. This is caused by inflammation around the epiphysis. Knee movements are normal but resisted extension is painful.

Xʀ

Radiographs are diagnostic, showing break-up of the tibial epiphysis (see Figure 7.6).

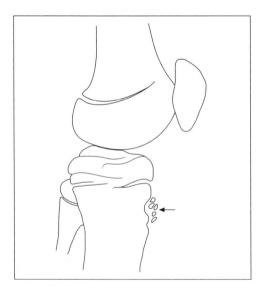

Figure 7.6 Osgood–Schlatter's disease (arrowed).

Tx

A tubular support bandage will provide symptomatic relief until an early orthopaedic outpatient consultation. Sport should be prohibited. Local injection of steroid may help but should be prescribed by and injected by a specialist. The condition always resolves when the epiphysis fuses just after puberty.

Sindig–Laarson's disease

This is of similar aetiology and involves the lower pole of the patella. Treatment is as for Osgood–Schlatter's disease.

Tumours and sepsis may occasionally present with knee pain, especially in children.

The lower leg

Two anatomical features provide potential complications for injuries to the lower leg:
1 The skin, thinly stretched over the tibia anteriorly, has a poor blood supply.
2 The muscles are enclosed in a rigid fascial envelope.
Consequently:
• many fractures of the tibia and fibula are compound;
• wounds of the skin in this area are slow to heal;
• muscle contusion or vascular damage in the calf may raise interstitial pressure sufficiently to occlude the circulation.

Fracture of the shaft of the tibia

Tibial shaft fractures follow a considerable amount of direct or indirect force. They are generally extremely painful injuries and render walking impossible. The fibula is usually also fractured, although a direct blow may break the tibia alone. In the latter case there will be minimal deformity and occasionally the patient is able to weight-bear with difficulty. Vascular damage should be suspected in all lower limb injuries, especially if there is either a crush or high-speed mechanism of injury. If present, early recognition and referral is essential.

Tx

For initial splintage see Box 7.9.

Box 7.9 Splinting the Lower Leg

Apply splintage under appropriate analgesia after removal of clothing and footwear but before radiography.
- Confirm the presence of foot pulses and toe movements.
- If there is gross ankle deformity, give nitrous oxide and quickly reduce the dislocation. This prevents pressure necrosis of overlying skin.
- If there is a compound fracture, remove gross contaminants and take an instant photograph before applying sterile iodine-soaked pads. Do not allow repeated examination – show the photograph instead. Start antibiotics.
- Apply an L-shaped splint or box splint.
- Check the pulses again and review the analgesia.
- Arrange for X-rays.

Most patients with a fractured tibia need admission, observation and internal fixation. Compound fractures must be debrided in theatre as soon as possible.

Some closed fractures can be managed on an outpatient basis but the decision should be left to the orthopaedic department. The application of a well-padded, above-knee plaster cast should not be delegated to the inexperienced. 'Check radiographs' in plaster are essential, even if the fracture initially appeared stable and undisplaced. Displacement can occur during application of plaster. Crutches and analgesia will be required as will early orthopaedic follow-up.

Tibial fractures in children

Children with these injuries present with a limp or failure to weight-bear. A history of trauma is by no means inevitable. There may be no swelling or deformity and tenderness (although present) may be difficult to localise. Knee and ankle flexion are usually unaffected, although ankle rotation may be painful. The diagnosis is thus elusive and if there is any doubt follow the procedure for the limping child as described in *Box 7.3*.

Xʀ

Radiographs may not show an obvious fracture. Look at both films for a faint, long, oblique, black line. In the so-called toddlers' fracture, X-rays are initially normal and the characteristic periosteal elevation is not seen for several days.

Tx

Obvious fractures should be immobilised in an above-knee cast. The child will need analgesia and fracture clinic follow-up. Toddlers' fractures can be treated with rest and either an elastic support bandage or a below-knee plaster of Paris cast depending on the degree of pain and discomfort. In cases of doubt, arrange for a second opinion as soon as possible.

Fracture of the shaft of the fibula

The shaft of the fibula may be broken by direct trauma. Although there is localised pain and tenderness, there is little swelling and the patient can weight-bear. Consequently, the injury is often missed.

Xʀ

The radiograph is diagnostic.

Tx

The fibula at this point does not transmit much force so a plaster cast is unnecessary. The patient requires an elastic bandage, analgesia, crutches and a fracture clinic follow-up.

Pretibial pain

Shin pain may develop acutely in athletes. The patient complains of intermittent discomfort over the front of the lower leg. There may be local tenderness, but the diagnosis is made chiefly from the history of gradually increasing pain associated with exercise. "Shin splints", as the condition is known, is probably caused by oedema within the anterior compartment.

Other possible diagnoses are chronic or acute osteomyelitis, bone tumour or hyperplasia of the anterior tibial cortex. This last condition occurs in footballers subjected to repeated skin injury and subperiosteal haematoma.

XR

Radiographs may show cortical thickening in some cases, but only a bone scan is diagnostic; this will also identify a stress fracture.

Tx

Management of these patients depends on symptoms and diagnosis. A referral to a physiotherapist or a sports injury clinic may be appropriate. Stress fractures should be immobilised in a cast. All patients should have follow-up arranged.

Calf muscle strain/tear

Disruption within the calf muscles or at the junction with the tendon may be caused by overuse or sudden stretching. There is acute localised pain, usually towards the medial side of the gastrocnemius muscle. Weight-bearing is painful as is passive ankle dorsiflexion. It is important to exclude rupture of the Achilles tendon, which gives a similar clinical picture. Deep vein thrombosis and ruptured Baker's cyst must be also be considered (*see pages 103 and 114*).

Tx

Patients need an elastic bandage, analgesia and crutches. Follow-up should be arranged, as should early physiotherapy.

Achilles tendon pain

Avascular degeneration of the tendon is common and may produce chronic pain on exercise. Despite the localised discomfort, there is full, active, plantar flexion. Inflammation of the tendon sheath produces more florid local signs but is less sinister as it never leads to rupture.

Tx

Tenosynovitis may benefit from local steroid injection into the sheath but tendonitis will be exacerbated. Steroid injection into the Achilles tendon may actually cause its rupture. The two conditions can easily be confused and so steroids should not be injected around the Achilles tendon in the ED. Rest, NSAIDs and physiotherapy may help. An orthopaedic opinion should be arranged.

Rupture of the Achilles tendon

Surprisingly, acute rupture may at first be dismissed by the patient as a trivial injury. The usual history is of sudden calf pain thought to have been caused by an object hitting the back of the leg. The acute pain subsides and the patient is able to walk flat-footed with difficulty but cannot run. On examination there is a palpable gap in the tendon, although this may be filled with inflammatory exudate. Plantar flexion is possible using the toe flexors, but is weak. Squeezing the calf fails to cause plantar flexion of the foot and is painful. This test is performed with the feet of the prone patient extending over the end of the couch and is always compared with the normal side.

Tx

Refer the patient to the orthopaedic department. Most patients will undergo early primary tendon repair, although immobilisation in equinus in a cast is another option. Recovery is often delayed because of pre-existing degenerative changes.

Partial rupture

Sometimes patients present with the hallmarks of acute rupture and a normal, but painful, calf-squeeze test. This may be caused by partial rupture of a degenerate tendon. Management is similar to that described for a complete rupture of the Achilles tendon.

Rupture of the musculotendinous junction

Injuries that are in this area, also merit an orthopaedic opinion.

The ankle

Inversion sprains

These are the most common injuries seen in an ED. They represent damage to the lateral ligament and tendon complex of the ankle and so are seen in a number of different varieties, depending on the particular structures torn (*see Figure 7.7*).

Some sprains will resolve quickly without treatment, many will heal more slowly and need routine outpatient care and a few require specialised management from the outset. It is important, but not always easy, to assign the patient to the appropriate treatment category as soon as possible.

Ask the patient about:
- history and mechanism of injury;
- extent and speed of appearance of pain and swelling;
- mobility;
- occupational and recreational demands.

The usual history is of ankle inversion while running, playing sports or slipping down a step. A crack may have been heard but this does not inevitably indicate bone injury. The initial pain settles and then gets worse again over the next few hours, causing difficulty in weight-bearing. This sequence is typical – but not diagnostic – of a soft-tissue injury.

Swelling and pain are often focused just anterior to the lateral malleolus – caused by injury to the anterior talofibular ligament – or over the side of the foot. Exclude ankle mortice instability by gripping the heel with one hand and the lower leg with the other. There should be no pain or movement when a sideways force is applied to the heel. In contrast, the patient will have acute pain on attempted inversion of the foot.

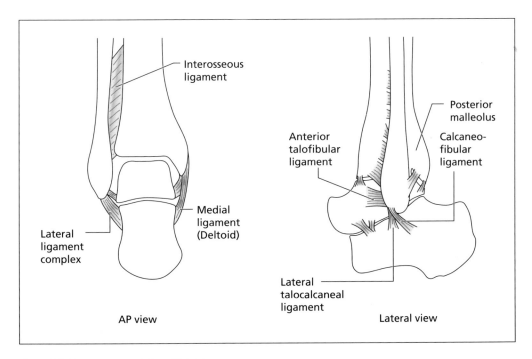

Figure 7.7 Ligaments around the ankle joint.

After examining the lateral side of the ankle, there are six places to feel for related injuries:

1 the medial malleolus and medial ligament complex;
2 the base of the little (fifth) metatarsal bone;
3 the calcaneum;
4 the Achilles tendon;
5 the neck of the fibula;
6 the mid-tarsal region.

The ankle must be palpated all around for bony tenderness, not just the swollen lateral side. Pain over the styloid process of the fifth metatarsal base may be caused by ligament or bone avulsion – a variation of ankle inversion injury. Fracture of the calcaneum and rupture of the Achilles tendon are injuries that are often wrongly diagnosed as ankle sprains on first presentation. The neck of the fibula should be examined because of its involvement in rotational injuries of the ankle (see below). Fracture dislocation at the tarso–metatarsal junction (Lisfranc's fracture) causes significant pain over the dorsum of the foot, especially medially.

XR

If indicated, plain radiographs of the ankle are taken to exclude significant fractures of the malleoli. They should be supplemented with other films (e.g. knee, heel and foot) if there are atypical findings on clinical examination. *For the indications for ankle X-rays see Box 7.10.*

Ankle sprains may be associated with an avulsed flake from the lateral malleolus or the dorsum of the talus. New flake fractures have a sharp, irregular outline without a complete marginal cortex. Do not forget to look at the calcaneum. Lisfranc's fracture may be difficult to diagnose on standard X-rays.

Some patients continue to have severe symptoms and signs despite normal initial X-rays. These patients should be reviewed by a senior doctor after 7–10 days; further X-rays may be required.

Tx

Exclude fracture or mortice instability and consider the need for X-ray (*see Box 7.10*).

If the patient has a classical inversion sprain and is able to weight-bear, then treat with:
• a compression bandage, ice packs and analgesia;
• initial rest and elevation, leading to graduated exercise;
• GP follow-up.

If the patient is unable to weight-bear or has an obviously more severe injury, add:
• crutches (partial weight-bearing);
• early physiotherapy;
• review after about 2 weeks to ensure satisfactory progress (physiotherapist or clinic).

Patients with very severe symptoms or signs should receive a second opinion. Stress views may be indicated to help choose optimum treatment. Plaster cast or operative repair may be appropriate.

Box 7.10 Indications for Radiography of the Ankle following Injury

Any of the following:
• history suggesting severe injury;
• severe pain;
• age over 55 years;
• inability to walk four steps unaided;
• obvious deformity;
• severe swelling of rapid onset;
• bony tenderness of the lateral malleolus especially posteriorly – anterior bone pain is common without a fracture;
• atypical features;
• return visit with no improvement.
The corollary of these indications is that an X-ray is not needed in:
• a younger patient;
• with a history of a simple inversion injury;
• who can partially weight-bear; and
• who has tenderness and swelling over the lateral ligament area (dorsolateral foot) only.

Flake fractures represent variants of ligament injuries and should be treated in the same way. However, their detection is useful as they often indicate that a more severe injury has occurred. The patient should be told of their presence to prevent a later misunderstanding.

Most patients with mild ankle sprains can expect a marked improvement by the end of a week and to be weight-bearing almost normally within 2–3 weeks.

Eversion sprains

These injuries produce pain and swelling below the medial malleolus. They are uncommon but may produce an unstable ankle joint.

Xʀ

Radiographs should be taken unless the patient can bear full weight without pain and has very little local swelling.

Tx

Evidence of fracture or incongruity of the ankle joint is an indication for orthopaedic referral. Less severe injuries usually resolve with a support bandage and a short course of physiotherapy. Analgesia and crutches may be necessary.

Ankle fractures

A fracture of the ankle may follow a mechanism of injury similar to a sprain. There is usually significant pain and swelling, although some patients may be able to weight-bear. Examination must again include the knee, calf, ankle, heel and foot.

Two or more separate lesions, whether of bone or ligament, will produce a potentially unstable joint and require specialist attention. Isolated fracture of the lateral malleolus, for example, may render the ankle mortice unstable if there is concurrent rupture of the deltoid ligament (between the medial malleolus and the calcaneum). Fracture of the medial malleolus may be associated with a spiral fracture of the neck of the fibula (Maisonneuve's fracture).

Xʀ

Radiographs of the ankle are usually diagnostic but should be supplemented with views of the knee, leg, heel and foot, as clinically indicated. Vertical fractures of the posterior part of the tibia (seen on the lateral view and extending down to the ankle joint) are conveniently but inaccurately termed fractures of the posterior malleolus. Thus a fracture may be described as bimalleolar or even trimalleolar.

Tx

Stable, undisplaced fractures of the lateral malleolus may be treated on an outpatient basis in a below-knee plaster cast. The patient should be seen at the next fracture clinic.

Unstable or displaced lateral malleolar fractures and all fractures involving the medial malleolus or distal fibula should be referred for an immediate orthopaedic opinion.

Posterior displacement of the lower tibial epiphysis

This may occur in children. Reduction under general anaesthesia is straightforward but overnight admission is usually required.

Dislocation of the ankle

The talus, and with it the foot, may be completely dislocated following severe local trauma. Usually, the skin remains intact but is stretched tightly over the bone. An accompanying fracture is common.

Xʀ

Radiographs should be delayed until after reduction.

Tx

Immediate reduction is essential to reduce pain and minimise the risk of tissue necrosis.
• Give IV analgesia and supplement it with nitrous oxide or midazolam during the procedure.

109

- Reduce the ankle with axial traction.
- Check the skin circulation and foot pulses.
- Apply a splint.
- Obtain X-rays.
- Refer the patient to the orthopaedic team.

The foot

For the relative positions of the bones of the foot see Figure 7.8.

Fracture of the talus

Talar fractures present in a similar way to ankle injuries. They often produce long-term disability because of disruption of the subtalar joint; sometimes avascular necrosis occurs.

X_R

These fractures can be missed on X-rays unless the area is carefully inspected.

T_x

The patient needs analgesia and orthopaedic referral.

Fracture of the calcaneum

Calcaneal fracture is usually caused by a direct fall on to the heel from a height such as a roof or a ladder. There is:

- pain and difficulty in weight-bearing;
- local tenderness and sometimes bruising;

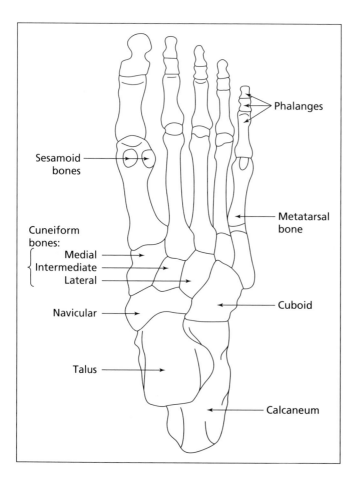

Figure 7.8 The bones of the foot.

• a possibility of associated, and perhaps masked, injuries elsewhere (e.g. lumbar spine).

A fracture of this region may also occur in osteoporotic bone, following relatively minor trauma. In this case, it may superficially mimic a soft-tissue injury of the ankle.

X_R

Radiographs should be obtained of the ankle, heel and foot. The X-ray shows a normal ankle mortice. Single or multiple fracture lines through the cancellous os calcis are often missed. The flattening of Böhler's angle is an important radiographic sign (*see Figure 7.9*).

Tx

Exclude associated injuries. Patients with this fracture need analgesia and orthopaedic referral.

The need for internal fixation may be decided by CT scanning.

Other tarsal injuries

Fractures of the tarsus may be produced by crushing and twisting forces. Pain and swelling are usually prominent.

X_R

Tarso–metatarsal dislocation with fracture of the second metatarsal base (Lisfranc's fracture) is important to recognise but may be overlooked on standard radiological views. A true lateral view of the area will reveal dorsal displacement.

Tx

Open reduction may be necessary. Specialist advice should always be sought.

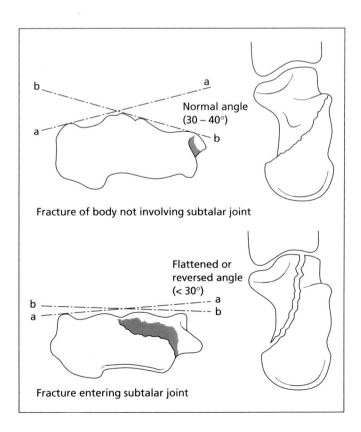

Normal angle (30 – 40°)

Fracture of body not involving subtalar joint

Flattened or reversed angle (< 30°)

Fracture entering subtalar joint

Figure 7.9 Loss of Böhler's angle.

Plantar fasciitis

The patient complains of pain on the sole of the foot, often worst in the morning and after exercise. Pain is exacerbated by the heel striking the ground. There is tenderness localised to the anteromedial part of the os calcis about 5 cm below and 1 cm in front of the medial malleolus. The condition is caused by degenerative changes in or overuse of the plantar fascia, as with jogging. This results in partial avulsion of the fascia from the os calcis. Chronic symptoms may be associated with a calcaneal spur.

XR

Radiographs are taken to exclude a fracture and to identify a spur.

Tx

The presence of a spur is not an indication for surgery, although its removal is occasionally necessary. Most cases can be effectively treated by prescribing an excavated heel cushion or a pad composed of an energy-absorbing hydrogel. NSAIDs and physiotherapy may be helpful. Local infiltration with a steroid is often effective but should be left to the discretion of the orthopaedic department.

Pain in the mid-foot

Köhler's disease

Osteochondritis of the navicular bone occurs mostly in teenage boys. They present with chronic pain on exercise. There may be a history of minor trauma. Midtarsal and subtalar joint movements are restricted.

XR

Radiographs show a collapsed sclerotic bone (*see Figure 7.10*).

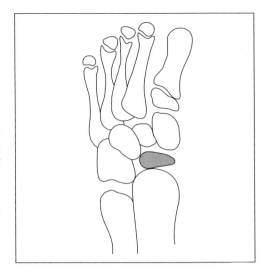

Figure 7.10 Avascular necrosis of the navicular bone.

Tx

The patient should be given a support bandage and referred to the next orthopaedic clinic.

Prominent navicular bone

Teenage girls may complain of pain over the inner aspect of the foot and relate the symptoms to exercise or injury. Anxious parents point to the prominent medial end of the navicular bone as the cause of the pain. If examination of the foot is otherwise normal they should be reassured. Periosteal inflammation may indeed make the bone appear prominent but most cases settle spontaneously. Attention should be directed to appropriate footwear.

Fractures of the forefoot

Metatarsal fractures are common but are only of importance when there is gross disruption or the bones of the first ray are involved. Most forces through the forefoot are transmitted along the first metatarsus. A stress fracture (March fracture) is most commonly seen in the index (second) metatarsal neck.

XR

Stress fractures may not be visible on an X-ray until callus formation has occurred. Bone scan may be diagnostic.

Tx

Multiple fractures of the metatarsal bones may require internal fixation. Patients with significant fractures of the first metatarsus should also be referred for an orthopaedic opinion. For most other metatarsal fractures, a below-knee plaster cast can be applied on an outpatient basis. The patient will require analgesia, crutches and follow-up in the fracture clinic.

Pain under the metatarsal heads

This is often chronic and degenerative (metatarsalgia). It may be relieved by providing a metatarsal pad. This should extend almost up to, but not under, the prominent bone.

Fractures of the toes

Fractures of the toes are common and usually result from a kicking or stubbing injury.

XR

Radiography is usually not necessary except where there is clinical deformity or the proximal phalanx of the big toe is involved.

Tx

Fractures of the proximal phalanx of the big toe may need a below-knee walking plaster and fracture clinic follow-up.

Angulated toes should be straightened under ring block and then neighbour-strapped. Check X-rays should be obtained and follow-up arranged.

Other toe injuries are treated symptomatically irrespective of the presence of a minor undisplaced fracture. Neighbour-strapping is helpful. Pain around the metatarsophalangeal joints may be helped by the application of a metatarsal pad. Bulky dressings prevent the use of normal footwear and should be avoided. Follow-up is not necessary if the patient is advised on care of the strapping and told that symptoms will abate over the ensuing month.

Vascular conditions of the lower limb

Arterial embolism

Thrombi, which embolise to peripheral arteries, may arise from several sites:

1 the left atrial appendage (usually in the presence of atrial fibrillation);
2 the left ventricle (invariably on an area damaged by a recent myocardial infarction);
3 an atheromatous plaque;
4 an aortic aneurysm;
5 a thrombosis in a deep vein in a patient with a patent foramen ovale (paradoxical embolism).

All of these possibilities should be considered although the first two are by far the most common.

Emboli tend to lodge at the sites of bifurcation of arteries. Their effects depend on the extent of the occlusion of the circulation and on the degree of collateral circulation that exists. Common sites that involve the lower limb are:

- the aortic bifurcation (bilateral ischaemia to the level of the knees);
- the origin of the deep femoral artery (ischaemia to the mid-calf);
- the bifurcation of the popliteal artery (ischaemia of the foot).

Sudden occlusion of the femoral artery causes the six 'Ps':

1 pain;
2 pallor;
3 pulselessness;
4 parasthesia;
5 paralysis;
6 perishing cold.

Tx

Embolism must be treated within 6 h of the onset of symptoms or else propagation of thrombus distal to the embolus will greatly worsen prognosis. Treatment includes:

- oral aspirin (300 mg);
- IV analgesia;
- IV fluids;
- referral to a vascular surgeon. Embolectomy or thrombolysis (usually with streptokinase) may be required.

Intra-arterial injection

Irritant substances may cause critical ischaemia if injected into an artery. Intravenous drug abusers are the most common sufferers from this problem and temazepam gel is the drug most usually involved. The ischaemia results from a mixture of vasospasm and multiple small emboli. Severe pain is the prominent symptom but the other signs described above (*see the six 'Ps'*) may be absent.

Tx

This is similar to that described above for arterial embolism. Drugs that cause arterial dilatation may be considered.

Venous thrombosis

Thrombosis of the deep veins of the lower limb or pelvis (deep vein thrombosis or DVT) may be caused by changes in:

1 blood coagulation (smoking, hormonal contraception, malignancy, recent surgery or major illness);

2 blood vessels (pregnancy);

3 blood flow (immobility, long-haul air or road travel, plaster casts).

> Thrombosis of veins distal to the popliteal vein ('below-knee DVT') is particularly common because of the venous sinuses present in the soleus muscle of the calf. At least 5% of below-knee DVTs spread to the proximal veins and a half of all above-knee venous thromboses embolise to the lungs.

The classical clinical features of DVT are:

- swelling and oedema distal to the occlusion;
- warmth, redness and deep tenderness of the thigh or calf.

These signs depend on venous occlusion. In contrast, there may be no signs in the presence of an extensive, non-occlusive but potentially lethal thrombus. Moreover, there is some evidence that non-occlusive thrombi float in the middle of the vein and thus break free very easily.

> Homans' sign cannot be relied upon – it is positive in less than 20% of patients with DVT of the leg.

The following conditions may all be mistaken for DVT:

- chronic venous obstruction (*see page 115*);
- superficial phlebitis (*see page 115*);
- post-thrombotic syndrome;
- acute or subacute arterial ischaemia (*see page 113*);
- cellulitis of the leg (*see page 400*);
- calf muscle tear (*see page 106*) or other soft tissue injury;
- ruptured Baker's cyst (*see page 103*);
- fracture of the lower limb;
- lymphoedema;
- hypoproteinaemia.

> In the United Kingdom, about a quarter of all women aged between 16 and 49 years (and almost half of all women in their 20s) use regular hormonal contraception. *For the relative risks of DVT and PE with combined oestrogen and progestogen contraceptive pills see Box 7.11.*

Investigation

The Well's scoring system for clinical DVT may be used to stratify patients into low, moderate or high-risk groups – see Box 7.12. Those patients with a low risk may be further subdivided by requesting a D-dimer blood test. (This protein is a cross-linked fibrin degradation product that is released into the blood stream from active blood clots and sites of wound healing.) A negative D-dimer has a greater than 95% negative predictive value for DVT whereas a positive result has less than 70% positive predictive value. D-dimer is

Box 7.11 Relative Risks of DVT & PE for Women taking Combined Oestrogen and Progestogen Contraceptive Pills

	Incidence of DVT or PE	Relative risk
No combined pill	5 per 100 000 women	1
Second generation combined pill	15 per 100 000 women	3
Third generation combined pill	25 per 100 000 women	5
Pregnancy	60 per 100 000 women	12

Box 7.12 Well's Scoring System for Clinical DVT

Clinical feature	Score
Cancer treatment on-going or within last 6 months	+1
Immobilisation of lower limb	+1
Bedriddden for more than 3 days	+1
Major surgery in last 4 weeks	+1
Entire leg swollen	+1
Calf swelling greater than 3 cm in diameter	+1
Increased pitting oedema in symptomatic leg	+1
Superficial collateral veins visible	+1
Alternative diagnosis as likely or more likely	−2

Total score = 0 or less;	Low probability of DVT
Total score = 1 to 2;	Moderate probability of DVT
Total score = 3 or more;	High probability of DVT

therefore a good test to rule out DVT in low-risk patients but is not a useful method of diagnosis.

First line imaging depends on local availability. Doppler ultrasound studies are replacing the traditional venogram in many centres. If neither investigation is immediately available the patient must be treated on clinical grounds alone. Pelvic imaging may be required at a later date to look for causative factors.

Tx

Once the diagnosis has been confirmed or provisionally suspected, most patients will be treated by rapid anticoagulation (usually as an outpatient). This may be achieved with either an intravenous infusion of standard unfractionated heparin (in hospital) or preferably, with a low molecular weight heparin (LMWH) given subcutaneously, for example, enoxaparin 1.5 mg per kg once a day. This should be altered to 1 mg per kg twice a day in pregnant patients (based on weight in early pregnancy) and 1 mg per kg once a day in patients with severe renal impairment. Heparinisation will be required for at least 5 days and consequently effective community liaison is essential for outpatients. Follow-up in a clinic should be arranged to occur within 48 h. Oral anticoagulants are substituted for the heparin as soon as possible and are usually continued for about 3 months. In some cases of rapidly progressing or life-threatening DVT, thrombolysis (with streptokinase) may be considered.

For the risk factors for venous thrombo-embolism see Box 12.12 on page 197.

For the diagnosis and management of suspected pulmonary embolism see page 197 and page 223.

Phlebitis

Inflammation of the long or short saphenous vein usually occurs in patients with varicose veins or those who have had IV therapy. The vein is red, hot and tender.

Tx

Phlebitis usually settles with topical therapy and oral NSAIDs. If there is a systemic pyrexia, an antibiotic (e.g. co-amoxiclav) can be added.

Venous disease in IV drug abusers

Repeated injection into the femoral vein causes chronic venous obstruction. There is swelling and oedema of the whole lower limb and dilatation of the superficial vessels; sinuses are often found in the groin. Thrombosis may occur, in which case the limb becomes hot, red and painful. This deep-vein thrombosis is potentially life threatening.

Acute compartment syndrome

Closed compartment syndrome is caused by swollen, contused muscle or bleeding inside a rigid fascial envelope. The onset may be delayed after injury and insidious. Early symptoms are pain – particularly on muscle stretching – and paraesthesia. The affected part may also, but not inevitably, be pale and cool with a slow capillary refill. Ischaemia results from compression of small blood vessels and so the presence of distal pulses is of no help in excluding the diagnosis.

Compartment syndrome can easily develop unseen under a plaster cast or below an eschar from a burn. The most common site to be affected is the lower leg, which has four anatomical compartments, but the syndrome is also seen in the forearm (three fascial compartments), the foot and the hand.

> In compartment syndrome, the limb may not be broken, distal pulses may be present and pulse oximetry may be normal.

XR

Arteriography will reveal arterial lesions but will not demonstrate compartment syndrome.

Tx

Suspicion of compartment syndrome is an indication for an immediate orthopaedic referral. Manometry is useful, particularly in patients with a depressed level of consciousness. There are four compartments in the lower leg and all may require extensive fasciotomy. This will produce significant fluid loss and transfusion may be necessary.

Chapter 8

The upper limb

For the general principles of the management of limb injuries see page 90.

Provide analgesia, support and splintage if necessary (*see Box 8.1*) before starting your assessment.

Box 8.1 Upper Limb Support and Splintage

Broad arm or triangular sling
Used to support the weight of the arm and restrict its movement. Useful for:
• fractures, dislocations and other painful conditions of the shoulder and clavicle;
• fractures and other injuries of the forearm, wrist and hand including support of plaster casts on these parts;
• painful conditions of the elbow and support of casts on the elbow.

The high arm sling
This is a variant of the triangular sling used to decrease swelling of the hand. It is of doubtful effectiveness as flexion of the elbow above 90° may decrease venous drainage of the distal parts.

Collar and cuff
Originally made from two leather bands joined by a cord but now made in the ED by securing a length of covered foam with a plastic clip. It uses gravity to restrict movement while applying slight traction at the elbow and is useful for injuries of the elbow and humerus. Flexion of the elbow of more than 20° above the right angle is painful and should be avoided. Check the radial pulse.

Advice to patients
• Wear the sling outside clothes.
• Remove the sling at night and support the injured part on pillows.
• Remember the importance of maintaining shoulder and hand mobility.

The shoulder and upper arm

If the patient can put his or her hand behind the head and into the small of the back without pain, then the shoulder on that side is unlikely to be significantly injured.

Fracture of the clavicle

The clavicle provides the only skeletal continuity between the upper limb and trunk. It is occasionally broken by direct trauma but usually breaks in the middle two-thirds as a result of transmitted violence from a fall on to the upper limb. Damage to adjacent neurovascular structures is very rare except with posterior sternoclavicular dislocation. In adults, fractures cause well-localised symptoms with obvious deformity and tenderness.

Children

Greenstick fractures are common after childhood falls. There may be little deformity and remarkably good movement of the arm and shoulder girdle. Alternatively, the child may refuse to use the whole arm on the affected side and thus mimic a pulled elbow.

XR

An anteroposterior (AP) radiograph confirms the diagnosis.

Tx

The weight of the arm should be supported in a broad arm sling. Figure-of-eight bandages, applied to achieve reduction, are usually more painful and do not succeed in their objective. Most displaced fractures settle to produce an acceptable cosmetic result. Prescribe appropriate analgesia and refer the patient to the next fracture clinic. Very painful, comminuted fractures may rarely require initial inpatient care, as do the occasionally occurring compound fractures.

Sternoclavicular joint disruption

This is rare and is the result of considerable indirect violence applied to the shoulder. Usually anterior dislocation with prominent bone is seen; posterior displacement is even more rare and may involve damage to major blood vessels, the trachea or the oesophagus.

Xr

Radiological confirmation is difficult. CT scan may be helpful.

Tx

This can be a major injury with potentially serious consequences. Orthopaedic advice should be sought.

Acromioclavicular joint disruption

This is much more common than the sternoclavicular joint disruption. The outer end of the clavicle is elevated at its articulation with the acromion. The weak fibres of the acromioclavicular joint are readily ruptured. The joint's normal stability is maintained by the conoid and trapezoid ligaments, binding the outer fifth of the clavicle down to the coracoid process of the scapula. It is the complete or partial rupture of these strong ligaments that results in an acromioclavicular dislocation or subluxation. Direct downward pressure will reduce the deformity rather painfully and transiently. Shoulder movements are restricted because of pain.

Xr

Radiographic confirmation, if required, is obtained by taking a wide-angled erect AP film to show both acromioclavicular joints with the patient holding weights in both hands. Slight subluxation may occur normally.

Tx

The raised outer end of the clavicle is accepted as a minor disability by most patients. Reduction is very difficult to maintain by closed methods and internal fixation, although successful, will leave an ugly prominent scar. A sling and analgesia are provided until the pain has settled. The shoulder will remain weak for some months. Manual workers may notice a very slight but permanent loss of power in the affected limb.

Supraspinatus tendinitis/subacromial bursitis

These two conditions are very difficult to separate. Both are caused by a combination of soft-tissue degeneration and a modest increase in activity. The patient presents with an injured shoulder often following an event such as lifting. Symptoms may occur suddenly or may be more gradual in onset. Movements are restricted, particularly abduction and forward flexion. Classically, there is a painful arc from about 20–90° of abduction but initially the pain may be intense and affect all movements. There may be specific tenderness in the supraspinatus fossa laterally.

Xr

Radiographs sometimes show calcification within the tendon, near its attachment to the joint capsule.

Tx

A broad arm sling and non-steroidal anti-inflammatory drugs (NSAIDS) should be prescribed; physiotherapy may also be helpful. Patients should be reviewed within a week, when steroid injection and orthopaedic referral may be considered. Surgical decompression may help in chronic cases.

Rotator cuff injury

The glenohumeral joint is stabilised by four muscles which surround it – the rotator cuff. These muscles are:

1 *subscapularis* – a medial rotator;
2 *supraspinatus* – which initiates abduction;
3 *infraspinatus* – a lateral rotator;
4 *teres minor* – another lateral rotator.

The rotator cuff muscles may be acutely injured or chronically inflamed, or both. This causes pain with shoulder movements, sometimes of the painful arc type. There may be a tender area anteriorly. The tendons of all the rotator cuff muscles may rupture or degenerate in a similar manner to the supraspinatus tendon (*see page 118*).
For frozen shoulder see page 122.

Tx

Analgesia, together with rest in a sling is required for a few days. Early physiotherapy is essential. The condition can be very slow to settle (up to 2 years), especially in older patients and in those with an acute onset.

Rupture of the long head of biceps

This is caused by a combination of tendon degeneration and powerful elbow flexion. The patient presents with the sudden appearance of a painless lump reminiscent of Popeye's biceps.

Tx

This is usually symptomatic, but a specialist opinion should be sought at the next fracture clinic.

Dislocation of the shoulder joint

This may occur after trivial injury in a predisposed individual or follow major violence to the shoulder girdle and be associated with other bone and soft-tissue injuries.

A full examination is mandatory to exclude associated injuries and distal neurovascular complications.

The dislocation is usually anterior and is easily detected clinically and radiologically (*see Figure 8.1*). Posterior dislocation is rarer and is associated with the muscle contraction that occurs during fits and electric shocks. Inferior dislocation is very rare – the patient presents with the arm erect. A fracture of the greater tuberosity or neck of the humerus may accompany a dislocation.

XR

Radiographs must be taken before reduction is attempted. Lateral radiographs are difficult to interpret; modified axial views are more useful. *Figures 8.2 and 8.3* demonstrate the normal appearances of the shoulder joint on lateral and apical radiographs.

> Posterior dislocation of the shoulder may not be obvious clinically and can easily be missed on the AP radiograph (*see Figure 8.4*).

Tx

The patient will need early parenteral analgesia. Reduction can be achieved without general anaesthetic by using one of a number of techniques to overcome muscle spasm. Prior analgesia helps but large amounts should not be necessary if the technique is good. The method of sedation will depend

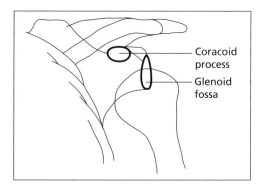

Figure 8.1 Anterior dislocation of the shoulder joint.

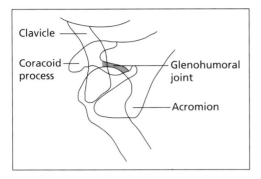

Figure 8.2 The normal appearance of the shoulder joint (apical view).

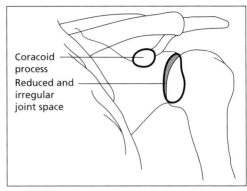

Figure 8.4 Posterior dislocation of the shoulder joint.

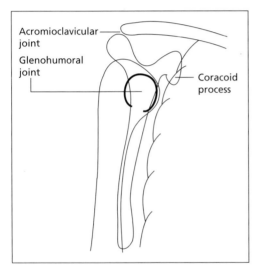

Figure 8.3 The normal appearance of the shoulder joint (lateral view).

Box 8.2 Reduction of a Dislocated Shoulder

● Explain the procedure to the patient.
● Ensure adequate sedation and analgesia are achieved and that appropriate resuscitation facilities are available.
● Gently hold the wrist on the dislocated side in both hands. Countertraction, if required, may be applied by a second person supporting the patient with a towel sling around the shoulder or by the operator's (unshod) toes in the axilla. The latter (Hippocratic) method requires the operator to stand on a low stool.
● Slowly (over a minute or two) abduct the arm out to 90°, keeping the elbow extended. As the arm is abducting, rotate it externally (i.e. so that the palm is facing upwards).
● Apply firm, constant traction along the patient's abducted, rotated arm. The shoulder joint is approaching its most unstable position. Gentle, uninterrupted traction with reassurance to maintain muscle relaxation is the key to success. Do not use excessive force as it may damage the axillary neurovascular structures. By slightly varying the angle of pull and the axial rotation of the arm the joint will usually relocate within about 5 min with minimal patient discomfort.

largely on the experience of the staff involved (*see page 17*). Many methods of reduction can be equally successful; a simple technique for anterior and posterior dislocations is described in *Box 8.2*.

Inferior dislocations usually reduce easily; the arm is gently brought down to a partially abducted position and then treated as an anterior dislocation.

Fracture of the greater tuberosity may accompany a dislocated shoulder. It will usually relocate easily as the shoulder dislocation is reduced.

Patients with a dislocation and a fracture of the neck of the humerus need immediate orthopaedic referral as do patients with a dislocation that is more than 24 h old.

After reduction, the arm is immobilised in a sling and a body bandage is applied to prevent abduction and external rotation. Radiographs are then repeated to confirm reduction and the arm is again examined to exclude neurovascular damage. The patient is then referred to the next fracture clinic with instructions to keep the wrist and hand mobile. Physiotherapy and gradual mobilisation will be necessary at a later date, possibly followed by surgical repair of the lax shoulder joint capsule if there has been recurrent dislocation.

Brachial plexus injuries

These injuries are caused by sudden traction on the arm (e.g. a window cleaner grasping the window ledge as the ladder slips) or by direct violence to the shoulder region (e.g. a motor cyclist struck from in front by an oncoming vehicle). They may also be seen in patients who have sustained prolonged pressure on the axilla while under the influence of alcohol. Proximal injuries may avulse the nerve roots from the spinal cord. Differing amounts of damage occur. There may be:

- *complete section* – neuroptmesis;
- *axonal damage* – axonoptmesis;
- *failure of transmission only* – neuropraxia;
- *a combination of the above.*

Neurological examination determines the areas involved. The presence of Horner's syndrome indicates pre-ganglionic damage. A histamine test on anaesthetised skin distinguishes lesions proximal (triple response) and distal (no response) to the dorsal root ganglion.

XR

Radiological examination should include the shoulder, cervical spine and thoracic outlet.

Tx

Early specialist referral will be required. Axonal regeneration down intact sheaths occurs at a rate of about 1 mm per day (or 1 inch per month). Surgical repair is rarely attempted and then mainly for distal lesions. No regeneration or repair is possible if part of the plexus has been avulsed from the spinal cord.

Fracture of the scapula

Fractures of the scapula are relatively uncommon and are usually the result of direct trauma. Significant force is required to break the scapula and so accompanying injuries must be excluded. Any part of the bone may be fractured including the body, spine, neck, acromion process and coracoid process. Local pain and tenderness are the main clinical features; shoulder movements may be relatively intact.

XR

Fractures of the scapula are often missed on X-ray. An oblique view of the shoulder (to show the scapula more clearly) may be requested in cases of doubt.

Tx

Displacement of a fracture of the spine or blade is rarely significant and management is conservative. The patient should be given a broad arm sling and analgesia and then referred to the next fracture clinic. The scapula has an excellent blood supply and usually heals very well.

Fracture of the humoral neck

This can occur at all ages, but is particularly common in the elderly. It is usually an isolated injury, caused by a low-speed impact. Displacement is common and may be gross, but is usually unimportant.

A full examination should be made to exclude other injury, particularly at the wrist. The axillary nerve may be damaged, causing deltoid paralysis and an area of anaesthesia over the outer aspect of the shoulder. The joint may sublux inferiorly because of this deltoid paralysis. The nerve will recover spontaneously over a period of a few weeks. Bruising is often very extensive and may extend down to the mid-forearm over the first few days. The patient should be warned that this rather frightening but harmless phenomenon might occur.

XR

An AP radiograph may be sufficient, but if shoulder dislocation is suspected an axial view will be required. In children, it is necessary to distinguish a greenstick fracture, with buckled cortex, from the normal epiphyseal line.

TX

A sling, analgesics and reassurance are all that are required initially. Fracture clinic referral is arranged; physiotherapy should follow.

Frozen shoulder

Adhesive capsulitis of the shoulder joint is most commonly seen in older patients. It may be spontaneous or follow the disuse associated with any type of upper limb injury. Early mobilisation after injury will help to prevent its development (e.g. for patients with Colles' fractures remove the sling every few hours so that the arm can be moved behind the back and the neck). Patients with established disease and no recent history of trauma may present to the ED. Cervical and thoracic outlet problems must be excluded. The patient often complains of pain at the deltoid insertion but is actually tender over the anterior capsule. Abduction and internal rotation are particularly restricted.

> When assessing glenohumoral movement, always put one hand on the scapula to exclude the scapulothoracic contribution to shoulder mobility.

XR

Radiographs may show an area of calcification in the shoulder joint capsule.

TX

This condition may be very slow (up to 2 years) to resolve spontaneously. The other shoulder may be affected just as the first is recovering. Physiotherapy is the mainstay of treatment. Steroid injection –

particularly into calcified areas of the capsule – and NSAIDs may be helpful. Manipulation under anaesthesia may sometimes be needed.

Thoracic outlet obstruction

The neurovascular outflow from the thorax and spine to the upper limb is constrained by a narrow-based triangle above the first rib. The lower parts of the brachial plexus and the subclavian artery may be compressed here if the shoulders are depressed by heavy backpacks or unaccustomed lifting. Symptoms are more likely if the brachial plexus is post-fixed (i.e. arises from the spinal cord more caudally than usual) or if there is a cervical rib. A tumour at the apex of the lung can spread upwards to involve the lower part of the brachial plexus.

The patient complains of a gradual onset of diffuse shoulder girdle pain, made worse by carrying shopping bags, etc. Symptoms can be reproduced by pulling down on the arm with the patient standing. The radial pulse may be obliterated if the arm is abducted to 90° and the patient turns his or her head to the opposite side. There may be weakness of the small muscles of the hand and paraesthesia in the hand extending up the inner border of the arm.

XR

Radiographs are taken of the cervical spine, the thoracic inlet and the chest.

TX

Always seek advice about management. If more sinister causes have been excluded, slow recovery usually occurs if traction on the shoulder can be avoided. Physiotherapy may help. Resection of the first rib may be necessary in severe cases.

Referred pain at the shoulder

Diaphragmatic irritation may produce shoulder-tip pain. Causes include cholecystitis, splenic injury, subphrenic abscess and pleurisy. Cardiac pain may present initially with a generalised ache in the shoulder joint.

Fracture of the humoral shaft

This fracture is unstable and painful and thus requires immediate splintage. The mechanism of injury and the possibility of damage elsewhere should always be considered. If little force was involved, pathological fracture is a possibility. The radial nerve is often damaged, but rarely divided, as it winds around the humoral shaft in the spiral groove; ensure ability to extend the wrist and fingers. The radial pulse should also be checked as brachial artery injury may sometimes occur.

XR

Radiographs should include the shoulder and elbow joints.

TX

Provide support and analgesia. Orthopaedic referral is indicated. Internal fixation is usually undertaken but external splintage with a U-slab of plaster and a collar and cuff is an alternative.

The elbow

The elbow may be injured by a direct blow or by transmitted forces. In children, the constantly changing epiphyses make the interpretation of radiographs rather difficult (*see Box 8.3 and Figure 8.5*).

> Full extension of the elbow (to a bony block) without pain makes the presence of a fracture very unlikely.

Pulled elbow

Sudden traction on a young child's arm may sublux the radial head through the soft annular ligament. A history of pulling may not be forthcoming. A fall may have occurred but picking the

---

> **Box 8.3 Elbow Radiographs in Children**
>
> Interpretation may be difficult in children but is aided by a knowledge of the times of appearance and fusion of secondary ossification centres (*see also Figure 8.5.*):
>
> | | | |
> |---|---|---|
> | C | 2 | Capitellum – present by age 2 years. |
> | R | 4 | Radial head – appears at 3–5 years of age. |
> | I | 6 | Internal or medial epicondyle – present by age 6 years. |
> | T | 8 | Trochlea – appears at age 7–9 years. |
> | O | 10 | Olecranon – appears at age 9–11 years. |
> | E | 12 | External or lateral epicondyle – present by age 11–14 years. |
>
> ● The epiphyses of the capitellum, the trochlea and the lateral epicondyle become one centre in the early teenage years.
> ● All the epiphyses fuse in teenage, usually a year or two later in boys than in girls.
> ● Comparative views of the other elbow, taken at the same angle, are occasionally helpful but should not be requested unless absolutely necessary.

child up afterwards is more likely to have caused the problem than the fall itself. The diagnosis should be suspected in a child who:

● is between 1 and 4 years old;
● has no history of significant trauma;
● is unwilling to use one arm;
● holds that arm limply by his or her side with the elbow semiflexed in mid-pronation;
● has no obvious swelling, bruising or tenderness;
● cries at attempts to elevate the arm.

XR

Radiographs are normal and initially it is unnecessary to take them.

TX

The subluxation is reduced by gentle but determined supination of the forearm with the elbow at 90° and a thumb over the radial head. A palpable click indicates success. Final reassurance for the doctor, and doubting parents, is obtained by letting the child play and watching normal movements return. This may take some time. Arms, which have been immobile for several hours, can be slightly swollen and more difficult to reduce.

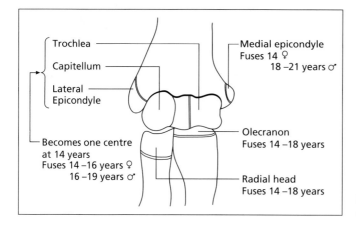

Trochlea

Capitellum

Lateral
Epicondyle

Becomes one centre
at 14 years
Fuses 14 –16 years ♀
16 –19 years ♂

Medial epicondyle
Fuses 14 ♀
18 –21 years ♂

Olecranon
Fuses 14 –18 years

Radial head
Fuses 14 –18 years

Figure 8.5 Secondary ossification centres around the elbow.

Do not attempt to reduce a pulled elbow if you are in any doubt about the diagnosis. You will probably not do any harm but the child's parents may be upset if you discover a fracture sometime later!

If the above procedure is unsuccessful at any stage, the whole arm should be re-examined and radiographed. If nothing abnormal is found, a collar and cuff should be supplied and the child reviewed within 48 h. Most cases settle spontaneously in a few days.

The parents can be reassured that although the condition may recur (in either arm), the ligaments

Box 8.4 The Management of the Child who is not Using an Arm

- Get a clear history.
- Watch the child playing with toys.
- Look for bruising, swelling or tenderness. Do not forget to examine the clavicle and wrist.
- Decide where the problem areas are. If there are no immediately obvious areas and the arm is held limply by the side, consider pulled elbow or fractured clavicle.
- Obtain radiographs of the whole arm, including the clavicle. If they seem normal, look again for buckle fractures of the wrist or clavicle and effusions of the elbow.
- If you are still no wiser, prescribe analgesia and a collar and cuff, reassure the parents and arrange for the child to be reviewed within 2 or 3 days.

will stiffen up after the age of 5 years and put an end to the problem (*See also Box 8.4*).

Supracondylar fracture

This injury occurs in older children (peak incidence at age 8 years) who fall on the outstretched arm. Severity varies from a hairline fracture to gross displacement, usually of the distal fragment posteriorly. All displaced fractures are associated with the risk of brachial artery injury; check distal pulses.

Fractures of this area in adults are often comminuted and involve the articular surface. The elbow is swollen and movement very restricted. Neurovascular damage may occur.

Tx

Reduction under general anaesthesia by the orthopaedic team and subsequent monitoring of distal neurovascular function is essential. Failure to do this may result in Volkmann's ischaemic contracture of the forearm muscles, with permanent disability in the hand. Internal fixation is often required especially if the articular surface is implicated. Some undisplaced fractures may be treated on an outpatient basis, but this decision should be left to the orthopaedic staff.

Fractures of the medial and lateral epicondyles

These fractures are caused by a varus or valgus strain at the elbow. Swelling may not be a major feature, but there is always a restriction of elbow extension and local bony tenderness. The medial epicondyle may be trapped in the joint; ulnar or median nerve injury may occur.

XR

Radiographs may show little more than an effusion (*see Figure 8.6*). Avulsion of an epicondyle in a child involves much more of the joint than the radiographs suggest, as most of the structure is cartilaginous.

Tx

An orthopaedic opinion is essential.

Fracture of the olecranon

This is sustained by falling on the point of the flexed elbow. Triceps action will distract the bone ends and a gap can usually be felt beneath

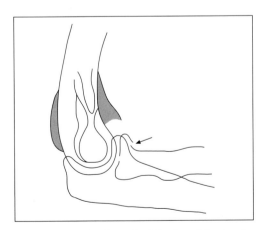

Figure 8.6 Lateral radiograph of the elbow joint showing anterior and posterior effusions (shaded) and fracture of the radial head (arrowed).

the rapidly developing haematoma and oedema. Active elbow extension is impossible. In the absence of an associated elbow dislocation, other movements particularly supination and pronation, are often quite good and pain-free.

Tx

The patient is given a sling whilst awaiting specialist advice. Inpatient care and internal fixation will be necessary.

Fracture of the head or neck of the radius

This common fracture is usually sustained by a fall on the outstretched arm. Elbow flexion may be full but extension is restricted. There is pain on palpation of the radial head, which is exacerbated during forearm rotation. Injury to the posterior interosseous nerve – which winds around the neck of the radius – is rare.

XR

Radiographs usually show an effusion (*see Figure 8.6*) but the fracture may be elusive. Further oblique views may be necessary.

> Radial head fracture is one of the most commonly missed limb injuries. It should be diagnosed clinically when there is:
> - an appropriate history;
> - local tenderness;
> - reduced extension and supination;
> - a positive fat pad sign on X-ray (anterior effusion).

Tx

Minor undisplaced fractures are treated conservatively with early mobilisation. The patient will need analgesia, a collar and cuff and referral to the next fracture clinic. More significant injuries may require internal fixation or excision of the radial head and should be referred immediately for specialist advice. (*See also Box 8.5*).

Dislocation of the elbow joint

This requires considerable force. Consequently, there are usually associated fractures of the coronoid process, olecranon, capitellum or trochlea. There may also be damage to the brachial artery, ulnar, median or radial nerves.

Tx

Analgesia and splintage should be provided prior to radiography and the radial pulse must be monitored. Reduction may be carried out in the ED by suitably experienced staff. Under sedation, axial traction is applied to the elbow while it is in about 30° of extension. Subsequent care is carried out by the orthopaedic department.

Epicondylitis: tennis elbow and golfer's elbow

Tennis elbow

This term describes pain around the lateral epicondyle of the humerus. The underlying 'epicondylitis' is most common between the ages of 40 and 60 years and is usually caused by repetitive hand and wrist movements. There is inflammation and sometimes partial avulsion of the common extensor origin, which may be tender. Nerve entrapment is occasionally responsible for the symptoms. Movements of the elbow joint are not usually reduced, although there may be slight restriction of pronation. Sudden passive flexion of the wrist, especially from the extended position, may reproduce the pain as may gripping and twisting movements.

XR

A radiograph may be taken to exclude fracture or bone disease. Ultrasound scan is also a useful investigation.

Tx

The inflammation is usually self-limiting although symptoms may persist for many months. In mild cases, an oral NSAID together with advice to modify activity at work or sport may be sufficient. A wrist brace may provide some symptomatic relief. Physiotherapy is of some value and local injection of steroid often helps. Surgical division of part of the extensor origin is occasionally necessary.

Golfer's elbow

This refers to a similar inflammation of the common flexor origin at the medial epicondyle of the humerus. There is chronic pain, which is worse on gripping. Treatment is similar to that for tennis elbow.

Degenerative disease of the elbow joint

Chronic osteoarthrosis of the elbow is usually secondary to imperfectly reduced fractures involving the articular surfaces. Symptoms may begin spontaneously or be triggered by further minor trauma. The main complaint is of an inability to extend the elbow fully with some restriction of forearm rotation. Loose bodies may cause locking. If the fracture occurred during childhood, inequalities of growth may have resulted in marked deformity.

A traction injury to the ulnar nerve may develop if cubitus valgus occurs after a lateral epicondyle fracture.

Xʀ

Radiographs may reveal more joint destruction than might be expected from clinical examination.

Tx

The elbow should be rested in a sling for a few days to allow any inflammation to settle. NSAIDs may also help. Physiotherapy often exacerbates elbow stiffness, whatever the aetiology. The patient should be referred to the orthopaedic department either directly or via the GP.

Olecranon bursitis

The patient presents with a large swelling over the olecranon, often following minor trauma. The elbow joint is not affected and is clinically normal except for pain on movement. The lump may be soft and fluctuant or tense and very painful if secondarily infected. Occasionally, the cause will be a crystal arthropathy.

Xʀ

Radiographs may reveal an underlying bony spur.

Tx

The inflammation usually settles with an elastic support bandage and NSAIDs. Antibiotics should be prescribed if there is evidence of spreading infection or if the patient is pyrexic. Rarely, incision and drainage will be required under adequate anaesthesia. The patient should be reviewed at a clinic after a few days. When the acute episode has resolved, consideration should be given to referring the patient for formal excision of the bursa and underlying spur. If crystal arthropathy is considered to be a serious possibility, then the patient should be discussed with a rheumatologist.

The forearm and wrist

Wounds to the forearm and wrist

Lacerations in this area frequently involve deep structures and accurate diagnosis is essential. The history is usually helpful, although many such injuries are either self-inflicted or sustained whilst intoxicated and so the patient's account may be misleading. Penetrating glass can cause nerve and tendon damage at a distance from the puncture wound and casual exploration under local anaesthesia will fail to reveal deep injuries. A full assessment of distal neurovascular function is essential. Test all tendons and nerves individually (*see Box 8.6*). Any positive finding of deep structure involvement must be discussed with a senior colleague at once. Further exploration must be carried out:

- in an operating theatre;
- under adequate anaesthesia (usually general);
- with a bloodless field;
- by an experienced surgeon.

> A divided nerve may continue to conduct some sensation for several hours if the nerve ends are touching.

Abductor pollicis brevis is paralysed in T1 root lesions but not in ulnar nerve lesions. To test this muscle the thumb is moved vertically upwards against resistance with the hand in a supine position.

> **Box 8.6 Median and Ulnar Nerve Supply to Muscles that are Involved in Movements of the Hand**
>
> *Nerve supply to the muscles of the anterior forearm.*
> The ulnar nerve supplies:
> 1 flexor carpi ulnaris;
> 2 half of flexor digitorum profundus.
> The median nerve supplies all the rest.
>
> *Nerve supply to the intrinsic muscles of the hand.*
> The median nerve supplies:
> 1 the lateral two lumbricals;
> 2 opponens pollicis;
> 3 abductor pollicis brevis;
> 4 flexor pollicis brevis.
> The ulnar nerve supplies all the rest.

Fractures of the midshafts of the radius and ulna

These injuries are of three types:

1 A direct blow to the forearm produces a transverse fracture of either the ulna or both bones at the same level.

2 Rotational or transmitted forces produce a spiral fracture of each bone at different levels.

3 Rotational forces produce a fracture of one bone and a dislocation of the other at either of the radio-ulnar joints (*see Figure 8.7*).

Clinical and radiological examination must thus include the elbow and wrist joints and neurovascular status must be carefully assessed. All of these forearm fractures are potentially unstable.

XR

One long X-ray plate, including both joints with the forearm bones, is inadequate as it produces oblique, atypical views of the joints, which are

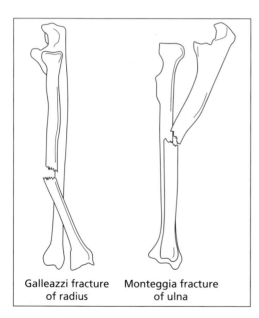

Galleazzi fracture   Monteggia fracture
of radius   of ulna

Figure 8.7 Fracture dislocations of the radius and ulna. *Galleazzi fracture dislocation*: Fracture of the RADIAL shaft with dorsal dislocation of the lower ulna from the inferior radio-ulnar joint.
Monteggia fracture dislocation: Fracture of the ULNAR shaft with volar dislocation of the radial head into the antecubital fossa.

difficult to interpret. Standard films of adjacent joints should be obtained.

Tx

Analgesia and splintage should precede orthopaedic advice. Closed manipulation of some fractures under general anaesthetic may be successful, but this should be carried out in a fully equipped operating theatre so that failure can be quickly followed by open reduction and internal fixation under the same anaesthetic.

Children

Children commonly sustain greenstick fractures of both forearm bones, in which case:

• there may be very little angulation;

• there is usually only a modest amount of pain;

• forearm rotation is always restricted;

• elbow and wrist movements may be full;

• neurovascular complications are unlikely.

For these reasons the fracture may be overlooked.

Tx for children

Management must be discussed with an experienced colleague. A well-padded, above-elbow plaster cast, a sling, oral analgesics and outpatient follow-up may be acceptable but significant displacement demands manipulation under general anaesthesia. This can be difficult. The greenstick fracture may have to be converted to a complete fracture before reduction can be achieved. Subsequent swelling caused by oedema formation and haematoma from the bone and damaged muscle always makes a second attempt technically more difficult. It is essential that the first attempt is successful and that the child is kept in hospital for 24 h with the arm elevated and the peripheral circulation carefully monitored.

Fractures of the distal radius

Fractures of the distal radius mostly occur in osteoporotic bone and so are most common in older women. These fractures are usually sustained by falling on the outstretched hand and consequently injuries higher up the arm should always be excluded. In adults, impaction of cancellous bone imparts some stability compared with the obvious instability of midshaft fractures. However, pain and deformity are usually obvious and supination is always restricted.

A Colles' fracture is actually defined as any fracture of the radius within 2.5 cm of the wrist joint but the term is usually taken to mean a wrist fracture with either dorsal displacement or anterior angulation. *For the six characteristic features of a Colles' fracture see Box 8.7.*

For management of fractures of the distal radius with volar displacement of the distal fragment see page 130.

Box 8.7 The Six Characteristic Features of a Displaced Colles' Fracture

1 Dorsal displacement
2 Anterior angulation
3 Impaction
4 Lateral (radial) displacement
5 Ulnar angulation
6 Rotational deformity
Avulsion of the ulnar styloid is a common accompanying feature.

XR

The degree of displacement or angulation, and therefore the need for reduction, can be estimated from the radiographs. The malposition is significant if either:

1 the articular surface of the distal radius on the lateral X-ray is not angulated in a volar direction, ie., if angle ABC as seen in *Figure 8.8* is less than 90°; or

2 radial shortening is seen on the AP view such that the ulnar articular surface is more than 2 mm distal to the radial articular surface.

Tx

For the purposes of management in the ED, there are three main types of Colles' fracture of the distal radius:

1 *Fracture with minimal or acceptable displacement in an older patient with osteoporotic bone*
● Confirm acceptable position (*see Figure 8.8*).
● Exclude other injuries.
● Exclude medical cause of fall.
● Apply padded forearm backslab.
● Provide sling and analgesia.
● Encourage shoulder and hand mobility.
● Ensure adequate domestic support.
● Refer to fracture clinic on the following day.

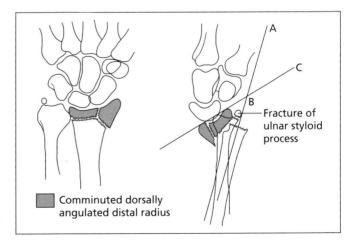

Figure 8.8 Comminuted Colles' fracture (with angle ABC identified).

A

C

B

Fracture of ulnar styloid process

Comminuted dorsally angulated distal radius

2 Displaced/angulated fracture in an osteoporotic wrist.

Treatment is as described in (1) above, but the fracture must be reduced under appropriate local, regional or general anaesthesia – *for one method of local anaesthesia see Box 8.8.* In some hospitals this will take place in the ED. Satisfactory home circumstances are then of even greater importance if post-operative discharge is anticipated.

Reduction is achieved by traction and slight hyperextension (to disimpact the fracture) and then flexion and ulnar deviation. Countertraction is applied by a colleague holding the upper arm. Unfortunately, the poor-quality dorsal cortex often allows the fracture to redisplace over the next 2 weeks. Re-manipulation may then be necessary. Good function is more important than good anatomical and radiological reduction, but this fact should not influence initial attempts to obtain perfection. The manipulated fracture is held in its reduced position by a plaster backslab, which extends from the metacarpal heads to the antecubital fossa, over the dorsoradial aspect of the forearm. Radiographs must be taken after reduction but before ending the anaesthetic, so that an inadequate manipulation can be corrected immediately (*see Figure 8.8*). Because of the difficulty in maintaining a good position after reduction, many orthopaedic surgeons prefer to manipulate these fractures in theatre and then fix the bones in position with wires.

3 Fracture in a younger patient.

After providing temporary splintage and analgesia, refer the patient to the orthopaedic team for reduction and plating of the fracture under general anaesthesia.

Box 8.8 Haematoma Block for Reduction of a Colles' Fracture

- Use an aseptic technique; clean the skin thoroughly.
- Inject a maximum of 20 mL of prilocaine 0.25% into the fracture haematoma. Approach from the dorsal aspect; the fracture site lies more proximally than you might expect.
- Also inject some local anaesthetic around the ulnar styloid.

Smith's fracture

A 'reversed Colles' fracture' in which the distal radial fragment is displaced in a volar direction and is tilted anteriorly (i.e. there is posterior angulation). It usually results from a fall onto the back of the hand. All such fractures should be discussed with the orthopaedic department.

Barton's fracture

A type of Smith's fracture in which only the anterior portion of the distal radius is involved. It should be referred to the orthopaedic team for fixation.

Significant injury to the wrist is very unlikely following minor trauma if:

1 full supination is possible without pain;
2 there is no tenderness in the anatomical snuff box.

Wrist fractures in children

In children three types of wrist fracture are commonly seen:

1) Distal radial epiphysis

The distal radial epiphysis may slip dorsally, usually taking with it a flake of metaphysis (*see Figure 8.9*).

Tx

Reduction is easily achieved by the orthopaedic staff under general anaesthetic and maintained by a forearm plaster backslab. Outpatient follow-up is appropriate. The patient is given a sling and oral analgesic.

2) Distal radial metaphysis

A complete fracture may occur through the distal radial metaphysis, often with significant displacement of the distal fragment (*see Figure 8.10*).

Tx

Reduction can be difficult and may even require open operation. Refer for orthopaedic advice.

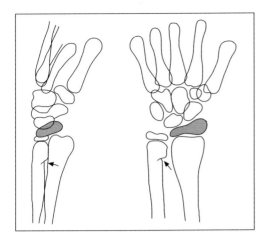

Figure 8.9 Posterior displacement of distal radial epiphysis (shaded) with buckle fracture of ulna (arrowed).

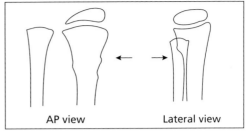

AP view   Lateral view

Figure 8.11 Buckle fracture of the distal radius (arrowed).

The radiological abnormality is often minimal *(see Figure 8.11)*.

Tx

These fractures rarely require manipulation and can be managed on an outpatient basis in a forearm plaster cast or wrist brace and sling.

Fracture of the radial styloid

This injury may mimic an undisplaced Colles' fracture or a scaphoid injury.

Tx

A Colles'-type plaster should be applied and the patient followed-up in fracture clinic.

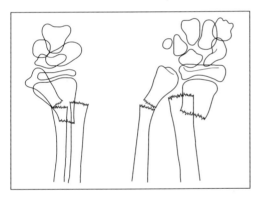

Figure 8.10 Metaphyseal (pronator quadratus) fracture of the distal radius and ulna.

Small chip fractures of the carpus

These are commonly seen after hyperextension or flexion injuries of the wrist.

Xr

The bone of origin is not always obvious.
For the relative positions of the carpal bones see Figure 8.12.

3) Lower radial metaphysis

A buckle (or torus) fracture of the lower radial metaphysis may be easily overlooked. The child always has limitation of supination by at least 10° and is tender over the lower radius. There may be almost no visible swelling.

> All children with wrist pain need an X-ray, even if their wrist looks normal.

Tx

The wrist usually needs support in a cast or splint for 3 or 4 weeks.

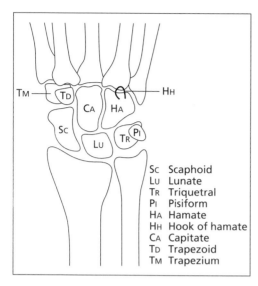

Figure 8.12 The carpal bones (AP view).

Sc Scaphoid
Lu Lunate
Tr Triquetral
Pi Pisiform
Ha Hamate
Hh Hook of hamate
Ca Capitate
Td Trapezoid
Tm Trapezium

Fracture of the scaphoid bone

The carpal bones lie in two rows but the scaphoid bone straddles both rows on the radial side. During trauma, considerable force may be transmitted through it, thus making it the most commonly fractured carpal bone (70% of all carpal fractures). *For the sites of fracture in the scaphoid bone see Figure 8.13.* Fracture of the scaphoid bone is most common in men aged between 20 and 50 years. The relative compressibility of the bone in children makes fracture uncommon under the age of 14 years, although it can occur in children as young as 8 years old. Early and accurate diagnosis of fractures of the scaphoid bone is essential to avoid the complications of avascular necrosis, non-union and radiocarpal arthrosis. The diagnosis should be suspected if there is:

1 An appropriate mechanism of injury – usually a fall onto the outstretched hand or a direct blow to the scaphoid area.
2 Tenderness in the anatomical snuffbox between the long and short extensors of the thumb and also on the dorsal and volar aspects of the scaphoid bone. In particular, the scaphoid tubercle may be tender when palpated on the palmar aspect of the wrist in radial deviation. Accompanying swelling is usually minimal.

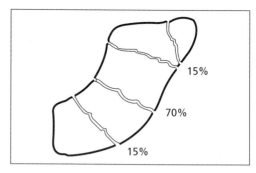

Figure 8.13 Sites of fracture in the scaphoid bone.

3 A well-preserved range of movements. Forced thumb abduction and extension are usually painful as are pronation and ulnar deviation of the wrist.
4 A positive compression test. (Hold the thumb and apply pressure along the thumb metacarpus; a positive test causes wrist pain.)

Unfortunately, many soft tissue injuries, fracture of the radial styloid process and osteoarthritis of the carpo–metacarpal joint may present a similar clinical picture.

> The extensive articular surface of the scaphoid bone restricts the sites of vascular supply. Consequently, avascular necrosis – and long-term disability – may follow a missed fracture. This can cause more long-term morbidity than many major trunk injuries.

Xr

Two special radiographs of the wrist (ie. scaphoid views = oblique and AP in ulnar deviation) should be obtained in addition to the standard two films. Even so, radiological evidence of the fracture may be elusive until bone resorption at 10–14 days has widened the fracture line. (The sensitivity of the first series of X-rays is only 65%.) Displacement of the fragments is uncommon. Magnetic resonance imaging is now replacing the traditional technetium bone scan (scintigraphy) as the definitive diagnostic modality for the carpus. ˙

Tx

Patients with definite fractures should have their wrists immobilised in a cast (extending from the thumb interphalangeal joint to the elbow) with specialist follow-up at 2 weeks. Prolonged immobilisation (up to 3 months) will be required until there is both clinical and radiological proof of union.

If the fracture has not been confirmed on X-ray, patients should be treated according to the severity of their symptoms. For most, this will entail support of the wrist in a splint but patients with severe pain will still require a cast. After 2 weeks, the wrist should be re-examined and further radiographs performed. Patients who have negative X-rays but who are still symptomatic must be reviewed at 2-week intervals. Magnetic resonance or scintigraphic imaging may be required to reach a diagnosis.

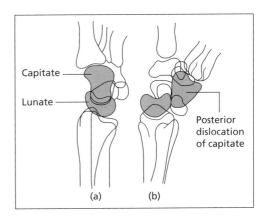

Figure 8.14 Lateral views of the wrist: (a) normal left and (b) abnormal right with perilunar dislocation.

Carpal dislocation

This uncommon problem is often missed on radiographs, although clinically there is obviously something wrong as swelling and pain are usually considerable. The lunate may be dislocated into the palm (anterior dislocation of the lunate) or the entire distal carpal row may dislocate dorsally (perilunar dislocation). In the latter case, there is often an associated fracture of the scaphoid. Other variations are also described. Median nerve signs may occur as a result of direct compression in the carpal tunnel.

XR

The lateral radiograph is diagnostic *(see Figure 8.14)*.

Tx

Immediate specialist referral is essential. Closed reduction under general anaesthesia may be successful. The injured part must be elevated and distal neurovascular function assessed.

Wrist sprain

Diffuse pain may follow either a fall on to the out-stretched hand or a hyperflexion injury. Tenderness is usually maximal over the dorsum of the carpus or at the inferior radio-ulnar joint. The degree of swelling is variable.

XR

Scaphoid views should be requested but will be normal in the presence of a sprain.

Tx

Suspicion of scaphoid injury should be treated accordingly. Most patients with a sprained wrist settle spontaneously if provided with a wrist brace for 10–14 days. However, occasionally significant ligamentous damage will have been sustained leading to carpal instability and long-term disability. Patients with symptoms of a wrist sprain that do not begin to resolve within 2 weeks, should be referred for specialist advice. Subsequent arthroscopy may identify specific lesions, which are amenable to surgical repair.

Carpal tunnel syndrome

The median nerve may be compressed because its tunnel has become smaller (e.g. after a carpal fracture) or because the nerve has become larger (e.g. in leprosy). However, the usual cause is that the

contents of the carpal tunnel have expanded and the most common reasons for this are:
- interstitial fluid retention in pregnant and middle-aged women;
- rheumatoid disease;
- myxoedema;
- acromegaly.

The condition is unusual, but not rare, in men.

The patient complains of paraesthesia in the hand and arm. The distribution varies but commonly includes the forearm and excludes the little finger. Symptoms classically awaken the patient in the early hours of the morning and are relieved by hand exercises or by hanging the arm out of bed. Examination reveals anaesthesia and thenar muscle wasting in advanced disease; otherwise, there is merely subjective impairment of touch. Pressure applied over the carpal tunnel may increase the symptoms. The upper limb should be examined to exclude pathology of the elbow, shoulder, thoracic outlet and cervical spine as nerve entrapment at these points can produce similar symptoms.

XR

Radiographs are taken to exclude previous carpal fracture.

Tx

Temporary relief of symptoms may be achieved by splinting the wrist with a removable brace in partial flexion at night. This is particularly useful in pregnancy. Other patients must be referred to the orthopaedic clinic for surgical release.

Peritendonitis crepitans

This condition is more common than de Quervain's tenosynovitis and involves the more proximal part of the extensor tendons where there is no synovial sheath. The patient, usually male, presents with pain on moving the wrist. There may be a recent history of unaccustomed or repetitive wrist movements. On examination there is a fusiform swelling over the radial side of the forearm, over which crepitus may be felt when the wrist is moved.

Tx

The wrist should be rested in a removable splint during the day and NSAIDs should be supplied. With this treatment the condition usually settles within a few days. In prolonged cases, physiotherapy with ultrasound treatment is helpful.

De Quervain's tenosynovitis

Inflammation of the tendon sheaths of extensor pollicis brevis and abductor pollicis longus (at the volar side of the anatomical snuff box) produces acute local tenderness. Pain extends over the dorsolateral aspect of the forearm and is made worse by thumb movements.

Tx

Immobilisation (thus stopping repetitive hand and wrist movements) will allow most cases to settle spontaneously. A replaceable splint is suitable. Referral back to the patient's GP is appropriate but some resistant cases may require steroid injection or surgical division of the stenosing tendon sheaths.

Avascular necrosis of the lunate

This condition is thought to be a long-term complication of minor wrist trauma without fracture. The patient presents with diffuse pain, which is worse on exercise; there is no recent history of injury.

XR

The radiograph is diagnostic, showing a relatively dense lunate in a porotic carpus.

Tx

A wrist splint should be supplied and an orthopaedic clinic appointment made; excision of the lunate bone may be necessary.

Osteoarthrosis of the wrist

This commonly involves the carpometacarpal joint of the thumb in older patients. It is often asymptomatic until minor trauma to the wrist causes pain in the joint. Symptoms suggest a scaphoid fracture, but this is unusual in the elderly.

XR

Degenerative changes in the joint are obvious on X-ray.

Tx

Symptoms are treated with a support bandage and NSAIDs and the patient is referred to the GP.

Sudek's atrophy

Rarely, a trivial injury to the hand or wrist may lead to this syndrome, which is characterised by vasomotor disturbance. Pain is the dominant symptom throughout. The skin is hot and dry at first and the hand and forearm are swollen. These signs settle after a few weeks but the patient continues to complain of discomfort.

The aetiology of Sudek's atrophy is unknown but the condition usually resolves spontaneously after many months. Early mobilisation after injury may prevent its occurrence.

XR

The affected areas may appear osteoporotic on X-ray.

Tx

Physiotherapy gives symptomatic relief. Orthopaedic referral is essential.

Chapter 9

The hand

The hand is a vital organ of function and is also important cosmetically. Its role in operating machines and using tools places it at a high risk of injury; 10–15% of all patients attending an ED have injured their hands.

Immediate assessment and management

- Check the patient's general condition – ABCs.
- Make a quick local assessment.
- Stop major bleeding by applying direct pressure.
- Remove rings and bracelets.
- Detect and document sensory loss.
- Inject local anaesthetic if necessary.
- Take a history of the injury.
- Take a brief past and social history.
- Begin a detailed examination.
- Obtain X-rays.

Swelling

Swelling, which accompanies soft-tissue injury, may produce venous occlusion under constricting bands such as rings and bracelets. The swelling will increase and eventually cause interruption of the arterial supply. Early removal of jewellery is essential, using ring-cutters if necessary.

Pain

Pain may be severe. It heightens anxiety. Early injection of local anaesthetic (after examination

of sensation) brings immediate relief. Subsequent cleaning and clinical and radiological examination can be carried out more carefully and therefore more accurately.

Cleaning

Cleaning can often be started by the patient. Industrial hand injuries are often extremely dirty. There is little point in applying a clean dressing to an oasis of sterile sutured skin that is surrounded by grease and grime.

History

The history may give important information on the extent of occult injury, for example, contusion and devitalisation caused by crushing, direction of wounding, retained foreign bodies or injection of material through high-pressure hoses.

Examination of the hand should follow the usual sequence of four four-letter words: *look, feel, move, X-ray*. Findings should be recorded with the aid of drawings. Digits must be identified by name, that is, index, middle, ring and little – never by number.

Wounds to the hand

For the general management of wounds see Chapter 21. In the hand, skin is at a premium and must be handled gently and conservatively;

toothed forceps should be avoided. The main obstacles to sound healing are haematoma, infection and tension.

- Dead tissue must be excised, but the normal blood supply is good and may maintain flaps that would die elsewhere.
- Cleaning must be thorough. Gentle use of a toothbrush or a scrubbing brush is effective.
- Lacerations over the dorsum of the hand, sustained in a fight, are often inflicted by the opponent's teeth. They are human bites and must be treated accordingly (*see page 394*).
- Patients with compound fractures should be given systemic antibiotics and referred for specialist care. Osteomyelitis or septic arthritis may not be radiographically apparent for the first 10 days after infection.
- All patients with hand wounds must be protected against tetanus. *See page 390.*
- The median nerve motor supply to the thenar muscles (*see page 127*) is very superficial and may be damaged by apparently minor wounds to the radial side of the palm.
- Adhesive, reinforced paper skin closures are not suitable for hand and proximal finger lacerations as they either restrict movement or impair blood supply.
- Sutures to the palm that are too large or badly placed adhesive strips, may cause skin overlap and a final unacceptable, proud wound.

Crush injuries

Inspection may not be a reliable guide to the extent of crushing. The history can give valuable additional information.

XR

This is almost always indicated.

TX

If the whole hand has been crushed, for example between rollers, admission and elevation are necessary even if the initial examination does not reveal extensive injuries.

Less extensive crushing injuries can be treated in the ED by:

- excluding injury to deep structures (X-ray and clinical examination);
- providing local anaesthesia;
- cleaning thoroughly (scrubbing brush or toothbrush);
- delaying closure for 3–5 days until the oedema has settled.

Amputation of the fingers

This type of damage to the fingers is common in many different types of workplace. The injury may be sharp or the finger may be crushed.

XR

This is necessary to exclude bony damage.

TX

Amputation of the digits proximal to the distal interphalangeal (DIP) joint may be suitable for re-implantation – *see page 389.*

Loss of more than the tip of the phalanx requires an orthopaedic opinion. Clean amputations through the terminal phalanx are best treated by primary closure. It may be necessary to trim the bone to allow flaps to be prepared without tension. The volar flap should be the longest, to achieve a dorsal suture line. Crush injuries producing amputation at this level must be left open.

Amputations through the finger tip can be left to close spontaneously. Cleaning must be vigorous and all dead tissue and dirt must be removed. The wound should then be covered with a non-adherent dressing and inspected not more than twice weekly. Antibiotics are not required unless there is bony involvement or infection is evident at the first dressing change. Exposed bone is best treated by referral for trimming.

> Finger tip injuries that remain red, tender or swollen for more than 10 days must be X-rayed to exclude osteomyelitis.

Partial avulsion of the finger tip

A combination of crushing and flexion of the finger tip (e.g. finger trapped by a door) may partially avulse the proximal end of the nail. There may be an associated crush fracture of the terminal phalanx (*see Figure 9.1*). This injury is very common in children.

XR

This should be obtained in all cases.

Tx

- Obtain adequate conditions for the repair. *For sedation of children see page 347.* General anaesthesia is always an option.
- Anaesthetise with a ring block.
- Clean the area thoroughly.
- Restore the normal alignment of the finger. It may sometimes be possible to replace a nail with a firm distal attachment under the proximal skin fold; otherwise remove it. Do not leave the nail in an avulsed position as it will splint the bone and/or finger pulp in the same position.
- Maintain the alignment with sutures to the lateral lacerations if needed but do not suture the nail bed (*see Figure 9.2*).
- Dress the finger with a non-adherent, antiseptic dressing.

- Provide adequate splintage. A Mallet splint may be slit dorsally for this purpose.
- Arrange follow-up.

The tip of the finger will swell but decompression will occur through the laceration.

Pressure hose injuries

Penetrating injuries may be inflicted by a variety of industrial tools. The most dangerous is the high-pressure hose, which can inject its contents (air, paint, grease, etc.) into the finger painlessly and leave an apparently normal digit. Symptoms appear after 24 h, when extensive soft-tissue destruction is apparent. *See also page 395.*

XR

This may reveal particles or an air track.

Tx

Orthopaedic referral is necessary for observation; debridement and decompression, if required.

Tendon injuries

Injuries to the tendons of the hand are common and are often overlooked. Even the smallest wound to the skin may sometimes have allowed sufficient penetration to damage a tendon. Wounds involving glass are particularly sinister in

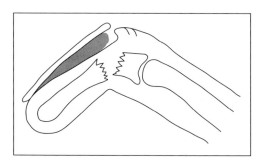

Figure 9.1 Crush-flexion injury to the finger tip.

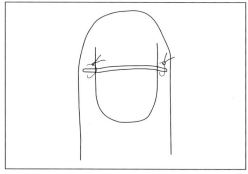

Figure 9.2 Position of sutures after removal of nail in crush-flexion injury.

this respect. Loss of function is the only reliable sign. Extensor tendon division is relatively easy to diagnose; for the detection of flexor tendon damage *see Box 9.1*. Also note the following:

- In the relaxed hand, the fingers tend to be held in increasing flexion from index to little finger. A pointing finger, which is out of line with this trend, suggests a flexor tendon or nerve injury.
- Partial division of a tendon may be overlooked initially but subsequent rupture may occur. Suspicion of a tendon injury warrants referral for exploration.
- The relationship between a tendon and the overlying skin varies with joint position. This means that the damage to a tendon may not be immediately visible through a skin wound. The tendon must therefore be inspected during finger or wrist movements.

XR

All wounds involving glass must be X-rayed.

Box 9.1 The Detection of Flexor Tendon Injuries

Anatomy. Flexor digitorum superficialis is used for fine movements. It has four fairly distinct muscle bellies. Each tendon inserts into the base of a middle phalanx. Flexor digitorum profundus is used for power grip. It arises as one muscle and is variably divided towards the musculotendinous junction. Each tendon inserts into the base of a distal phalanx.

Theory. Hyperextension of one finger tip will stretch all the profundus belly and preclude it from initiating flexion of any of the other fingers. Flexion of the unrestrained fingers can only be achieved at the proximal interphalangeal (PIP) joint by action of the more independent superficialis tendon.

Testing. For profundus assess active flexion at the DIP joint. For superficialis assess active flexion of the whole finger while the other fingers are hyperextended. Normally, flexion will occur at the PIP joint with the DIP joint remaining flaccid (profundus inactivated). If superficialis is divided, the whole finger will be flaccid.

TX

Extensor tendons on the back of the hand may be repaired in the ED if a clean theatre and appropriate skill are available. Patients with other tendon injuries must always be referred. Minor degrees of tendon damage, involving less than one-third of the diameter of the tendon, may be managed conservatively but this needs experienced judgement.

Injuries to digital nerves

Like tendon injuries, nerve injuries may not be immediately apparent. In both cases, deceptively small wounds can be sufficiently large to allow underlying damage. Distal sensation should always be tested and any complaint of changed sensation should be taken seriously. Sometimes the patient complains of paraesthesia in the affected digit but retains crude awareness of touch as a result of apposition of the severed nerve ends. The affected skin becomes dry 24 h later and is evidently anaesthetised. Patients often describe the sensation of absent nerve conduction in terms of their last experience of it – as being injected by the dentist with local anaesthesic.

TX

Neural injury distal to the PIP joint rarely warrants repair. Any resulting area of anaesthesia will become smaller with the passage of time as ingrowth occurs from other nerves.

The digital nerve is more commonly damaged in its superficial position near the metacarpophalangeal (MCP) joint. Repair is indicated, especially if the anaesthesia is on the ulnar border of the little finger, the radial aspect of the index finger or on the thumb. If in doubt, the patient should be referred for a specialist opinion.

Metacarpal fractures

Spiral fracture of the shaft of the metacarpus

This injury is produced by rotational forces on the finger. Rarely, it may be compound or multiple. The fracture is stable and usually undisplaced as a result of the integrity of the transverse metacarpal ligaments. Tendon and neurovascular damage is rare.

XR

Anteroposterior and oblique views of the hand usually show the fracture clearly. Overlapping soft-tissue shadow or nutrient artery may be misinterpreted as an undisplaced spiral fracture.

TX

Encourage movement but give a little support initially to alleviate pain. Follow-up should be in the fracture clinic.

Very rarely, rotational instability will result in persisting rotation of the finger, which is more easily detected on clinical than radiological examination. An immediate orthopaedic opinion is then necessary.

Transverse fracture of the metacarpal shaft

This injury is the result of direct trauma. It is often multiple and may be compounded with extensive soft-tissue damage. The inherent stability of the metacarpal arch is lost and so displacement is common.

XR

Epiphyseal lines may be partially developed at the proximal end of the index finger metacarpus and are commonly misinterpreted as linear fractures.

TX

This fracture requires immediate specialist attention. Internal fixation may be necessary to achieve stable reduction.

Fracture of the metacarpal neck

This is often termed the boxer's fracture, although most patients do not admit to fighting or, more usually, to missing their opponent and hitting a brick wall. The fracture is usually of the little metacarpus but injury to the ring or other metacarpal bones may also be seen.

> If the overlying skin is injured, it should be assumed that this is caused by contact with the opponent's teeth. This compound fracture has the potential to develop the serious complications of a human bite (*see page 394*).

In the absence of a bite injury, associated damage to deep structures is unusual. The metacarpal head may be angulated into the palm by up to 90°. Pain and angulation cause an associated lag in extension of the corresponding finger.

XR

The fracture is confirmed on oblique films of the hand, but may be missed on an anteroposterior film.

TX

Various manoeuvres have been described to achieve reduction of the displaced metacarpal head. These usually fail to maintain a good position and, indeed, are unnecessary because remodelling will achieve good long-term function despite gross initial displacement. The patient should be warned that inability to extend the affected finger fully will persist for a few months, but that normal function can be guaranteed if the joints are mobilised as soon as possible. This explanation is an important part of the treatment. Most long-term complications are a direct result of immobilisation.

A crepe bandage and oral analgesia are supplied for use in the first few days and the patient should then be reviewed to ensure appropriate mobilisation.

Bone and joint injuries to the fingers

Dislocation of the metacarpophalangeal joint

Dislocation without fracture may occur in either direction. The metacarpal head may 'button hole' through the articular capsule, which then becomes closely applied to the metacarpal neck and prevents closed reduction.

Tx

This dislocation should be referred for specialist advice. Open reduction may be necessary. The prognosis is usually good.

Ligament injuries of the metacarpophalangeal joint

Ligament injuries may occur at the index and little finger MCP joints caused by sudden sideways forces.

XR

Such injuries may be associated with minor flake fractures of the proximal phalanx – representing avulsion of the attachment of the collateral ligament – or with fractures of the base of the phalanx (see below).

Tx

These injuries resolve with conservative management unless the joint is grossly unstable, when open repair is indicated. Strapping the finger to its neighbour is sufficient. This allows flexion but prevents abduction. Follow-up by the orthopaedic department is advisable.

Fracture of the base of the proximal phalanx

This is most commonly seen, as a greenstick or buckle injury, in the little finger of children (*see Figure 9.3*).

XR

The fracture is often overlooked on X-ray. Post-reduction films are indicated if manipulation is attempted.

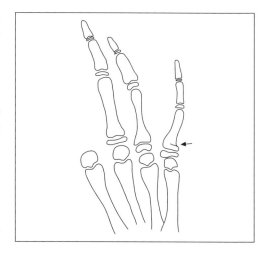

Figure 9.3 Greenstick fracture of the base of the proximal phalanx of the little finger.

Tx

Reduction may be achieved under local anaesthesia by inserting a pencil into the cleft between the little and ring fingers and pushing the little finger towards the ring finger. Neighbour strapping is then applied and follow-up arranged.

Other fractures of the proximal phalanx

Proximal phalanx fractures may occur through the base, shaft or neck. When compound, they must be referred immediately for specialist treatment. Antibiotics should be started in the ED and antitetanus cover provided. Fractures into the joint also require orthopaedic care.

Spiral fractures

These may produce rotational deformity, which is not always evident on X-ray. Rotation is best detected clinically by noting the relative positions of the finger nails when the fingers are fully flexed into the palm. All the nails should lie in approximately the same plane with the fingertips pointing towards the palpable part of the radial artery. Rotational deformity, if found, requires orthopaedic correction.

Fractures at the metaphyses

Fractures at the metaphyses through cancellous bone are usually stable and, if not significantly displaced, can be treated conservatively by neighbour-strapping. Displaced metaphyseal fractures may be reduced under local anaesthetic by manipulation over a pencil.

Fractures in the cortical diaphysis

These are more often displaced and very unstable. Delayed displacement of apparently stable fractures may occur. They may require internal fixation and should be referred immediately to the orthopaedic department.

Injury to the proximal interphalangeal joint

The PIP joint deserves careful consideration because:
1 it has the largest range of movement;
2 long-term stiffness is a major disability;
3 initial injury is often overlooked;
4 delayed displacement of the extensor tendon can occur.

The extensor hood, volar plate and collateral ligaments may all be damaged without joint dislocation and assessment can be difficult.

> The ability to extend fully, or even slightly hyperextend, all of the joints (especially the PIP joint) of an injured finger is associated with a good recovery. Failure to achieve a straight finger must be followed up as the flexion may become permanent.

XR

Initial radiographs may look normal, even in the presence of a serious injury. Volar plate fractures are often missed.

Tx

A patient with a PIP joint that is swollen or has a reduced range of movements, should be followed up in clinic. Swelling can take several months to settle.

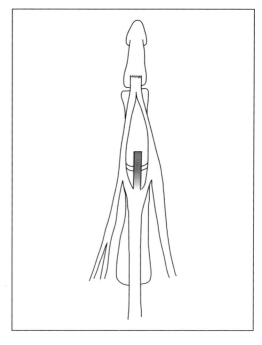

Figure 9.4 The extensor tendons of the finger. The central slip to the middle phalanx is shaded.

The boutonnière deformity

Extensor hood and central slip rupture may go unrecognised (*see Figure 9.4*). Extension may be possible initially because the lateral bands remain intact but, if the finger is not splinted, these gradually migrate laterally and within a few days lie anterior to the axis of the joint. The extensor mechanism now flexes the proximal joint, and by a compensatory device hyperextends the distal joint. This is a boutonnière deformity. To prevent this serious complication all significant proximal interphalangeal joint injuries should be immobilised in extension and advice sought.

Dislocation of the proximal interphalangeal joint

Dislocation may occur in either direction. Buttonhole entrapment of the head of the proximal phalanx in the disrupted volar plate (capsule) is particularly difficult to reduce and requires expert surgical skill to repair.

XR

Radiographs should always be taken before reduction of any finger dislocation.

TX

Manipulation may be attempted under local anaesthesia but if the dislocation does not reduce easily on the first attempt, specialist advice must be sought. Repeated attempts at closed reduction will increase soft-tissue damage and make open repair more difficult. If closed reduction is immediately successful and examination does not reveal major ligamentous instability, the finger is held fully extended in a volar splint and strapped to its neighbour. The MCP joint must be left free to allow 90° of flexion. The patient is referred to the next fracture clinic.

Fracture of the intermediate phalanx

Fractures of the middle phalanx often extend into either joint and thereby produce an inherently unstable finger with a tendency to increasing deformity.

TX

These injuries must be referred for specialist advice, however small the fracture and however minimal the apparent displacement.

Dislocation of the distal interphalangeal joint

The DIP joint has a smaller range of movement than the more proximal joints and injury to it is less often associated with major disability.

Dislocation of the DIP joint may be accompanied by a flake fracture from adjacent bone. This may indicate collateral ligament injury if it is lateral, or long-tendon avulsion if more central.

XR

Radiographs must precede attempts to reduce the dislocation and repeat clinical examination must follow successful reduction.

TX

Reduction is achieved by axial traction, without excessive force. Follow-up is required to ensure return of full movement.

Mallet finger

Extensor tendon avulsion from the terminal phalanx produces a Mallet deformity. Passive movements are full and pain-free, but there is no active extension at the DIP joint.

XR

Radiographs should be taken to exclude other fractures. The presence of a small dorsal flake fracture improves the prognosis – the repair potential of bone is better than that of the extensor tendon.

TX

This is conservative. The DIP joint is held in full extension continuously for 6 weeks by a small plastic (Mallet) splint. The proximal joint can be left free. Painting the area under the splint with iodine helps to reduce subsequent maceration of the skin. Follow-up should be arranged in the fracture clinic.

The splint may be changed occasionally to allow skin cleaning but the finger must not be allowed to flex whilst unsplinted. After 6 weeks the splint is worn only at night and during heavy manual work for a further month.

Full return of active extension cannot be guaranteed. Functional disability is minimal even if no treatment is given, although there is also a cosmetic consideration. Some patients prefer to accept this outcome rather than suffer the restrictions imposed by a finger splint.

Fracture of the distal phalanx

These fractures are usually produced by crushing forces and are often comminuted. They may cause problems at the DIP joint when they extend across the articular surface but this is unusual. Bleeding is

143

restricted by the fibrous loculi of the pulp space and by the nail to produce a subungual haematoma. Interstitial pressure quickly rises and the pain is severe.

Tx

Trephining the nail with a red-hot paper clip brings instant relief to the patient who has a haematoma under the nail. It is not contraindicated in the presence of a fracture. The nail is insensitive and the blunt paper clip produces a wide sterile hole compared with that produced by the tip of a drill.

A simple fracture of the terminal phalanx can be treated in a Mallet splint for 2–3 weeks until the pain has settled. More commonly, there is a soft-tissue injury, which demands more careful attention (*see page 138*).

Injuries to the thumb

Thumb injuries produce greater disability than similar injuries to the other digits because of impairment of pinch and grip. Principles of treatment are similar, but particular attention is given to maintenance of length after terminal injury and the ability to oppose and rotate the thumb against the other fingers.

> A thumb that can be flexed to touch the palm of the hand at the base of the little finger is unlikely to be severely injured.

Fracture of the thumb metacarpus

These fractures are often the result of an oblique abducting force and may be disabling. They usually occur through the proximal part or the base of the metacarpus. There is a painful swollen deformity at the base of the thumb but associated deep, soft-tissue injuries are uncommon.

Xr

Epiphyseal lines may be partially developed at the distal end of the thumb metacarpus and are commonly misinterpreted as linear fractures.

Tx

If the fracture enters the carpometacarpal (trapezometacarpal) joint (Bennett's fracture), displacement is significant and reduction is then difficult. The patient should be referred to the orthopaedic department as internal fixation may be necessary. Closed manipulation may succeed but must be carried out by an experienced doctor. The fracture is usually held in a modified scaphoid plaster cast with the thumb abducted.

The more usual fracture through the metacarpal base, not involving the joint, is adequately treated in a scaphoid plaster cast. Reduction is not usually necessary.

Injury to the MCP joint of the thumb

Injury to the MCP joint of the thumb may be incapacitating as functional impairment is associated with thumb instability. The collateral ligaments or the MCP joint capsule may be extensively torn by forced extension or abduction. The ulnar collateral ligament is the most frequently damaged structure. Chronic injury to this ligament was common in gamekeepers. Nowadays skiers sustain an acute injury by pulling the thumb back in the ski stick strap or artificial ski slope matting during a fall – hence the term skier's thumb.

Examination reveals specific tenderness over the palmar and web aspects of the MCP joint and pain on attempted abduction. There is usually a haematoma in the thenar area. The laxity of the joint may be compared with that of the opposite thumb. Instability is not always apparent because of the protective action of the thenar muscles.

Xr

Stress views may show subluxation of the joint. Local anaesthetic around the metacarpus may be required to enable this procedure.

Tx

Operative repair or plaster cast immobilisation may be indicated for significant ligamentous injury; specialist advice should be sought. Injuries to the MCP joint without either laxity or haematoma can be treated with a bandage thumb spica and review in clinic.

Dislocation of the MCP joint of the thumb

Reduction can be achieved by axial traction. The patient should then be referred to the orthopaedic department because instability may accompany the dislocation.

Other injuries to the thumb

Fractures of the proximal phalanx of the thumb

Unstable or angulated fractures should be referred for reduction and fixation. This will include all fractures of the shaft. Undisplaced fractures of the base of the proximal phalanx can be treated with a bandage thumb spica and clinic review.

Dislocation of the interphalangeal joint of the thumb

This can be reduced with axial traction. A Mallett splint is then applied and fracture clinic review arranged.

Fracture of the distal phalanx of the thumb

This usually follows a crushing type of injury. Associated soft-tissue injury predominates. The treatment is the same as that for distal phalangeal injuries of the other fingers (*see page 143*).

Chapter 10

Burns

The skin is the largest organ of the body and constitutes a vital barrier against disease. It is also a major sense organ and one of the main determinants of beauty. Its damage is thus dangerous, painful and distressing. Thermal injuries may also involve the respiratory tract.

For management of radiation casualties see page 298.

Large burns

Immediate assessment and management

- Ensure an adequate airway. Give a high concentration of oxygen.
- Remove the source of the burn. Cut off clothes. Flood the affected area with cold water if there is still evidence of heat transfer.
- Look for evidence of inhalation injury (*see later*). If there is wheezing, give nebulised salbutamol.
- Measure the arterial blood gases and carboxyhaemoglobin level.
- Estimate the extent of the burn (*see page 147*). If more than 15% of skin area (or more than 10% in a patient under 10 or over 70 years), set up an intravenous (IV) infusion and take blood for Hb, PCV, urea, electrolytes and glucose.
- Monitor the pulse, BP and SaO$_2$.
- Assess the level of consciousness; if depressed consider carbon monoxide poisoning – *see page 288*.

- Obtain brief details of the incident and the patient.
- Give adequate IV analgesia.
- Assess the depth of the burn (*see page 147*). If there are extensive, deep burns, cross-match blood and begin colloid infusion.
- Cover burns with sterile towels, dry dressings or cling film.
- Insert a urinary catheter and measure the output of urine.
- Consider the possibility of other injuries.

Inhalation injury

Inhalation of hot smoke and fumes is common in patients exposed to house fires. This may cause:
- direct thermal injury to the respiratory tract;
- bronchospasm;
- delayed pulmonary oedema;
- systemic poisoning.

Direct thermal damage to the respiratory tract is uncommon in the otherwise minimally injured victim of a fire. In a more seriously burned patient, it may lead to severe oedema and a rapid onset of airway obstruction. This may also result from delayed sloughing of tracheal or bronchial mucosa. Such cases may need fibre-optic bronchoscopy.

Fumes may contain gases that impair surfactant activity and irritate the respiratory mucosa. Early bronchospasm may occur but there may be no obvious evidence of damage until pulmonary oedema develops some hours later.

Incapacity, which occurs quickly in domestic and industrial fires, is caused by a combination of hypoxia, carbon monoxide poisoning (caused by incomplete combustion) and hydrogen cyanide poisoning. Soft furnishings are a particular hazard, producing many toxic substances, including highly irritant and lethal hydrogen chloride.

Inhalation is likely to have occurred if two or more of the following apply:
- history of exposure to fire in enclosed space;
- decreased ability to respond to fire, as with small children, handicapped or intoxicated patients;
- history of impaired consciousness or confusion at any time;
- symptoms or signs of respiratory distress, including irritation of mucous membranes;
- stridor, hoarseness or aphonia;
- production of carboniferous (black) sputum;
- burns around the lips, mouth, throat or nose, including singeing of nasal hairs.

Tx

- Consider the need for early intubation – before oedema of the upper airway makes this difficult or impossible. Request anaesthetic advice. Endotracheal tubes should be left long and uncut to allow for swelling of the face and airway.

> Suxamethonium may cause a dangerous rise in serum potassium in patients with burns.

- Give high-concentration oxygen.
- Give nebulised salbutamol for wheezing.
- Estimate arterial blood gases and carboxy-haemoglobin.

> Beware of conventional blood gas analyser readings in patients who may have high carboxy- or methaemoglobin levels. The oxygen electrode measures oxygen dissolved in plasma only and oxygen saturation is then calculated assuming all haemoglobin to be normal. PaO_2 and oxygen saturation may thus appear to be satisfactory despite very low total blood oxygen content.

- Save blood for forensic tests.
- Request a Chest X-ray.
- Admit for 24 h observation even if burns appear minimal.

For treatment of carbon monoxide poisoning see page 288.

For treatment of cyanide poisoning see page 292.

Assessment of a burn

Extent

The extent of a burn is estimated by using the Rule of Nines in adults (*see Figure 10.1*). In children, the Lund–Browder chart is used to take account of the relatively larger head and smaller legs (*see Figure 10.2*). As a useful guide, the surface area of the patient's own outstretched hand is around 1% (0.8%) of the total body surface area.

> Do not take areas of superficial erythema into account when calculating the area of a burn. Make a note of these areas separately.

There is only a slight difference between the volume of fluid lost through partial- and full-thickness burns, although the extent of erythrocyte destruction is greater in the latter.

Depth

The depth of a burn is a function of:
1 the temperature of the agent causing the burn;
2 the length of time it is in contact with the skin (i.e. the amount of energy transferred). Scalds are associated with a water temperature greater than 50° C.

> It is often very difficult to estimate confidently the depth of a burn in the first few days.

The circumstances leading to the cause of the burn may help. A motorbike exhaust pipe burning through a leather boot is likely to inflict a superficial burn. An epileptic or alcoholic who falls into a fire will sustain deep burns. Elderly patients and those with peripheral neuropathy (e.g. diabetics) are at special risk. Electrical burns are usually very deep.

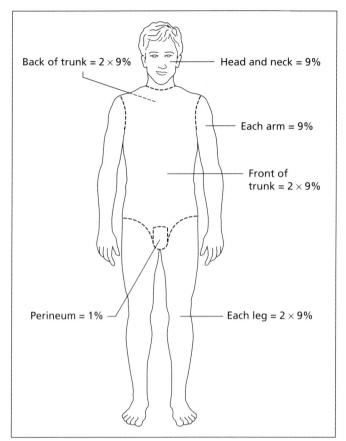

Figure 10.1 The 'Rule of Nines'.

Clothes closely applied to the skin, such as underwear, socks, belts and collars, tend to trap fluids and potentiate the severity of the burn locally.

Superficial burns expose intact nerve endings and are painful. Deep burns destroy nerve endings and are painless – hence pinprick testing. The skin often resembles thick, dry, cream-coloured parchment, unlike the red, angry skin of a superficial burn.

> Infection can easily convert a partial-thickness burn to a full-thickness injury.

Treatment of burns

Flooding with cold water

The damage inflicted by hot fluids may be diminished by flooding the affected part with cold water. Pain is simultaneously reduced. Immediate irrigation for up to 5 min may limit the extent of the burn, but beware of hypothermia, especially in small children.

> Never apply neutralising fluids to acid or alkali burns – the resulting chemical reaction is exothermic.

Analgesia

Analgesia should be given early and always before transfer to another unit. It is usually underprescribed. The beneficial effects of morphine in small children greatly outweigh any haemodynamic side effects, but it is essential to calculate the initial dose using the patient's weight. Do not be afraid to give further doses as dictated by the state of the patient (*see page 328*).

> Most significant burns need IV analgesia.

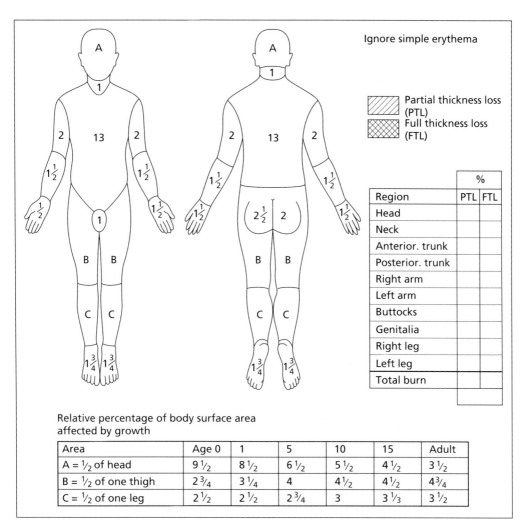

Figure 10.2 The Lund–Browder Chart.

Ignore simple erythema		

	Partial thickness loss (PTL)
	Full thickness loss (FTL)

	%	
Region	PTL	FTL
Head		
Neck		
Anterior. trunk		
Posterior. trunk		
Right arm		
Left arm		
Buttocks		
Genitalia		
Right leg		
Left leg		
Total burn		

Relative percentage of body surface area affected by growth

Area	Age 0	1	5	10	15	Adult
A = ½ of head	9½	8½	6½	5½	4½	3½
B = ½ of one thigh	2¾	3¼	4	4½	4½	4¾
C = ½ of one leg	2½	2½	2¾	3	3⅓	3½

Intravenous fluids

If the burn involves more than 15% of the skin (10% in children and the elderly) or involves the face making oral feeding difficult, an IV line must be set up. It will be required for a few days and must be reliable and easy to maintain. Reduced immunological competence increases the risk of infection after burns. An aseptic technique must be used.

The priming fluid can be isotonic saline. Thereafter a colloid is used. The choice includes synthetic sugars, gelatin and starch, albumin, plasma protein fraction and reconstituted plasma. Most departments use a gelatin solution initially but check the local burns unit's preference. Whole blood will be required if there is a significant element of full-thickness skin loss. *For a method of calculating fluid requirements see Box 10.1.*

Calculated fluids are required in addition to normal metabolic requirements.
Fluid loss begins at the time of the burn.

Box 10.1 Fluid Replacement for Burns

- Intravenous fluids required if more than a 15% surface burn (10% in those under 10 or over 70 years).
- Isolated areas of erythema are not included in the calculation but cannot be ignored.
- No distinction is made between areas of full- and partial-thickness loss initially.
- Fluid can be considered to be lost in equal amounts in the following time-bands (measured from time of burn):

> 0–4 h
> 4–8 h
> 8–12 h
> 12–18 h
> 18–24 h
> 24–36 h

- Fluid given in the first time-band has to be given at a faster rate if there is a delay between time of burn and time of arrival at hospital.
- The absolute amount required to replace the burn loss in each of these time-bands is:

$$\frac{[\text{Weight (kg)} \times \%\text{burn}]\ \text{mL}}{2}$$

- An additional amount will be required to satisfy the patient's normal fluid requirements (about 1500 mL per day for a 70 kg man). This will be raised if there is pyrexia.
- Equal amounts of crystalloid and colloid should be used initially. Isotonic saline and gelatin are appropriate. Later transfusion of blood will be required if there is a significant element of full-thickness burning.

Definitive care of large burns

Patients with large burns must not be kept in the ED for longer than it takes to:
- initiate resuscitation;
- exclude, or treat, other major injuries;
- establish monitoring and investigations;
- agree a treatment plan with the local burns unit;
- prepare for controlled transfer to the appropriate area.

The indications for admission are based on the extent and site of the burns.
- Burns over 15% (over 10% in children and the elderly) produce haemodynamic changes, which demand inpatient treatment.
- Burns to the perineum, around the mouth and to the airway will require specialised nursing care.

- Some small burns can only be managed safely and effectively if the patient is in hospital. These include circumferential limb burns and full-thickness loss around the eyes, nose and ears (these are discussed in the next section).

Local arrangements will influence whether admission is to a general surgical ward, an intensive care unit or a specialised burns unit. The latter is often some distance from the ED and usually has a limited number of beds. It is inappropriate to refer very severely burned elderly patients to specialised units if they are expected to die.

> If age + % burn ≥ 100, survival is most unlikely even with optimum care.

Before transfer check that:
- airway control is immaculate, and unlikely to deteriorate;
- IV access is adequate and cannula fixed well in place;
- fluid regime is agreed and running;
- monitoring equipment is suitable;
- charts, notes and laboratory results are with the patient;
- analgesia is satisfactory and can be topped up;
- level of nursing/medical care required en route has been considered.

Small burns

Most burns under 10% of the body surface area can be managed on an outpatient basis. Exceptions are discussed in the section on special burns. *See page 152.*

Initial assessment and management

Initial action includes:
- the removal of the source of the burn;
- flooding with cold water;
- analgesia;
- assessment of size, site and depth (a drawing is useful) *see page 147.*

A temporary dressing, without medication, is applied once the burn area has been exposed and the patient is waiting for definitive care. Analgesia must be given as soon as possible, especially to children.

> Simple erythema is extremely painful. Even patients expected to go home after treatment may need parenteral analgesia.

The pattern of burning should be considered in the light of the history available. A scald from spilt water will produce a cascade effect, with streaks of burnt skin following the path of the falling fluid, possibly with increasing depth of injury where its flow has been held up by constricting clothes such as waistbands or socks. A scald with a glove or stocking distribution is unusual; either the patient has impaired peripheral or central pain perception or the limb was held under water. In children, this type of appearance suggests abuse (*see Box 10.2 and page 348*).

The depth of the burn influences long-term treatment and should be determined as soon as possible. Superficial erythema is initially painful whereas full-thickness burns will be insensitive because the nerve endings have been destroyed. Most areas of most burns fall between these extremes and are termed partial-thickness.

If most of the dermal papillae and all of the skin appendages (hair follicles and sweat glands) are intact there is a very good potential for spontaneous regeneration. The term 'deep dermal' is used to describe partial-thickness burns with only a few epidermal remnants remaining – usually around the necks of sweat glands and hair follicles. If the wound becomes infected, these cells may

Box 10.2 Features of a Burn that Suggest Non-Accidental Injury

Glove or stocking distribution, especially if bilateral.
Involvement of buttocks or perineum.
Scalds with a clearly demarcated edge with no peripheral splash marks.
Small, even, rounded (cigarette tip) burns.
General features of history and presentation suspicious of abuse.

die, resulting in full-thickness skin loss. Prevention of infection is thus of paramount importance in deep dermal burns.

There is frequently a combination of partial- and full-thickness burning. The patient may consider the whole area sensitive and it is often difficult to determine depth at the first examination. However, the distinction is usually unimportant in the very early stages of treatment. Most areas of full-thickness loss, which require grafts, are evident by 5–10 days. Electrical burns may be suitable for the specialised technique of immediate excision and grafting.

Dressing and follow-up of simple superficial burns

Skin debris and foreign material are removed with dilute antiseptic and cotton-wool balls.

> Small blisters should be left alone. Large ones can be slit open at the dependent edge to allow drainage. Complete deroofing is unnecessary and leaves a painful base.

A sterile, non-adherent dressing is then applied. Antiseptic substances are not needed for most burns but are often used (e.g. silver sulphadiazine or mupirocin cream). Healing will occur more rapidly in a moist environment, but excess exudate should be kept away from the wound surface. A moist wound surface reduces damage to the new epithelium when the dressing is changed and is less painful. Specialised dressings are available that retain excess exudate and allow gas exchange but they are expensive. Technique and experience are as important as dressing material.

The wound dressing is covered with a more robust gauze for added protection. Limb burns should be elevated, but the patient encouraged to move the burned part as much as possible. Stiffness will develop quickly and is slow to resolve once established. Routine prophylaxis with antibiotics is not indicated.

The burn should be reassessed within 36–48 h. Dressings should be changed no more than three times in the first week and less frequently thereafter. Most patients can be taught to dress small burns at home. Elderly patients can be treated at home by the district nurse or at the local health centre. All burns to special areas and full-thickness burns should be reviewed in the ED.

Once the wound has fully epithelialised, and has thus become dry, it should be exposed to a clean environment but protected from dirt and friction by temporary dry dressings. A moisturising cream can be applied to replace the sweat gland secretions, which are often deficient for some months after burning. The patient should be warned that the skin will be especially sensitive to ultraviolet light throughout the following summer.

Skin grafting of burns

Some electrical burns are most effectively treated by initial excision and early grafting and are best referred immediately to a burns unit. However, most small, simple burns treated on an outpatient basis in an ED should be managed conservatively for at least the first 10 days.

Wounds under 2 cm in diameter usually contract and close spontaneously, even if there is full-thickness skin loss. Larger wounds will show evidence of marginal and focal epithelialisation. It should be possible to distinguish deep-dermal burns from full-thickness burns within 10 days of the injury. If the former remain sterile, thereby avoiding destruction of the epithelial remnants, they will heal spontaneously. The latter will require split-skin grafts. The technique is described on *page 389*.

Special burns

Burns to the face

Inhalation burns must be excluded (*see page 146*). The patient may have deceptively good function when first assessed but can deteriorate over 24 h. Swelling is a major problem.

- Patients with burns to the eyelids and cornea must be admitted to a specialised eye unit. Lid retraction may cause major problems. Apply an antibiotic (e.g. chloramphenicol) eye ointment before transfer.
- Burns around the mouth cause feeding problems. Inpatient care is usually required. The burns unit should be contacted for advice.
- Deep burns involving the nose and ear may destroy underlying cartilage and should always be referred for specialised care.
- Partial-thickness burns of other areas of the face can be adequately treated on an outpatient basis. Silver sulphadiazine cream is applied very sparingly and repeated by the patient at home, once or twice per day. The area may blacken and be unsightly, but this is not harmful. No other dressing is required. Chloramphenicol ointment should be prescribed if the burns have encroached on the periorbital area.

Burns to the hands

The fingers quickly stiffen up and conventional bandages become very dirty, with an increased risk of infection. These complications are avoided if plastic gloves are used initially instead of standard dressings. Silver sulphadiazine cream is applied and a loosely fitting examination glove is fitted in place with tape around the wrist. The gloves tend to burst, so patients must be given a supply to apply by themselves.

Patients are encouraged to move the hand as much as possible. The skin becomes macerated and the exudate and silver sulphadiazine produce an aesthetically unpleasant sight. Coloured gloves overcome some of the patient's understandable anxieties but reassurance should be given that the maceration will resolve rapidly once the glove is removed.

Burns to the perineum

The perineum must be examined carefully. It is a common site for non-accidental burns. Any burns to the top of the thighs or on the buttocks, which cannot be adequately dressed, and all those nearer the perineum, which cannot easily be kept clean, must be managed in hospital. A short-stay ward may be appropriate, but extensive or full-thickness burns should be referred to the burns unit.

Circumferential burns

If a partial- or full-thickness burn extends completely around a limb the distal circulation may become impaired. Minor degrees of venous obstruction can be treated by admission and elevation. Deep burns, which will quickly contract, may cause more serious obstruction. Similar complications may occur on the trunk causing respiratory distress. Escharotomy may be required. This is associated with significant fluid loss and must not be undertaken without expert advice.

Chemical burns

No attempt should be made to neutralise chemicals on the skin (except hydrofluoric acid *see later*). Most neutralising reactions are exothermic and would cause an additional thermal injury.

Dilution by continuous irrigation with water for at least 5 min is the mainstay of treatment. Prolonged irrigation with cold water also reduces pain significantly. Caution must be exercised with young children who quickly become hypothermic.

Systemic absorption of some chemicals (e.g. phenol) may be significant. Toxicological advice should be sought.

Hydrofluoric acid burns

Hydrofluoric acid (hydrogen fluoride) is used extensively in industry and horticulture. Skin contact causes severe local tissue damage with a great deal of pain. The burn is deep and slow to heal. With solutions containing less than 50% hydrofluoric acid there may be a delay until the burn develops as follows:

- anhydrous or > 50% concentrations – immediate damage
- 20–50% concentrations – up to 8 h delay
- < 20% concentrations – up to 24 h delay.

Even concentrations of acid as low as 2% may cause burns after prolonged skin contact.

Investigations

Significant absorption of fluoride ion through the skin may cause hypocalcaemia. Cardiac arrest may occur in the extensively burned patient. The serum calcium should be checked in all patients with larger burns resulting from contact with hydrogen fluoride.

Tx

Immediate irrigation of the contaminated area is essential and may be as effective as any other local treatment. Pain, tissue destruction and hypocalcaemia can be reduced by converting the acid to its calcium salt. This is achieved by repeated application of calcium gluconate gel (marketed as hydrofluoric acid burn jelly). There is no exothermic reaction. The injection of 10% calcium gluconate around and under the burn is sometimes advocated for persistent pain in well-localised lesions.

Chemical burns from giant hogweed

The plant *Heracleum mantegazzianum* – better known as giant hogweed – is a public health hazard and an environmental nuisance. In addition to its toxicity, this aggressive foreign invader prevents native plant species from growing and increases soil erosion. Under the Wildlife and Countryside Act 1981 and the Wildlife (Northern Ireland) Order 1985, it is an offence to 'plant or otherwise cause giant hogweed to grow'. Despite this, the species in common in the British Isles and is found alongside roads, railway lines, rivers and footpaths, often in areas of wasteland. The plant is characterised by its size. Over a period of 4 years, it may grow up to 5 m in height and looks rather like an overgrown cow parsley. It has a reddish purple stem and spotted leaf stalks with fine spines that make it appear furry. The leaves may be up to 1.5 m in width with large flowering heads. These characteristics make the giant hogweed plant irresistible to children who make swords and umbrellas from it.

Unfortunately, giant hogweed exudes a clear watery sap from its leaves and also from the stem in even greater quantities. This sap contains a glucoside called furanocoumarin, which renders the skin photosensitive to ultraviolet light. Exposure to sunlight following contact with the sap results in large painful blisters, burns and linear inflammation. This reaction usually appears within 15 to 20 h of contact although it can occur up to 48 h later. Damaged skin heals very slowly over at least 2 weeks, leaving residual pigmentation that can develop into chronic phytophotodermatitis. Inflammation may recur in sunlight for many months.

Tx

In the event of contact with giant hogweed sap, the skin should be washed immediately with soap and water and then covered to reduce the exposure to sunlight. Application of topical steroids, if started early in the inflammatory process, can reduce the severity of the developing burns. Otherwise, partial thickness lesions are treated with dressings and analgesia until healing occurs. Advice about subsequent UV light exposure should be given to all patients.

Burns from hot tar

Hot bitumen solidifies on contact with the skin. Water should be applied at the site to hasten hardening and limit heat transfer. Bitumen on blistering skin should be removed with the blister. Adherent bitumen should be left in place and covered with paraffin gauze. This will help to dissolve and separate it. Earlier excision would inflict more damage.

Sunburn

Unprotected exposure to UV radiation can cause extremely painful, blistering, oedematous skin. In general, the treatment is as for any other burn. However, the pain of the intense erythema, which so often results, can be greatly alleviated by the regular application of 1% hydrocortisone cream.

Electrocution

High-voltage injury (including lightning)

Injuries following a high-voltage electric shock may result from:
- falling or being thrown to the ground, causing secondary injuries;
- tetanic muscle contraction, causing fractures of long bones, crushed vertebrae, torn muscles;
- spontaneous ignition of clothing, causing burns;
- conduction of electricity through the body, causing entry and exit wounds and internal injuries;
- current passing along the surface of the body to earth, causing very deep burns over a large area of skin;
- current jumping from one part of the body to another, causing secondary exit and entry wounds.

The patient may have a respiratory or cardiac arrest. If this is successfully reversed or if the patient presents without having had a life-threatening cardiac dysrhythmia it is unlikely that one will develop subsequently. Supraventricular tachycardia has been reported, but more commonly the ECG shows right bundle branch block and/or ST changes. These may last many weeks. Treatment is based on symptoms and clinical signs in the normal way. Cardiac markers will be raised irrespective of cardiac damage and so their measurement is not helpful.

If the current travels through the body it naturally follows the path of least resistance. Nerves and blood vessels are good conductors. Increasing resistance is offered by muscle, skin, tendon, fat and bone in that order. Structures with high resistance will generate the greatest heat but, clearly, some tissues are more readily damaged by heat than others. Nerves, blood vessels, muscles and skin sustain most of the injury.

The entry point is typically charred and depressed. It becomes swollen very quickly, with the accumulation of extracellular fluid. The exit point has an explosive appearance – round or oval grey craters with no inflammatory changes. These increase in size over the first few days.

In the peripheral nerves, axons are distorted and Schwann cells break down and coalesce. Spinal cord lesions are surprisingly common, often producing partial transections. Brain damage is unusual unless the head has been directly involved.

Blood vessels sustain endothelial damage and media degeneration. Thrombosis and late rupture can occur at sites distant from the entry point. Visceral lesions, which are often unrecognised, probably have a vascular aetiology.

Muscle involvement is typically patchy, with swelling, necrosis and the later development of deep sepsis.

Acute tubular necrosis is common. Inadequate volume replacement, myoglobinuria and direct damage to renal vessels probably all contribute to its development.

Cataracts are a well recognised, late complication.

Late death is commonly caused by overwhelming sepsis.

For characteristic signs in patients struck by lightning see Box 10.3. However, there is only a 1 in 2 000 000 chance of being killed by lightning in the United Kingdom!

Tx

Treatment in the ED is directed towards stabilisation of any life-threatening dysrhythmia and the early transfusion of crystalloid. Fluid loss cannot be calculated by burns formuli. The volume required is titrated against central venous pressure (CVP), pulse and blood pressure to maintain a high urine output. Blood gases and plasma urea and electrolytes (including creatinine) should be measured. Acidosis is common in patients with extensive electrocution injuries and bicarbonate is often required.

The care of all patients who have been electrocuted must be discussed with a senior member of staff. Extensive soft tissue injuries will be assessed in the main theatre. Tissue loss can be minimised by very early fasciotomy and removal of dead tissue. However, because of the patchy nature of the muscle involvement, this process is not as easy as with muscle damage resulting from direct injury. Occult visceral damage must also be considered.

Antitetanus prophylaxis is required for all patients.

Low-voltage injury

Low-voltage burns of the type sustained from the domestic electricity supply are not usually associated with the above complications. However, the local burn is almost always full-thickness and much deeper than it appears. The area of tissue necrosis may extend over the first few days. Senior advice should be sought; early excision and grafting is often favoured by specialised burns units. Continuous ECG monitoring is not required.

Chapter 11

Cardiac arrest and cardiac dysrhythmias

This chapter covers the essential theoretical and practical aspects of cardiac arrest and dysrhythmia management. However, it does not claim to equip the reader with all the skills necessary for leading a resuscitation team. To achieve such competence, it is essential to have participated in an Advanced Life Support or similar course.

The protocols and algorithms used in this chapter are taken from the guidelines published in 2005 by the Resuscitation Council (UK). As such, they are consistent with the European Resuscitation Council (ERC) Guidelines for Resuscitation 2005 and are based on the publication by the International Liaison Committee on Resuscitation (ILCOR): *2005 International Consensus on Cardiopulmonary Resuscitation and Emergency Cardiovascular Care Science with Treatment Recommendations* (CoSTR).

For resuscitation of the newborn infant see also Box 17.2 on page 313.

For the Resuscitation Council (UK) algorithm for life support of the newborn infant see Figure 17.2 on page 314.

For cardiac arrest in hypothermic patients see also page 250.

For choking see page 205.

For the Resuscitation Council (UK) algorithms for the treatment of choking in adults and children see Figures 13.1 and 13.2 on pages 205 and 206.

Cardiac arrest

In 20% of people with cardiac arrest there is no previous history of ischaemic heart disease.

The heart is a pump with an electrical controlling system. Its power supply comes from burning fuel with oxygen. It stops functioning in three main ways:

1 Failure of the oxygen supply causes asystole (or extreme bradycardia). There is no electrical activity and no pumping.

2 Failure of electrical control causes ventricular fibrillation (VF) or pulseless ventricular tachycardia (VT). There is no effective electrical activity and no effective pumping.

3 Failure of the pump mechanism causes pulseless electrical activity (PEA) (also known as electro-mechanical dissociation or EMD). There is electrical activity but no pumping.

Asystole is the final rhythm in all cases. The underlying causes of the three arrest rhythms are described below.

Asystole

Like any other pump, the heart slows and stops when deprived of its power supply. This results from:
- hypoxia or;
- a condition leading to hypoxia (e.g. hypovolaemia).

Tachycardia during hypoxia is the result of the influence of the autonomic nervous system. Left to its own devices, the hypoxic heart contracts more slowly (terminal bradycardia) and then arrests in asystole.

Ventricular fibrillation

Ventricular fibrillation is caused by direct damage or irritation of the heart. This may be because of:
- myocardial ischaemia or infarction;
- poisoning;
- gross electrolyte imbalance;
- hypothermia and near-drowning;
- electrocution;
- penetrating trauma;
- iatrogenic causes (e.g. cardioversion and cardiac catheterisation).

In adults VF is most commonly seen in patients with ischaemic heart disease while in children, poisoning with tricyclic antidepressants should always be considered. Pulseless VT is a similar condition to VF in both causation and treatment. Unfortunately, these 'shockable' rhythms occur less than half the time, accounting for only 40% of pre-hospital cardiac arrests and 25% of arrests in hospital.

Pulseless electrical activity (also known as electromechanical dissociation)

Pulseless Electrical Activity (PEA) is that state when the pump (the myocardium) is unable to function despite a relatively normal electrical stimulus (the ECG signal). This can be because of primary damage to the muscle:
- extensive myocardial infarction;
- ruptured cardiac aneurysm;
- papillary muscle rupture;
- extreme direct trauma;

or because of various secondary causes (some of which may be treatable):
- tension pneumothorax;
- cardiac tamponade;
- pulmonary embolism;
- hypovolaemia;
- hypothermia;
- poisoning;
- electrolyte imbalance.

In adults, myocardial infarction is the most common cause of PEA, while hypovolaemia should be suspected in children. PEA should not be confused with an agonal rhythm (*see page 168*).

> Many patients with diagnosed PEA will, in fact, be suffering from a very low output state rather than complete circulatory arrest.

The chain of survival

Survival from cardiac arrest is most likely if:
- the arrest is witnessed;
- the initial rhythm is VF (or VT).

Thereafter, the chain of survival depends on the patient receiving:

1 basic life support at scene;

2 defibrillation as soon as possible;

3 advanced life support from trained health professionals.

Complete failure of the circulation for more than 3 or 4 min leads to irreversible brain damage.

There are only three interventions which are known to increase the survival from cardiac arrest: chest compression, defibrillation and airway management. The aim of life support must be to deliver these three treatments to the patient in the shortest possible time.

> Even after a cardiac arrest in hospital, less than 20% of adults will survive to go home.

Cardiac arrest in children

Childrens hearts usually arrest as a result of hypoxia (secondary to respiratory distress or depression) or hypovolaemia (fluid loss or maldistribution). These conditions lead to asystole, which has a very poor prognosis. Coronary artery disease and thus VF is extremely uncommon in children.

For cardiac arrest protocols for children see below.

For drug dosages and equipment sizes for children see page 323.

For intraosseous access see Box 18.5 on page 326.

Basic life support

For the Resuscitation Council (UK) algorithm for Basic Life Support (BLS) for adults see Figure 11.1.
For the Resuscitation Council (UK) algorithm for Basic Life Support (BLS) for children see Figure 11.2.
For choking and airway obstruction see page 205.

The manual methods of BLS (Schafer's, Silvester's and Holger–Nielsen's procedures) were replaced by exhaled air resuscitation in the late 1950s. In 1960, Kouwenhoven, Jude and Knickerbocker reminded the world of the efficacy of closed chest compression and thus modern BLS was born. There are four elements:

1 initial assessment;
2 airway clearance and maintenance;
3 rescue breathing;
4 chest compression to support the circulation.

Basic life support is not very effective - even optimal chest compressions do not achieve more than 30% of the normal blood flow to the brain and 15%

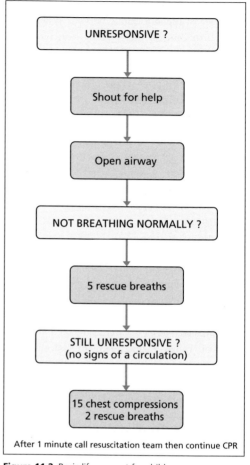

Figure 11.2 Basic life support for children

of the normal coronary blood flow. It is thus essential to restart the heart within a few minutes - *see above* (chain of survival).

In adults, arrest is usually a primary cardiac event and so most effort relates to obtaining a defibrillator as soon as possible, even if this means leaving a pulseless patient to go to a telephone before starting chest compressions. In children, more attention is given to the correction of hypoxia and so resuscitation, starting with 5 rescue breaths, should be performed for about 1 minute before an isolated rescuer goes for help. Adults who are victims of drowning should also be given 5 breaths and a short period of CPR before seeking assistance. BLS for adults is now taught assuming one rescuer who will perform sequences

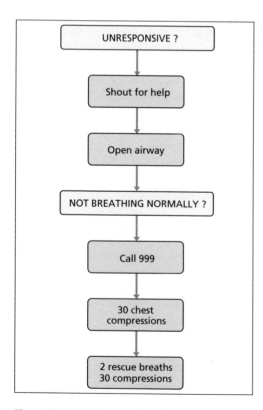

Figure 11.1 Basic life support for adults

of 30 compressions to two ventilations. Two-rescuer CPR (using the same compression:ventilation ratio of 30:2) is taught to professionals only. For children, the 30:2 ratio is taught to lay rescuers but two or more health professionals should use a 15:2 sequence. The only exception is neonates where a 3:1 ratio of compressions to ventilations is advocated. After successful endotracheal intubation, the synchronisation of compression and ventilation is abandoned and the two operations are performed independently.

Initial assessment

- Make sure that the victim, any bystanders and yourself are safe.
- Shake and shout 'Are you alright?'
- If the patient is responsive, leave them in the position found (or in the recovery position if safer), try to find out what is wrong and get help. Review the situation regularly.
- If the patient is unresponsive, call for help (or go for help if alone). Turn the victim onto their back, open the airway and, in less than 10 seconds, look for chest movements, listen at the mouth for sounds and feel for air flow on your cheek.
- If the patient is breathing normally, turn them into the recovery position, get help and continue monitoring the situation.
- If the patient is not breathing, call for help (or go for help if alone) and then start chest compressions.

Chest compression

> Chest compression is more important than ventilation in BLS and, as a single therapy, gives far better results than inactivity. (Chest compression-only CPR may be effective for up to 5 min!) The Resuscitation Council (UK) 2005 Guidelines emphasise the importance of chest movements at the expense of rescue breathing.

Even the best external chest compression provides poor core circulation. Squeezing the chest results in cardiac valve deformation and incompetence which allows regurgitation of blood into the inferior vena cava. Retrograde flow up the superior vena cava is reduced by a valvular effect where the superior vena cava enters the chest. Forward flow to the brain is thus more likely to occur than forward flow to the trunk. In contrast, coronary artery perfusion, which normally only occurs in diastole against a closed aortic valve, is very poor during BLS. A coronary perfusion pressure of less than 15 mmHg has been shown to be unlikely to lead to a return of spontaneous circulation and the average coronary perfusion pressure during manual CPR is only around 12.5 mmHg.

For mechanical chest compression see page 167.

The mechanism by which BLS produces cardiac output remains unclear; there is probably a combination of direct cardiac compression and intrathoracic pressure fluctuations. Their relative importance may vary between individuals, depending on the shape and elasticity of the chest. At the present time, Resuscitation Council teaching assumes that direct cardiac compression is the most important factor – hence the emphasis on correct site and adequate depth. A compression rate of about 100 per minute is recommended for both adults and children. The weight of the resuscitator's body is transmitted through the arms to achieve a compression of 4–5 cm in normal adults or about one-third of the depth of the chest in children. The compression to release ratio should be 1:1. The 2005 guidelines aim to reduce the interruptions in chest compression that occur for 'rescue breaths' by increasing the ratio of compressions to ventilation to 30:2. Pauses for ventilation should be limited to one second per breath only. For children, the same ratio of 30:2 is taught to lay rescuers but two or more health professionals should use a 15:2 sequence. The only exception is neonates where a 3:1 ratio of compressions to ventilations is advocated. After successful endotracheal intubation, the synchronisation of compression and ventilation is abandoned and the two operations are performed independently.

Ventilation

Two effective initial 'rescue breaths' are recommended for both adults and children and the guidelines permit up to five attempts to achieve this in the case of children. Breaths should only take one second so as to maintain constant chest compressions. Mouth to mouth-and-nose ventilation is required for infants. A Pocket Mask may be used by occasional resuscitators to avoid direct patient contact; professional rescuers should use bag, valve and mask units initially but aim for endotracheal intubation as soon as practically possible. Airway adjuncts such as the oesophageal obturator airway and Combitube are not recommended - there are more disadvantages to their use than advantages. However, the laryngeal mask airway (LMA) is increasingly accepted as the airway of choice for first responders.

Advanced life support

These protocols apply, by definition, to healthcare professionals trained in advanced life support techniques. The significant changes in the international 2005 guidelines were driven by emerging evidence and the need for simplification.

For the Resuscitation Council (UK) algorithm for Advanced Life Support (ALS) for adults see Figure 11.3. For the Resuscitation Council (UK) algorithm for Advanced Life Support (ALS) for children see Figure 11.4.

A display of the ECG must be obtained as soon as possible to guide treatment. Monitoring via defibrillator paddles may be adequate initially but

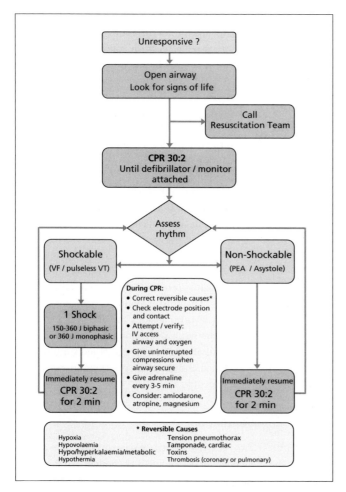

Figure 11.3 Advanced life support for adults

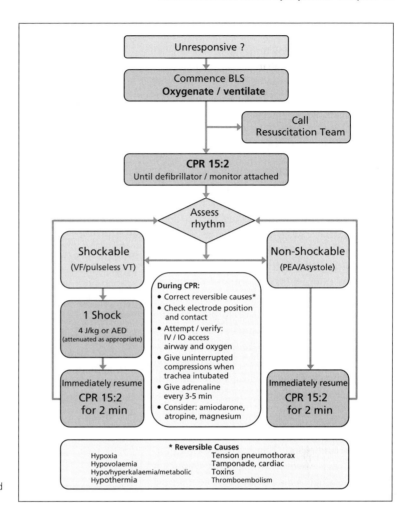

During CPR:
- Correct reversible causes*
- Check electrode position and contact
- Attempt / verify:
  IV / IO access
  airway and oxygen
- Give uninterrupted compressions when trachea intubated
- Give adrenaline every 3-5 min
- Consider: amiodarone, atropine, magnesium

* Reversible Causes

Hypoxia	Tension pneumothorax
Hypovolaemia	Tamponade, cardiac
Hypo/hyperkalaemia/metabolic	Toxins
Hypothermia	Thromboembolism

Figure **11.4** Advanced life support for children

should be replaced by adhesive chest electrodes once ALS is established. Endotracheal intubation must be achieved as soon as practically possible and early central venous access is also desirable. Once the airway has been secured with a cuffed endotracheal tube, compressions should not be interrupted for ventilations. From then on, ventilation of the lungs should be performed asynchronously at a rate of approximately 10–12 breaths per minute. To ensure effective chest compressions, the person responsible for this tiring part of the resuscitation should be changed every two minutes.

For mechanical chest compression see page 167.

With the aid of the ECG rhythm, the algorithms divide patients into two categories: those who have VF or pulseless VT and those who do not have VF or VT. VF is not the most common arrest rhythm but is the most survivable by far. The only effective treatment for it - defibrillation - was introduced into clinical practice by Zoll and colleagues in 1956. In most circumstances, no other intervention must take precedence over defibrillation. However, there is some evidence that if BLS has not taken place, two minutes of chest compression before defibrillation may increase the success rate. Therefore, after prolonged (more than 5 min) cardiac arrest out of hospital, CPR should be performed for two minutes prior to defibrillation. This is not recommended in hospital practice.

Precordial thump

This supplies energy which may abort VT or even VF but in the unstable heart it may also possibly convert sinus rhythm into VF. Therefore, its use is recommended only in witnessed arrests when ALS skills are available.

Gastric decompression

Inflation of the stomach is inevitable during BLS. It causes splinting of the diaphragm and may impair cardiac output. For this reason, it is appropriate to decompress the stomach with a large-bore orogastric (lavage-type) tube as soon as possible during all resuscitations. This should not be attempted until the airway is protected by intubation. The stomach may be emptied of both air and fluids in order to decrease the risk of aspiration. At autopsy, nearly half of all patients who have died after attempted resuscitation are found to have full stomachs. Contamination of the respiratory tract is evident in 30%. Airway protection is ensured by early endotracheal intubation; the LMA is an effective alternative for first responders.

Relatives

Honest, accurate and frequent communication with relatives is essential throughout all resuscitations. Increasingly, relatives are being encouraged to come into the resuscitation room, even if it is only for a very short period. Staff may feel threatened by their presence but relatives are reassured by the experience; however, cluttered and confusing the resuscitation area may appear, the reality is often less frightening than their imaginings. A dedicated member of staff should accompany relatives in the resuscitation room at all times.

Drugs in advanced life support

Adrenaline

The vasoconstrictor adrenaline (epinephrine) is known to enhance both myocardial and cerebral perfusion, although there is no evidence that it increases the survival to hospital discharge in cardiac arrest. It has a very short half-life and so repeated IV doses (1 mg for adults) are given every 3–5 min during CPR. In children, the corresponding IV/IO dose is 10 µg per kg. Very high IV doses of adrenaline (5 mg for adults or 100 µg per kg for children) are of unproven value even in refractory asystole and are no longer recommended. The endotracheal doses of adrenaline are 3 mg for adults and 100 µg per kg for children, diluted with saline. Adrenaline may be contraindicated in arrests secondary to solvents, cocaine or other sympathomimetic drugs. Vasopressin is sometimes used as an alternative to adrenaline.

Atropine

Atropine may help in asystole occurring as a primary event caused by parasympathetic overload. More commonly asystole is the end stage of a dying heart. Nevertheless, a single IV dose of 3 mg of atropine is given routinely in ALS to adult patients with either asystole or PEA with a rate below 60 complexes a minute. Pulseless patients with extreme bradycardia or isolated P waves may benefit from pacing (*see page 167*). Atropine is only given in children when bradycardia is unresponsive to improved ventilation and circulatory support. The dose is 20 µg per kg with a minimum

---

Box 11.1 Doses of Adrenaline for Adults and Children in Cardiac Arrest (to be given every 3–5 min)

	IV dose	Endotracheal dose
Adult	1 mg	3 mg
Child	10 µg per kg	100 µg per kg

10 µg per kg of adrenaline = 0.1 mL per kg of 1 in 10000 solution.
100 µg per kg of adrenaline = 1 mL per kg of 1 in 10000 solution (or 0.1 mL per kg of 1 in 1000 solution).
10000 solution (or 0.1ml per kg of 1 in 1000 solution).
- IV doses may be given via the intra-osseous route.
- Peripheral IV or intra-osseous doses should be flushed in with saline.
- Endotracheal doses should be diluted to a relatively large volume.

dose of 100 μg to avoid a paradoxical effect at low doses.

Bicarbonate

Bicarbonate therapy is contraindicated in early resuscitation. Acidosis develops but aids oxy-haemoglobin dissociation; temporary buffering of pH is achieved by hyperventilation. Sodium bicarbonate is reserved for cardiac arrests that are associated with:

1 severe metabolic acidosis (pH <7.1 or base excess <–10);
2 hyperkalaemia (*see page 253*);
3 poisoning with tricyclic antidepressants (*see page 276*).

The initial dose is 50–100 mmol (or 1–2 mmol per kg). *For more details about bicarbonate therapy see Box 14.20 on page 257.* Prolonged arrest (i.e. over 20–25 min) causes profound intracellular acidosis and so may also be treated with alkalizing agents, especially in children. Bicarbonate must not be given by the endotracheal route.

Amiodarone

Amiodarone is used for refractory VF/pulseless VT. It stabilises cell membranes and thus increases the duration of the action potential and refractory period in both atrial and ventricular myocardial cells. As an anti-arrhythmic agent, it prolongs the QT interval and slows conduction through both the AV node and any accessory pathways. Amiodarone has less negative inotropic effects and less pro-arrhythmic actions than most similar drugs. An initial IV bolus of 300 mg should be given if VF or VT persists after three shocks. Central venous injection is preferable, although in cardiac arrest peripheral veins are often used. The IV/IO dose for children is 5 mg per kg. A further dose of 150 mg may be given for refractory or recurrent VF/VT, followed by an infusion of 900 mg over 24 h.

Lidocaine

Lidocaine (lignocaine) reduces ventricular auto-maticity and ectopic activity and increases the

threshold for the development of VF. However, it also causes an increase in:

• the energy required for defibrillation;
• the incidence of post-shock asystole.

In addition, it is a negative inotrope. For these reasons, it is not routinely used for refractory VF/VT unless amiodarone is unavailable. The initial IV/IO dose for both adults and children is 1 mg per kg to a maximum total dose of 3 mg per kg in the first hour. Lignocaine and amiodarone should not be used together.

Magnesium

Magnesium is an important intracellular cation and co-factor. It should be given for refractory VF that could be associated with low serum magnesium levels – for example, in a patient known to be taking potassium-losing diuretics. Similar indications include arrests following episodes of torsades de pointes or in patients with digoxin toxicity. The usual dose of magnesium sulphate is 8 mmol (2 g or 4 mL of a 50% solution). For children, the dose is 25–50 mg per kg by IV infusion over several minutes.

For further information about magnesium see Box 11.9 on pages 178 and 255.

Calcium

Calcium influx occurs at the time of cell death and thus it is illogical to give calcium to patients in cardiac arrest. Exceptions occur during resuscitation from PEA when there is thought to be one of the following conditions:

1 hyperkalaemia;
2 hypocalcaemia;
3 poisoning with calcium antagonists;
4 overdosage with magnesium (e.g. during treatment of eclampsia).

The initial IV dose in these situations is 10 mL of 10% calcium chloride (6.8 mmol of calcium ions), repeated as necessary. This must not be given via an endotracheal tube. For children the dose of 10% calcium chloride solution is 0.2 mL per kg. Calcium may form a precipitate if given in the same IV line as bicarbonate and is dangerous in the digitalized patient. Calcium antagonists have not fulfilled their early promise and do not improve outcome after cardiac arrest.

For further information about calcium see page 255.

Drugs in cardiac arrest following hypothermia

Drug metabolism is reduced in hypothermia and toxic accumulation of drugs may thus occur. For this reason, it is usually recommended that adrenaline and other drugs are withheld until the patient's core temperature reaches 30°C. At this point, the interval between drug doses is doubled (adrenaline is given every 6–10 min) until at least 32°C has been reached.

For hypothermic patients with no detectable cardiac output see also page 250.

Access to the central circulation

During circulatory arrest, drugs must be delivered into the central veins in order to reach their target site with sufficient speed. *For cannulation of the subclavian and internal jugular veins see Box 11.2.* Central venous access via the subclavian vein is:

- unaffected by neck movements and by the presence of a cervical collar;
- well-tolerated in conscious patients;
- good for transvenous pacing (the natural curve of the pacing wire takes it into the right atrium).

Jugular venous access carries less risk of pneumothorax but is not as comfortable for a conscious patient and provides a more difficult curve for a pacing wire to negotiate. It is, however, often recommended in cardiac arrest as it is relatively undisturbed by actions of chest compression. Cannulation of the femoral vein is safer and easier than either of the above routes in children and is a useful alternative in adults. *For intra-osseous access see Box 18.5 on page 326.*

If a peripheral vein is used, drugs should be flushed into the central circulation with at least 20 mL of saline. The endotracheal route is of unproven value in resuscitation and cannot be used for calcium or bicarbonate. A long endobronchial catheter gives the best chance of spread and absorption. Doses must be higher than with IV administration (up to triple for adults and 10-fold

---

> **Box 11.2 Central Venous Cannulation**
>
> *If possible, cannulation of central veins should take place under ultrasound guidance.*
>
> - Position the patient slightly head-down to fill the veins and minimise the risk of air embolism.
> - Take whatever aseptic precautions are reasonable for the urgency of the situation.
> - Use a cannulation set which is familiar to you. A Seldinger-wire/long-line approach is ideal but a simple cannula-over-needle can be inserted more quickly.
> - Attempted cannulation of the right side is preferable as it avoids damage to the thoracic duct (which lies on the left), and the apex of the pleural cavity (which is more inferior on this side).
> - Local anaesthetic should be used in the conscious patient.
>
> **Cannulation of the subclavian vein**
>
> Introduce the needle in the concavity below the clavicle, one-third of the way along from the tip. Advance the needle under the clavicle while withdrawing on the attached syringe. Aim for an index finger placed in the suprasternal notch. The vein is usually entered about 4–6 cm from the entry point. Coughing suggests pleural penetration.
>
> **Cannulation of the internal jugular vein**
>
> Turn the patient's head away from the vein. Identify the triangle which is made by the bifurcation of the lower end of the sternocleidomastoid muscle into its two insertions. Insert the needle at the apex of this triangle. Palpate the carotid artery; the jugular vein lies lateral to it. Advance the needle towards the ipsilateral nipple at about 30° to the horizontal and the sagittal planes, while withdrawing on the syringe. The vein lies about 2–3 cm from the skin.
>
> - When blood is aspirated, slide the cannula into the vein and withdraw the needle simultaneously.
> - Connect the cannula to a three-way tap and secure it in place.
> - Request a chest X-ray to check the cannula position and to exclude pneumothorax.

---

for children). Five large ventilations should be given after each endotracheal dose of a drug.

Ventricular fibrillation and pulseless ventricular tachycardia

In adults, VF/VT is the most treatable cause of cardiac arrest. Cardioversion by DC shock is most likely to be successful if carried out within 90 sec of cardiac arrest. Thereafter, the chances of success decline at a rate of about 7–10% per minute. Nevertheless, repeated shocks are delivered until sinus rhythm is established or resuscitation is abandoned. The first and all subsequent shocks are delivered with an energy level of 360 J (or 4 J per kg) from a monophasic source. However, when using a biphasic defibrillator, fixed or escalating energies of between 150 and 360 J (4 J per kg for children) may be used – *see Box 11.3*

The largest possible size of paddle (electrode) should be used for all DC shocks. There are three diameters currently available – *see Box 11.4*. Size is limited by the two following criteria:

1 *The curve of the chest* - there must be good contact over the entire paddle area.

2 *The width of the chest* - the two paddles must be well separated.

Self-adhesive electrode pads are likely to replace defibrillator paddles completely in the near future.

Single shocks are given every two minutes. After administering a shock, there should be no delay in resuming CPR. It will not harm the patient if the defibrillation has been successful and the circulation has returned. The central pulse is checked only

if the clinical condition of the patient changes or if the ECG shows a rhythm which is compatible with a cardiac output. (The carotid pulse is used in adults and children over 12 months old but in infants the brachial pulse is more appropriate.) After two unsuccessful shocks, adrenaline should be given. Further doses are given every 3–5 min throughout the resuscitation, immediately before alternate shocks - *for doses see Box 11.1.*

After three unsuccessful shocks, an anti-arrhythmic drug such as amiodarone 300 mg (5 mg per kg for children) IV may be given; lidocaine 100 mg (1 mg per kg) IV is an alternative. For recurrent or refractory VF/VT, a further dose of amiodarone 150 mg IV may be given followed by an infusion of 900 mg over 24 h. Potentially reversible causes of cardiac arrest must always be considered - *see Box 11.5*. Underlying non-cardiac causes of VF are more likely to be found in children than in adults. Magnesium should be considered if there is any suspicion of hypomagnesaemia – *see page 163*; Bicarbonate may be indicated for prolonged arrest. If attempts at defibrillation remain unsuccessful, a change of paddle positions or a change of machine should be considered. Alternatives to the traditional anteroapical (AA) positioning of electrodes include anteroposterior (AP) and bi-axillary (LL) placement. The latter positions (LL) should always be employed in patients with a pacemaker *in situ*.

After successful defibrillation

After successful defibrillation (if it has not already been utilised), amiodarone may be given to stabilise

---

Box 11.3 Doses of Electricity for Adults and Children in VF or Pulseless VT

	Monophasic all shocks	Biphasic first shock	Biphasic second shock
Adult	360 J	150–200 J	150–360 J
Child	4 J per kg	4 J per kg	4 J per kg

Box 11.4 Suggested Paddle Diameters for DC Shock

Size of patient	Diameter of paddle
Infants (i.e. weight <10 kg)	4.5 cm
Children under 8 years old (i.e. weight <25 kg)	8 cm
Adults and children over 8 years old	13 cm

Box 11.5 Potentially Reversible Causes of Cardiac Arrest (4 x Hs and 4 x Ts)

Hypoxia.
Hypovolaemia.
Hypo- or hyperkalaemia, hypocalcaemia, acidaemia and other metabolic disorders.
Hypothermia.
Tension pneumothorax.
Tamponade of the heart.
Toxic substances.
Thrombo-embolism (pulmonary embolus or coronary thrombosis).

the myocardium and prevent a return to VF/VT. The dose is 300 mg IV over 20–60 min followed by an infusion of 900 mg over 24 h. Lidocaine (which also raises the fibrillation threshold) is a further option. The dose is 100 mg for an average adult followed by an infusion of 2–4 mg per minute.

Safety of staff

This is paramount during attempts at defibrillation and requires:
- a good knowledge of the equipment;
- a warning shout of 'stand clear' and a visual check before each discharge.

The use of adhesive electrode pads makes the procedure much safer and better controlled.

Defibrillation in cardiac arrest following hypothermia

VF may not respond to defibrillation if the patient's core temperature is less than 30°C. Thus it is usually recommended that if there is no response to the initial three shocks, subsequent attempts at defibrillation are delayed until the core temperature rises above 30°C.

For hypothermic patients with no detectable cardiac output see also page 250.

Developments in defibrillation

1 Conventional defibrillators produce a damped sinusoidal waveform but a biphasic discharge has both theoretical and empirical advantages and so almost all newer defibrillators are incorporating this technology into their design. In practice, biphasic shocks delivered with an energy of 150 J seem to be more effective than monophasic currents with higher energies, although the optimal level for either type is uncertain. A biphasic shock crosses the heart and then returns along the same pathway as the phase inverts. This returning current catches the fibrillating myocytes that the first current missed (in much the same way as a double-bladed safety razor removes stubborn remaining hairs with its second blade). There are three different biphasic waveforms which are commonly used. The two most effective are truncated

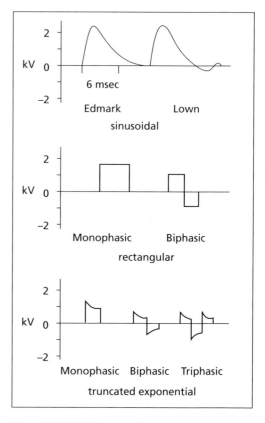

Figure 11.5 Defibrillator waveforms.

exponential and rectilinear waves. *For some typical defibrillator waveforms see Figure 11.5.* The exact equivalence of biphasic and monophasic shocks depends on the waveform that is generated but, as a rough rule, 1 J of biphasic discharge equates to 1.5 J of monophasic discharge.

2 Successful defibrillation depends on the passage of an appropriate current through the chest rather than on the administration of a preset energy. This current is around 30 A for an average adult (about 0.4 A per kg). New current-preset defibrillators, which measure transthoracic impedance and then give a pre-determined current, may replace traditional energy-preset machines in the future.

3 Myocardial current density is the ultimate determinant of both efficacy of defibrillation and cellular damage. The positioning of the treatment electrodes (paddles) is the main variable which can be used to alter the distribution of the current

in the chest and heart. Oesophageal electrodes which can be positioned directly behind the heart have been described; transoesophageal defibrillation may one day become accepted practice.

Asystole

Before a diagnosis of asystole is made, the leads, 'gain' control and switches on the monitor/defibrillator must be checked. 'Fine VF' is no longer an indication for defibrillation and has a poor prognosis. In confirmed aystole, 2-min cycles of CPR are performed between rhythm checks. Adrenaline is given during alternate cycles (*for doses see Box 11.1*) and a single dose of atropine (3 mg for adults) is also given. Potentially treatable causes for the arrest must be sought - *see Box 11.5*. Prolonged arrest may be an indication for bicarbonate – *see page 162*. Cardiac pacing for asystole (see below) is only of benefit in cases with complete heart block where P waves are present.

> Most patients who present in asystole are dead, having been in VF for some time and having suffered irreversible hypoxic damage as a result. In a few cases, the primary rhythm change is extreme bradycardia and it is these patients who are most likely to respond to therapy.

Pulseless Electrical Activity

In PEA (also known as EMD), 2-min cycles of CPR are performed between rhythm checks. Adrenaline is given during alternate cycles) (*for doses see Box 11.1*) and a single dose of atropine (3 mg for adults) is given if the heart rate is less than 60 complexes per minute. If the ECG changes and organised electrical activity continues, a central pulse should be checked. (The carotid pulse is used in adults and children over 12 months old but in infants the brachial pulse on the inner aspect of the upper arm is more appropriate.) Potentially treatable causes for the arrest must always be considered (the four Hs and four Ts - *see Box 11.5*). For *a discussion of the significance of these reversible causes of PEA see page 157*. The administration of either IV fluids or bicarbonate is particularly relevant for children.

Emergency pacing

External cardiac pacing is the method of choice in an ED; it is available as an additional feature on most advanced defibrillators. The external pacing electrodes must be placed on the front and the back of the chest to ensure good contact. The pacing voltage is increased until capture of the ECG is obtained. While establishing pacing, the patient's general condition and central pulse should be monitored. 'Blind' transvenous pacing in the ED is rarely successful - there is a risk that the pacing wire may loop and knot in the right ventricle or in the pulmonary artery. In the absence of any form of pacing equipment, external cardiac percussion (fist pacing) may sometimes maintain a satisfactory heart rate. Blows are delivered to the left central side of the chest at a rate of about 100 per minute.

Alternative techniques of cardiac compression

Several alternative techniques of external chest compression have also been described. None has found widespread acceptance yet in the UK.

Mechanical chest compression

This has been around for over 30 years, but recently, there has been a long overdue resurgence of interest. Three main types of devices are now on the market:
1 Mechanical arms which directly compress the anterior chest (gas-driven)
2 Pneumatic vests which inflate to squeeze the entire chest (electric)
3 Encircling bands which tighten around the mid-chest (electric)

Studies have shown that these machines give an increased cardiac output and are reliable and constant when compared with a human resuscitator who generally tires after only a couple of minutes. Mechanical CPR is particularly desirable during transfers and for prolonged resuscitations. It is ideal for chest compression in the back of an ambulance.

Active compression and decompression

Active compression and decompression of the chest can be achieved with a sucker attached to the pre-cordium (the AMBU ACD device). The active decompression which occurs when the chest is pulled upwards by the suction device has been claimed to improve cardiac filling and hence cardiac output. However, the instrument is very tiring to use and in most controlled trials has not been shown to improve survival. It is more likely to be effective when coupled with mechanical CPR as in (1) above.

Internal cardiac massage

This achieves a much better output than external chest compression. Access to the pleural cavity is gained via a fourth left interspace thoracotomy; the pericardium may be left intact. The heart is squeezed up against the sternum with the extended fingers. *(For emergency thoracotomy see page 83.)*

When to stop life support

> A person with a cardiac arrest should not be declared dead inside an ambulance at the door of the ED. The full cardiac arrest procedure should be initiated. The decision to abandon resuscitation can be made when there is no response and all of the relevant information is available.

The team leader must decide when it is appropriate to abandon attempts at resuscitation. This will require consideration of:
- the patient's past medical history;
- the history of the current collapse and resuscitation;
- the clinical and ECG findings;
- the views of the other team members, including paramedics.

Recovery is very unlikely in asystole from a primary cardiorespiratory cause that does not respond to 15 min of ALS.

For medicolegal aspects of death see page 381.

Agonal rhythm

The wide, rounded or M-shaped complexes which are characteristic of a dying heart are not capable

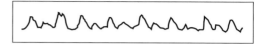

Figure 11.6 Agonal rhythm

of stimulating myocardial contraction (*see Figure 11.6*). Thus, this agonal rhythm is not a form of PEA although the two are often confused.

Post-resuscitation care

Recovery from cardiac arrest depends on the maintenance of an adequate circulation to protect the brain and then on the restoration of spontaneous cardiac output as soon as possible. The arbiter of success is thus satisfactory tissue perfusion and not electrical activity on an ECG. Neurological recovery from cerebral ischaemia may take more than 24 hours and so isolated signs such as the state of the pupils are of little prognostic value in the first few hours after cardiac arrest. Fits may occur in up to 25% of patients and are also unrelated to eventual outcome. On the whole, however, rapid return of normal function equates with a good outcome, especially regular spontaneous ventilation and improving level of consciousness. Coma persisting for more than 6 hours post-arrest is associated with a high probability of severe neurological damage and only 10% of such patients will return to an independent existence. After three days in coma, absent pupillary light reflexes and absent motor responses to pain are independent and specific predictors of a poor outcome (death or vegetative state).

Tx

When spontaneous cardiac output returns 'reanimation' becomes 'resuscitation' and intensive care must begin. The patient has been effectively dead for a short period of time.
- Continue with oxygen therapy/ventilation.
- Ensure good venous access; usually both peripherally and centrally.
- Consider therapy with amiodarone (or lidocaine) in order to prevent a recurrence of VF.

- Monitor pulse, BP, SaO_2 and ECG.
- Obtain a 12-lead ECG and a chest X-ray.
- Take blood for arterial blood gases, blood chemistry and FBC.
- Obtain a detailed history and perform a full examination.
- Catherise the patient and monitor the urinary output.
- Consider the possibility of immediate coronary reperfusion by either thrombolysis or PCI *(see page 188)*.
- Treat pyrexia with antipyretics and cooling. (Body temperatures above 37°C worsen prognosis after cardiac arrest.)
- Control the blood glucose with an insulin infusion if necessary. (High blood glucose levels are strongly associated with a poor neurological outcome after cardiac arrest.)
- Arrange admission to CCU or ICU. Ventilation will be necessary in the absence of adequate spontaneous breathing or satisfactory tissue oxygenation. Some authorities advocate at least 24 h of controlled ventilation for all post-arrest patients, irrespective of their respiratory state, although there is little evidence that this improves outcome.

Inotropic and vasopressor support may be required *(see Box 14.10 on page 243)* as haemodynamic instability is common after the return of spontaneous circulation. A blood pressure of greater than 80–90 mmHg is necessary to maintain coronary perfusion, which occurs mainly during diastole. Intra-arterial BP monitoring is essential in this situation. Treatment may also be needed for pulmonary oedema *(see page 217)* and cardiac dysrhythmias *(see page 170)*. The intensivist will aim for a pulmonary capillary wedge pressure (PCWP) of less than 18 mmHg, measured with a pulmonary artery or Swan–Ganz catheter. This may require the administration of IV fluids, vasodilators or diuretics.

Therapeutic hypothermia

Mild hypothermia (32–34°C) is thought to suppress many of the chemical reactions associated with reperfusion injury. A period of 12–24 h is sufficient. It is now recommended for unconscious adult patients with return of spontaneous circulation after out-of-hospital VF arrest. There are no conclusive data to support the use of induced hypothermia in other situations. Shivering must be avoided (by sedation and neuromuscular blockade) as it causes a marked increase in metabolic demands.

Unsuccessful resuscitation

The care of the bereaved is as important as any other care in the ED *(see below)*. After some resuscitations, staff may be distressed and in need of either formal or informal support.

For brainstem death see page 381.

For organ donation see page 382.

For notification of death to the coroner or procurator fiscal see page 381.

Care of the suddenly bereaved

Death of a patient from a cardiac arrest is always sudden and thus is generally unexpected by the next-of-kin who may be ill-prepared for it. The same is true of other, less common, causes of death in an ED such as trauma and sudden infant death syndrome. *(For cot death see page 350.)* Certain principles of care may make this terrible experience more bearable:

- Relatives should be contacted promptly and dealt with as soon as they arrive at the ED. A designated (named) nurse should stay with the family throughout and act as a liaison with the rest of the medical and nursing team. In an on-going resuscitation, this nurse must make every effort to obtain up-to-date information for the relatives.
- Special facilities should be available for bereaved relatives, including a quiet, private room with a telephone, access to drinks and a toilet.
- Spiritual support may be needed for all denominations and religions. The hospital chaplains should be welcomed into the ED as a part of the team.
- When bad news is broken, it should be imparted gently and honestly, avoiding euphemism and over-involved medical explanations. Presumptions as to the cause of death should not be made. The family can be left to assimilate the news but should have another opportunity to ask further questions later on. Although the medical staff must be

involved in the contact with the relatives, the breaking of bad news can be undertaken by any experienced member of the team.

• Both verbal and written information must be provided for the relatives concerning:

– what to do next;

– coroner's procedures and the possibility of a post-mortem examination;

– helpful telephone numbers;

– a named contact in the ED with a phone number;

– details about any follow-up by a nurse or counsellor specialising in bereavement care *(see below)*.

• Arrangements must be made for relatives to get home safely and for care for those who are alone.

• Other agencies must be informed including:

– the deceased patient's GP;

– the next of kin's GP;

– the medical records department;

– the health visitor for a child under 5 years of age and the school nurse for an older child.

• Staff support and training should be available. All staff need access to a staff care or counselling scheme; this may involve contact with the hospital chaplains or psychologists. Debriefing can include both clinical and emotional aspects. Feedback from the relatives should be reviewed.

The bereavement nurse

A person specialising in the care and counselling of suddenly bereaved people can be invaluable to an ED. Such a person, who is usually a specially trained nurse, can visit the next-of-kin soon after death to provide information, answer questions and offer comfort. This visit also serves to reinforce the caring nature of the ED's work and to provide an outlet for any anger or misunderstandings. A second visit, after about 6 weeks, serves the same purposes later on in the grieving process and may identify the emergence of long-term problems in the bereaved relative.

Cardiac dysrhythmias

For all rhythms where the patient does not have a palpable pulse see cardiac arrest on page 156.

For the specific treatment of tachydysrhythmias as a result of poisoning with tricyclic antidepressant drugs see page 276.
For the management of palpitations see page 245.

General principles

Treatment of all cardiac dysrhythmias should include:

• attention to the ABCs;

• high-concentration oxygen;

• venous access;

• monitoring of SaO_2, ECG and BP;

• obtaining a 12-lead ECG as soon as possible;

• observing the patient in a high-dependency area.

The ECG should be examined to determine:

1 the ventricular rate;

2 whether the QRS rhythm is regular or irregular (fast AF may look deceptively regular);

3 the presence of atrial activity (P waves may be hidden; atrial activity includes AF);

4 the relationship between atrial and ventricular activity;

5 whether the QRS complex is normal or prolonged.

The clinical condition of the patient, especially the presence of a central pulse, is the most important factor in any treatment decision. Pallor and sweating are always bad signs.

> In patients with otherwise normal hearts, serious symptoms and signs are unusual if the ventricular rate is above 40 or less than 150 contractions per minute.

Assessment and management of bradycardia

The need for emergency treatment depends on the following:.

1 The presence of adverse clinical findings:

• symptoms of low cardiac output (dizziness and faintness);

• hypotension (systolic BP less than 90mmHg);

• heart rate less than 40 beats per minute;

• heart failure;

• presence of ventricular escape dysrhythmias which require suppression.

2 The presence of features which suggest that there is a significant risk of asystole:
• previous asystolic episodes;
• Mobitz type 2 or fixed 2:1 AV block;
• pause greater than 3 seconds;
• complete heart block (especially with a wide QRS complex or initial rate below 40 per minute).

> Bradycardias with wide QRS complexes are likely to be caused by blocks below the level of the AV node. They are usually unresponsive to atropine and relatively unstable. An AV junctional ectopic pacemaker is more reliable and may provide a reasonable heart rate with a narrow QRS.

Tx

Bradycardias which do not fall into the above criteria may be observed. Other bradycardias should be treated with IV atropine (in 500 μg increments up to a maximum of 3mg for an adult) and then expert advice sought immediately. Interim measures while awaiting emergency transvenous pacing (*see page 167*) include:
• Transcutaneous external pacing;
• Adrenaline by IV infusion (at a rate of 2–10 μg per minute for an adult);
• A range of other chronotropic drugs – aminophylline, isoprenaline and dopamine. Glucagon is used for bradycardia in poisoning with beta-blockers and calcium antagonists. Glycopyrrolate is an alternative to atropine.

For the Resuscitation Council (UK) algorithm for the treatment of bradycardia in adults see Figure 11.7.

Bradycardia in children may be a pre-terminal finding secondary to hypoxia or hypovolaemia. It is treated with a combination of:
• Resuscitation with oxygen and fluids;
• Atropine by IV/IO bolus (20μg per kg);
• Adrenaline by IV/IO bolus (10μg per kg);
• Adrenaline by IV infusion (0.05 to 2 μg per kg per minute).

Sinus bradycardia

Sinus rhythm with a heart rate of less than 60 per minute may follow:
• a myocardial infarction, usually inferior;
• a vasovagal attack;
• the use of some drugs (e.g. beta-blockers).

Hypotension, accompanied by symptoms of faintness and malaise, does not usually occur until the heart rate falls below about 40–45 beats per minute.

Tx

At heart rates above 40 in asymptomatic patients, the bradycardia can be observed without treatment. Below this rate, it can be corrected with small increments of IV atropine (i.e. doses of 100–200μg for an adult) depending on the response. Tachycardia may reduce coronary perfusion while increasing oxygen demand and is thus to be avoided.

Complete (third degree) heart block

Impairment of conduction of electrical impulses from the atria to the ventricles is usually a result of:
• myocardial ischaemia;
• poisoning (including digitalis);
• chronic heart diseases, especially aortic stenosis and congenital lesions; or
• some acute infectious diseases, including rheumatic fever.

In inferior infarction, complete AV block results from localised occlusion of the right coronary artery; the AV nodal artery is one of its branches. However, in anterior infarction complete AV block usually represents massive septal necrosis with additional damage in the territory of the circumflex artery.

The heart rate is around 35–45 beats per minute in complete heart block and thus symptoms are likely. However, if there is narrow complex junctional escape rhythm, there may be a heart rate which is both adequate and regular.

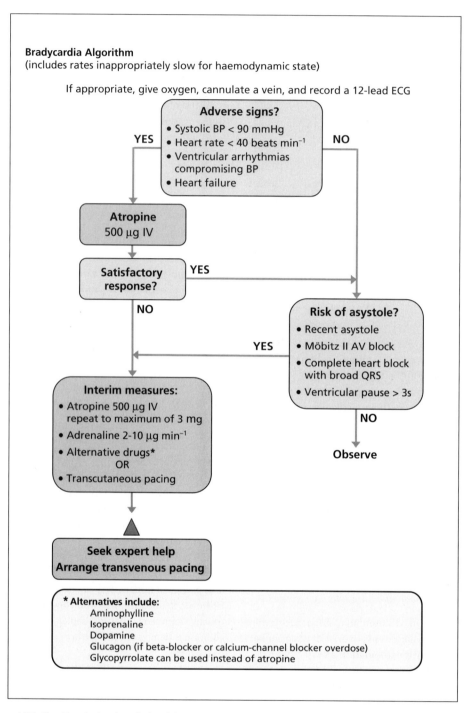

Bradycardia Algorithm
(includes rates inappropriately slow for haemodynamic state)

If appropriate, give oxygen, cannulate a vein, and record a 12-lead ECG

Adverse signs?
- Systolic BP < 90 mmHg
- Heart rate < 40 beats min⁻¹
- Ventricular arrhythmias compromising BP
- Heart failure

YES   NO

Atropine
500 μg IV

Satisfactory response?   YES

NO

Risk of asystole?
- Recent asystole
- Möbitz II AV block
- Complete heart block with broad QRS
- Ventricular pause > 3s

YES

NO

Interim measures:
- Atropine 500 μg IV repeat to maximum of 3 mg
- Adrenaline 2-10 μg min⁻¹
- Alternative drugs*
  OR
- Transcutaneous pacing

Observe

Seek expert help
Arrange transvenous pacing

* **Alternatives include:**
  Aminophylline
  Isoprenaline
  Dopamine
  Glucagon (if beta-blocker or calcium-channel blocker overdose)
  Glycopyrrolate can be used instead of atropine

Figure 11.7 Algorithm for bradycardia in adults.

Tx

The Resuscitation Council (UK) algorithm for bradycardia should be followed *(see Fig.11.7)* and the patient referred to a cardiologist for assessment and temporary pacing.

Chronic complete AV block causing Stokes–Adams attacks

This is usually caused by fibrosis around the bundle of His (Lenegre's disease). There is a widened QRS complex. Pacing abolishes symptoms and prolongs life.

> Lyme disease should be considered as a possible cause in a young person with a new onset of heart block. *Borrelia burgdorferi* may cause a myocarditis which involves the heart's conducting tissue, especially the AV node.

Incomplete heart block

This may be caused by ischaemic heart disease, acute carditis, drugs or metabolic disturbance.

First-degree heart block

This causes prolongation of the PR interval so that it is greater than 0.2 seconds (one large square). After myocardial infarction, 40% of patients with first-degree AV block will go on to develop second- or third-degree blocks and so close observation of these patients is required.

Second-degree heart block

This is said to exist when there is an intermittent failure of conduction through the AV node or the bundle of His. There are three variations:
1 *Wenckebach phenomenon (Mobitz type 1 block).* There is progressive lengthening of the PR interval and then a failure of conduction. This is followed by a conducted beat with a normal PR interval and the lengthening process then starts again. The conduction deficit is in the AV node.
2 *Mobitz type 2 block.* The majority of beats are conducted with a normal and constant PR interval

but occasionally a P wave is not followed by a QRS complex—a dropped beat. The problem lies distal to the AV node.
3 *Fixed second-degree (2:1 or 3:1) block.* There are intermittent conducted and non-conducted atrial beats giving a ratio of P waves to QRS complexes of 2:1 or 3:1.

Tx

Mobitz type 2 block and fixed 2:1 AV block may herald complete heart block and so require prophylactic pacing.

The Wenckebach phenomenon is usually benign and transient; it is caused by drug toxicity, high vagal tone, or an inferior myocardial infarction involving the AV nodal artery. The heart rate may be increased by atropine. When Wenckebach second-degree block occurs after an anterior infarction, temporary pacing is indicated.

Bundle branch block

Bundle branch block of recent onset after myocardial infarction is associated with a less favourable prognosis and, in the case of LBBB, is an ECG indication for thrombolytic therapy—*see page 187.* As a rough guide, a broad RSR (M-shaped) pattern in V1 is caused by RBBB and a similar pattern in V6 indicates LBBB. (*For more details on ECG diagnosis of BBB see Box 11.6.*) The further interpretation of bundle branch block requires an expert opinion.

Box 11.6 ECG Diagnosis of Bundle Branch Blocks	
RBBB	**LBBB**
QRS > 120 m sec	QRS > 120 m sec
Secondary R wave in V1, V2 and V3	Broad monophasic R wave and absence of Q wave in I, V5 and V6
Wide S wave in I, V5 and V6	ST and T in opposite direction to QRS

Bifascicular block

This results when only half of one bundle branch is conducting normally. There is most usually a combination of RBBB with left anterior hemiblock, which appears as left axis deviation on the ECG. A quick way to check for this common type of bifascicular block is to look for a broadened M pattern in V1 and a deep S wave which is bigger than the R wave in lead II. This conduction disturbance may cause drop attacks in the same way as complete heart block. Patients with evidence of either trifascicular or bifascicular disease after myocardial infarction may need to be prophylactically paced.

Intraventricular abnormalities of conduction

These may cause notching of the QRS complex but do not require treatment.

Supraventricular tachycardia

The main causes of SVT are:
- ischaemic heart disease, often at the time of acute myocardial infarction or in the peri-arrest situation;
- congenital abnormalities of conduction (which cause paroxysmal attacks);
- drugs;
- metabolic disturbances.

There are two main types of SVT which are outlined below:

1 Junctional tachycardias

Atrioventricular nodal re-entry tachycardia (AVNRT)

This is the commonest type of regular narrow-complex tachyarrhythmia and also the commonest paroxysmal SVT. It often occurs in patients with otherwise normal hearts and is thus relatively benign. The cause is a re-entry circuit within the AV node. *For an explanation of AV nodal re-entry circuits see Box 11.7.* The ECG is regular with no visible atrial activity.

> **Box 11.7 AV Nodal Re-Entry Circuits**
>
> In the normal AV node there are two pathways along which the atrial impulse can travel – a slow pathway with a short refractory period and a fast pathway with a longer refractory period. The two unite to become the Bundle of His. During normal sinus rhythm, the atrial impulse travels along both pathways but completes its journey via the fast pathway only because the slow pathway has already become refractory. In atrioventricular nodal re-entry tachycardia a premature atrial beat occurs at a crucial time and the impulse finds the fast pathway to be still refractory and so travels along the slow pathway. When it gets to the point where both fast and slow pathways join to form the bundle of His, the fast pathway has recovered from its refractory period and the impulse travels backwards up it. This establishes a re-entry circuit and is the mechanism in 90% of patients with AV nodal tachycardia. In the other 10% of patients, a premature ventricular beat is the source of the problem and a slow-fast circuit is set up – the reverse of the situation described above. Because of the normal anatomy involved, affected individuals are often young and healthy with no detectable heart disease.

Atrioventricular re-entry tachycardia (AVRT)

Re-entry involves an accessory pathway such as the bundle of Kent in Wolff-Parkinson–White (WPW) syndrome. There is usually no visible atrial activity on the ECG. After resolution of the tachycardia, the ECG may show a short PR interval and a delta-wave (a slurred upstroke denoting pre-excitation) at the start of the QRS complex.

2 Atrial tachycardias

Atrial tachycardia

An ectopic atrial focus causes an atrial rate of 150–250 beats per minute. Often the rate is between 160–170 beats per minute with a 1:1 response but at faster rates 2:1 block may occur.

Atrial flutter

The atria flutter at around 300 beats per minute and 2:1 or 3:1 block occurs to give rates of up to 150–160 complexes per minute—*see below*. It may be difficult to identify flutter waves on the ECG.

Atrial fibrillation

The heart rate is irregular.
For fast atrial fibrillation see page 177.

It is unwise to assume that haemodynamic disturbance accompanying tachycardia inevitably points to a ventricular origin for the dysrhythmia.

Irregular or broad-complex SVT

SVT usually appears as a narrow-complex tachycardia on ECG but, if there is aberrant (i.e. abnormal) conduction such as bundle branch block, then broad complexes may be seen. In the peri-arrest situation, SVT may precipitate VF. An irregular narrow-complex tachycardia is most likely to be fast AF.

Infants with SVT

Infants with a tachydysrhythmia may present with a sudden onset of poor feeding, tachypnoea, pallor and lethargy. SVT is the commonest non-arrest arrhythmia of infancy and may give rise to cardiogenic shock. Heart rates range from 220 per minute to as high as 300 complexes per minute.

Tx

For the Resuscitation Council (UK) algorithm for the treatment of tachycardia in adults (with a pulse) see Figure 11.8.

Fast atrial fibrillation is a difficult situation requiring expert advice (*see page 177*).

• Vagal manoeuvres such as carotid sinus massage, orbital pressure, Valsalva, iced water to the face, etc. can be attempted—with care—in most patients. Infants can have their faces immersed in iced water for 5 seconds.

• Adenosine is effectively a 'chemical shock'—immediate effect, short-acting and relatively safe in both stable and unstable patients. The initial dose is 6mg for an adult which is given as a rapid IV bolus. If this proves to be ineffective, up to two further doses (each of 12 mg) may be given at two minute intervals. Patients after heart transplantation are very sensitive to the effects of adenosine and should be given an initial dose of 3 mg. Undesirable effects from adenosine may be seen in

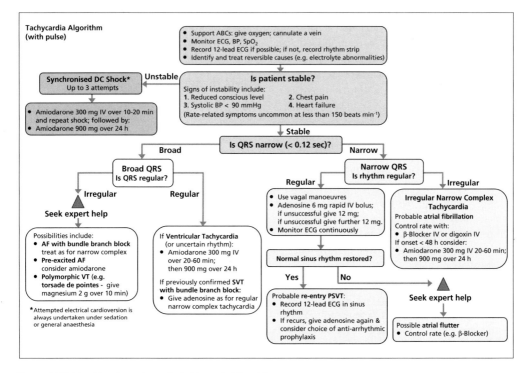

Figure 11.8 Algorithm for tachycardia (with a pulse) in adults.

patients with WPW syndrome or in those who are taking dipyridamole or carbamazepine. Adenosine (or vagal manoeuvres) will terminate almost all AVNRTs or AVRTs within seconds. Failure to terminate a regular narrow-complex tachycardia with adenosine suggests the presence of an atrial tachycardia such as atrial flutter.

Patient with signs of cardiac or cerebral compromise

(i.e. Systolic BP < 90mmHg, LVF, chest pain, heart rate >200 beats per minute, impaired consciousness)
• *Sedation and synchronized cardioversion* (starting with 120–150 J biphasic or 200 J monophasic shocks);
• *Amiodarone* 300mg IV over 20–60 min followed by 900mg over 24 h and repeated shocks if SVT persists.

Stable, alert patient

(There is a choice of drugs).
• *Verapamil* (5–10 mg IV). Verapamil is hazardous in WPW syndrome, some SVTs of childhood, ventricular tachycardias and in conjunction with beta-blockers. It must not be used in infants.
• *Esmolol.* Esmolol is an ultra short-acting cardioselective beta-blocker with a half-life of 9 min; it is contraindicated in shock, heart failure, heart block, asthma and after verapamil. In SVT when time for titration is available, a loading dose of 40 mg (500 µg per kg) is given IV over 1 minute, followed by an infusion of 50–100 µg per kg per minute until the desired effect is achieved. Esmolol may also be used for the treatment of symptomatic sinus tachycardia.
• *Digoxin* (up to 500 µg IV over 30 min, repeated if necessary).
• *Amiodarone* (300 mg IV over 20–60 min followed by 900mg over 24 h).
• *Flecainide.* Flecainide is a potent sodium channel blocker which is indicated in the special SVTs associated with accessory pathways (e.g. WPW syndrome) and AF. The dose is 100–150 mg (2 mg per kg for children) given IV over 20–30 min.

Overdrive pacing is a further option (not for AF). In patients who have ventricular pre-excitation (due to WPW syndrome) together with AF or atrial flutter, drugs which block the AV node must be avoided as they cause an increase in pre-excitation. These drugs include adenosine, verapamil, diltiazem and digoxin.

Children with narrow-complex tachycardias

Children are treated along much the same lines as adults. *For the doses of adenosine and electricity for children see Box 11.8.*

> **Box 11.8 Adenosine and Synchronised DC Shock for Narrow-Complex Tachycardia in Children**
>
> *Adenosine*
> 50 µg per kg, then 100 µg per kg and then 250 µg per kg
> (To maximum total dosage of 500 µg per kg or 300 µg per kg for infants under one month old)
>
> *Synchronised DC shock*
> 0.5 J per kg, then 1 J per kg and then 2 J per kg

Atrial flutter

The atria flutter at a rate of between 280 and 320 contractions per minute. 2:1 or 3:1 AV block occurs, resulting in a ventricular response of around either 150 or 100 beats per minute. The ECG shows a characteristic saw-tooth pattern (best seen in lead II) which is accentuated by increasing the degree of AV block (e.g. by carotid sinus massage). An irregular narrow-complex tachycardia may result from atrial flutter with a variable AV block.

Tx

An isolated attack of atrial flutter is best treated by cardioversion. It is the cardiac dysrhythmia which is most likely to convert to sinus rhythm. Only relatively small DC shocks are usually required: 70–120 J biphasic or 100 J monophasic. If necessary, the ventricular rate can be slowed with either beta-blockers or digoxin (*see page 177*). Paroxysmal flutter is controlled with drugs.

Fast atrial fibrillation

Atrial fibrillation (AF) is the most common sustained cardiac dysrhythmia. Its prevalence doubles with each advancing decade of life after the age of 50, rising to 9% in patients over 80 years old. It is also the most common dysrhythmia to cause hospitalisation. AF is associated with a 1.5 fold increase in mortality in males and 1.9 fold increase in females. The fibrillation is a non-specific response to atrial distension and so may occur acutely in conditions such as:
- myocardial infarction (AF occurs in up to 10% of cases);
- pulmonary embolism;
- sudden and excessive ingestion of alcohol.

> The factors which would cause a sinus tachycardia in a patient in sinus rhythm may result in fast AF in a patient who is already fibrillating.

Chronic AF is seen with:
- ischaemic and hypertensive heart disease;
- mitral valve disease;
- ventricular failure;
- cor pulmonale;
- cardiomyopathy;
- thyrotoxicosis.

Recurrent bouts of AF (paroxysmal AF) may also occur. There is usually no identifiable underlying cause and episodes settle spontaneously.

In AF chaotic depolarisation of the atria results in a loss of atrial contraction and a fast, irregular ventricular rhythm. There is a consequent reduction in cardiac output and a risk of systemic embolism. Symptoms of AF include palpitations, dyspnoea, fatigue and chest pain. The main need for treatment of AF in the ED arises when a fast heart rate is causing signs of haemodynamic disturbance or is contributing to left ventricular failure (LVF).

Tx

For the Resuscitation Council (UK) algorithm for the treatment of tachycardia in adults (with a pulse) see Figure 11.8.

For AF, there are three main treatment options:
1 Control of the ventricular rate by drugs
2 Control of the atrial rhythm by pharmacological cardioversion
3 Control of the atrial rhythm by electrical cardioversion

It is important to treat the underlying causes of both the fibrillation and the tachycardia. In addition, some complications must be prevented (eg. thrombo-embolism) and some must be treated (e.g. heart failure).

Paroxysmal AF usually reverts spontaneously to sinus rhythm within 48 hours and so cardioversion is seldom required.

In patients with AF complicating heart failure, digoxin is used to slow AV conduction and thus control the ventricular rate. It has no effect on the underlying dysrhythmia. It may be given orally or IV depending on the urgency of the situation. A suitable IV dose of digoxin is 0.75–1 mg made up to 50 mL and infused over two or more hours. Too rapid infusion causes nausea and dysrhythmias. Oral digitalisation can be achieved by giving 1–1.5 mg of digoxin in divided doses over 24 h.

> In AF, the optimum ventricular rate at rest is about 90 beats per minute.

In a patient with AF complicating an acute illness, sinus rhythm usually returns spontaneously when the underlying disease, together with any aggravating factor such as hypokalaemia, resolves. Cardioversion is usually unnecessary unless AF is causing haemodynamic instability. Fast heart rates causing breathlessness or poor perfusion can be controlled with digoxin, verapamil, diltiazem or beta-blockers, the choice of drug and the route of administration depending on the underlying condition and the urgency of the situation. Magnesium has also been advocated for this purpose (*see Box 11.10*).

Cardioversion for AF

Electrical cardioversion is usually successful in AF of recent onset (less than 48 hours) and may be required urgently in the presence of chest pain or critical perfusion. Under sedation or general anaesthesia, synchronised DC shocks are delivered with escalating energies starting with 120–150 J (biphasic) or 200 J (monophasic). Following successful cardioversion, there are several drugs which can be used to maintain sinus rhythm; the choice depends on the underlying condition and is a matter for a cardiologist. However, amiodarone (300 mg given IV over 20–60 min followed by 900 mg over 24 h) is a safe and common choice.

If the anaesthetic skills needed for the administration of a DC shock are not available, then chemical cardioversion is also an option in acute AF of under 48 h duration. The best drug (for a relatively healthy heart) is probably IV flecainide 2 mg per kg (to a maximum of 150 mg) given over 20 min. Amiodarone can also be used (300 mg IV over 20–60 min followed by 900 mg over 24 h) and is better than flecainide for a diseased heart. Both drugs may worsen haemodynamic disturbance and so should only be administered by the experienced practitioner. Patients who have been in AF for more than 48 h should not be cardioverted, either electrically or pharmacologically, until they have been anticoagulated for at least three weeks.

Anticoagulation for AF

Thrombi may form in the atria within 48 hours of the onset of AF. They may also form after successful cardioversion as the atria may not empty well for several days due to 'atrial stunning'. All patients should therefore be considered for prophylactic heparinisation.

Ventricular tachycardia

This is a sign of a heart which is 'irritable' or has disordered conduction caused by intrinsic damage, electrolyte disturbance or drugs. High rates may cause a variable loss of cardiac output although this feature alone does not distinguish VT from SVT. The ECG shows a regular broad complex tachycardia (QRS >120 ms) at a rate of over 120 beats per minute. Independent P waves may

be seen which are unrelated to the QRS complexes; fusion beats can also occur. VT may be monomorphic or polymorphic depending on the origin. Torsades de pointes is a form of polymorphic VT (*see page 179*).

Tx

VT always has the potential to degenerate into VF and so treatment must not be delayed.
For the Resuscitation Council (UK) algorithm for the treatment of tachycardia in adults (with a pulse) see Figure 11.8.
For magnesium therapy see Box 11.10.

Patient with no pulse

Go to the VF protocol.

Patient with signs of cardiac or cerebral compromise

(i.e. Systolic BP < 90 mmHg, LVF, chest pain, heart rate >150 beats per minute, impaired consciousness)
- *Sedation and synchronised cardioversion* (starting with 120–150 J biphasic or 200 J monophasic shocks);
- *Consider treatment for hypokalaemia* if the serum potassium is known to be low (with IV potassium and magnesium);
- *Amiodarone* 300 mg IV over 20–60 min followed by an infusion of 900 mg over 24 h;
- *Further shocks as required* and consider treatment with other drugs (e.g. lidocaine, procainamide, flecainide or sotalol) or overdrive pacing.

Stable, alert patient

- *Consider treatment for hypokalaemia* if the serum potassium is known to be low (with IV potassium and magnesium);
- *Amiodarone* 300 mg IV over 20–60 min followed by an infusion of 900 mg over 24 h. An alternative is lidocaine (100 mg by slow IV bolus for an average adult, followed by an infusion of 4 mg per minute for 30 min, then 2 mg per minute for 2 h and then

1mg per minute. Intravenous lidocaine has a short duration of action (15–20 min). If an infusion is not immediately available, the initial IV bolus can be repeated once or twice at intervals of not less than 10 min.

• *Synchronised DC shock* if VT persists, then amiodarone and further shocks if necessary.

Broad-complex supraventricular tachycardia

This arises when SVT occurs in conjunction with delayed conduction through the ventricles (aberrant conduction). The commonest causes of aberrant conduction are bundle branch blocks and pre-excitation from accessory pathways. Fast AF with pre-existing LBBB is especially easy to mistake for VT.

Broad-complex tachycardia of uncertain origin

Unlike verapamil, which may be dangerous, adenosine can be given to a patient with a broad-complex tachycardia of uncertain origin. This constitutes a useful diagnostic test—in SVT the ventricular rate will usually slow after adenosine whereas in VT the heart rate will continue unchanged. However, in fast AF or flutter occurring in patients with an accessory AV pathway, there may even be a worsening of the tachycardia as the anomalous pathway is left unchallenged by normal conduction.

Broad-complex tachycardia that is irregular

This is most likely to result from AF with bundle branch block or, in patients with WPW syndrome, AF with ventricular pre-excitation *(see page 175)*. A third cause is polymorphic VT (e.g. torsades de pointes *see below*).

Children with broad-complex tachycardias

Children with broad-complex tachycardias are treated in much the same way as adults.

Adenosine may be used as described above to determine the source of the tachycardia. It can sometimes be impossible to deliver a synchronised DC shock in VT as synchronisation relies upon the ability of the defibrillator to recognise a QRS complex within the ECG signal. In many cases of VT, especially in children, there is no recognisable complex and so the defibrillator will not discharge whilst in the synchronised mode. For this reason, non-synchronous shocks are sometimes recommended for VT in shocked or otherwise unstable children. However, it is best to attempt to use synchronous shocks at first as these are less likely to produce VF than asynchronous ones. If the defibrillator fails to discharge, then it should be desynchronised immediately. *For the doses of amiodarone, lidocaine and electricity for VT in children see Box 11.9.* Procainamide is sometimes used in stable children with VT (15mg per kg given IV over 30 min).

Box 11.9 Amiodarone, Lidocaine and DC Shock for Broad-Complex Tachycardia in Children

Amiodarone
5 mg per kg IV over 30 min

Lidocaine
IV boluses of 0.5 mg per kg and then 1mg per kg followed by an infusion of 10–50 μg per kg per minute

DC shock
0.5 J per kg, then 1 J per kg and then 2 J per kg

Torsades de pointes

This is a variety of polymorphic VT where the fast ventricular complexes vary from beat to beat, as if the electrical axis is twisting around a fixed point *(see Figure 11.9)*. There is usually an underlying prolongation of the QT interval, caused by drugs (especially antidepressants) or electrolyte disturbance (e.g. hypokalaemia). The condition may occur in patients who have taken the antihistamine terfenadine in overdosage or in combination with any of the following interacting substances:

• erythromycin, clarithromycin or related macrolide antibiotics;

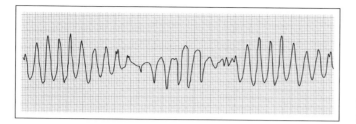

Figure 11.9 ECG trace of torsades de pointes

- ketoconazole, itraconazole or related imidazole antifungal drugs;
- concentrated grapefruit juice.

Patients with cardiac or hepatic disease are especially at risk.

Tx

Episodes of torsades de pointes are usually self-limiting but may progress to VF. Treatment is with IV magnesium (*see Box 11.10*) or beta-blockers. Anti-arrhythmic drugs such as lidocaine, quinidine, sotalol or amiodarone may further increase the QT interval and thus worsen the condition. Overdrive pacing may be required to prevent rapid relapse.

Box 11.10 MagnesiumTherapy

Intravenous magnesium may sometimes be helpful in the control of certain resistant ventricular dysrhythmias such as:
- VT secondary to hypokalaemia
- VT which is resistant to DC shock
- Torsade de pointes
- Some tachycardias which are secondary to the effects of drugs including digitalis, anti-arrhythmics and occasionally tricyclics

The dose is 4–8 mmol of magnesium (diluted to 20 mL with saline) administered IV over 5–10 min. One gram of magnesium sulphate contains 4mmol of magnesium ion; a 50% solution contains approximately 2 mmol per ml. Transient flushing—sometimes accompanied by hypotension—is to be expected in almost all patients. The total dose of magnesium may be up to 16 mmol, followed by an infusion of 2.5 mmol per hour.

Children: Magnesium sulphate 25–50 mg per kg IV over several minutes; maximum dose 2g

---

Box 11.11 Acquired Causes of a Long QT Interval

Drugs (antiarrhythmics, antidepressants, antihistamines, antimalarials, phenothiazines, organophosphates)
Electrolyte disturbances (hypokalaemia, hypocalcaemia or hypomagnesaemia)
High protein liquid diets and other dietary factors
Coronary ischaemia, myocarditis and severe heart failure

Long QT syndromes

A long QT interval may be acquired or, in very rare cases, congenital. *For a list of the commoner acquired causes of a long QT syndrome see Box 11.11.* Consequent ventricular dysrhythmias may cause palpitations, syncope or even sudden death. The QT interval must be corrected for heart rate and is then called the QTc. This calculation is usually performed automatically by modern ECG machines. The normal QTc is 0.38–0.46 seconds. To make a confident 'eyeball' diagnosis, the QT interval should be around half a second (0.48s or 12 small squares on the ECG).

Ectopic beats

During a 24-hour period, over 50% of apparently normal subjects will have ectopic beats within their ECG; in some cases these will be multifocal. The causes of extrasystoles include:
- fatigue;
- anxiety;
- excessive smoking, alcohol or caffeine intake;
- idiopathic causes;
- myocardial ischaemia;
- heart diseases with atrial enlargement (*see atrial fibrillation on page 177*);

- digitalis and other drugs;
- hyperthyroidism.

The treatment (if any) is dependent on identifying the likely causation. Multifocal ectopics, with differing waveforms, and runs of ectopic beats are more significant than isolated extrasystoles as they are more likely to develop into VT and VF. *For palpitations see page 245.*

Identification of pacemakers

The increasing complexity and diversity of pacemakers has necessitated the use of an identification system. An original three-letter code, which was agreed by the International Association of Pacemaker Manufacturers, has been expanded into a five-letter code to enable description of newer programmable units – *see Box 11.12.* The most common pacemaker in the UK is described by the code VVI (ventricular pacing which is inhibited by sensed ventricular impulses).

Box 11.12 Pacemaker Code	
Position of letter	**Meaning of letter**
1st	Identifies chamber(s) paced (V = ventricle; A = atrium; D = dual)
2nd	Identifies chamber(s) sensed (V = ventricle; A = atrium; D = dual; 0 = none)
3rd	Describes the pacemaker's response to sensed impulses (T = triggered; I = inhibited; D = dual; R = reverse)
4th	Describes programmable functions
5th	Describes tachydysrhythmia control functions

Chapter 12

Chest pain

Pain in the area of the chest is a worrying symptom for both the doctor and the patient. The patient knows that chest pain occurs in a heart attack. The doctor is aware that the symptoms of myocardial infarction and pulmonary embolism can be very different from the classical descriptions in the textbooks.

> Patients with chest pain account for more than 20% of all medical admissions in the United Kingdom.

Immediate assessment and management

- Assess ABCs as outlined in Chapter 1.
- Reassure the patient.
- Allow the patient to sit or lie in whatever position is most comfortable.
- Obtain a 12-lead ECG immediately (within 5–10 min of arrival) and interpret it at once. If there are changes which, when combined with the clinical picture, indicate the need for reperfusion therapy (ST-segment elevation myocardial infarction left bundle branch block or posterior myocardial infarction) proceed without delay – *see page 187.*

In any case, if there are any immediately obvious symptoms or signs of serious illness or if the patient looks unwell:

- Administer high-concentration oxygen by mask.

- Connect the patient to monitoring devices – ECG, BP and SaO_2.
- Obtain venous access and take blood for routine tests. Samples for cardiac markers should be taken at times dictated by local protocols – *see page 192.*
- Request an urgent chest X-ray.
- Consider the need for early analgesia.

> Pallor and sweating usually indicate serious illness. Beware of the middle-aged man who wants you to make a diagnosis of indigestion.

Further assessment

Ask about
- Duration of pain.
- Nature of pain including radiation and whether constant or intermittent.
- Relationship of pain to breathing, coughing or moving.
- Precipitating or relieving factors, including glyceryl trinitrate (GTN).
- Similarity of pain to previous events (e.g. MI or angina).
- Accompanying symptoms such as sweating, nausea, vomiting, flatus or general malaise.
- Shortness of breath.
- Collapse or blackout, however transitory.
- Family and smoking history.

Look for
- Pallor, sweating or cyanosis.
- Abnormal pulse or BP.

• Raised jugular venous pressure (JVP) or dependent oedema.

• Added heart sounds.

• Tracheal deviation – a difficult and unreliable sign.

• Changed respiratory rate and pattern.

• Low SaO$_2$ on air.

• Reduced air entry and abnormal breath sounds.

• Abdominal tenderness – especially epigastric and renal (which may mimic chest pain) and hepatic discomfort (congestive heart failure).

Myocardial Infarction and the acute coronary syndromes

Coronary heart disease (CHD) is the most common cause of death and the single main cause of premature death in both men and women in the United Kingdom. It accounted for over a quarter of all deaths in England and Wales in 2004. By 2020, it is projected to be both the number one cause of death and the leading cause of life years lost on a global scale. The three major risk factors for CHD are smoking, hypertension and hyperlipidaemia. The disease progresses faster in the presence of diabetes and obesity and doubles in incidence in those who are physically inactive. However, its victims are not all overweight, unfit individuals; MI strikes all shapes and sizes of people at almost all ages. 30% of people die from their first MI.

Only 10% of the British population are free from all the major risk factors for CHD. Asians in the United Kingdom are at a particularly high risk. People with no obvious risk factors are still more likely to die of MI than from any other cause.

CHD begins several decades before the acute event with the formation of atherosclerotic plaques. 75% of fatal coronary thromboses occur when there is a sudden rupture of the thin fibrous cap covering an inflamed, lipid-rich plaque. Mechanisms such as plaque erosion account for the rest. The initial flow obstruction is due to platelet aggregation followed by vasospasm. This process is accelerated by the secretion of substances such as thromboxane A2, ADP and 5-HT

from entrapped platelets. Activation of the coagulation cascade then leads to the conversion of fibrinogen to fibrin, which is responsible for the subsequent stabilisation of the fragile thrombus. Within 30 min of complete coronary occlusion, MI develops, progressing from the subendocardium to the subepicardium.

The term 'acute coronary syndromes' describes a continuum of conditions that are associated with acute myocardial ischaemia as a result of interruption of the coronary blood supply. The syndromes range from unstable angina to full-thickness MI. ST-segment elevation myocardial infarction (STEMI) exists as a distinct diagnostic entity because patients with specific ECG changes derive a unique benefit from immediate reperfusion therapy [thrombolysis or percutaneous coronary intervention (PCI)]. Patients with other manifestations of ACS are treated with low molecular weight heparins and antiplatelet therapy instead of fibrinolytic drugs – *see later*.

Every year, nearly a quarter of a million people in England and Wales have an acute MI. Up to 50% of them die in the first month. Half of these deaths occur in the first 2 h.

Diagnosis of acute coronary syndromes and evolving MI

Symptoms

The pain is classically experienced in the central chest and described as crushing or heavy. Some patients say it feels like a tight band around their chest; others describe it as like someone is sitting on them. It is common for the patient to clench his or her fist as an aid to description. The pain usually lasts longer than 20 min. The radiation, if any, may be to the left arm, neck or jaw. There is some suggestion that in right coronary artery blockage the jaw is the site of radiation while in left-sided occlusions the pain is felt in the arm.

Accompanying symptoms such as sweating, pallor, nausea or general malaise are almost as helpful in making a diagnosis as the character of the pain. Coronary thrombosis may also present without pain ('silent MI'), with atypical pain, with complications of MI (e.g. LVF) or with an acute confusional state in the elderly.

Symptoms of 'indigestion'

Be aware of the middle-aged man with 'indigestion', especially if he has no past dyspeptic history of significance. A few days of vague retrosternal pain is not a history of dyspepsia. It is much more likely to be the warning pains that often predate an MI. Recurrent belching is a sign of autonomic disturbance and as such may accompany an infarction. Even symptomatic relief from antacids should not be relied upon to point away from the heart.

Some patients present with very atypical pain, both in site and character. Examples of this would be pain localised to the abdomen or to the left shoulder or arm alone.

> Many experienced doctors have sent patients home who have later proved to have an MI; sudden death may be this proof.

Signs

There are no invariable signs. Cardiogenic shock, acute pulmonary oedema or dysrhythmia make the diagnosis much easier but physical examination of the patient is often normal. Pallor and sweating should never be ignored; they point to autonomic disturbance. The heart rate may be fast, slow or average. Likewise, the blood pressure may be raised or low but is often normal. A slow heart rate often occurs in an inferior MI since the right coronary artery which supplies this area also supplies the conducting system. (In addition, it delivers blood to the posterior myocardium and the right ventricle, although in some patients the circumflex branch of the left coronary artery is responsible for much of this territory. The anterior and lateral myocardium is invariably supplied by the left anterior descending artery).

Investigations

● Immediate ECG (within a few minutes of arrival) is essential. Repeat ECG after 30–60 min may also be helpful.

For ECG diagnosis of STEMI and indications for thrombolysis see page 185.
For ECG changes in other acute coronary syndromes see page 187.
For cardiac dysrhythmias see page 170.

> A normal ECG does not exclude an MI.

● Chest X-ray is usually normal.
● Routine blood tests should be taken, especially a blood glucose to identify the need for a glucose and insulin infusion in ACS and MI.
For the use of cardiac markers in ACS see page 192.
● A reduction in pain following the administration of GTN may be a helpful test but unfortunately this effect also occurs in oesophageal spasm.

More advanced methods of diagnosis of myocardial ischaemia exist and some are undergoing clinical trials:
● multi-lead 'vest' ECGs, which use over 80 chest electrodes;
● high-resolution CT scanning;
● two-dimensional echocardiography – regional motion abnormalities of the myocardium develop seconds after coronary occlusion;
● technetium scanning – a normal resting technetium-99 myocardial perfusion scintigram effectively excludes major MI. However, an abnormal scan is not diagnostic.

ECG diagnosis of coronary thrombosis and evolving infarction requiring immediate reperfusion therapy

Complete coronary occlusion causes an evolving MI that can be averted by timely reperfusion therapy. However, only when chest pain is accompanied by three specific ECG patterns has immediate reperfusion been shown to be of benefit. These three patterns are:
1 STEMI
2 True posterior MI
3 New LBBB.
(The term STEMI is useful in the acute situation to determine treatment and is analogous to older descriptions such as Q-wave MI and transmural infarction.)

1) ECG changes in STEMI

ST-segment elevation signifies complete occlusion of a major coronary artery and accounts for 30–40% of classical MIs. The occlusion/infarction sequence classically begins with subtle alterations in the T wave. These hyperacute T waves are tall, peaked and broadened with a loss of clear demarcation from the ST segment (*see Figure 12.1*). Elevation of the ST segment ('convex-upwards') soon follows in leads that face the area of injury; reciprocal ST depression may also occur (*see Figure 12.2*). Abnormal Q waves, which signify myocardial necrosis, may be present in the first ECG but in most cases do not appear for hours or even days after presentation. These pathological Q waves are wide (0.04 s – one small square – or more) and deep (4 mm or a quarter of the size of the subsequent R wave). They result from potentials that are transmitted through an electrical window of inexcitable myocardium and so suggest the presence of complete (transmural) rather than

partial-thickness (subendocardial) damage – *see later*. Severe intracellular disturbance may cause a similar picture. Finally, as the ST segment returns to the baseline, symmetrically inverted T waves appear. The timing and magnitude of all of these ECG changes varies greatly from patient to patient.

The site of a typical transmural infarction may be localised from the position of the ECG changes:

Anterior   V1, V2, V3, V4
Lateral   V5, V6
High lateral   I, aVL
Inferior   II, III, aVF [additional ST elevation in V4R (a right-sided V4) suggests infarction of the right ventricle – *see Box 12.1 and page 196*.]

ECG changes must meet defined criteria for the diagnosis of STEMI and the initiation of reperfusion therapy:

1 ST elevation of at least 2 mm in two adjacent precordial (chest) leads (V2–V6) or

2 ST elevation of at least 1 mm in two limb leads (I, II, III, aVL or aVF).

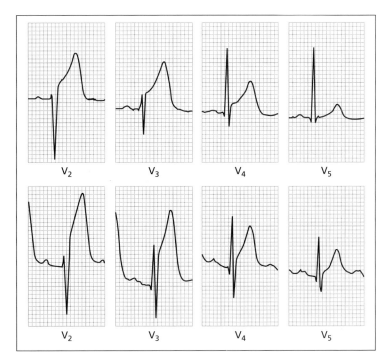

Figure 12.1 Two examples of hyperacute T waves in acute MI.

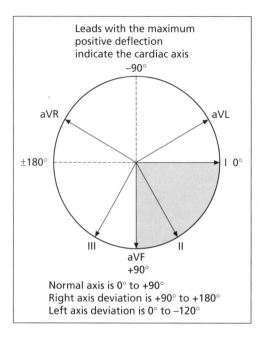

Leads with the maximum positive deflection indicate the cardiac axis

Normal axis is 0° to +90°
Right axis deviation is +90° to +180°
Left axis deviation is 0° to −120°

Figure 12.2 The ECG limb leads and the cardiac axis.

Box 12.1 ECG Signs of True Posterior and Right Ventricular MI

Posterior infarction
- tall R wave in the anterior leads (V1–V3);
- ST depression in the anterior leads (V1–V3), that is, there is a mirror image of the usual Q wave and ST elevation pattern (*see Figure 12.3*);
- ST elevation in posterior chest leads (*see Figure 12.4*).

Right ventricular infarction
- ST elevation in V4R;
- ST elevation in V1–V3 (and eventually Q waves in these leads);
- ECG changes of inferior MI.

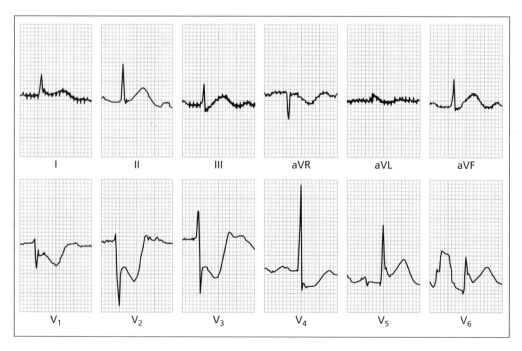

Figure 12.3 12-lead ECG of a true posterior infarction.

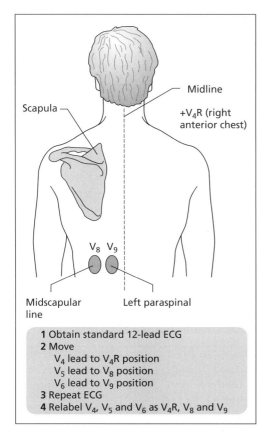

Scapula

Midline

+V₄R (right
anterior chest)

V₈ V₉

Midscapular
line

Left paraspinal

1 Obtain standard 12-lead ECG
2 Move
 V₄ lead to V₄R position
 V₅ lead to V₈ position
 V₆ lead to V₉ position
3 Repeat ECG
4 Relabel V₄, V₅ and V₆ as V₄R, V₈ and V₉

Figure 12.4 How to record a 15-lead ECG.

2) ECG changes in true posterior MI

Like conventional STEMI, true posterior infarction results from complete occlusion of a major coronary artery and, if untreated, leads to irreversible myocardial necrosis. The term 'true' refers to the isolation of the infarct to the posterior myocardium as opposed to being part of a posterolateral or inferoposterior picture.

For the ECG signs of true posterior and right ventricular MI see Box 12.1.

Figure 12.3 shows a 12-lead ECG of a posterior infarction. However, although an isolated posterior infarct may be hard to diagnose on a conventional 12-lead ECG, it can be more reliably seen on a 15-lead or a 17-lead ECG. A 15-lead ECG has been described that utilises V4R and two posterior leads – *see Figure 12.4.* This technique increases the detection of ST elevation in MI by about 10%. The extra three leads should be obtained when the standard 12-lead ECG shows either ST depression in the anterior chest leads or equivocal right-sided or inferior changes. Low voltage ST elevation of just 0.5 mm in the posterior chest leads is sufficient to diagnose a posterior STEMI and initiate reperfusion therapy.

3) ECG changes in LBBB with MI

Patients with LBBB have a much worse prognosis with acute MI than patients with normal ventricular conduction, whether the LBBB is pre-existing or new. However, these patients (who account for around 0.5% of all patients with infarcts) have been shown to benefit greatly from reperfusion therapy. Consequently, in the presence of LBBB, it is essential to diagnose an MI promptly. This is difficult because the normal sequence of ventricular activation is altered and there is ST elevation because of the LBBB itself. Three ECG criteria (the 'Sgarbossa criteria') have been shown to have independent value in the diagnosis of MI in patients with LBBB – *see Box 12.2.* Unfortunately, these criteria have to be scored and added to be useful and do not apply to all MIs with LBBB. Therefore, all patients with chest pain and proven or suspected new LBBB should be treated with PCI or fibrinolytic therapy without delay. *For diagnosis of LBBB see Box 11.6 and page 173.*

Treatment of STEMI

The following section applies to new LBBB and posterior MI as well as to STEMI.

Having made the diagnosis of an evolving MI requiring immediate reperfusion therapy, the emergency treatment detailed below must not delay preparations for thrombolysis or PCI.

Box 12.2 ECG Diagnosis of MI in the Presence of LBBB

Three ECG criteria have been shown to be useful in the diagnosis of MI in patients with LBBB:
1 ST-segment elevation of 1 mm or more that is concordant with (in the same direction as) a positive QRS complex
2 ST-segment depression of 1 mm or more in lead V1 or V2 or V3 (concordant change)
3 ST elevation of 5 mm or more that is discordant with (in the opposite direction from) a negative QRS complex

Proceed immediately to reperfusion therapy without completing the following list.
• *Oxygen by mask and IV access.*
• *Continuous monitoring* of vital signs and ECG.
• *Analgesia* – diamorphine 2.5–5 mg IV with an antiemetic (e.g. metoclopramide 10 mg IV).
• *Antiplatelet therapy* – aspirin 300 mg by mouth and oral clopidogrel.
Aspirin is as effective as (and additive to) fibrinolysis in reducing death rates in STEMI. After an MI, it is continued for life in a dose of 75 mg daily. There are few contraindications to aspirin – known hypersensitivity, bleeding peptic ulcer and severe liver disease. Clopidogrel 300 mg by mouth should also be given to all patients with STEMI, including many of those in whom aspirin is contraindicated. It seems to have a synergistic effect with fibrinolytic drugs. For those patients who are having primary PCI, many centres routinely prescribe clopidogrel 600 mg by mouth and IV abciximab.
• *Nitrates* – nitrates are used for persistent pain. Buccal GTN is a convenient and effective alternative to IV nitrates. The initial dose is 2 mg but this may be increased to 3–5 mg if necessary in the carefully monitored patient. A sublingual aerosol spray of GTN can be useful for a quick effect (two puffs = 800 μg).
For GTN infusions see page 218.
• *Glucose and insulin infusion* – diabetic patients with MI have double the mortality of non-diabetics. In addition, there is experimental and limited

clinical evidence that routine administration of glucose and insulin may improve metabolism in ischaemic myocardium. This treatment is inexpensive and should be given to all patients with either known diabetes or a blood sugar greater than 11 mmols per L on admission. *For a suitable variable rate IV insulin regimen see Box 14.11 on page 247.*
• *Beta-blockers* – if not contraindicated, early administration of a beta-blocker is recommended for all patients with MI. Atenolol 5 mg IV is given over 5 min and the dose repeated after 10–15 min; 25 mg by mouth is an alternative. IV metoprolol is also licensed for this indication.
For thrombolysis see page 189.
For details of inpatient treatment of MI and ACS see page 195.

Reperfusion therapy for STEMI

This section applies to new LBBB and posterior MI as well as to STEMI.

There are three possible first-line reperfusion treatments for STEMI:
1 *Immediate thrombolysis* – see page 189. Thrombolysis should start within 20–30 min of arrival in hospital ('door to needle' time) or within 60 min of first contact with the emergency services ('call to needle' time). This is both effective and achievable. Even better results can be obtained with faster times or prehospital thrombolysis. Ideally, PCI should be performed during the following 24 h–48 h.
2 *Primary PCI.* Coronary angioplasty should be taking place within 90 min of arrival in hospital ('door to balloon' time) or within 120 min of first medical contact ('call to balloon' time). As a treatment standard, PCI should not be delayed for more than 60 min after the time that thrombolysis could have been given. PCI is a very effective therapy but system constraints tend to limit its delivery. Percutaneous Transluminal Coronary Angioplasty (PTCA) is an older name for balloon-assisted PCI.
3 *Facilitated PCI.* Immediate thrombolysis as in (1) above is followed by PCI within no more than

12 h. This is achievable and may well deliver the benefits of both independent treatments (although it is still under investigation). Glycoprotein IIb/IIIa receptor inhibitors (abciximab) have also been used for facilitation of PCI – *see page 196*. Early PCI (where immediate thrombolysis is followed by PCI within 24–48 h) is another interesting variant of treatment, which is being investigated at present.

Local factors and protocols will control which of the above three treatments is recommended for a particular patient. The availability of interventional cardiac cathetherisation facilities is usually a major limiting factor in the United Kingdom (where, in 2005, the ratio of thrombolysis to PCI was more than 10 : 1). PCI is the treatment of choice in cases where thrombolysis is contraindicated or has obviously failed. If the patient's chest pain started more than 3 h before arrival, (a delayed 'pain to needle' time), then primary PCI is more effective than thrombolysis. PCI is contraindicated in severe thrombocytopenia. In the prehospital situation, fibrinolytic drugs offer the only possible means of reperfusion.

> There is a 'golden hour' for reperfusion therapy, which starts at the onset of pain.

PCI is better at opening closed arteries than thrombolysis. It achieves TIMI ('Thrombolysis in Myocardial Infarction') grade 2 or 3 flow in over 95% of cases whereas fibrinolytic drugs have a maximum success rate of around 55% at completely opening up the artery responsible for the STEMI (TIMI grade 3 flow). Primary PCI is also associated with lower rates of stroke and non-fatal reinfarction than thrombolysis and goes some way to treating the underlying condition. It is definitely superior for patients with cardiogenic shock. When compared to tenecteplase or alteplase given within 2 h of symptom onset, very early PCI saves the lives of about 10 patients per 1000 treated. However, the added time to accomplish angioplasty often negates this advantage. Fibrinolytic drugs are most effective within 2–3 h of symptom onset. Within 6 h of the onset of chest pain, their administration prevents 30

deaths per 1000 patients treated (with aspirin increased to 50 per 1000 patients). Between 7 and 12 h, this reduces to 20 lives saved per 1000 patients treated. After 12 h, the risk/benefit ratio for fibrinolytic drugs is less certain. Thrombolysis increase mortality if given more than 24 h after symptom onset or to patients with ST depression or T-wave inversion without ST elevation.

> The rate of intercranial hamorrhage with thrombolysis is less than 1% but half of these bleeds are fatal.

Fibrinolytic drugs cause around four extra strokes per 1000 patients treated. These occur in the first 24 h, two patients dying and two surviving, one of whom will be disabled. The risk of stroke is predicted by advanced age, low body weight, female gender, previous cerebrovascular accident and hypertension, especially hypertension on admission. Major non-cerebral bleeds occur in 7 per 1000 patients treated and are most commonly procedure-related. Again advanced age, low body weight and female gender are associated factors.

> Reduction in ST elevation of more than 50% within 45–60 min of thrombolysis suggests a patent artery and preserved myocardium.

The resolution of chest pain and reduction in ST elevation suggest reperfusion as does the emergence of arrhythmias. Failed reperfusion (i.e. less than 50% reduction in ST elevation within 45–60 min of starting the treatment) is an indication for rescue PCI. There is little evidence for re-thrombolysis except after the less effective drug streptokinase. Coronary Artery Bypass Graft (CABG) surgery is becoming more common as an emergency procedure in the United Kingdom.

Thrombolytic therapy for STEMI

This section applies to new LBBB and posterior MI as well as to STEMI.

Fibrinolysis is an endogenous process whereby the insoluble fibrin that binds a blood clot together is broken down into soluble fragments (fibrin degradation products or FDPs). It is initiated by plasminogen activators such as tissue plasminogen activator (tPA), which are secreted into the circulation by the vessel wall. These substances convert plasminogen, a protein normally present in the plasma, into plasmin that digests fibrin. Free circulating plasmin is inactivated by α2-antiplasmin. Fibrinolytic drugs exert their effect by activating plasminogen to form plasmin, which degrades fibrin and so breaks up thrombi.

The criteria for the administration of thrombolytic therapy are:

1 history compatible with MI;

2 onset of symptoms within the last 12 h;

3 diagnostic ECG changes as below (see also page 184):

- ST elevation of at least 2 mm in two adjacent precordial leads (V2–V6);
- ST elevation of at least 1mm in two limb leads (I, II, III, aVL or aVF);
- LBBB (presumed or proven to be new);
- evidence of true posterior infarction (see Box 12.1 and Figure 12.3). Low voltage ST elevation of just 0.5 mm in the posterior chest leads would be sufficient to diagnose STEMI;

4 no contraindications to thrombolysis – see Box 12.3.

Patients who present more than 12 h after the onset of symptoms (but not more than 24 h) may still be considered for thrombolysis if there are signs or symptoms of continuing ischaemia. Thrombolytic therapy is contraindicated in a considerable number of patients (see Box 12.3). The contraindications are mostly those conditions that might result in severe or life-threatening bleeding. In some cases, there is a possibility of pre-existing thrombus (e.g. with aneurysms or atrial fibrillation) and so there is a risk of causing an embolism by dissolution of the clot.

Heparin is given with all fibrinolytic drugs except streptokinase. An IV bolus of 5000 units is followed by an IV infusion for 24–48 h – see Box 12.4. The heparin does not improve clot lysis but seems to help maintain coronary patency in the following hours and days. Low molecular

---

Box 12.3 Contraindications to Thrombolytic Therapy

This is not an exhaustive list.

Absolute contraindications

Known coagulation defects or bleeding diatheses

Recent haemorrhage, significant trauma or surgery (including dental extraction)

Haemorrhagic stroke or stroke of unknown causation at any time

Ischaemic stroke in last 6 months

History of CNS damage, aneurysm or neoplasm

Intracranial surgery or significant head injury within last 3 weeks

Severe uncontrolled hypertension

Acute pericarditis or bacterial endocarditis

Active pulmonary disease with cavitation

Aortic dissection

Active peptic ulceration

GI bleeding within last 4 weeks

Acute pancreatitis

Severe liver disease

Oesophageal varices

Visceral neoplasm with increased risk of bleeding

Heavy vaginal bleeding

Coma

Previous allergic reaction to drug (streptokinase)

Cautions/relative contraindications (*balance risk/ benefit for each individual patient*)

Current oral anticoagulant therapy

Recent non-compressible arterial or central venous puncture sites

Traumatic resuscitation

TIA in last 6 months

Diabetic retinopathy (small risk of bleeding only; therefore not a major contraindication)

Hypertension (systolic BP > 180 mmHg)

Abdominal aortic aneurysm

GU bleeding in last 10 days

Pregnant or less than 1 week post-partum

---

weight heparins (LMWH) are sometimes used in place of standard unfractionated heparin but the risk of bleeding in elderly patients has not yet been fully evaluated.

To be of maximum benefit, thrombolysis must be commenced as soon as possible and certainly within 20–30 min of hospital arrival. *Prehospital thrombolysis* is a logical way of improving 'call to needle' times yet further (often yielding time gains of up to 1 h). It has been shown to save an additional 16 lives per 1000 patients treated when compared to conventional inhospital thrombolysis. A recent study found that prehospital thrombolysis reduced mortality by the same amount as primary PCI.

Box 12.4 Thrombolytic Regimens for STEMI

Tenecteplase (TNK-tPA)

Single IV bolus given over 10 s + heparin for 24–48 h. Weight-adjusted (500 to 600 μg per kg):
- 30 mg if weight less than 60 kg;
- 35 mg if weight 60 kg to under 70 kg;
- 40 mg if weight 70 kg to under 80 kg;
- 45 mg if weight 80 kg to under 90 kg;
- 50 mg if weight 90 kg or more.

Alteplase (tPA)

IV bolus followed by infusion to maximum dose of 100 mg over 90 min + heparin for 24–48 h.

If not using a special programmable syringe driver:
- Draw up 50 mg of alteplase into each of two 50 mL syringes.
- Give a 15 mg bolus IV from the first syringe.
- Infuse 50 mg (the entire contents of the second syringe) over 30 min, using an infusion pump.
- Infuse the remainder of the first syringe (35 mg) over the next 60 min.

For patients < 65 kg give a 15 mg IV bolus, then 0.75 mg per kg over 30 min and then 0.5 mg per kg over 60 min.

Reteplase (rPA)

Double IV bolus of 10 units + 10 units given 30 min apart + heparin for 24–48 h. Reteplase is not adjusted for weight.

Streptokinase

Infusion of 1.5 million units over 1 h. Heparin is not required (but may be given).
- Dilute the contents of a 1.5 million unit vial in 10 mL of 5% dextrose.
- Add this to a further 50 mL of 5% dextrose in a 60 mL infusion pump syringe.
- Run at 1 mL per min.

Heparin

Maximum benefit is obtained if heparin is given in conjunction with tissue plasminogen activators.
- Give 5000 units of unfractionated heparin as an IV bolus.
- Continue with a heparin infusion for a minimum of 24 h. Infuse at 1250 units per h initially. The clotting time (APTT) should be measured within 12 h and the heparin infusion adjusted to keep the value at twice normal. These doses should be adjusted for patients with a low body weight (i.e. less than 60 kg).

Choice of thrombolytic drug

For contraindications to thrombolysis see Box 12.3.

Tenecteplase (TNK-tPA) is the best drug for all patients with STEMI as it combines maximum efficacy with ease of administration. It is given as a single weight-adjusted IV bolus over 10 s – *see Box 12.4*. It is always accompanied by IV heparin to prevent re-thrombosis. An IV bolus of 5000 units of unfractionated heparin is followed by an IV infusion for 24–48 h – *see Box 12.4*. Tenecteplase is the end result of a long research programme to find an 'ideal' fibrinolytic agent and was created by recombinant DNA modification of standard tissue-type plasminogen activator – *see Box 12.5*. A longer half-life allows for single bolus treatment and increased fibrin specificity targets the plasminogen on the clot surface while minimising systemic plasminogen activation. This latter property leads to a decrease in non-cerebral bleeding complications and the need for blood transfusions.

The three other standard fibrinolytic drugs are alteplase, reteplase and streptokinase. Alteplase and reteplase are both plasminogen activators but streptokinase is not a naturally occurring substance in humans. Although it is cheap, it is antigenic and causes allergy and hypotension. Infusions of streptokinase are often discontinued or slowed down because of these side effects – a

---

Box 12.5 Genetic Modification of tPA to create TNK-tPA

Both alteplase and tenecteplase molecules consist of 527 amino acids organised into five distinct modules. However, tenecteplase (TNK-tPA) has three modifications to specific areas of alteplase (standard tPA), which improve its pharmacokinetics:

1 Threonine (T) replaced with asparagine at position 103 (increases the half-life).

2 Asparagine (N) replaced with glutamine at position 117 (reduces plasma clearance and so increases the half-life).

3 Lysine (K), histidine and two arginines replaced with four alanines at positions 296–299 (increases fibrin specificity and gives an 80-fold greater resistance to plasminogen activator inhibitors such as PAI-1).

Box 12.6 Comparison of the Four Main Fibrinolytic Drugs

	Tenecteplase	Alteplase	Reteplase	Streptokinase
Molecular weight (Daltons)	70 000	70 000	39 000	47 000
Plasma half-life (min)	20–24	4–7	15–18	23–29
Fibrin specificity	+++	++	+	—
Usual dose	0.53 mg per kg as a single bolus	100 mg over 90 min	Two 10 iu boluses 30 min apart	1.5 million iu over 60 min
Ease of use	+++	+	++	+
Reduction in mortality	++	++	+(+)?	+
Risk of haemorrhagic stroke	++	++	++	+
Antigenicity	—	—	—	++
Likelihood of hypotension	—	—	—	++

Urokinase is a direct plasminogen activator, which is produced by human kidney cells and so is non-antigenic. It is given as an IV infusion of 2 million units over 15 min but is not routinely available in the United Kingdom.

problem which is concealed by auditing 'door to needle' times in isolation. Streptokinase is much less effective than tPA in patients under 75 years old with anterior infarcts and, in addition, should not be given to patients who:

1 have received streptokinase or anistreplase (a related drug) ever before;

2 have had a recent, proven, streptococcal infection;

3 have a systolic BP of less than 90 mmHg;

4 may need an urgent invasive procedure (e.g. pacing or PCI).

Overall, the use of tenecteplase or alteplase rather than streptokinase has been shown to save around 9 lives per 1000 patients treated.

For a comparison of the four main fibrinolytic drugs see Box 12.6.

For standard regimens for all of the four main fibrinolytic drugs and heparin see Box 12.4.

For the treatment of complications of thrombolytic therapy see Box 12.7.

Biochemical markers of myocardial damage

The biochemical markers of ischaemic injury include the traditional cardiac enzymes [especially creatinine kinase-myocardial band (CK-MB)] and more recently, the cardiac proteins myoglobin and troponin. The exact use of these tests depends on local protocols; only the troponins are discussed in detail in this section. *For the timing of the release of the three main cardiac markers into the bloodstream after ischaemic chest pain see Figure 12.5.*

The cardiac specific troponins T and I (cTnT and cTnI) are proteins that are released into the bloodstream by damaged heart muscle. They are polypeptide components of the tropomyosin complex in myofibrils, which mediate actin/myosin interaction and consequent muscle contraction. The cardiac isoforms of both troponins are specific and are not found in skeletal muscle or other tissues. They are used for three main purposes:

1 To confirm or exclude the diagnosis of an acute coronary syndrome.

2 To quantify the extent of myocardial damage and thus allow for risk stratification.

3 To assess reperfusion and reinfarction.

Troponins have diagnostic sensitivities for acute MI, approach 100%. The maximum sensitivity occurs 12 h after the onset of symptoms and thus this is the point at which a blood sample for troponin should be taken. A normal troponin level at this time indicates a very low risk of cardiac complications in the following 30 days. However, it does not exclude the possibility of underlying CHD or that the patient's symptoms were due to myocardial ischaemia. Raised troponins (especially if elevated early in the ischaemic process) are associated with reduced ejection fractions and

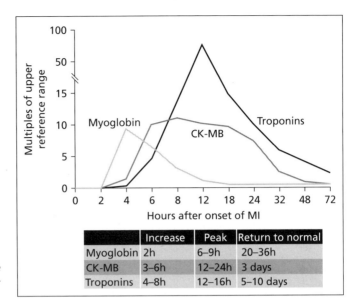

	Increase	Peak	Return to normal
Myoglobin	2h	6–9h	20–36h
CK-MB	3–6h	12–24h	3 days
Troponins	4–8h	12–16h	5–10 days

Figure 12.5 The release of the three main cardiac markers into the bloodstream after MI.

Box 12.7 Treatment of Complications of Thrombolysis

Bleeding

Apply pressure, if possible, to any bleeding sites and, if the bleeding is severe then:

- stop the infusion;
- start careful volume replacement;
- give cryoprecipitate 6 units or FFP 2 units;
- consider antifibrinolytic drugs (tranexamic acid 10 mg per kg by slow IV injection or, exceptionally, aprotinin 500 000 units by slow IV injection).

Reperfusion arrhythmias

- observe if transitory or minor;
- for the treatment of peri-arrest arrhythmias *see page 170*.

Mild allergic reaction (to streptokinase)

- give hydrocortisone IV 100–200 mg;
- give chlorphenamine (chlorpheniramine) IV 10–20 mg;
- continue the fibrinolytic drug with careful observation.

Severe allergic reaction (to streptokinase)

- stop the infusion;
- give hydrocortisone and chlorphenamine as above.

In addition, if indicated give:

- nebulised bronchodilators;
- Adrenaline IM/IV.

Hypotension (following streptokinase)

- interrupt the infusion temporarily;
- elevate the legs if necessary;
- in extreme cases consider starting a low-dose noradrenaline infusion.

Box 12.8 Troponin T Levels

The values given below are intended as a guide only; individual laboratories will set their own diagnostic ranges.

Troponin T less than 0.03 mg per L. Although this does not rule out underlying coronary heart disease, a Troponin T value in this category conveys no additional prognostic information. However, values between 0.01 and 0.03 µg per L are abnormal and indicate either an acute coronary syndrome or an alternative condition.

Troponin T 0.03–0.1 mg per L. This indicates minimal myocardial damage. Higher values are associated with greater degrees of myocardial cell loss and thus an increased likelihood of the patient developing complications.

Troponin T 0.1–0.2 mg per L. Troponin T levels above 0.1 µg per L suggest that significant myocardial damage has occurred. This group of patients has the greatest benefit from antiplatelet therapy.

Troponin T greater than 0.2 mg per L. This is the level associated with classical MI with all the attendant implications for prognosis.

---

increased morbidity and mortality in subsequent months. Troponin T remains elevated for 12–14 days after a large MI; troponin I for 3–7 days. *For the diagnostic significance of raised levels of Troponin T see Box 12.8.*

Discharge of patients from hospital. A patient who has a low clinical probability of cardiac pain, no ECG changes, a full resolution of symptoms and a normal 12 h troponin level can be safely discharged from hospital with (or sometimes without) outpatient follow-up. Use of troponins in this way has been shown to reduce the length of hospitalisation for patients with chest pain by around 33%.

False positive troponin levels. Increased troponin levels can occur in patients who do not exhibit the clinical features of an acute coronary syndrome. These false positive results can lead to situations where a raised troponin is difficult to interpret. *For the other clinical conditions in which raised troponins have been identified see Box 12.9.*

Box 12.9 Other Conditions Associated with a Raised Troponin Level

Cardiac conditions

myocardial contusion (raised troponin is not a sensitive indicator of trauma but has a high positive predictive value);

heart failure and septic shock;

cardiac arrhythmias;

myocarditis and cardiomyopathy;

cardiac surgery and post-transplantation;

cardiac electrophysiological procedures (not DC cardioversion).

Non- cardiac conditions

renal failure (commonest reason for a false positive);

pulmonary embolism (associated with large emboli and RV damage);

non-cardiac surgery.

Acute coronary syndromes without persistent ST elevation

The acute coronary syndromes without ST elevation comprise a continuum from unstable angina (UA) through to non-ST elevation MI (NSTEMI). Sensitive markers of myocardial damage (such as troponins) have revealed that there is no real qualitative difference between the various diagnostic labels. There is an underlying critical but incomplete occlusion of one or more coronary arteries. The ECG may show ST depression and/or T wave inversion but is often completely normal. ST depression carries a worse prognosis. *For the significance of T wave inversion on a 12-lead ECG see Box 12.10.* The diagnosis of myocardial necrosis may be made from the ECG alone (especially in the case of certain patterns such as subendocardial infarction – *see below* but more commonly depends on the presence of raised levels of serum cardiac markers. The most commonly used cardiac markers are CK-MB, myoglobin, troponin T and troponin I – *see page 192.* With the aid of troponin levels, unstable angina may be somewhat arbitrarily differentiated from NSTEMI – *see Box 12.8.* In addition, the injury may be quantified in terms of myocardial cell loss (i.e. size of infarct). Unfortunately, troponins do not reach their maximum sensitivity until 12 h after the onset of symptoms and so vigorous treatment must be initiated for all patients with suspected ACS.

Subendocardial infarction

Although the pathological and electrical findings do not correlate exactly, established MIs may be classified by ECG into two broad groups: Q wave and non-Q-wave infarctions. Patients with ECGs in the latter group have smaller infarcts and a lower initial mortality although they have a high risk of further (usually Q wave) infarctions. Transmural damage to the myocardium

---

Box 12.10 Significance of T wave Inversion on a 12-Lead ECG

Abnormal T wave inversion may be due to ischaemia, strain or pericarditis

Leads with T wave inversion	Significance
AVR only	Normal
V1 only	Occurs in 20% of normal adults and most children
V1 and V2	Occurs in 5% of normal adults and many children
V3–V6	Always abnormal in adults
I and II	Always abnormal in adults
AVL, AVF and III	May be normal if the T wave axis is similar to the QRS axis

---

> **Box 12.11 ECG Signs of Subendocardial Infarction**
>
> - ST segment depression (earliest change);
> - reduction in size of R wave;
> - deep symmetrical negative T wave.
>
> Unlike the more common transmural infarction, subendocardial infarction does not result in Q waves. The ECG changes are usually reflected in multiple leads but are especially frequent in the precordial leads. Exact location of the infarct site is difficult or impossible.

(e.g. untreated STEMI) is usually associated with the development of Q waves and/or the loss of R-wave voltages, whereas incomplete infarction of the ventricular wall leads to prolonged ST and T-wave changes – *see Box 12.11*. This subendocardial infarction accounts for about 25% of all classical infarcts and represents the most severe end of the ACS spectrum, just before STEMI. It results from either diffuse three-vessel disease or a single severe stenosis.

Tx of ACS without ST elevation

- *Oxygen and IV access*
- *Continuous monitoring* of vital signs and ECG
- *Analgesia* – diamorphine 2.5–5mg IV with an antiemetic (e.g. metoclopramide 10 mg IV)
- *Antiplatelet therapy* – aspirin 300 mg and clopidogrel 300 mg by mouth. *For GP IIb/IIIa inhibitors see page 196.*

Aspirin induces a long-lasting functional defect in platelets by blocking the arachidonate metabolism (thromboxane A2-dependent platelet aggregation). After ACS, it is continued for life in a dose of 75 mg daily. There are only a few contraindications to aspirin – known hypersensitivity, bleeding peptic ulcer and severe liver disease.

Clopidogrel is a thienopyridine that inhibits ADP-induced platelet aggregation. In patients with ACS, it provides an additional 20% relative risk reduction over and above aspirin for MI, CVA and death. The loading dose is 300 mg, followed by 75 mg a day for 12 months. The onset of action of clopidogrel is delayed for 2–4 h.

- *Antithrombin therapy*

Enoxaparin 1 mg per kg subcutaneously.

Low molecular weight heparins (LMWH) are more effective in ACS than standard unfractionated heparin. They have a higher plasma availability and better Factor Xa inhibition. The prolonged half-life and more predictable kinetics allow them to be given subcutaneously without monitoring of clotting parameters. The best evidence is for enoxaparin – 1 mg per kg subcutaneously immediately and then twice daily for 6 doses or, if the pain is ongoing, until the patient has been pain-free for 24 h. This dosage is reduced to 1 mg per kg once daily in severe renal impairment (i.e. creatinine clearance less than 30 mL per min).

- *Nitrates*

Nitrates are given for persistent pain. Buccal GTN is a convenient and effective alternative to IV nitrates. The initial dose is 2 mg but this may be increased to 3–5 mg if necessary in the carefully monitored patient. A sublingual aerosol spray of GTN can be useful for a quick effect (two puffs = 800 µg). *For GTN infusions see page 218.*

- *Glucose and insulin infusion*

Diabetic patients with MI have double the mortality of non-diabetics. In addition, there is experimental and limited clinical evidence that routine administration of glucose and insulin may improve metabolism in ischaemic myocardium. This treatment is inexpensive and should be given to all patients with either known diabetes or a blood sugar greater than 11 mmols per L on admission. *For a suitable variable rate IV insulin regimen see Box 14.11 on page 247.*

- *Beta-blockers*

If not contraindicated, early administration of a beta-blocker is recommended for all patients with MI or other ACS. Atenolol 5 mg IV is given over 5 min and the dose repeated after 10–15 min; 25 mg by mouth is an alternative. IV metoprolol is also licensed for this indication. Beta-blockers may be used for persistent or recurrent chest pain. Calcium antagonists are an alternative if beta-blockers are contraindicated.

Inpatient treatment. All patients with MI or suspected ACS require admission to hospital for monitoring, 12 h troponin measurement and specialist assessment. Risk factor modification, optimisation of BP control and lipid-lowering therapy will then be considered. Ideally, an exercise ECG test and coronary angiography should be performed within 24 h.

ACE inhibitors. These drugs are of benefit to all patients with MI who have no contraindications, especially those with hypertension or poor LV function. Treatment with an ACE inhibitor should be started within 24 h of the acute episode and continued for at least 6 weeks. A raised troponin is strongly associated with a reduced ejection fraction and so is used in some centres as an indication for ACE inhibitor therapy.

Glycoprotein IIb/IIIa inhibitors. Platelets are a key element of the thrombus formation in ACS. Their initial aggregation is caused by the formation of fibrinogen bridges between surface receptors. The glycoprotein (GP) IIb/IIIa inhibitors (abciximab, eptifibatide and tirofiban) are the most potent inhibitors of platelet aggregation available and work by blocking the binding of fibrinogen to these receptors. Abciximab is a monoclonal antibody, which binds to GP IIb/IIIa receptors, and should only be used once in an individual patient. This group of drugs are used, under specialist advice:
• in acute coronary syndromes without persistent ST elevation;
• as an adjunct to primary PCI (especially in patients with diabetes or undergoing complex procedures);
• in facilitated or delayed PCI.
Unfortunately, GP IIb/IIIa inhibitors have been shown to cause increased bleeding when combined with fibrinolytic drugs.

Treatment of complications of MI

The outcome after acute MI is in part determined by the characteristics of the patient. Advanced age, diabetes, renal insufficiency and previous MI or CVA are all contributors to a less favourable outcome.

Right ventricular infarction. This accompanies around a third of inferior MIs and causes the non-specific triad of hypotension, raised JVP and clear lung fields. ST elevation in V4R is very suggestive of the diagnosis; ST elevation in V1–V3 is also often present (*see Box 12.1*). Echocardiography may confirm the diagnosis. RV preload must be maintained with IV fluids and vasodilators should be avoided.

Sinus bradycardia. This is common with inferior infarction because the inferior myocardium shares its blood supply with the right ventricle, the posterior left heart and the conducting system. (The SA node is supplied by the right coronary artery in 55% of patients and by the circumflex artery in the remaining 45%. The AV node is served by the right coronary artery in 90% of cases with just 10% of patients having a circumflex supply.) At heart rates above 45 bpm, sinus bradycardia is best just observed, but below this it starts to cause hypotension and faintness. Atropine IV is effective (adult dose: 200–2000 µg depending on the response). Tachycardia may reduce coronary perfusion while increasing oxygen demand and is thus to be avoided.

Left ventricular aneurysm. This occurs in 5% of MIs (usually large transmural anterior infarcts). Unsurprisingly, it decreases cardiac output and increases mortality by a factor of 6. Thrombus may form inside the aneurysmal sac. Chest X-ray may show cardiomegaly and there may be persistent ST elevation on the ECG. Echocardiogram is required for a definitive diagnosis. Treatment is symptomatic together with anticoagulation.

Free wall rupture of the ventricle. This is seen after 5% of MIs, 90% of cases occurring within 14 days of infarction. Acute tearing chest pain is followed by collapse, profound shock, pulseless electrical activity (PEA) and death. Ruptured ventricle is thought to be responsible for 10–20% of post-MI deaths. Subacute free wall rupture causes a rapid onset tamponade.

Ventricular septal rupture (acute VSD).
This occurs in 1% of MIs, usually in the first week.
The patient experiences a sudden onset of chest
pain and shortness of breath. On examination,
there is biventricular failure and shock. A harsh
pan-systolic murmur is present in 90% of cases
with a systolic thrill in 50%. Echocardiogram
confirms the diagnosis. Treatment of the heart
failure is aimed at keeping the patient alive while
waiting for immediate surgical repair of the defect.

Acute mitral regurgitation. This occurs in
1% of MIs, usually in the first week. It is caused
by LV dilatation, papillary muscle dysfunction or
papillary muscle rupture. The clinical
presentation ranges from tachycardia and LVF
to shock and PEA. There is usually a soft pan-
systolic murmur. Chest X-ray shows pulmonary
oedema; echocardiogram confirms the diagnosis.
Temporary medical management of the heart
failure should precede immediate valve
replacement surgery.
For dysrhythmias see page 170.
For cardiac arrest see page 156.
For LVF and acute pulmonary oedema see page 217.
For cardiogenic shock see page 243.
For pericarditis see page 200.

Other common causes of chest pain

Pulmonary embolism

The overall incidence of pulmonary embolism
(PE) in the United Kingdom is 60–70 per 100 000
people per year with an inhospital mortality of
around 10%. The incidence of venous thrombo-
embolism rises exponentially with increasing age
above 40 years but age may not be an independent
risk factor. *For the recognised risk factors for venous
thrombo-embolism see Box 12.12.* A positive family
history causes a variable increase in risk of venous
thrombo-embolism; the risk associated with cigarette smoking is still uncertain. About 50% of PEs
occur in patients in hospital or long-term care,
25% occur in patients with other recognised risk
factors and the final 25% are idiopathic. Without
prophylaxis, up to 50% of patients undergoing

major orthopaedic surgery, around 25% of general
surgical patients and nearly 20% of general medical patients will have a venous thrombo-
embolism. Thromboprophylaxis with heparin
reduces these figures by around 50%. *For the relative risks of PE and DVT for women taking combined
oestrogen and progestogen contraceptive pills (and in
pregnancy) see Box 7.11 on page 115.*
For DVT see page 114.

Over 90% of patients with PE are breathless
or have a raised respiratory rate (more than 20
breaths per min). Only 3% will not have dyspnoea,
tachypnoea or pleuritic chest pain. Haemoptysis
occurs in around 10% of cases of PE but, in the
absence of respiratory symptoms, a patient's pleuritic chest pain or haemoptysis is usually due to
another cause. A fifth of patients with a PE have a
cough. Tachycardia is also fairly common but

**Box 12.12 The Risk Factors for Venous
Thrombo-Embolism**

Major risk factors *(relative risk = 5 to 20 fold)*:
late pregnancy or puerperium;
caesarian section;
major abdominal or pelvic surgery (usually procedures
  lasting more than 30 min);
major orthopaedic surgery (e.g. hip or knee replacement);
post-operative intensive care;
malignancy (especially advanced or metastatic or in the
  abdomen / pelvis);
lower limb fracture (especially with cast);
previous proven venous-thrombo-embolism;
varicose veins;
reduced mobility (hospitalisation or other institutional
  care).
Minor risk factors *(relative risk = 2 to 4 fold)*:
oral contraceptives and hormone replacement therapy
  (see also Box 7.11 on page 115);
heart disease (congenital disease, cardiac failure, acute
  MI);
hypertension;
other chronic diseases (e.g. COPD, renal dialysis and
  neurological disability);
thrombotic disorders;
central venous catheter *in situ*;
previous superficial venous thrombosis;
obesity;
long-distance sedentary travel (both by air and by road).

other symptoms and signs are very variable. Areas of crepitus or a pleural rub are sometimes heard, as is a pulmonary flow murmur. Thrombosis of the deep veins may be present but is usually occult.

PE is present in less than 10% of patients with a low clinical probability of the condition. The clinical features compatible with PE are breathlessness and tachypnoea +/− chest pain +/− haemoptysis. In the presence of these symptoms, two further features help to determine the patient's clinical probability of having a PE:

1 There is no other likely explanation for the patient's symptoms.

2 The patient has a major risk factor. (*For the major risk factors for venous thrombo-embolism see Box 12.12 on page 197.*)

Both 1 and 2 = high clinical probability. Either 1 or 2 = intermediate clinical probability. Neither 1 nor 2 = low clinical probability.

Massive pulmonary embolism

Sometimes, the presenting symptoms of PE are collapse, syncope, hypotension, shock or even cardiac arrest. A diagnosis of massive PE is likely in the presence of unexplained hypoxia, engorged neck veins and a right ventricular gallop rhythm. An overwhelming urge to defaecate may herald the onset of the illness. Urgent treatment is vital – see later.

> Massive PE accounts for 10% of patients arriving at an ED in cardiac arrest and up to 50% of those arriving with PEA or asystole. The prognosis in these cases is very poor.

Investigations

● Routine FBC/WCC ('? infection') and blood chemistry should be requested.

● A negative D-dimer assay may be used to exclude PE in patients with low or intermediate clinical probability. (D-dimer is a breakdown product of cross-linked fibrin.)

● Blood gases and SaO_2 may show hypoxia on air but this is not invariable with small pulmonary emboli. Measurement of the blood gases is not indicated if there is a normal SaO_2 on air.

● Around one-third of patients with a moderate or large pulmonary embolus have a raised troponin level. This is associated with right ventricular damage and may in the future be used as an indication for thrombolysis in PE.

● Investigations for occult cancer in idiopathic venous thrombo-embolism (present in 7–12% of such patients) are only indicated if the presence of malignancy is clinically suspected or suggested by Chest X-ray or blood tests. Tests for thrombophilia are indicated in patients under 50 years old with recurrent PEs or a strong family history of thrombo-embolic disease.

● ECG may be normal; any changes are the result of right heart strain – see Box 12.13.

● Chest X-ray is often unremarkable – *for possible changes in PE see Box 12.14.* After upper abdominal surgery, PE may be confused on Chest X-ray with segmental collapse of the lung or pulmonary infection.

● Identification of a DVT will help in the diagnosis of PE (*see page 114*). Venography will identify twice as many thromboses as ultrasound in this situation. Ultrasound scanning is obviously adequate if a DVT is clinically identified.

● Definitive imaging should take place within an hour in massive PE and within 24 h in all other cases. Ventilation/perfusion (V/Q) scan of the

> **Box 12.13 ECG Signs of PE**
>
> Sinus tachycardia (most common positive finding)
> New atrial fibrillation
> S1, Q3, T3 (an S wave in lead I and a Q wave with T wave inversion in lead III)
> ST depression and T wave inversion in the right chest leads

> **Box 12.14 Chest X-ray Signs Seen in PE**
>
> Segmental collapse
> Pleural effusion
> Area of peripheral infarction ('sail' shadow)
> Raised hemidiaphragm
> Prominent pulmonary artery
> Localised absence of vascular markings

lungs is the classical investigation for suspected PE but is often unavailable in the acute situation. Moreover, although a normal isotope scan can reliably exclude PE, a significant proportion of results are false positives. Isotope scanning is even less reliable in the presence of an abnormal chest X-ray or concurrent cardio-respiratory disease. CTPA (computed tomographic pulmonary angiography) is gradually replacing it as the first-line investigation in PE. Patients with a good quality negative CTPA do not require further investigation or treatment for PE. Echocardiography may be diagnostic in massive PE where the patient cannot be safely moved to a CT scanner.

Tx

- *Initial treatment.* Includes high-concentration oxygen, monitoring and analgesia.
- *Anticoagulation with heparin.* Should be started before imaging in patients with anything more than a low clinical probability of PE. Enoxaparin 1.5 mg per kg is given subcutaneously immediately and then daily for at least 5 days (and until oral anticoagulation is established). In pregnancy, a regimen of 1 mg per kg stat and then 1 mg per kg twice daily is used (based on weight in early pregnancy). The dose of enoxaparin should be reduced to 1 mg per kg once daily in patients with severe renal impairment (i.e. creatinine clearance less than 30 mL per min). Standard unfractionated heparin is a less convenient and less effective alternative to LMWHs with more unwanted effects. An initial IV loading dose of 80 units per kg is followed by a continuous IV infusion of 15–25 units per kg per h (1000–2000 units per h). An IV bolus dose of unfractionated heparin (80 units per kg) should also be given (instead of LMWH) to unstable patients, to those with massive PE or in situations where rapid reversal of anticoagulation may be required.
- *Thrombolysis.* May be considered for massive life-threatening emboli. Alteplase 10 mg IV is given over 1–2 min followed by an IV infusion of 90 mg over 2 h (maximum dose 1.5 mg per kg in patients less than 65 kg). The accelerated MI regimen for alteplase *(see Box 12.4)* can also be used. Streptokinase is a less effective alternative to

alteplase. Thrombolysis is followed by unfractionated heparin after 3 h. An IV bolus of alteplase 50 mg can be administered during cardiac arrest, which is most likely due to PE or if cardiac arrest is thought to be imminent. A few units have the facility for clot fragmentation via a pulmonary artery catheter. Elsewhere, contraindications to thrombolysis should be ignored in life- threatening PE.

- *Oral anticoagulation.* (eg. warfarin) is commenced once the diagnosis of PE is confirmed. The target INR is 2.0–3.0 and when this is achieved, heparin can be discontinued. Warfarin is given for 4–6 weeks to patients with temporary risk factors, for 3 months to patients with a first idiopathic thrombosis and for at least 6 months to most other patients. Oral anticoagulants are teratogenic and so should not be given to pregnant patients (although they are not contraindicated during breast feeding). Pregnant patients must be anticoagulated with heparin, which should be reduced a few hours before expected delivery and then restarted after the baby has been born.
- *Admission to hospital.* This is required for the majority of patients with PE. A proportion of patients can be managed in the community but this depends upon local protocols and services.

Isolated dyspnoea

The diagnosis of PE may be overlooked in patients with shortness of breath as their only symptom. Recurrent small pulmonary emboli are very often forgotten as a cause of a stepwise increase in dyspnoea. PEs in elderly patients or in those with preexisting cardio-respiratory disease are similarly misdiagnosed.

Isolated pleuritic chest pain

Young adults (e.g. women on oral contraception) frequently present to ED departments with a single complaint of pleuritic chest pain. They have a very low risk of PE if they are under 40 years old with:

1 no major risk factors for thrombo-embolism (oestrogens are only a minor risk factor);
2 no clinical features of DVT;
3 a respiratory rate of less than 20 per min;

4 a normal SaO_2 on air;

5 a normal chest x-ray.

A D-dimer assay may be used to rule out PE in this situation.

Angina pectoris (stable angina)

> Cardiac pain occurring at rest is always worrying. A couple of attacks of resting pain (i.e. unstable angina) commonly occur a few days before a fatal infarction.

The pain of angina pectoris is cardiac pain and thus is identical to that described above for MI. Even the intensity of the pain apparently overlaps that experienced in some infarctions. Angina arises from heart muscle, which is working too hard for its available blood, and hence oxygen, supply. As such it must be differentiated from the pain felt in myocardium that is losing its blood supply, ie., infarcting.

> A patient with cardiac pain that has lasted for more than 20 min should be admitted to hospital.

To diagnose stable angina confidently the following should be confirmed.

- The patient is known to suffer from angina.
- The pain only lasts a few minutes.
- There are no atypical accompanying features, eg, sweating.
- There is no increase in the frequency of the attacks, ie, the patient is not developing crescendo angina.
- The pain is precipitated by the usual factors, (eg, exercise) and it is not becoming unstable angina.
- Relief from the pain is spontaneous or by GTN.
- The ECG is unchanged.
- Everything is the same as usual.

> If this episode is so typical, why did the patient come to hospital? Resolve this question before discharge.

Tx

For the treatment of unstable angina see 'acute coronary syndromes' on page 194.

Patients with stable angina of short duration can be allowed to go home if the above criteria are met. GP follow-up should be arranged.

Dissecting aneurysm of the thoracic aorta

This presents with severe pain radiating to the back. There may be evidence of hypertension, pregnancy, aortic coarctation or Marfan's syndrome. Pulses may be absent or unequal and acute aortic incompetence is sometimes found.

Investigations

Chest X-ray changes are often seen – *see Box 12.15. For other (benign) causes of a widened mediastinum see page 84.*

> A normal radiograph does not exclude the diagnosis of aortic dissection.

For radiographic changes after injury to the great vessels see page 83.

> **Box 12.15 Chest X-ray Signs of Thoracic Aortic Dissection**
>
> Wide superior mediastinum
> Left pleural effusion
> Left pleural 'cap'
> Trachea moved to right
> Aortic outline blurred
> Left main bronchus moved down

Tx

Immediate consultation with a thoracic surgeon is indicated. Meanwhile, treatment should include oxygen, monitoring and IV access. The patient should be given IV analgesia and blood samples sent to the laboratory for routine tests and cross-matching. Treatment will be required for any concomitant hypertension – *see page 244.*

Pericarditis

Pericarditis presents as sharp, persistent mid-sternal chest pain, which varies in intensity with body position. The pain may be worsened by inspiration, swallowing and lying down. It is usually said that the pain is relieved by sitting and leaning forwards. However, the authors have known the reverse to occur – exacerbation of the pain with flexion of the trunk. Radiation of the pain to the area of the trapezius muscle is very suggestive of pericarditis. A rub is sometimes heard during part of the cardiac cycle and is often loudest at the left sternal border.

Investigations

The ECG may show widespread ST elevation (in all leads except aVR and V1), characteristically 'concave upwards'. There is no accompanying ST depression. Diffuse PR segment depression is also often seen, especially in lead II. Echocardiography may detect an effusion.

Tx

Treatment of viral pericarditis (the most common form) is with NSAIDS and rest to avoid the development of myocarditis. Tenoxicam 20 mg IV/IM may be given in the ED.

Post-infarction pericarditis is seen in 5–20% of patients with transmural MI. The incidence is halved by the use of fibrinolytic drugs. There may be a low-grade fever and echocardiogram may show an effusion. Post-infarction pericarditis is treated with high-dose aspirin. (NSAIDs and steroids can interfere with myocardial healing.)

Dressler's syndrome occurs in 1–5% of patients 2–3 months post-MI. It is thought to have an autoimmune origin. Pericardial effusion is rare in Dressler's syndrome. This type of pericarditis is also treated with aspirin.

For myocarditis and endocarditis see page 245.

Pneumothorax

Spontaneous pneumothorax is most commonly seen in two groups of patients:
1 young adults who are otherwise healthy and thus can tolerate a large air leak (primary pneumothorax);

2 older patients with emphysema, pulmonary fibrosis or other underlying lung disease in whom even a small pneumothorax can precipitate respiratory failure (secondary pneumothorax).

Up to 5% of people with HIV infection will develop a pneumothorax, usually with either TB or PCP (*Pneumocystis carinii* pneumonia) as the underlying cause.

Spontaneous pneumothorax is usually caused by rupture of a small area of abnormal lung tissue such as a bulla or subpleural bleb. This may be precipitated by increases in intra-alveolar pressure such as may occur with exertion or coughing. The patient complains of a sudden onset of pleuritic pain but this may not be severe. The degree of shortness of breath depends on the size of the pneumothorax. There may be a history of a previous episode. The signs – resonance to percussion and diminished air entry over the affected lung – also depend on the amount of pulmonary collapse.

Tension pneumothorax causes life-threatening dyspnoea. It is more common after trauma. *For the diagnosis and management of tension pneumothorax see page 77.*

Investigations

Standard PA chest X-ray confirms the diagnosis. Special films taken in expiration are no longer recommended. Look at the border of the lung fields, especially in the upper outer corner. Occasionally, the pneumothorax is only visible medially, in the cardiophrenic angle. If the chest X-ray is normal despite a high degree of clinical suspicion, then a lateral chest or lateral decubitus radiograph should be requested. CT scanning is used to differentiate a pneumothorax from complex bullous lung disease or when the lung fields are obscured by surgical emphysema. It is also useful for the localisation of misplaced chest drain tubes!

Using the chest X-ray, the size of a pneumothorax is described as either 'small' or 'large', depending on the distance between the lung edge and the chest wall. If this gap is less than 2 cm across, then the pneumothorax is classified as small; a rim of 2 cm or more defines a large pneumothorax. Other descriptions are now obsolete and percentage estimations of lung collapse are meaningless. However, a 2 cm pneumothorax has been calculated as being equivalent to a 50% loss of lung volume.

Blood gas measurements are often abnormal but are only useful in distressed patients with secondary pneumothoraces.

Tx

For the technique of aspiration of a pneumothorax see Box 12.16.

For insertion of a chest drain tube see Box 6.1 on page 78.

Box 12.16. Pneumothorax Aspiration Technique

- Locate the second intercostal space in the mid-clavic-ular line. (An axillary approach is an alternative.)
- Infiltrate local anaesthetic down to the pleura.
- Enter the pleural cavity with a cannula and withdraw the needle. (The cannula should be 16 FG or larger and at least 3 cm long.)
- Connect the cannula to a 50 mL syringe via a 3-way tap.
- Begin aspirating air from the pleural cavity. Aspiration should be discontinued if the patient becomes distressed or coughs excessively or if more than 2.5 L (50 mL × 50) is aspirated.
- Obtain a repeat chest x-ray.

Most patients with a primary pneumothorax do not have a persistent air leak. Moreover, it has been shown that the risk of recurrence is less if a chest drain tube is not inserted. For these reasons – and to minimise patient discomfort – simple aspiration is recommended as the initial treatment for primary pneumothoraces. If this fails, a second aspiration attempt is successful in one-third of cases. Small-bore catheter aspiration kits with integral one-way valves are convenient and may reduce the need for repeated insertion of needles. Simple aspiration is less likely to succeed in secondary pneumothoraces (50% success rate versus 75% for primary pneumothoraces). It is also less successful with increasing age of the patient (more than 50 years) and size of the pneumothorax

(more than 3 L). Persistent air leak is more likely in patients with underlying lung disease and so all patients with a secondary pneumothorax should be admitted to hospital.

There is no evidence that large chest drainage tubes (20–24 F) are any better than smaller tubes (10–14 F) in the management of pneumothoraces. Therefore, smaller tubes should be used; catheter over guidewire (Seldinger technique) sets are now available in these sizes. The instillation of intrapleural local anaesthetic has been shown to reduce the pain caused by a chest tube *in situ*. Lidocaine 1% 20–25 mL (200–250 mg) is injected after insertion of the tube and then 8-hourly as required.

Patients with pneumothoraces that fail to expand or who have a continuing air leak after 48 h should be referred to a respiratory physician. This is an indication for suction to be applied to the drainage bottle (high volume, low pressure up to -20 cm H_2O). If the same problems continue for 4–5 days, then a thoracic surgeon should be consulted.

Spontaneous absorption of pneumothoraces does occur but can take several weeks as the pleura is, for obvious functional reasons, resistant to gas exchange in either direction. Around 1.5% of the volume of each pleural cavity can be absorbed per 24 h. High flow oxygen increases this rate by a factor of 4 (but only during the period of administration).

Tx of primary pneumothorax (no underlying lung disease)

1 *Small primary pneumothorax (less than 2 cm rim on Chest X-ray).* If the patient is not breathless, observation without admission is appropriate. The patient can be discharged from hospital with outpatient review and instructions to return immediately if they become short of breath.

2 *Large primary pneumothorax (2 cm rim or more on Chest X-ray) or patient breathless.* This should be treated by aspiration – *for a description of the technique see Box 12.16*. If this is unsuccessful, a second aspiration should be attempted, providing that less than 2.5 L of air was aspirated during the first

attempt. After a successful aspiration, the patient may be discharged pending outpatient review with instructions to return to hospital if they become breathless. If a second attempted aspiration is unsuccessful, then an intercostal chest drain will be required, followed by observation in hospital. The chest tube can be removed 24 h after full re-expansion of the lung and cessation of any air leakage.

Tx of secondary pneumothorax (significant underlying lung disease)

1 *Very small secondary pneumothorax (less than 1 cm rim on Chest X-ray or isolated apical pneumothorax) and patient asymptomatic.* Observation in hospital should be arranged.

2 *Small secondary pneumothorax (less than 2 cm rim on Chest X-ray), patient minimally breathless and under 50 years old.* One attempt at aspiration may be made, followed by admission to hospital for 24 h. If this fails to expand the lung or there is a continuing air leak, then a chest drain will be required, followed by admission to hospital until 24 h after resolution of symptoms.

3 *Large secondary pneumothorax (2 cm rim or more on Chest X-ray) or patient breathless or over 50 years old.* Intercostal tube drainage should be the initial treatment, followed by admission to hospital until 24 h after full re-expansion of the lung and cessation of any air leakage.

Pneumomediastinum

This is an under-recognised condition caused by the same factors as give rise to pneumothorax. The two may coexist. The most common symptom is discomfort in the neck, although chest pain is also frequently experienced. Hamman's sign, a pathognomonic crunching sound in phase with the cardiac cycle, is heard in less than 50% of cases.

Investigations

Diagnosis is by Chest X-ray. Pneumomediastinum is usually unilateral whereas air in the pericardium is seen all around the heart border.

Tx

This consists of mild analgesia and observation while awaiting spontaneous resolution.

Pleurisy

Inflammation of the pleura causes a characteristic, unilateral, sharp pain, which is worse with movements of the lungs (i.e. deep breathing and coughing). Patients often describe it as being like a knife. Pyrexia is common; a pleural rub is not.

Investigations

Chest X-ray is often normal but may show an area of underlying pneumonia or an accompanying pleural effusion.

Tx

Antibiotic therapy is given as for other chest infections – *see page 215*. Analgesics will be required; NSAIDs may sometimes help.

Tracheitis

In adults, tracheitis causes central chest pain of a burning nature, which is worse with deep breathing. A similar pain may be experienced after periods of hyperventilation. The patient may be pyrexial and purulent phlegm may be expectorated.

Tx

This is directed at the underlying infection.
For bacterial tracheitis in children (a much more severe illness) – see page 331.

Oesophagitis

Reflex oesophagitis and oesophageal spasm cause central chest pain, which is sometimes relieved by GTN. Relief also occurs with simple antacids, suppression of acid production being the main treatment. Unfortunately, there is often no easy way to differentiate this condition from MI and thus caution is always needed – *see page 184*.

Shingles

Shingles is the infection of a peripheral sensory nerve by the chickenpox virus. It spreads from the dorsal root ganglion where it has lain dormant since primary infection.

> A patient with shingles can infect others – causing chickenpox. Shingles is the result of autoinfection and thus cannot be 'caught'.

The burning pain of herpes zoster infection always predates the characteristic vesicular rash. A thoracic nerve is often affected by shingles and initially the diagnosis can be very elusive. A vague red patch may sometimes be seen in the early stages of the disease.

Tx

Treatment with acyclovir should be started as soon as possible. The adult dose is 800 mg five times daily for 7 days. Such treatment is expensive but reduces the severity of post-herpetic neuralgia, a difficult and time-consuming condition to treat. There is some evidence that amitriptyline given concurrently may reduce the severity of the neuralgia still further.

Precordial catch/transitory pains of young adults

Sudden, excruciating pain in the chest is often experienced by young adults. It is usually left-sided and may cause a doubled-up posture and pain with breathing. Symptoms only last for a few minutes and then disappear apart from a slight residual ache. The pain is not accompanied by nausea or sweating. The cause of the condition is unknown.

Tx

Treatment consists of reasonable examination and investigation (ECG, Chest X-ray) followed by reassurance.

Musculoskeletal pain

Pain in the chest wall is usually worsened by movements of the trunk such as sitting up and by deep breathing and coughing. It may also be related to movement of the arm at the shoulder joint. Sometimes the pain radiates down the arms but systemic features are usually absent. Areas of tenderness are common but by no means inevitable.

The problem may emanate from the muscles (viral myalgia or Bornholm disease) or from the costal cartilages (Tietze's syndrome). Rib and muscle injuries can also present as unexplained chest pain. Such injuries often go unnoticed during sporting activities or periods of intoxication. Prolonged coughing is another cause of rib fractures.

Tx

Treatment of musculoskeletal pain consists of analgesia and reassurance.
For rib fractures see page 80.

Other causes of chest pain

Upper abdominal conditions such as pancreatitis, peptic ulceration, cholecystitis and renal colic can sometimes present as pain in the chest. In contrast, in communities where cocaine abuse is widespread this is one of the most common causes of chest pain (*see page 281*).

The upper airway

The upper airway is very vulnerable to both infection and obstruction. Its clearance and maintenance are the primary concern in any patient with respiratory distress.

Choking and complete upper airway obstruction

Choking is the result of complete or near-complete obstruction of the upper airway by foreign or ectopic material. It is most common in children and the elderly.

> Most elderly patients who present with inhalation of foreign material have had a stroke while eating.

The patient may grip the throat with one hand and the wrist with the other hand ('the universal choking sign'). Sudden collapse with cyanosis while eating may mimic myocardial infarction (the 'cafe coronary').

Tx

Get help. Encourage coughing in the responsive patient. *For the Resuscitation Council (UK) Algorithms for the treatment of Choking in Adults and Children see Figures 13.1 and 13.2.*

Advanced life support entails careful judgement and an ascending hierarchy of treatment:
1 suction and finger sweeps;

2 back blows and chest thrusts;

3 the Heimlich manoeuvre;

4 direct laryngoscopic removal of foreign material; and

5 surgical bypass of the obstruction.

Complete airway obstruction that does not result from foreign material will always require an artificial airway. Notes on 1–5 above:

1 Blind probing with a finger is contraindicated in a child as it may force a foreign body further down the narrow respiratory tract and cause impaction in the conical laryngeal inlet.

2 Swift blows to the back and thrusts to the chest or abdomen may raise intrathoracic pressure sufficiently to cause foreign material to be ejected from the airway. In children, back blows can be administered with the child prone and the head lower than trunk. In adults, the most suitable position is with the patient standing upright. Sequences of five blows or thrusts are recommended.

3 An obstructing foreign body may be expelled by means of the Heimlich manoeuvre (abdominal thrusts that work by increasing the intrathoracic pressure) – *see Box 13.1*. The liver and spleen are less well protected by the ribs in infants, making the Heimlich manoeuvre relatively dangerous.

4 Direct laryngoscopy may allow visualisation of the obstruction and then its removal by suction or with Magill's forceps.

5 The cricothyroid membrane is the recommended site for an emergency surgical airway as

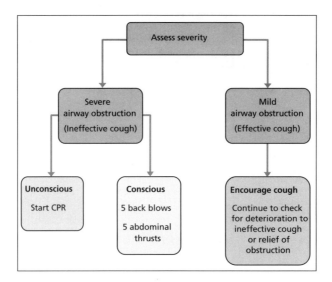

Figure 13.1 Treatment of a Choking Adult.

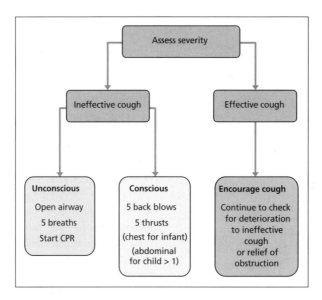

Figure 13.2 Treatment of a Choking Child.

tracheostomy is difficult and time-consuming to perform. Damage to the first tracheal ring may cause intractable stenosis. In children under the age of 12 years, needle cricothyroid puncture is preferable to direct surgical cricothyroidotomy. However, ventilation can then only be achieved with high-pressure oxygen and not with a bag and mask.

For the technique of cricothyroidotomy see page 23.

For the technique of needle cricothyroid puncture see page 24.

Post-asphyxial care

All patients who have had an episode of choking should be admitted, often to ICU. Those who remain dyspnoeic or who have a depressed level

> **Box 13.1 The Heimlich Manoeuvre**
>
> *Patient standing*
>
> Place your arms around the patient's waist from behind. Grip your wrists together directly beneath the xiphisternum and then give five short, sharp 'bear hugs' up into the epigastrium.
>
> *Patient lying*
>
> Stand or kneel astride the patient's pelvis. Place the heel of one hand in the epigastrium and reinforce it with the other hand. Then give five short sharp thrusts upwards and backwards.

of consciousness should be ventilated. Cerebral oedema is common after severe asphyxia; treatment with dexamethasone remains controversial.

Stridor and partial upper airway obstruction

Partial obstruction of the extrathoracic airways – at or above the cricoid ring – causes stridor, which is a harsh, high-pitched noise during inspiration. Intrathoracic obstruction causes wheezing. Characteristically, the patient is sat perched forward with the arms extended backwards (the 'tripod position'). Other signs of partial obstruction of the upper airway are:
- drooling of saliva;
- hoarseness;
- rattling noises in the upper airway; and
- snoring (in the unresponsive patient).

Pulmonary oedema may complicate prolonged obstruction. *See also Chapter 1, pages 1–3.*

> Absence of stridor may indicate sudden complete obstruction.

The causes of partial obstruction of the upper airway are:
- inhaled foreign body;
- allergic swelling of the airway, including insect stings;
- burns to the airway;
- other direct trauma to the airway (rare) (NB. dislocation of the cricoid cartilage may occur in children)

- infection of the larynx, including the epiglottis, or trachea;
- infection of the mouth, tonsils or pharynx;
- infection superimposed on congenital abnormality in a small infant. Congenital abnormalities of the airway usually present in the first few weeks of life but should be considered up to the age of 6 months.

Xr

Radiographs should only be obtained in a stable, calm, well-oxygenated patient with an uncertain underlying diagnosis. The only appropriate films are anteroposterior chest and lateral soft-tissue view of the neck, performed in the ED.

A widened soft-tissue shadow on the lateral view of the neck may represent a retropharyngeal abscess or a swollen epiglottis. A coin in the trachea will have passed through the vocal cords in the sagittal plane and will thus appear end-on as a linear shadow on an anteroposterior Chest X-ray. In contrast, a coin in the oesophagus usually lies in the coronal plane.

Special problems in children

1 The flow in any tube is proportional to the fourth power of the radius. Hence, any reduction in the size of the child's small upper airway will have a much greater effect on airflow than a similar reduction in an adult.

2 Any stimulus is likely to cause increased distress, crying and consequent clinical deterioration. Therefore interventions such as venepuncture should not be undertaken until specialist help has arrived. Pulse oximetry may be useful in the interim.

Tx

If there is marked stridor and cyanosis:
- Call for expert help immediately (anaesthetic and ENT).
- Notify theatre.
- Reassure the patient and allow any position of comfort.

• Give 100% oxygen or, better still, Heliox (70% helium with 30% oxygen). (Helium has better flow characteristics than nitrogen or oxygen and may carry the oxygen through a small remaining passage).

• Try nebulised adrenaline (5 mg) as a temporary measure.

• Consider parenteral adrenaline for allergic swelling.

> Do not examine the mouth or throat – any stimulus will increase the risk of complete obstruction.

If no help is available and the patient is about to die:

• Attempt laryngoscopy and endotracheal intubation – this is dangerous. Foreign material can be removed with suction and Magill's forceps. If the anatomy of the pharynx is distorted by oedema, ask a colleague to squeeze the chest; escaping air bubbles will help to identify the position of the upper larynx.

• Be prepared to perform cricothyroidotomy or needle cricothyroid puncture – *see pages 23 and 24.*

In less urgent cases:

• Reassure the patient and allow a position of comfort.

• Give 100% oxygen.

• Obtain radiographs of the chest and lateral cervical spine in the resuscitation area.

• Ask for ENT or paediatric advice. Be content not to make an immediate diagnosis in every case – looking for one may precipitate complete airway obstruction.

Management of specific conditions

Epiglottitis occurs in both children and adults but is often misdiagnosed in the latter. The Hib vaccination programme has led to a marked fall in the incidence in children but will have no effect on the adult disease which is caused by different pathogens, such as staphylococci and streptococci. The clinical course can be dramatic and fatal.

For epiglottitis in adults see page 418.
For allergic swelling of the upper airway see page 295.
For stridor in children see page 330.
For peritonsillar infections see page 418.
For Ludwig's angina see page 418.

For retropharyngeal abscess see page 418.
For inhalational burns see page 146.
For *diphtheria see page 417.*

The lower airways and lungs

The restoration of adequate breathing is a priority, which is second only to the maintenance of a clear airway.

Respiratory arrest

Isolated respiratory arrest or failure of ventilation in the presence of a clear airway and a central pulse occurs in four main circumstances:

1 poisoning with narcotic analgesics – *see page 280*;
2 general brainstem depression (e.g. drugs, CVA, head injury);
3 respiratory failure with CO_2 narcosis – *see page 224*;
4 neuromuscular paralysis.

It may also herald cardiac arrest in conditions such as pulmonary embolism. The treatment is artificial ventilation with 100% oxygen until the underlying cause can be remedied.

Initial assessment and management of acute breathlessness

• Ensure that airway obstruction is not the cause of the dyspnoea.

• Give oxygen by mask (*see Box 13.2*).

• Consider the need to support the ventilation:

  1 with a bag, valve and mask (a temporary measure that does not protect the airway);

  2 by intubation and ventilation, (but intubation may be extremely difficult in the patient who has not yet arrested);

  3 by requesting immediate anaesthetic support.

Box 13.2 Initial Oxygen Therapy in a Patient with Respiratory Distress

Is the patient known to have had previous episodes of hypercapnic respiratory failure?

Is the patient drowsy?

No to both	Give 100% oxygen
Yes to either	Give 24–35% oxygen until more information is available, keeping the SaO_2 around 90–92%

• Check that the circulation is adequate, otherwise the situation is that of cardiorespiratory arrest.

• Sit the patient up, loosen clothing and briefly examine the chest.

• Obtain IV access.

• Monitor SaO_2, ECG and BP.

• Score the level of consciousness (AVPU or GCS).

• Get a brief history.

• Obtain a Chest X-ray and ECG and check the blood gases – *see later*.

• Consider immediate therapy for wheezing or pulmonary oedema.

Like pain, shortness of breath must be relieved as soon as possible after initial assessment.

Investigations in respiratory distress

Chest X-ray (PA if possible)

An anteroposterior chest X-ray taken on the trolley in the resuscitation room may be necessary in a critically ill patient but is a poor substitute for a PA erect film as:

• the mediastinum and heart size is magnified;

• fluid levels are not identified;

• the penetration is often inappropriate;

• the film is often rotated or incomplete; and

• there is a potential radiation hazard to staff.

For changes in the lung fields on Chest X-ray see Box 13.3.

On a supine chest X-ray, an effusion or haemothorax may mimic diffuse lung changes – *see page 76*.

Twelve-lead ECG

A rhythm strip from a three-lead electrocardiogram is insufficient for diagnostic purposes in a patient who may have subtle changes of myocardial ischaemia or pulmonary embolism.

Pulse oximetry

Measurement of SaO_2 is extremely valuable but has some drawbacks.

• It does not assess pH and $PaCO_2$, which may be abnormal in the presence of normal oxygen saturation.

Box 13.3 Changes in the Lung Fields on a Chest X-ray

Shadows in the lung fields may be focal, multifocal or diffuse. Causes of focal and multifocal abnormalities include:

• metastases;

• lung abscesses;

• carcinoma of the lung;

• pulmonary infarcts;

• TB;

• rheumatoid nodules;

• hydatid cysts.

Diffuse changes may be of two main types (1) alveolar or (2) interstitial. The presence of an air bronchogram indicates alveolar pathology and this may be cardiac or non-cardiac in origin. The alveoli may be filled with:

• *blood* – lung contusion;

• *fluid* – pulmonary oedema;

• *consolidated pus* – pneumonia.

Interstitial lung disease is more complex and less relevant to emergency medicine. Lung field changes caused by it may be:

• *nodular* – small in pneumoconiosis, larger in silicosis and sometimes miliary in TB;

• *linear* – fibrosis (usually lower zone), asbestosis, connective tissue disease and cryptogenic;

• *cystic* – seen in the lower zone in bronchiectasis and cystic fibrosis and in the upper zone in histiocytosis X.

• The steep fall of the oxy-Hb curve means that $SaO_2 < 95\%$ is abnormal (cf. PaO_2).

• SaO_2 is inaccurate in the presence of carboxyhaemoglobin (COHb), which is not uncommon in respiratory distress (house fires, faulty gas heaters, heavy smokers).

Blood gas samples should be taken from the radial artery of the non-dominant hand.

Arterial blood gases

See Box 13.4.

For the rules of compensation in acid–base disorders see Box 14.22 on page 258.

To convert partial pressures of gases expressed in kPa to mmHg multiply by 7.6 and vice versa.

Box 13.4 Estimation of the Expected Partial Pressure of Oxygen in an Arterial Blood Gas Sample

With healthy lungs, the PaO_2 in mmHg should be approximately equal to five times the percentage of oxygen in the inspired gases:

i.e. expected PaO_2 (mmHg) = 5 × FIO_2 (%)

For example, breathing air with healthy lungs: expected PaO_2 = 5 × 21% = 100 mmHg.

Similarly, the PaO_2 in kPa should be around two-thirds of the inspired percentage of oxygen.

For example, breathing air with healthy lungs: expected PaO_2 = 00.66 × 21% = 13.5 kPa.

Foreign bodies in the lower airways

Sudden onset of coughing and wheezing may accompany aspiration of a foreign body into the lower airways. Young children are especially vulnerable to this problem; a history of aspiration may be lacking. The right main, intermediate or lower bronchi are the most likely sites for obstruction to occur. Peanuts and toy fragments are the most commonly inhaled objects in children; bony food particles, broken teeth and small dental instruments predominate in adults. The presence of a unilateral wheeze, recurrent infection or other atypical symptoms and signs should always suggest the possibility of an intrathoracic foreign body.

XR

The foreign body is invariably radiolucent but the obstructive emphysema or absorption collapse that it causes may often be seen. Inspiratory and expiratory chest X-rays should be requested to demonstrate the ball valve effect of a partial obstruction upon the lung volume.

Tx

All patients with a possibility of a foreign body in the airways should be referred for bronchoscopy. This would include those with suspicious histories, signs or X-ray changes.

For foreign bodies in the upper airways see page 205. For foreign bodies in the oesophagus and gastrointestinal tract see page 415.

For allergic reactions causing lower airway obstruction and respiratory distress see page 295.

Asthma in adults

Asthma continues to be a major health problem in the United Kingdom, affecting an estimated 1.4 million children and 3.7 million adults. It is responsible for the deaths of over 1500 people each year. Throughout Western Europe, there is an average prevalence of asthma of 13% in children and 8.4% in adults with a 2–4% annual increase in prevalence over the last 15–20 years. The reasons for this increase are uncertain but possible explanations include:

- A rise in the house dust mite population
- Increased diesel particulate emissions
- A decrease in exposure to bacterial pathogens in childhood
- Changes in diet (more polyunsaturated fats and less antioxidants).

Patients with severe asthma and one or more adverse behavioural or psychosocial factors have a higher risk of death. *For the risk factors for developing near fatal or fatal asthma see Box 13.5.* However, around 90% of asthma attacks that are severe enough to require admission to hospital, develop relatively slowly over a period of 6 hours or more. Therefore, there is usually enough time for effective action.

The clinical features of asthma result from a reversible inflammatory obstruction of the lower airways, which has three main components:

1 hyper-reactivity and spasm of the bronchial smooth muscle;

2 oedema of the walls of the bronchi;

3 increased production and retention of secretions.

It is caused by an allergic response to a wide variety of substances but there is usually an underlying sensitivity to house dust mite. A viral infection is a common trigger for an acute exacerbation; exercise is responsible for around 40% of attacks.

A pneumothorax may occasionally be the cause of an acute deterioration.

Dyspnoea and wheezing are the predominant features. Bronchodilators may control these

Box 13.5 Patients at Risk of Developing Fatal or near Fatal Asthma:

Patients with a combination of one of more indicators of severe asthma:
Previous near fatal asthma (e.g. required ventilation or had respiratory acidosis)
Previous admission for asthma (especially if in the last year)
Repeated attendances at ED for asthma (especially if in the last year)
Asthma treatment requiring three or more classes of medication
Heavy use of beta-2 agonists
Brittle asthma

and one or more adverse behavioural or psychosocial factors:
Non-compliance with treatment, failure to attend appointments or self-discharge from hospital
Psychiatric illness including depression and self-harm
Current or recent major tranquilliser usage
Alcohol or drug abuse
Learning difficulties
History of abuse in childhood
Employment and income problems
Severe domestic, marital or legal stress
Social isolation
Denial of illness
Obesity

symptoms, but it is steroids that modify the underlying inflammatory processes.

Ask about
• When this attack started
• Improvement or deterioration in symptoms
• The patient's assessment of severity
• What triggers an attack and how often
• Recent hospital admissions
• Any ICU admission
• Why this time was chosen to come to hospital; this is an important discriminator when considering discharge
• Previous and current drug use, especially steroids and theophyllines
• Other conditions, including upper respiratory tract infections and pregnancy.
If nebulised drugs were given prior to hospital arrival by the paramedics, precise details and initial peak flow rate should be noted.

Examination begins while taking the history and setting up the nebuliser.

Look for
• Difficulty with speech – spontaneous sentences or single words?
• Reduced peak expiratory flow rate (PEF). *For predicted values of PEF for adults see Figure 13.3 and Box 13.6*
• Tachycardia and tachypnoea
• Indrawing of ribs, flaring of nostrils and use of accessory muscles
• Wheezing and signs of pneumothorax
• Agitation, confusion or drowsiness
• Exhaustion
• Pyrexia
• Cyanosis.

Less wheezing than expected on auscultation may indicate less air movement, not less asthma.

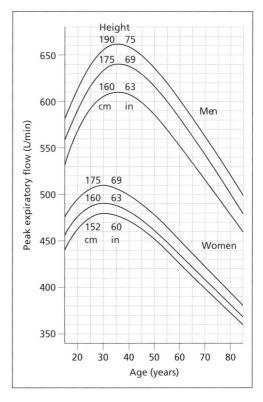

Figure 13.3 Predicted peak expiratory flow rates in adults.

Box 13.6 Predicted Peak Expiratory Flow Rates for Adults of Average Height (in L per min)

Age (years)	15	20	30	40	50	60	70
Male		550	590	630	630	610	580	540
Female		460	480	500	480	460	430	410

The standard deviation for men is 48 L per min and for women is 42 L per min.

Values of PEF up to 2 standard deviations less than predicted are within normal limits.

Investigations

Chest X-ray is not indicated routinely in acute asthma. It should only be requested in cases of suspected pneumothorax, pneumomediastinum, pneumonic consolidation or inhaled foreign body. Patients with life-threatening asthma or failure to respond to treatment will also require a Chest X-ray as will those who have been intubated and ventilated.

Arterial blood gas analysis is only required in patients with features of life-threatening asthma and in those with a SaO_2 (on pulse oximetry) of less than 92%. There is usually a low $PaCO_2$ as a result of hyperventilation and a low PaO_2 caused by ventilation–perfusion mismatch. A normal $PaCO_2$ is worrying and a high $PaCO_2$ (over 40–45 mmHg or 5.3–6.0 kPa) indicates respiratory muscle fatigue and impending respiratory failure. Measurement of blood gas tensions should be repeated after 2 h in all patients in whom the initial PaO_2 was below 60 mmHg (8 kPa) unless the SaO_2 has risen above 92% in the meantime. Electrolyte estimation is important – hypokalaemia can occur – but haematological investigation is often unnecessary. A raised white cell count is to be expected with catecholamine and steroid therapy. Theophylline levels should be measured in patients who are taking regular methylxanthines at home.

The peak expiratory flow rate (PEF) should be measured in all patients and used as a guide to treatment. PEF expressed as a percentage of the patient's previous best value is the most useful clinical parameter. In its absence, PEF expressed as a percentage of the patient's predicted value is a reasonable guide. *For predicted values of PEF for adults see Figure 13.3 and Box 13.6.*

Life-threatening asthma (PEF < 33% best or predicted)

Features include:
- unable to talk;
- silent chest, cyanosis, feeble respiratory effort;
- bradycardia, dysrhythmia or hypotension;
- exhaustion, confusion or coma.

Pulse oximetry and arterial blood gas analysis show:
- SaO_2 below 92%
- $PaCO_2$ within the normal range of 35–45 mmHg (4.6–6.0 kPa) or higher in near fatal asthma
- PaO_2 below 60 mmHg (8 kPa) irrespective of oxygen therapy
- Low pH.

Tx

- Obtain anaesthetic / intensive care help immediately in life-threatening asthma.
- Give a high concentration of oxygen (at least 60%) via a well-fitting facemask. The aim is to keep the SaO_2 above 92%.
- Monitor SaO_2, ECG and BP.
- Give salbutamol 5 mg (or terbutaline 10 mg) made up to 5 mL with normal saline and nebulised by oxygen with a flow rate of at least 6 L per min. Add ipratropium 500 µg to the same nebuliser. (This anticholinergic drug has been shown to produce additional bronchodilation to that produced by beta-2 agonists alone, leading to faster recovery times and shorter durations of admission).
- Give prednisolone 40–50 mg by mouth. If the patient cannot swallow oral medication or is vomiting, give hydrocortisone 100–200 mg IV 6 hourly. (Prednisolone 10 mg is roughly equivalent to hydrocortisone 40 mg). Steroids should be continued for at least 5 days or until full recovery.
- Repeat the salbutamol / terbutaline and ipratropium nebulisers after 15 min. (The beta-2 agonists can be administered almost continuously; the ipratropium may be repeated at 4–6 h intervals).
- Commence IV fluids.
- Give a single dose of magnesium sulphate 1.2–2 g by IV infusion over 20 min. *For more information on magnesium see page 255.*

- Consider continuous administration of nebulised beta-2 agonists (i.e. repeated doses at 15–30 min intervals).
- Consider the use of IV salbutamol 200 μg or IV terbutaline 250 μg (given slowly over 10 min) for those patients in whom inhaled therapy cannot be used reliably.
- Consider (after consultation with senior staff) the use of IV aminophylline. This may benefit occasional patients with life-threatening asthma who are resistant to standard therapies. A loading dose of 5 mg per kg is given over 20 min under ECG control. This is followed by an infusion of aminophylline of 0.5–0.7 mg per kg per h. The loading dose (and possibly the idea of using aminophylline at all) should be abandoned in patients who are already taking oral methylxanthines. Caution is needed when giving aminophylline to patients who are hypoxic.

> Failure to recognise and act on the need for ventilation is the main preventable cause of death in asthma.

Intubation and ventilation may be required. All patients who are failing to respond to treatment should be referred to ICU. This includes patients with worsening PEF, deteriorating blood gases or acidosis, exhaustion, confusion or drowsiness.

IV adrenaline is sometimes used in a critical situation. Despite theoretical reasons for its efficacy, Heliox (helium and oxygen mixture in a ratio of 70 : 30) has not been shown to be of conclusive benefit in asthma. Similarly, non-invasive ventilation (NIV) is not recommended for the unstable situation of acute asthma.

Severe asthma (PEF between 33 and 50% best or predicted)

Features include:
- inability to complete a sentence in one breath;
- respiratory rate > 25 breaths per min;
- pulse rate > 110 per min.

Tx

The patient should be treated as described for 'life-threatening asthma' above, although IV magnesium should only be given if there is a poor response to inhaled bronchodilators. Aminophylline is unlikely to be considered. Admission is always required; the patient must be accompanied by a doctor or a nurse at all times.

Moderate asthma (PEF between 50 and 75% best or predicted)

The patient can finish a sentence and has no features of severe asthma.

Tx

- Give salbutamol 5 mg (or terbutaline 10 mg) made up to 5 mL with normal saline and nebulised by oxygen with a flow rate of at least 6 L per min.
- Monitor SaO_2, ECG and BP.
- Wait 15–30 min after the initial nebuliser and then repeat the PEF.
- If the patient is worse and the PEF is <50% treat as severe asthma. If better and the PEF is >75% consider discharge (*see below*). If the PEF is still between 50 and 75% repeat the salbutamol or terbutaline nebuliser and give prednisolone 40–50 mg orally. Then wait a further 30 min.
- If the patient is worse and the PEF is <50% treat as severe asthma. If better and the PEF is >75% consider discharge (*see later*). If the same (PEF 50–75%) wait a further 60 min whilst monitoring the SaO_2, heart rate and respiratory rate.
- If, at this point, the PEF is <50% treat as severe asthma. If the PEF is >50% *and* the patient is stable or improving consider discharge (*see later*).

Mild asthma (PEF > 75% best or predicted)

The patient can talk normally.

Tx

The patient should be given his or her usual bronchodilator and then kept under observation for at least 30–60 min. If the PEF remains above 75% consider discharge (*see later*). If the PEF falls, treat as described in the appropriate section above.

Discharge of a patient with asthma

Most patients who are sufficiently ill to request emergency help with their chronic condition will require oral steroids (as well as inhaled steroids and bronchodilators as part of a long-term management plan). Prednisolone 40–50 mg given orally for 5 days is usually adequate. (If used within an hour of ED arrival, steroid tablets are effective at preventing admission and reducing the risk of relapse in the ensuing 21 days. Despite this, they are not always prescribed by ED staff). There are several alternatives for high-dose inhaled steroids:

- beclometasone (beclomethasone) (400–500 µg bd);
- budesonide (400–500 µg bd);
- fluticasone (250 µg bd).

These doses are halved for children.

Over 15% of patients with asthma who are discharged from an ED or hospital ward reattend within 2 weeks.

Patients who return to the ED after discharge should be automatically admitted. Referral for specialist review after ED attendance has been shown to improve outcomes significantly for most patients with asthma. The patient's GP should be informed of the attendance and arrangements made for primary care follow-up within 48 h.

For a predischarge checklist for moderate and mild asthma see Box 13.7.

Box 13.7 Predischarge Checklist for Moderate and Mild Asthma

Moderate asthma

The patient is stable over at least 1 h of observation.

The PEF is at least 75% of normal for the patient at 1 h or 50% at 2 h and improving.

The patient has both oral steroids and inhaled bronchodilators to take out.

The patient understands his or her condition and treatment and can use the inhalers satisfactorily.

Follow-up is arranged (e.g. by the GP within 48 h) and the patient has the telephone number of the ED.

There is good home support.

The patient has a letter for the GP (who must be informed within 24 h of attendance).

Mild asthma

Oral steroids are not necessary. Otherwise as for moderate asthma.

Box 13.8 Relative Contraindications to Discharge of a Patient with Asthma

Remaining significant symptoms

Concerns about compliance

Psychological problems or learning difficulties

Physical disability

Poor social circumstances or lives alone

Presentation at night

Previous ICU admission for asthma

Previous severe attacks needing hospitalisation

Diagnosed brittle asthma

Already on steroids

Pregnancy

Drug-induced attack

For the relative contraindications to the discharge from hospital of a patient with asthma see Box 13.8.

For asthma in children under 5 years of age see page 331.

Acute exacerbations of chronic obstructive pulmonary disease

Chronic obstructive pulmonary disease (COPD) is characterised by reduced respiratory function as a result of a combination of destruction of alveoli and obstruction of bronchioles by a chronic inflammatory process. The airflow obstruction is usually progressive, not fully reversible and relatively unchanged over a period of several months. COPD is predominately caused by smoking. Most patients have a chronic productive cough, which is worse in winter. There is no single diagnostic test for COPD but airflow obstruction is defined as a forced expiratory volume in 1 s less than 80% of the predicted value for that patient.

Acute deterioration that precipitates ED attendance is usually associated with:

- Increased dyspnoea
- Purulent sputum
- Increased sputum volume.

This is frequently the result of superadded infection. Other causes include minor chest injury, inappropriate sedation and uncontrolled oxygen therapy. A cough fracture may also precipitate deterioration.

Patients with COPD have varying combinations of chronic bronchitis and emphysema. However, the two classical descriptions of 'blue bloaters' and 'pink puffers' are no longer thought to describe the extremes of this spectrum of lung pathologies. Instead, they represent patients with different physiological responses to abnormal blood gases – 'blue bloaters' tolerate high CO_2 levels, 'pink puffers' do not. The former is cyanosed and oedematous with signs of CO_2 retention (peripheral vasodilatation, retinal engorgement, staring eyes, confusion); the latter maintains a normal CO_2 level by hyperventilation. Most patients present with a mixture of these features, attempting to hyperventilate but failing to maintain a normal $PaCO_2$. Wheezes and rattles are heard on auscultation in bronchitis but there may be minimal chest signs with severe emphysema. Exhaustion is a common feature, with the patient sitting up using accessory muscles of respiration. Confusion and shortness of breath may make a clear history difficult to obtain.

> The risk of dying from an exacerbation of COPD is closely related to the development of a respiratory acidosis, the presence of other serious illnesses and the need for ventilatory support.

Cor pulmonale is suggested by the combination of peripheral oedema, raised venous pressure, a systolic parasternal heave and a loud pulmonary second heart sound.

Investigations

• Peak expiratory flow rate should be measured. A PEF of less than 100 L per min indicates a severe exacerbation.
• Pulse oximetry will demonstate a low oxygen saturation in most patients with COPD. Some patients may have a resting SaO_2 below 90% even when stable.
• Analysis of blood gases will usually confirm hypoxia with rising hypercapnia and respiratory acidosis. The blood gas analysis should be repeated after 30–60 min of treatment.
• Full blood count, electrolytes, Chest X-ray and ECG must be obtained together with the past medical notes.

• Plasma theophylline levels should be measured in all patients who are taking regular methylxanthines.
• Sputum should be sent for microscopy and culture in patients with purulent sputum.

Tx

Immediate treatment: The patient should be sat up and given controlled oxygen by facemask to keep the SaO_2 above 90% – *see Box 13.2.*

Bronchodilators: Nebulised beta-2 adrenoceptor agonists (salbutamol 5 mg or terbutaline 10 mg, made up to 5 mL with normal saline) will treat any reversible element of the COPD. Nebulised ipratropium bromide 500 μg is also helpful. This antimuscarinic bronchodilator has a delayed onset of action of up to 30 min but lasts for 3–6 h. The sympathomimetic nebulisers may be repeated at short intervals if they prove to be beneficial. After consultation with senior staff, IV aminophylline may be considered for patients who have a poor response to nebulised bronchodilators. A loading dose of 5 mg per kg is given over 20 min under ECG control. This is followed by an infusion of aminophylline of 500 μg per kg per h. Aminophylline should not be used in patients who are already taking oral methylxanthines at home and great caution is required when giving it to patients who are hypoxic. (Aminophylline is a stable mixture of theophylline and ethylenediamine, which is 20 times more water soluble than theophylline alone. The plasma theophylline concentration for optimum response is 10–20 mg per L; there is a very narrow margin between the therapeutic and the toxic dose).

Oxygen: The administration of a high concentration of oxygen in patients with COPD may cause increased respiratory depression, CO_2 narcosis and worsening hypoxia. It used to be said that the normal hypercarbic drive to respiration could be abolished by chronic hypercarbia and the theory ran that the patient was then reliant on the less sensitive hypoxic drive to stimulate respiratory effort. In actual fact, the clinical deterioration that may follow oxygen therapy is almost certainly due to a loss of physiological hypoxic vasoconstriction, which is partially protecting the patient from the effects of areas of gross alveolar hypoventilation. However, the patient has presented to an ED because of dyspnoea, increasing hypoxia will ensure further deterioration. Immediate oxygen therapy is thus determined by the presence of drowsiness or known previous hypercapnic respiratory failure – *see Box 13.2*. For most patients, the target should be an SaO$_2$ of between 85 and 92%. The PaO$_2$ should certainly not fall below 50 mmHg (6.6 kPa; equivalent to an SaO$_2$ of approximately 80%). (A PaO$_2$ of less than 60 mmHg (8 kPa) is regarded as respiratory failure – *see page 224*). The aim of controlled oxygen therapy is to raise the PaO$_2$ above 50 mmHg without worsening the acidosis.

Steroids: It is now recognised that almost all patients with an acute exacerbation of COPD benefit from high dose steroids (prednisolone 30 mg daily) for 1–2 weeks. For patients who are unable to take tablets in the ED, hydrocortisone 200–300 mg IV should be given.

Antibiotics: In the presence of purulent sputum, antibacterial therapy is required. *Haemophilus influenzae*, *Streptococcus pneumoniae* and *Moraxella catarrhalis* are typical pathogens in COPD and so amoxicillin 500 mg tds or tetracycline 250 mg qds are suitable first line antibiotics. Trimethoprim 200 mg bd is also often used. Because of increasing antibiotic resistance, co-amoxiclav or quinolones (e.g. ciprofloxacin 500 mg bd) are given after 3 days if there is a failure to respond to first line treatment. Patients with consolidation on Chest X-ray should be treated as pneumonia – *see page 218.*

Admission to hospital: The decision to admit a patient with COPD to hospital depends on a variety of both clinical and social factors as well as the availability of a specialist home care team. *For factors that suggest that a patient with an exacerbation of COPD should be admitted to hospital see Box 13.9.* Regular physiotherapy is of great benefit to patients with retained sputum.

Respiratory support: Subsequent therapy depends on the clinical findings, further history and the results

Box 13.9 Factors Which Suggest that a Patient with COPD Should Be Admitted to Hospital

Difficulty coping at home, living alone or in poor social circumstances
Poor or deteriorating general health
Poor activity or confined to bed
On long-term oxygen therapy
Significant co-morbidity (especially cardiac disease and insulin-dependent diabetes)
Rapid rate of onset of exacerbation
Severe breathlessness or cyanosis
Worsening peripheral oedema
Acute confusion or otherwise impaired level of consciousness
SaO$_2$ < 90%, pH < 7.35 or PaO$_2$ < 7 kPa
Chest x-ray changes

of blood gas analysis. The presence of an acidosis (pH < 7.35) in these often well-compensated patients is usually a bad sign and is now regarded as an indication for non-invasive ventilation (NIV). Bi-level pressure support ventilators (delivering bi-level positive airway pressure or BiPAP) are usually used for this purpose. The respiratory stimulant, doxapram, is sometimes used if NIV is unavailable – *see Box 13.13*. If the pH falls below 7.25 or the PaCO$_2$ rises above 80 mmHg (10.6 kPa) or if the patient becomes drowsy or exhausted, ICU specialists should be involved with a view to performing intubation and intermittent positive pressure ventilation (IPPV).

For respiratory failure see page 224.
For bronchiolitis in children see page 334.

Acute exacerbations of bronchiectasis

Around 1 in 1000 adults in the United Kingdom has bronchiectasis, usually as a result of childhood infections, cystic fibrosis, immunodeficiency or rheumatoid disease. However, in 50% of patients no cause or associated condition is found. It is believed that the bronchi are dilated and destroyed by a cycle of recurrent infection, inflammation, excessive production of mucous and reduced mucous clearance. Patients have chronic symptoms of dyspnoea and a productive cough; their sputum is mucopurulent. Some patients may present to an ED with an acute exacerbation, usually brought about by infection. Symptoms include worsening breathlessness, increased coughing and sputum production, haemoptysis (usually not severe), chest pain, fever, malaise and lethargy. Chest signs may be minimal; low-pitched crackles may be heard. In severe disease, finger clubbing and respiratory failure are seen.

Investigations

Chest X-ray shows the characteristic changes of bronchiectasis in only 50% of patients:
• Thickened bronchial walls seen as parallel 'tramlines' or ring-shaped opacities
• Cystic lesions with fluid levels
• Areas of collapse and scarring.
High resolution CT scan or bronchoscopy may be required.

Tx

Treatment includes oxygen, physiotherapy (postural drainage and percussion) and antibiotics. If likely pathogens are not known from previous sputum cultures, amoxicillin 500 mg tds is given for 14 days. Steroids may be used to reduce inflammation. For more severe exacerbations, blind prescription of broad spectrum anti-pseudomonal antibiotics should be considered. Intubation and ventilation may be required. Excessive secretions tend to limit the effectiveness of non-invasive ventilation (NIV) in bronchiectasis.

Pulmonary oedema

Fluid may collect in the lung tissue for a variety of reasons, the most common being left ventricular failure. Pulmonary oedema may also be associated with:
1 over-transfusion and excessive fluid therapy;
2 smoke and other noxious gas inhalation *(see page 291)*;
3 acute traumatic brain injury (neurogenic pulmonary oedema – *see page 38*);
4 intracranial haemorrhage (neurogenic pulmonary oedema – *see page 234*);
5 shock, from any cause (adult respiratory distress syndrome);

6) ascents to high altitudes *(see page 242)*.
Acute pulmonary oedema causes symptoms and signs of hypoxia:
• rapidly increasing shortness of breath, which is worse on lying down;
• tachypnoea and laboured breathing (stiff water-logged lungs);
• pallor and sweating (characteristic);
• tachycardia;
• anxiety and distress;
• depression of consciousness (mostly caused by CO_2 narcosis).
The hypoxia leads to a vicious cycle of worsening myocardial performance and increasing oedema. On auscultation there are widespread crackles. These make the diagnostic gallop rhythm difficult to hear. Classical pink, frothy sputum is uncommon. Peripheral oedema and a raised jugular venous pressure indicate associated right heart failure. There may be a history of ischaemic heart disease, orthopnoea or paroxysmal nocturnal dyspnoea. Chest pain results from either angina secondary to the hypoxia or from an MI that precipitated the left ventricular failure.

'Cardiac asthma' describes the wheeze that these patients may develop if oedema causes significant airway obstruction. The history and presentation will usually distinguish it from bronchial asthma but confusion can occur, especially in patients with both conditions.

Box 13.10 Radiographic Changes in Pulmonary Oedema

Widened vascular markings in the upper lung fields as a result of diversion of blood (upper lobe diversion)
Air bronchogram
A widened mediastinum with spreading (bat's wing) shadows
Horizontal lines in the lower lobes (Kerley B lines)
Small pleural effusions
Cotton wool shadows throughout the lung fields
Cardiomegaly

Investigations

Arterial blood gases will show a variable degree of hypoxia, hypercapnia and acidosis.

Box 13.11 Alternative Routes for GTN Administration in Left Ventricular Failure

1 GTN spray 1–2 puffs (= 400–800 µg) or equivalent tablet sublingually, followed by a GTN 10 mg transdermal patch.

2 GTN 5 mg buccal tablet, followed by a second tablet in the opposite buccal sulcus, if necessary, after 3–5 min.

3 GTN infusion 10–200 µg per min – *see Box 13.12.*

Box 13.12 Intravenous Infusion of GTN

● Make 50 mg of GTN solution up to 50 mL with normal saline in a large syringe in an infusion pump (i.e. mix a 1 mg per mL solution). The syringe and the giving-set should be made of polyethylene as PVC absorbs glyceryl trinitrate

● The IV dose of GTN is from 0.6–12 mg per h (equivalent to 10–200 µg per min)

● Start the infusion at 1.5–3 mL (1.5–3 mg) per h and adjust this dose by a factor of two every 15–30 min according to the patient's clinical condition

---

B-type natriuretic peptide (BNP) is a cardiac hormone produced by the heart in response to ventricular stretching from volume expansion and pressure overload. It is a marker for ventricular dysfunction, the circulating BNP concentration increasing with the severity of the heart failure. BNP can also be used as a diagnostic test to help differentiate congestive cardiac failure from COPD. A BNP level in excess of 100 picograms per mL has a high specificity for CCF.

For radiographic changes in pulmonary oedema see Box 13.10 on page 217.

Tx

● Sit the patient up, with the legs dependent if possible.

● Give high-concentration oxygen by mask or via a continuous positive airway pressure (CPAP) circuit at 5 cm H_2O pressure initially.

● Establish IV access.

● Start monitoring SaO_2, ECG and BP.

● Request a Chest X-ray and ECG. Arterial blood gases may be taken, but unless the results are instantly available, they are unlikely to affect initial treatment.

● Give diamorphine (2.5–5 mg IV) with prochlorperazine (12.5 mg IV) to relieve distress and to start venodilatation.

● If the patient has a history of fluid retention (CCF), give furosemide (frusemide) 1–2 mg per kg IV and consider the need for a urinary catheter.

● Start nitrate therapy to further reduce venous return. Several alternative routes are effective – *see Boxes 13.11 and 13.12.* GTN must be used with care as it may worsen hypotension and tachycardia.

Inotropes such as dobutamine are indicated in low output states (forward failure) – *see page 243.* When the clinical picture is dominated by wheezing (cardiac asthma), nebulised salbutamol may be given. (Aminophylline is no longer used in LVF). CPAP is useful in pulmonary oedema (see before) but the role of non-invasive ventilation (e.g. BiPAP) is less certain. Conventional positive pressure ventilation (IPPV) may be required in a rapidly deteriorating patient.

Pneumonia

This is the most common serious infection seen in adults in the ED and may be fatal even in people who have been previously healthy. The outcome is greatly improved by very early treatment with appropriate antibiotics. The patient with pneumonia presents with a short history of fever and productive cough ('rusty' sputum with *Streptococcus pneumoniae* infection). There may be tachycardia, shortness of breath and pleuritic chest pain. Findings on examination vary from obvious lobar consolidation to minimal crepitations. Lethargy and confusion are often the first signs in the elderly. Children may present with abdominal pain – *see page 334.* Pneumonia is defined as severe if two or more of the following criteria are present:

● age > 65 years;

● new confusion;

● respiratory rate > 30 breaths per min;

● systolic BP < 90 mmHg or diastolic BP < 60 mmHg;

● PaO_2 < 60 mmHg (8 kPa);

● urea > 7 mmol per L.

Community-acquired pneumonia

Previously fit people are most likely to have been infected by pneumococci although previously esoteric causes of pneumonia are becoming more common. Pneumonia caused by *Mycoplasma pneumoniae* occurs in epidemics every 3–4 years. Extra-pulmonary manifestations of mycoplasma infection include skin rashes, musculoskeletal pain, GI upset, haemolytic anaemia and neurological disease. TB and AIDS may both present as an acute community-acquired pneumonia.

For TB see page 223.

For HIV infection/AIDS see page 265.

For Legionnaires' disease see page 221.

For Q fever see page 221.

For acute infection complicating chronic obstructive pulmonary disease see page 216.

For pneumonia in children see page 334.

Hospital-acquired pneumonia

This is defined as a pneumonia that occurs after at least 3 days in hospital and so should be of no direct relevance to an ED. However, patients may present themselves from institutions such as nursing homes where hospital-type opportunistic organisms abound. Pathogens gain access by inhalation or aspiration, directly via the bloodstream or by local spread.

Every sick or badly injured patient who passes through the ED is at risk of subsequent nosocomial (i.e. hospital-acquired) infection. This can be reduced by:

1 Using sterile techniques when siting IV lines and catheters

2 Ensuring that all airway equipment, including suction, is completely clean

3 Maintaining good tissue perfusion (i.e. promptly treating shock)

4 Humidifying inspired gases (dry gases damage the airways, thereby impairing normal respiratory defence mechanisms).

Patients at an increased risk of pneumococcal infection

Patients who have had a splenectomy, no matter how long ago, are at a high risk of developing overwhelming pneumococcal infection. Similarly, some other conditions may cause a functional hyposplenism:

- sickle cell disease and thalassaemia;
- coeliac disease;
- systemic lupus erythematosus;
- lymphoma and leukaemia;
- other immunodeficiencies.

Such patients should have received pneumococcal vaccine and must be regarded with a high level of suspicion whenever they develop a pyrexia or acute respiratory symptoms.

Investigations

Chest X-ray may show a variable picture; a classical lobar atelectasis is unusual. *For the appearances of lobar collapse–consolidation on Chest X-ray see Figure 13.4.* The distinction between pneumonia and an exacerbation of COPD depends on the pres-

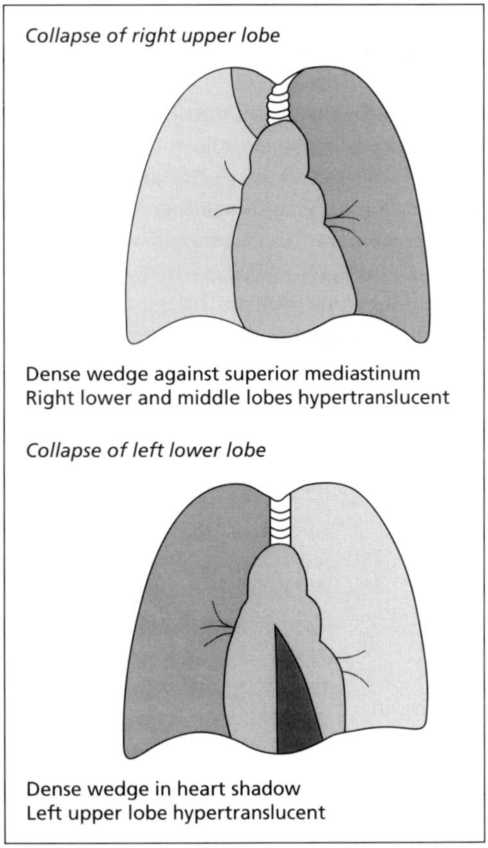

Collapse of right upper lobe

Dense wedge against superior mediastinum
Right lower and middle lobes hypertranslucent

Collapse of left lower lobe

Dense wedge in heart shadow
Left upper lobe hypertranslucent

Figure 13.4 Appearance of lobar collapses on Chest X-ray.

ence or absence of the radiological signs of pneumonia; patients with consolidation on Chest X-ray should be treated for pneumonia. Identification of the causative organism will be aided by the culture of blood (taken before the administration of antibiotics), sputum, pleural aspirate and bronchial lavage fluid. Blood specimens should also be taken for full blood count, blood chemistry and arterial blood gases. A urine sample may be obtained to look for pneumococcal antigen in patients with severe pneumonia.

Tx

- Sit the patient up and give a high concentration of humidified oxygen.
- Start rehydration.
- Monitor SaO_2, ECG and BP.
- Consider immediate transfer to ICU if the PaO_2 cannot be maintained above 60 mmHg (8 kPa). (This level of desaturation is regarded as respiratory failure – see page 224).

Almost all patients who present to hospital with pneumonia will require admission. Intravenous antibiotics should be started in the ED for those patients who have severe infections (see page 218 for the definition of severe pneumonia) or who are obviously frail. Physiotherapy is contraindicated in pneumonia unless the patient is producing large amounts of sputum (usually because of underlying COPD).

Community-acquired pneumonia is often caused by Streptococcus pneumoniae or Mycoplasma pneumoniae although a variety of atypical pathogens may also be responsible. If the infection is not severe (see before) and the patient has not been previously treated in the community, amoxicillin 500 mg–1g tds by mouth is an appropriate antibiotic. For patients who are allergic to penicillins, erythromycin 500 mg qds can be used. If there is no response after 2 days, then erythromycin is added to the amoxicillin (or cefadroxil 1g bd to the erythromycin). For patients who have already been treated in the community, the combination of amoxicillin and erythromycin (or erythromycin and cefadroxil) is used immediately. All patients

with a severe community-acquired pneumonia (see page 218 for definition of severe) should be given cefotaxime 1–2 g IV bd with erythromycin 1g IV bd from first presentation. Cefuroxime is an alternative to cefotaxime.

Hospital-acquired pneumonia may be caused by a wide variety of pathogens including Gram-negative bacilli and Streptococcus pneumoniae. Cefotaxime 1–2 g IV bd is a suitable antibiotic for seriously ill patients; an anti-pseudomonal penicillin is an alternative. For other patients, oral therapy is appropriate: amoxicillin 500 mg–1 g tds by mouth, or cefadroxil 1 g bd if allergic to penicillins. Ciprofloxacin 500 mg bd is a useful second line antibiotic in this situation.

Post-influenza pneumonia is caused by secondary bacterial infection of inflamed lung tissue. The mortality associated with staphylococcal superinfection is particularly high. Consequently, the condition is treated with cefotaxime 1–2 g IV bd with the addition of flucloxacillin 1–2 g IV qds Pneumonia following measles infection is also treated with this combination of antibiotics.

Pneumocystis carinii pneumonia is invariably associated with AIDS – see page 265. Chest X-ray shows diffuse interstitial changes. The diagnosis may be confirmed by culture of sputum or broncho-alveolar lavage specimens. Pneumocystis pneumonia is treated with co-trimoxazole 120 mg per kg per day in 2–4 divided doses either by mouth or IV.

Aspiration pneumonia may occur in emergency patients with impaired airway reflexes from a wide variety of causes including depressed consciousness, neurological disease and general debilitation. Radiographic changes are often inconclusive or delayed for several hours after aspiration. Consolidation appears most usually in the right upper or middle zones. Pathogens in this situation include Streptococcus pneumoniae, Klebsiella pneumoniae and anaerobic bacteria. Cefotaxime 1–2 g IV bd is given together with metronidazole 500 mg IV tds. For less serious cases, ciprofloxacin 500 mg orally bd can be used. There is little evidence for the efficacy of steroids in aspiration pneumonia.

For clearance and protection of the airway see pages 2 and 3.

For prophylaxis of gastric acid aspiration in pregnant patients with major trauma see page 32.

For respiratory failure see page 224.

Legionnaires' disease

This atypical pneumonia is caused by infection with the Gram-negative organism *Legionella pneumophilia*, which is harboured in institutional water systems. The disease is spread by airborne droplets, most commonly to middle-aged men in warm conditions. There may be a history of a recent stay in a hotel, hospital or other large building. Legionnaires' disease starts with a flu-like illness and then develops into a severe chest infection, often with accompanying gastrointestinal features. Symptoms and signs include:

• fever and rigors;
• pleurisy and haemoptysis;
• abdominal pain, diarrhoea and vomiting;
• a relative bradycardia.

Investigations

These may reveal:

• raised white cell count with neutrophilia and lymphopenia;
• low plasma sodium (<130 mmol per L);
• proteinuria and haematuria;
• unilateral patchy shadowing (often confined to a lower lobe) and pleural effusions on Chest X-ray.

Tx

Patients in whom the diagnosis of legionellosis is suspected should be admitted to hospital. Erythromycin 500 mg qds by mouth is the first line antibiotic; ciprofloxacin 500 mg bd is an alternative. Severe infections may require the addition of rifampicin 600 mg bd by mouth.

For further treatment of pneumonias see page 218.

Q fever

This highly infectious zoonosis occurs throughout the world and is caused by the bacterium *Coxiella burnetti*. Humans become infected by inhaling or ingesting infected dust. (A single organism can cause disease if inhaled by a susceptible individual). The primary vector of *Coxiella burnetti* is the ticks that infest large, domesticated animals and so there is usually a history of recent contact with cattle, sheep or goats. Abattoir workers, meat packers and farmers are mostly affected; the peak incidence in the United Kingdom is associated with the spring lambing season. The incubation period of Q fever is 7–30 days. It has two main manifestations:

1 Pyrexia, sweating, fatigue, headache and malaise (an influenza-like illness). Retro-orbital pain is very suggestive of Q fever.

2 Chest pain and cough (atypical pneumonia with patchy basal consolidation on Chest X-ray).

Q fever is treated with doxycycline or tetracycline for 10–14 days.

For further treatment of pneumonias see page 218.

Influenza

Every winter in the United Kingdom, during a 6–8 week period, influenza is associated with a sharp increase in both mortality and requests for medical attention. At this time, consultations for respiratory illness may increase up to 10 fold. In an average year, an estimated 2000–3000 people die in Britain from influenza-related causes; in years with major epidemics there have been over 20,000 excess deaths. People at an increased risk from influenza (and who should be immunised against it) include those who are 65 years old or more, residents in long-term care and people with certain chronic illnesses including:

• respiratory disease (especially COPD and asthma)
• heart disease
• renal disease
• immunosuppression (from any cause and including asplenia)
• diabetes.

The symptoms of influenza are relatively non-specific – pyrexia, malaise, anorexia, myalgia, nausea and unproductive coughing.

Tx

The treatment of influenza is mostly symptomatic – fluids and antipyretic analgesics. However, during an epidemic, high risk patients in the groups listed above who present within 36 h of the onset of symptoms should be considered for antiviral therapy. For adults and children over 40 kg, oseltamivir 75 mg is given by mouth bd for 5 days. An alternative for patients over 12 years old is zanamivir 10 mg by inhalation bd for 5 days. These anti-viral compounds (neuraminidase inhibitors) are licensed for the treatment of both influenza A and B but are not suitable for pregnant or breast-feeding women.

Avian influenza (bird flu) is a disease of birds caused by influenza viruses closely related to human influenza viruses. It is an important disease economically for farmers because of losses in poultry flocks. Transmission to humans in close contact with poultry or other birds occurs rarely and only with some strains of avian influenza (e.g. subtype H5N1). The potential for transformation of avian influenza into a form that both causes severe disease in humans and spreads easily from person to person is a great concern for world health. During a pandemic, it is estimated that 1 in 4 of the population could become ill and that the deaths could number over 50,000 in the United Kingdom alone. *For infection control principles in respiratory epidemics see 'SARS' on page 222.*

For the treatment of post-influenza pneumonia see page 220.

Severe Acute Respiratory Syndrome

SARS (Severe Acute Respiratory Syndrome) is the term used to describe an emerging disease that first appeared in Southern China at the end of 2002 and has since been described in many countries around the world. It is a serious respiratory infection, which may lead to pneumonia and respiratory distress syndrome. The causative organism is the SARS coronavirus (SARS-CoV), a newly discovered member of the coronavirus family. (Coronaviruses are the second most common cause of a cold – after rhinoviruses). The SARS-CoV has been isolated from wild animals native to the Guangdong Province and other parts of China. It appears to be less infectious than the influenza

viruses, with a short incubation period of 2–10 days (usually less than a week). Transmission occurs through close contact with an infected person, probably by droplet spread. Many of the outbreaks have been in hospital workers or close family members of known cases. The reported death rate for probable cases of SARS is 4–10%. The main features of the disease are similar to severe influenza – high fever, sore throat, headache, myalgia, dry cough and dyspnoea. Chest X-ray changes suggestive of pneumonia may occur. The WHO clinical case definition of SARS has been developed for public health purposes:

1 Respiratory illness severe enough to warrant hospitalisation
2 Fever of ≥38° C (documented or reported)
3 One or more symptoms of lower respiratory tract illness (cough, difficulty breathing, shortness of breath)
4 Radiographic evidence of lung infiltrates consistent with pneumonia or Respiratory Distress Syndrome (RDS) or autopsy findings consistent with the pathology of pneumonia or RDS without an identifiable cause
5 No alternative diagnosis to fully explain the illness.

Investigations

- Routine blood tests and Chest X-ray
- Blood (30–40 mL) for serology (ELISA antibody test and PCR for SARS-CoV)
- Nasopharyngeal and throat swabs
- Urine and stool specimens

Tx

There is no specific treatment or vaccine against SARS-CoV. Control of SARS (and similar infective pathogens) depends on:

1 Early recognition of the symptoms and signs of the disease
2 Immediate isolation of suspected cases
3 Effective means to reduce cross-infection, by means of exceptional standards of environmental hygiene
4 No inappropriate re-use of equipment that has been used on or near a suspected case

5 Early involvement of infection control staff.
For respiratory failure see page 224.

Tuberculosis

TB was known as the 'white plague' in Europe during the industrial revolution and has continued to ravage third world countries ever since. For the major part of the twentieth century, it was well-controlled in the developed world but 20 years ago (in 1986) it began to increase in the United States and Europe. The reasons for the increase are complex but include social changes, immigration, new diseases (AIDS) and changing antimicrobial resistance in mycobacteria. The causative organism of TB, *Mycobacterium tuberculosis*, is an obligate parasite with no free-living saprophytic forms. It is capable of both intracellular and extra cellular existence. Other mycobacteria (e.g. *Mycobacterium avium-intracellulare*) are increasingly recognised as pathogens, which cause both pulmonary and systemic disease. High risk groups for TB (and some other mycobacterial infections) include:

- Children and young adults
- Immigrants from the developing world
- People with poor socio-economic status
- Residents of prisons, nursing homes and other institutions
- Alcoholics and IV drug abusers
- People with AIDS and other causes of immunodeficiency
- People with some chronic illnesses (e.g. diabetes)
- People on long-term steroid therapy
- Health care providers.

Patients with pulmonary TB may present to an ED with chronic respiratory symptoms, general illness and weight loss, complications of TB or superadded infection. Sometimes TB may be an incidental finding on Chest X-ray.

> A person with undiagnosed smear-positive pulmonary TB infects around 10 other people each year.

Investigations

The Chest X-ray in primary TB is likely to show changes in the lower lobes with mediastinal or hilar lymphadenopathy and sometimes, a pleural effusion. Post-primary TB is caused by either reinfection or reactivation of a primary lesion. (Tubercle bacilli can remain dormant but viable in the body for many years). The altered immune response of the host results in a different radiographic picture:

- Disease in the upper lobe or superior segments of the lower lobes
- Pleural effusions and cavitating lesions
- Pneumonic consolidation, nodules or miliary spread

In immunodeficient patients (e.g. those with AIDS) mycobacterial infection causes lymphadenopathy or minimal changes on Chest X-ray. In almost all patients, a tuberculin skin test confirms the diagnosis.

Tx

Patients with suspected TB should be referred to a respiratory physician for specialist treatment. In the United Kingdom, antimicrobial therapy with three drugs (rifampicin, isoniazid and pyrazinamide) is recommended with the addition of a fourth drug (ethambutol) if there is a risk of isoniazid resistance. After 2 months, rifampicin and isoniazid are given alone for another 4 months. TB is a notifiable disease throughout the United Kingdom.

Collapse of the lung (atelectasis)

Segmental collapse is generally a result of sputum retention or infection. Lobar collapse occurs with pneumonia, TB, malignancy and foreign body aspiration. The treatment of collapse is that of the primary condition. *For the radiographic appearances of lobar collapses see Figure 13.4 on page 219.*

Pulmonary embolism

PE (pulmonary embolism) is easily missed:
1 If the only symptom is breathlessness ('isolated dyspnoea')
2 In elderly patients
3 In the presence of co-existing cardiorespiratory disease.

A patient with increasing breathlessness, low SaO_2 and little else to find on clinical examination may be suffering from recurrent pulmonary emboli. The SaO_2 can sometimes improve dramatically with oxygen therapy. Pulmonary embolism may also cause a variety of other clinical presentations:

1 chest pain;

2 haemoptysis;

3 new onset of atrial fibrillation (*see page 177*);

4 collapse +/− hypotension;

5 shock;

6 cardiac arrest.

The diagnosis of PE is relatively unlikely in patients under 40 year old with no major risk factors who are not breathless or tachypnoeic.

For the major risk factors for venous thrombo-embolism see Box 12.12 on page 197.

Oestrogen therapy is only a minor risk factor for venous thrombo-embolism.

For the relative risks of PE and DVT for women taking combined oestrogen and progestogen contraceptive pills (and in pregnancy) see Box 7.11 on page 115. For DVT see page 114. For further details on the diagnosis and management of pulmonary embolism see page 197.

Respiratory failure

This is developing when the patient's conscious level begins to fall and the PaO_2 cannot be maintained above 60 mmHg (8 kPa). A normal $PaCO_2$ in the presence of tachypnoea, which should reduce it, is a worrying feature. Anaesthetic/ICU help should be requested at once.

Type I respiratory failure

Low PaO_2 (<60 mmHg or 8 kPa) with a normal or low $PaCO_2$ may result from any of the many pathological causes of maldistribution of ventilation and perfusion in the lungs. The definitive management is intubation and mechanical ventilation (IPPV) whilst treating the underlying cause. Continuous positive airway pressure (CPAP) is a technique that uses a tight-fitting face mask to deliver oxygen at pressure throughout the ventilatory cycle and thus improve oxygen delivery to underventilated areas.

Type II (ventilatory) respiratory failure

Low PaO_2 (<60 mmHg or 8 kPa) with a raised $PaCO_2$ (>45 mmHg or 6 kPa) most commonly results from COPD – *see page 214*. Other causes include:

• paralysis of the respiratory muscles;

• chest deformity, especially with superadded infection;

• depression of the respiratory centre by sedative or narcotic drugs.

Non-invasive ventilation (NIV) is very effective in ventilatory failure. It is indicated when the pH is less than 7.35. NIV is also known as non-invasive positive pressure ventilation (NIPPV). Bi-level pressure support ventilators are the commonest machines to be used for NIV. They deliver two levels of positive airway pressure over the respiratory cycle (BiPAP). The analeptic and respiratory stimulant drug, doxapram, is sometimes used if NIV is unavailable. Its main functions are:

1 to reduce oxygen-induced CO_2 retention

2 to treat a patient who is not thought to be suitable for assisted ventilation

3 as a holding measure whilst awaiting anaesthetic help.

For the use of controlled oxygen therapy with doxapram in type II respiratory failure see Box 13.13.

Intubation and conventional intermittent positive pressure ventilation (IPPV) remain the definitive treatment of both types of respiratory failure.

Box 13.13 Doxapram and Oxygen Therapy for Ventilatory Failure

PaO_2 > 45 mmHg (6 kPa) – 28% oxygen and observe.
PaO_2 <45 mmHg (6 kPa) – 24% oxygen and if:
• the PaO_2 fails to improve; or
• the $PaCO_2$ is rising more than 10 mmHg or 1.5 kPa in less than 1 h then doxapram should be commenced as follows:
4.0 mg per min × 15 min
3.0 mg per min × 15 min
2.0 mg per min × 30 min
1.5 mg per min thereafter.
Control of the CO_2 rise may enable a change to 28% oxygen.

Hyperventilation syndrome

Although some people are prone to attacks of hyperventilation, it is rare for significant psychiatric disease to be the cause. There is usually underlying anxiety and social stress.

The patient becomes increasingly frightened by an apparent inability to breath adequately. Attempts to breath rapidly result in dizziness and further anxiety. Tachypnoea blows off CO_2 and the resultant respiratory alkalosis causes a fall in ionised calcium. Paraesthesia in the fingers and around the mouth are common consequences but tetany with carpopedal spasm is unusual – see page 254.

Tx

Investigation should accompany treatment; the confirmation of normality with warm reassurance is essential. Organic respiratory problems, such as spontaneous pneumothorax, pulmonary embolus or salicylate poisoning must be ruled out. This will certainly entail physical examination and pulse oximetry; ECG, chest X-ray and blood gas analysis may also be needed in some cases.

If no organic cause can be found, then rebreathing into a closed bag and mask system without oxygen supplement may be helpful. Requests for tranquillisers should be resisted. The patient should either be discharged home with relatives and a note sent to the GP or else, in severe cases, admitted for further assessment. Outpatient psychiatric review, via the GP, may be required for patients who suffer from frequent attacks.

Other causes of respiratory distress

A wide range of other conditions may lead to respiratory distress, including shock from any cause, trauma, poisoning and metabolic upset.

For spontaneous pneumothorax see page 201.
For myocardial infarction see page 183.
For inhalation of fumes, smoke and other gases see pages 288 and 291.
For ketoacidosis see page 246.
For salicylate poisoning see page 274.

Haemoptysis

Patients may present with haemoptysis as an isolated symptom. The blood is usually coughed up in a small quantity mixed with sputum. History and examination must aim to exclude serious illnesses such as chest infection, left ventricular failure, pulmonary embolism, TB or malignancy. Full blood count, ECG and Chest X-ray should be performed on all such patients with the same aim. Patients who are then found to have no other apparent abnormalities or stable conditions can be referred back to their GP for further management. The majority of haemoptysis in young people is idiopathic.

For pulmonary embolism see pages 197 and 223.

Chapter 14

Collapse and sudden illness

Collapse

The term collapse is generally used to describe a sudden deterioration in health. As such, it covers a wide spectrum of disease. To collapse implies a change of such magnitude that an upright posture cannot be maintained; it does not necessarily refer to a depression in the level of consciousness. However, some collapsed patients will be comatose and many will have a history of having been unresponsive at some time. The priorities are to:

• start resuscitation;
• seek out easily reversible conditions and treat them;
• begin a structured assessment.

Assessment and management of the collapsed patient

For details of immediate assessment and management applicable to all emergency patients see Chapter 1.
The same structured system can be used to assess collapsed patients further.

A – Airway

• Clear the airway with suction or other physical means.
• Maintain the airway by positioning or by using airway adjuncts.
• Protect the airway by positioning the patient in the recovery position and having suction available.

• Consider the need for endotracheal intubation.
• Protect the cervical spine at all times if the history is unknown, vague or suggests the possibility of trauma.
• Consider specific treatment for foreign body obstruction (*see page 205*) or anaphylaxis (*see page 295*).

B – Breathing

• Give a high-concentration of oxygen.
• Briefly look at the adequacy of respiration.
• Consider the need for immediate ventilation.
• Establish monitoring (SaO_2, BP and ECG).
• If the SaO_2 is low or if there is a suggestion of CO_2 narcosis, check the blood gases.
• Commence therapy to relieve hypoxia and dyspnoea; consider specific treatment for:
  – cardiorespiratory problems (severe left ventricular failure, COAD, asthma, pneumonia, pulmonary embolism and spontaneous pneumothorax – *see Chapter 13*);
  – CO_2 narcosis – *see page 224*;
  – anaphylaxis – *see page 295*.

C – Circulation

• Establish venous access and give IV fluids as necessary.
• Examine the cardiovascular system.

- Consider the possibility of bleeding into the abdomen or the gut (abdominal + PR examination). Look for melena or coffee ground vomit and vaginal or rectal bleeding.
- Consider specific treatment for:
  - cardiothoracic problems (MI, pulmonary embolism – *see Chapter 12*; dysrhythmia – *see Chapter 11*);
  - abdominal problems (gastrointestinal bleed, intra-abdominal bleeding or sepsis – *see Chapter 16*);
  - anaphylaxis – *see page 295*.

D – Disability

- Record the level of consciousness.
- Look at the pupils, muscle tone and reflexes and record any localising signs.
- Run your hands over the scalp to discover any swelling or bleeding.
- Look in the ears for signs of base of skull fracture.
- Look in the fundi for preretinal haemorrhage (from a subarachnoid bleed).
- Look for photophobia, neck stiffness, Kernig's sign and purpura.
- Listen for neck bruits (cerebral ischaemia).

> A decreased level of consciousness indicates that something is wrong with the brain or its fuel supply. It may be:
> **1** Poisoning or gross metabolic disturbance (including CO_2 narcosis and hypothermia).
> **2** Cerebral injury or pathology (head injury, intracranial bleeding, thrombosis, embolism, infection, swelling, tumour, fitting, etc.).
> **3** Failure of the brain's fuel supply (hypoxia, hypovolaemia, cerebral ischaemia or hypoglycaemia).

For common causes of sudden collapse with coma see Box 14.1.

Box 14.1 Common Causes of Sudden Collapse with Coma

Subarachnoid haemorrhage
Brainstem CVA
Hypoglycaemia
Poisoning (e.g. tricyclics)
Head injury

E – Environment and exposure

- Take the temperature (tympanic or rectal).
- Remove clothing (but keep warm), and examine the whole patient – front and back. Search the clothing for treatment cards, drugs, suicide notes and identification. Consider forensic needs.
- Protect the eyes.
- Consider specific treatment for:
  - hypothermia – *see page 248*;
  - infection;
  - hyperpyrexia – *see pages 250 and 270*.

F – Fits

- Control any tonic–clonic activity with benzodiazepines (*see page 237*).
- Protect the tongue from the teeth with a Guedel airway.

G – Glucose

Check the blood sugar in any patient who is unresponsive or behaving strangely and administer IV glucose if necessary.

H – History

- Get as much detail as possible from bystanders, ambulance crew and relatives. The essentials are AMPLE (*see page 9*).
- Obtain hospital records or details from the GP by telephone.

I – Immediate analgesia and investigations

- Give analgesia, if required, and look for the cause of any pain.
- Request a Chest X-ray.
- Obtain an ECG.
- Take blood for Hb, white cell count, urea, electrolytes, sugar and serum osmolality. The osmolar gap is a useful and easily available indicator of toxic and metabolic disorders – *see Boxes 14.2 and 14.3*.

Box 14.2 The Osmolar Gap

This is useful as a screening test for osmotically active poisons in the bloodstream and in the search for a cause for a metabolic acidosis.

Osmolar gap is the difference between measured serum osmolality and calculated serum osmolality.

Measured serum osmolality is normally 280–300 mOsm per L (easily measured by freezing point osmometry).

Calculated serum osmolality is twice the serum sodium concentration plus the glucose and the urea levels (in mmol per L).

Calculated osmolality $= (2 \times Na) + glucose + urea$

This is a simplification of a more accurate formula:

Calculated osmolality
$= (1.86 \times Na) + glucose + urea/0.93$

If the osmolar gap is greater than 10 mOsm per L then there are probably abnormal osmotically active substances in the bloodstream such as:

- ethanol
- methanol
- ethylene glycol
- mannitol

These are all substances with a small molecular weight. Even in poisoned patients, most other drugs do not achieve a high enough molar concentration to contribute to osmolality, which depends purely on the number of molecules present.

Box 14.3 The Anion Gap

The anion gap refers to the concentration difference between the measured serum cation (sodium) and the measured serum anions (chloride and bicarbonate). It is normally 12 mmol per L (±2). An anion gap of >20 is definitely abnormal.

Anion gap$=Na-(Cl+HCO_3)=10-14$ mmol per L

- Insert a nasogastric tube and a urinary catheter in all unresponsive patients.
- X-ray the hips and pelvis in any older person who has collapsed or has been found on the floor.

Vaso-vagal attacks

Vaso-vagal attacks may follow unpleasant psychological stimuli or occur in early pregnancy but often no cause is found. Many patients who attend an ED after this type of collapse are in the

prodromal phase of a viral infection and thus sometimes a mild pyrexia is found.

Before this diagnosis is made, other causes of syncope must be excluded. This will entail a careful history and examination and, in all but young patients, an ECG.

Poisoning

For treatment of poisoned patients see Chapter 15.

Unexplained collapse with generalised or bizarre signs must always raise the possibility of poisoning, even if this is strenuously denied. In unresponsive patients, a gastric lavage may yield useful information and remove toxic substances from the stomach.

An increased anion gap suggests an underlying metabolic acidosis – usually as a result of poisoning, renal failure or excess production of lactate or ketones.

In metabolic acidosis, excess acids are titrated by bicarbonate, the level of which then falls. This causes an increase in the calculated anion gap. *For metabolic acidosis see page 257.*

Collapse in children

Collapse in children usually accompanies overwhelming pathology such as shock, respiratory failure or intracranial infection.
For paediatric resuscitation see page 157.
For meningococcal septicaemia see page 336.
For miscellaneous paediatric conditions see Chapter 18.

Collapse in the elderly

Collapse in the elderly is common because of the following:

1 A relatively small change in health can cause sudden decompensation of an already failing system.

2 Lack of social support may prevent timely interventions that could have avoided gross deterioration.

3 Elderly patients are often taking a multiplicity of drugs.

4 Symptoms and signs tend to be less focused, so that the patient presents with global vague

problems rather than specific and localised abnormalities.

The cause of a sudden deterioration in an elderly patient may not be immediately apparent from the history or clinical examination. For this reason, most collapsed older patients will need investigation before discharge to exclude diagnoses such as:
- MI (myocardial infarction) or pulmonary embolism;
- heart block or other dysrhythmia;
- pneumonia, pyelonephritis or other infection;
- gastrointestinal bleeding or other blood loss;
- anaemia or renal failure;
- chronic subdural haemorrhage or cerebrovascular accident (CVA);
- fractured neck of femur.

This requires full blood count, urea and electrolytes, glucose, ECG and Chest X-ray as a standard screen; plasma calcium is also a useful test in non-specific illness.

Patients who have been found on the floor in the morning are often cold, dehydrated and frightened; they need admission – *see crush injuries on page 255 and hypothermia on page 248.*

Prevention of pressure sores

Pressure sores cause a great deal of morbidity amongst hospitalised patients and are difficult and expensive to treat. They will begin to form or worsen during a period of immobility on an ED trolley, especially if the time is over 2 h. Thus all patients who are recumbent should be assessed for risk factors using a predetermined scoring system. There are general risk factors that include:
- obesity or low body weight;
- thin, oedematous, sweaty or damaged skin;
- reduced or restricted mobility, including that caused by pain or splintage;
- incontinence of urine or faeces;
- low intake of food and drink;
- increasing age (above 50 years old);
- female gender;

and problems that carry a special, and very high risk of skin breakdown such as:
- cachexia;
- cardiovascular disease;
- neurological disease;
- major trauma;
- history of lying on the floor;
- hypothermia;
- treatment with steroids and cytotoxics.

Patients who are found to be at risk of developing pressure sores should receive pressure area care and be moved to a ward bed as soon as possible.

Prevention of deep vein thrombosis

Deep vein thrombosis (DVT) is not just a problem in surgical patients; sick patients of all types are susceptible. Up to 20% of general medical patients are believed to suffer from (often undiagnosed) venous thrombosis. For this reason, many physicians recommend prophylaxis against DVT for all medical patients who have no contraindications to heparins. A suitable regimen is enoxaparin 40 mg daily by subcutaneous injection, started in the ED. Exceptions include patients who present with a condition that might be haemorrhagic in origin or who:
- are under 40 years old and fully mobile;
- are known to have a bleeding disorder or are already on anticoagulants;
- are known to have pericarditis or diabetic retinopathy;
- have a history of haemorrhagic stroke or subarachnoid haemorrhage;
- have a history of GI bleeding.

For risk factors for DVT see Box 12.12 on page 197.
For diagnosis and treatment of DVT see page 114.

Driving after a collapse or sudden illness

Patients who are suffering from conditions that may result in a sudden and dramatic change in health are not fit to drive or operate dangerous machinery – *see page 372.* An escort home should be arranged for all such patients and they should be warned of the possible dangers to themselves and others. *For advice on driving after a CVA or TIA see page 236.*

Neurological problems

For acute confusional states see page 353.

The ambulant patient with a headache

The discomfort described as a headache may result from the following:

- Muscular tension (tension headache).
- Arterial dilatation (hypertension, nitrates).
- Traction on arteries (raised intracranial pressure).
- Traction on venous sinuses (low pressure headache following cerebrospinal fluid leak or dehydration).
- Inflammation (meningitis, arteritis).
- Referred pain (sinusitis, glaucoma).

For some of the more common pathological causes of a headache see Box 14.4.

Worrying features in the history of a patient with a headache include:

- sudden onset of symptoms;
- neck stiffness;
- loss of consciousness, however transient;
- fit or other collapse;
- visual loss or other visual change;
- other neurological symptoms;
- change in personality, memory or mental ability;
- pain worse on waking or straining;
- worst-ever headache;
- first severe headache in a patient of age >35 years.

The minimum examination of an ambulant patient with a headache should record:

- cortical functioning/GCS;
- gross neurological state;
- pupillary signs;
- fundoscopy;
- the presence or absence of meningism or neck tenderness;
- temperature;
- the presence or absence of rashes;
- otoscopy;
- BP;
- palpation of the scalp and sinuses for tenderness.

Xᴿ

Computed tomography (CT) scan is the most useful first-line investigation of a headache unless lumbar puncture is needed to exclude meningitis. It is usually performed on patients who have already been admitted for observation. A negative scan does not rule out subarachnoid haemorrhage (SAH).

Tx

Patients with a headache who have symptoms or signs suggestive of serious pathology should be referred to the physician on-call.

Box 14.4 Causes of a Headache

Tension headache
Migraine/cluster headache
Subarachnoid haemorrhage
Other intracranial bleed
Post head injury
Intracranial infection
Systemic febrile illnesses
Space-occupying lesion
Temporal arteritis
Malignant hypertension
Paget's disease
Hypercapnia/hypoxia
Poisoning (CO_2, nitrates)
Glaucoma
ENT infection and nasal trauma
Dental problems
Neck problems
Cerebrospinal fluid leakage
Dehydration
Psychogenic factors, including anxiety and depression

Consider the possibility of SAH in all patients with a headache:
- 50% of patients with SAH have a warning headache in the week before a big bleed;
- 50% have a warning headache without major physical signs;
- nearly 50% have seen a doctor about the headache;
- 50% with missed initial bleeds die.

The history is the key to the diagnosis of SAH.

Head injury

For management of patients with head injuries see Chapter 3 on page 34.

Head injury must always be considered as a cause of collapse and may often coexist with it. Where there is doubt as to the relative influences of intracranial injury and other conditions, then a CT scan should be performed.

Subarachnoid haemorrhage

Primary SAH occurs in one in 1000 adults. Rupture of small intracerebral aneurysms is the most common cause; only 5% of patients have bled from an arteriovenous malformation. In 20% of cases no cause is ever identified and these patients have the best prognosis. Overall, 10% of patients with SAH die in the first few hours and this rises to 50% in the first few weeks. Bleeding recurs in one in five patients, usually at the end of the first week. Secondary SAH may occur from extension of an intracerebral bleed or after trauma.

SAH usually presents as:

1 sudden collapse with a depressed level of consciousness with or without convulsions and/or vomiting;

2 sudden onset of severe occipital headache with or without other neurological features. There may be a history of recent 'warning' episodes of sudden headache. The patient may be feeling much better at the time of ED examination.

• Meningism is often present even in the comatose patient although neck pain and photophobia are not essential for the diagnosis.

• Lateralising signs are usually 'soft' or absent.

• Fundoscopy of comatose patients with SAH may reveal preretinal (subhyaloid) haemorrhages; this sign is pathognomic. Tropicamide mydriatic drops may be used to dilate the pupils; pupillary signs must be recorded first.

> Beware of the patient who collapses with SAH but sustains a coincidental traumatic brain injury.

Investigations

CT scan has replaced lumbar puncture as the first-line investigation.

> A negative scan does not exclude SAH.

When the history is suggestive of SAH, the patient should be referred for inpatient investigation. Lumbar puncture will usually be indicated.

Tx

• ABCs.
• Terminate convulsions.
• Check the blood sugar.
• Refer the patient to the general physicians/neurosurgeons.

Calcium antagonists (nimodipine) are used to prevent the development of secondary cerebral ischaemia. This occurs in 50% of patients, usually in the first 5–10 days after the bleed.

Intracranial infection

Impaired consciousness and pyrexia suggest intracranial infection. Meningitis is the most common cause and may be associated with infection elsewhere. Encephalitis (usually herpetic) may present as confusion, disorientation, drowsiness or bizarre behaviour.

For the features and treatment of both bacterial and viral meningitis see pages 335 and 336.

For prophylaxis of meningitis contacts see pages 338 and 339.

For encephalitis see page 336.

> Neck stiffness is absent in up to 30% of cases of bacterial meningitis.

Meningococcal disease is especially important for ED personnel to recognise as very early treatment (with IV cefotaxime, fluids and ventilation) improves the prognosis. In the United Kingdom, cases of meningococcal infection, both meningitic and septicaemic, usually rise in the autumn and reach a peak early in the new year. This annual rise in cases starts in students in colleges of higher education, although the highest incidence rates are in children under 2 years of age. Muslim visitors to Saudi Arabia for the Hajj or Umrah pilgrimages are also at a high risk of meningococcal infection. *For the features and treatment of meningococcal disease see page 336.*

Temporal arteritis

Cranial or giant cell arteritis is a panarteritis of unknown aetiology, which affects medium-sized vessels, particularly those of the scalp. Affected arteries are thickened and tender and thrombosis may occur. The condition is related to polymyalgia rheumatica and is predominantly seen in the elderly. Recovery can take several months and recurrence is always a possibility.

Temporal arteritis – the most common manifestation – starts with an acute onset of headache. There is a sharp, burning pain over the temporal artery, which may be locally tender. Neurological signs are caused by ischaemia in the territory of other inflamed arteries:
- *visual impairment* – which may progress to blindness or ischaemia of the optic nerve and retina;
- *ophthalmoplegia* – ischaemia of the ocular motor nerves;
- *pain on eating* – masseter claudication;
- *TIA/stroke* – involvement of branches of the vertebral or carotid arteries.

Investigations

A raised erythrocyte sedimentation rate (ESR) may confirm the diagnosis but a normal ESR does not exclude it. Serial ESRs and biopsy of the temporal artery may be required.

Tx

> The primary aim of treatment in temporal arteritis is to prevent the occurrence of permanent neurological damage, especially blindness.

As soon as the diagnosis is suspected, prednisolone 40 mg should be given (60 mg if there are

visual symptoms) with soluble aspirin (300 mg). Analgesia and admission for observation will also be required.

Migraine

The first severe attack of migraine usually occurs in the teenage years or early twenties. There may be an isolated unilateral throbbing headache (common migraine) or a more complicated syndrome preceded by some form of aura (classical migraine). In the latter case, the headache may be accompanied by:
- gross malaise;
- pallor and tremor;
- nausea and vomiting with gastric stasis;
- visual disturbance;
- abdominal pain;
- focal neurological signs such as paraesthesia and numbness or even hemiparesis.

Over half of all patients with migraine have a family history of the condition and many have suffered from travel sickness as children.

Episodes of migraine may last for hours or even days. Those attacks that are atypical in severity or duration should be given special consideration.

Tx

A severe headache can often be avoided if simple analgesics are taken early enough in the course of an attack. Unfortunately, by the time most patients present to an ED, the opportunity for this has passed and vomiting then makes oral drugs

> **Box 14.5 Use of Sumatriptan**
>
> Oral dose = 100 mg, can be repeated if symptoms return (maximum oral dose = 300 mg in 24 h)
> Subcutaneous dose = 6 mg, can be repeated after an hour if symptoms recur (maximum subcutaneous dose = 12 mg in 24 h)
> Sumatriptan may cause:
> - lethargy
> - dizziness or vertigo
> - sensations of warmth
> - feelings of pressure or heaviness in any part of the body

---

Box 14.6 Contraindications to Sumatriptan

Known hypersensitivity to the drug
Ischaemic heart disease
Conditions predisposing to ischaemic heart disease
Prinzmetal's angina
Poorly controlled hypertension
Renal or hepatic impairment
Hemiplegic migraine
Patients taking monoamine oxidase inhibitors, selective 5-HT reuptake inhibitors or lithium
Pregnancy or lactation
Children
Age over 65 years

---

useless. A parenteral NSAID (e.g. tenoxicam 20 mg IV/IM) can be given together with an antiemetic injection. Sumatriptan (Imigran) is a specific treatment for migraine (*see Boxes 14.5 and 14.6*) but it is only effective in about 75% of patients.

Neurological symptoms should be treated by oral aspirin and admission for observation. Most severe attacks finally terminate when the sufferer falls asleep. Not surprisingly, a feeling of euphoria may accompany the subsequent relief.

Cluster headache (migrainous neuralgia)

This is a related condition that is more common in men. Severe unilateral headache occurs in clusters of episodes, often months apart. There is facial pain, lacrimation and rhinorrhoea. It is treated in a similar way to migraine.

Tension headache

This is the most common cause of a headache, occurring more often in females than in males. Symptoms may persist for several days and occur up to 14 days per month. The pain is usually described as a tight cap or band pressing over the head. The distribution of the sensation is that of the occipitofrontalis muscle and tension in this muscle is probably the cause of the pain. Nausea and difficulty getting to sleep may also be experienced. The muscular tension may be precipitated and maintained by:

• personal worries and difficulties;

• constant unremitting stress (e.g. mother with young children);
• depression;
• a minor injury (e.g. whiplash-type).

Tx

The patient has often found that simple analgesics have not relieved the pain. NSAIDs may help as may psycho- and physiotherapy. Tricyclic antidepressants are sometimes prescribed in relatively low doses (e.g. amitriptyline 50–100 mg at night). Referral should be made to the GP. SAH must be excluded – *see page 231.*

Other headaches

Most other patients with headaches should also be referred back to the GP but those with neurological signs should be admitted for investigation.

Brainstem cerebrovascular accident

Sudden catastrophic collapse may be caused by haemorrhage into or infarction of the brainstem. There will be:

• coma;
• small fixed pupils (exclude narcotic poisoning);
• few, if any, lateralising signs.

Respiration continues but other brainstem functions and reflexes are attenuated. The prognosis is grave.

Xr

It is important to make an accurate diagnosis as soon as possible to avoid inappropriate and distressing life support measures. CT scan may be needed for this purpose.

Tx

As soon as the prognosis is assured, the relatives must be gently informed. The patient should be admitted to a bed and kept comfortable while nature takes its course.

For bereavement counselling see page 169.
For diagnosis of brainstem death see page 381.

Cerebrovascular accident

Cerebrovascular disease is one of the most common causes of death in the United Kingdom and accounted for 25% of all cardiovascular deaths in England and Wales in 2004. After a stroke, approximately 23% of people die within 30 days and, of the initial stroke survivors, only 30–40% are alive after 3 years. Stroke is also the leading cause of disability in the United Kingdom and other Western countries, with about 25–30% of stroke survivors remaining permanently disabled. In Europe, people of West Indian origin are at a particularly high risk from CVA.

Collapse associated with unilateral abnormal neurological signs is most commonly caused by a stroke or a transient ischaemic attack (TIA) (*see later*). The distinction between the two overlapping conditions is impossible in patients who are not already recovering when seen. Most CVAs (80%) are a result of thrombotic or embolic cerebral infarction. Emboli usually result from atrial fibrillation or MI while atherosclerosis causes both intracerebral thrombosis and thromboembolism in the carotid vessels. Cerebral infarction leads to a progressive neurological deficit. Signs may be minimal at first with subjective weakness or paraesthesia only. The CVAs that result from intracerebral haemorrhage (the remaining 20%) are more sudden in onset with headache and rapidly established signs.

> A patient who complains of vague unilateral symptoms must be taken seriously.

A stroke causes loss or disturbance of motor and sensory function. The exact clinical picture depends on the territory of the blood vessel involved (*see Box 14.7*). Posterior lesions may affect conscious level (*see page 233*) or more rarely there may be cerebellar signs. In the very early stages, spinal reflexes are usually depressed although the plantar response may be extensor. Severe hypertension may be present but intervention to lower it in the ED is contraindicated as this may precipitate further cerebrovascular damage.

> **Box 14.7 Symptoms of a TIA**
>
> TIA in the carotid territory (80% of TIAs)
> - Unilateral paresis
> - Unilateral sensory loss
> - Aphasia
> - Monocular visual loss
>
> Vertebrobasilar TIA
> - Bilateral or alternating weakness or sensory loss.
> - Bilateral visual loss/hemianopia
> - Two or more of the following: vertigo, diplopia, dysphagia, dysarthria, ataxia

Investigations

Routine blood tests, Chest X-ray and ECG should be performed. Coincidental hip fracture must be considered and excluded. Brain imaging should be undertaken as soon as possible in all patients, certainly within 24 h of the onset of symptoms unless there are good clinical reasons for not doing so. The brain scan must be performed urgently if the patient has:
- a known bleeding tendency or is taking anticoagulants;
- a depressed level of consciousness;
- a severe headache at the onset;
- an uncertain diagnosis or atypical features (most doctors would consider age <60 years as atypical);
- unexplained, progressive or fluctuating signs;
- papilloedema, neck stiffness or fever;
- indications for thrombolysis or early anticoagulation (*see later*).

Elderly people often fall at the onset of a stroke, but this history may be lacking. Traumatic intracranial blood (acute or chronic subdural or even extradural) may mimic a CVA. Sudden deterioration, in particular with a fixed, dilated pupil, raises the suspicion of an expanding lesion. CT scan is indicated to confirm the suspected sequence of events.

Tx

- Give oxygen.
- Monitor vital signs.
- Check the blood sugar.
- Establish IV access.

- Treat complications (e.g. fits).
- Admit the patient to hospital for assessment and rehabilitation – usually in a specialist stroke unit.

Patients have a risk of a further stroke within 5 years of between 30% and 43% and also an increased risk of other cardiovascular events. Therefore, consideration needs to be given to lifestyle factors (smoking, diet and exercise), blood pressure and cholesterol reduction. Stroke patients should have an annual vaccination against influenza.

Anticoagulants are usually prescribed for all patients with persistent or paroxysmal AF. There is a 68% reduction in the risk of stroke for patients with AF on warfarin compared to a 25–30% risk reduction with aspirin. Other patients with an ischaemic stroke require antiplatelet therapy such as low-dose aspirin (75 mg a day), clopidogrel (75 mg a day), or a combination of low-dose aspirin and modified-release dipyridamole (200 mg bd). Dipyridamole has both antiplatelet and vasodilating properties and is thought to inhibit the uptake of adenosine (a potent inhibitor of platelet activation and aggregation) into platelets and vascular cells. Dipyridamole may also inhibit the breakdown of cyclic guanosine monophosphate. *For the actions of other antiplatelet drugs see page 195.*

Thrombolysis for CVA

There is increasing evidence that patients with an acute ischaemic stroke may benefit from thrombolysis. The aim is to limit the size of the cerebral infarct and thus improve the functional outcome. However, the administration of fibrinolytic drugs must begin within 3 h of the onset of symptoms as an absolute maximum. Alteplase (tPA) is given IV over 60 min in a dose of 900 µg per kg (to a maximum of 90 mg). The initial 10% of the dose should be given by bolus injection and the remaining 90% by infusion. Thrombolysis is not recommended for patients over 80 years old. This treatment is not yet standard in the United Kingdom and depends on rapid confirmation of the diagnosis (ischaemia rather than haemorrhage) by CT scanning.

> By 6 months after their stroke, 50% of all patients will need some help with daily living, 15% will have communication problems and over 50% will have some residual weakness. Many will also have mood or cognitive problems. Their carers also suffer.

Transient ischaemic attack

A transient ischaemic attack (TIA) is defined as an abrupt loss of focal cerebral or monocular function with symptoms lasting less than 24 h which, after adequate investigation, is presumed to be caused by embolic or thrombotic vascular disease.

> There is no qualitative difference between a TIA and an ischaemic stroke.

The risk of having a stroke after a hemispheric TIA is up to 20% in the first month, with the greatest risk occurring in the first 72 h. In addition, a TIA is a marker for general vascular disease (*see Box 14.8*). Half of all TIAs are caused by the thromboembolic complications of arteriosclerosis in the arteries that supply the brain; emboli from the heart account for a further 20%.

The diagnosis of TIA is based on the history. Symptoms – usually loss of function – are of sudden onset and are maximal from the start (*see Box 14.7*). As TIAs are focal events, global symptoms such as light headedness, dizziness and syncope are rarely consistent with the diagnosis. The following predisposing factors should be sought:

- atrial fibrillation or other source of cardiac embolism;
- hypertension;
- carotid disease (bruits);
- history of smoking;
- hypercholesterolaemia.

Box 14.8 Risk of Other Diseases after a TIA

The average annual risk of stroke is about 7% (seven times the normal population's risk).
The greatest risk of a stroke is in the first year.
The annual risk of MI is 2–3%.
The annual death rate from CVA, MI or other vascular death is about 9%.

Investigations

All patients should have a routine screen (full blood count, ESR, urea and electrolytes, LFTs (liver function tests), glucose, random cholesterol, ECG and Chest X-ray). An urgent CT scan of the brain should be considered for patients under 60 years old and for those with atypical features, reasons for bleeding or an uncertain diagnosis. Carotid duplex scan is usually requested from clinic by investigating physicians.

Tx

Once the symptoms are clearly resolving, oral aspirin (300 mg) should be given to all patients in whom it is not contraindicated. Patients should be admitted to hospital if they have any of the following:

1 residual symptoms or signs;
2 a likely source of emboli;
3 a history of more than one TIA in a week.

Other patients may go home, provided that there are arrangements for assessment by a specialist service within 7 days of the TIA. The GP must be notified and aspirin (300 mg daily for 2 weeks and then 75 mg a day) prescribed for all patients. (Aspirin therapy reduces the incidence of CVA in patients who have had a TIA by around 3% per annum.) Patients who are intolerant of aspirin (hypersensitivity or severe dyspepsia induced by low-dose aspirin) should receive clopidogrel 300 mg stat and then 75 mg daily. In the specialist clinic, the patient will be prescribed modified-release dipyridamole 200 mg bd in addition to aspirin or be changed to treatment with clopidogrel. If a patient is found to be in AF (and not anti-coagulated), they should be prescribed aspirin 300 mg a day until seen in clinic.

Driving after a CVA or TIA

The UK (DVLA) rules on fitness to drive state that a patient with a diagnosis of CVA or TIA must not drive for at least one month. He may resume driving after this time if his clinical recovery is judged to be satisfactory and he has not had any fits. There is no need to notify the licensing authority (DVLA) unless there is a residual neurological deficit one month after the episode. A patient with multiple TIAs will require an attack-free period of 3 months before resuming driving and must notify the DVLA. This advice has obvious implications for patients discharged from an ED with a diagnosis of TIA.

Labyrinthitis (vestibular neuronitis)

Presumed viral infection of the inner ear or its nerve supply may cause an unpleasant condition closely related to motion sickness. The symptoms are the same:

- profound nausea and vomiting;
- vertigo and ataxia;
- pallor, sweating and gross malaise.

The vertigo is positional and is usually worsened by movements of the head and reduced by keeping still. Nystagmus may be present (fast component towards the affected side) but there is no hearing loss.

Tx

Other conditions must be excluded before treatment is initiated. Bed rest is essential and affected patients cannot go home alone. The symptoms may persist for several days or even weeks, during which time the patient must not drive. (In its duration and dubious aetiology, vestibular neuronitis resembles another common cranial mononeuropathy, Bell's palsy.)

If not contraindicated, the most effective drugs by far are:

1 The sedative anticholinergic hyoscine hydrobromide. This is also known as 'scopolamine' and is different from the antispasmodic hyoscine butylbromide ('Buscopan'). It is given in an initial dose of 0.4 mg IM but may also be administered as a tablet or a transdermal patch.
2 The phenothiazine-derived antihistamine promethazine ('Phenergan'), given in a dose of 25–50 mg IM or orally. This drug also (and uniquely) seems to help 'reset' the labyrinthine mechanisms to their new state.
3 Sedative antihistamine tablets such as meclozine (marketed for motion sickness).

Standard phenothiazines (e.g. prochlorperazine) and 5HT$_3$ antagonists (e.g. metoclopramide) are totally ineffective for vestibular conditions.

Other vestibular or cerebellar signs

Sudden onset of ataxia must generally be referred to the physicians for investigation. Sometimes chronic alcoholics with known cerebral degeneration present with an apparent disproportionate worsening of the cerebellar component of this disease. They should be admitted as the combination of alcohol, ataxia and the environment is often fatal.
See also CVA and TIA on pages 234 and 235.

Convulsions (seizures)

For treatment of fits in children see page 339.
Fits occur when there is:
• *Deprivation of cerebral fuel supply (anoxic convulsion):*
  hypoglycaemia or hypoxia;
  transient dysrhythmia or cardiac arrest;
  syncope.
• *Cerebral irritation:*
  head injury;
  cerebral tumour or infection;
  poisoning;
  fever (viraemia) in children;
  primary epilepsy.
• *Withdrawal of sedatives:*
  alcohol or drug withdrawal.
A fit causes a dramatic increase in the cerebral metabolic demand for oxygen and also partial airway obstruction and decreased ventilation. Hypoxia must be prevented by urgent airway control and rapid treatment of the fit before elucidation of the underlying cause can be undertaken.

Tx

• Protect or remove the patient from harm.
• Give high-concentration oxygen by facemask. Never attempt to force open the airway by inserting a wedge in the mouth – use a Guedel airway once the jaw has relaxed.
• Obtain venous access.

• Give diazepam emulsion IV (initially 5–20 mg for adults in incremental doses). If IV access cannot be obtained, then diazepam can be given rectally. Midazolam or lorazepam, both at approximately one third of the dose recommended for diazepam, are useful alternatives.
When the fit has stopped:
• place the patient in the recovery position;
• monitor vital signs;
• check the blood sugar;
• start investigating the circumstances that led to the fit and perform a full physical examination.

> If the fit is not terminated within 30 min, the patient has status epilepticus (permanent damage is common, 10% mortality). Call for urgent help – an anaesthetist may be needed – and then consider the following therapies.

• Paraldehyde – 5–10 mL (up to 5 mL by deep IM injection into each buttock). This is useful if IV access is problematical.
• Phenytoin – immediate loading dose of 15 mg per kg by IV infusion at a rate of no more than 50 mg per min (or 1 mg per kg per min). Fosphenytoin sodium is a prodrug, which is converted to phenytoin immediately after administration. It is prescribed in milligram PE (phenytoin equivalents). Unlike phenytoin sodium, it dissolves freely in aqueous solutions and can be infused intravenously at rates up to three times faster than the parent drug (i.e. 100–150 mg PE per min). In the case of both drugs, the ECG must be monitored throughout the infusion and for at least 30 min afterwards.
• Phenobarbital – 15 mg per kg by IV infusion at a rate of not more than 100 mg per min.
• Clomethiazole (chlormethiazole) infusion – initially 40–120 mg (5–15 mL) per min up to a maximum total dose of 800 mg (100 mL) then 4–8 mg (0.5–1 mL) per min according to response.

As soon as it becomes apparent that more than one drug is required, consideration should be given to the need for general anaesthetic techniques. This usually entails either sedation with thiopental (up to 5 mg per kg) and then a thiopental infusion (1–3 mg per kg per h) accompanied by

ICU monitoring or full anaesthesia, paralysis and ventilation.

Status epilepticus must be distinguished from serial seizures without full recovery. If the patient stops tonic–clonic seizures but does not regain full consciousness consider 'absence' or complex partial seizures. These are difficult to detect but important to stop as on-going cerebral ischaemia is a strong possibility.

A fully recovered, known epileptic may go home if:

- there are no unusual features in this episode;
- he or she remains well after 2 h observation;
- there is continuous social support both en route and at home;
- the GP is informed of the discharge;
- the usual drug supply is available.

Pseudo-fits

The possibility of pseudo-fits must be considered. These are an attention-seeking device, often manifest in a public arena. They can be distinguished from genuine convulsions because:

- the patient is rarely injured;
- there is no incontinence or tongue biting;
- the plantar response remains flexor;
- pulse oximetry remains normal, as opposed to the marked fall in saturation seen in a genuine fit.

Nevertheless, these patients cannot simply be dismissed. The pseudo-fit represents abnormal behaviour, often prompted by chronic and complex social problems. Discharge and follow-up should be discussed with the GP over the telephone.

Peripheral neuropathies and similar conditions

There are many causes of failure of conduction of the peripheral nerves including drugs, diabetes, infections, vitamin deficiencies and alcoholism. Many cases are idiopathic. Guillain–Barré syndrome is the most common type of acute polyneuropathy in the United Kingdom – *see later.*

Isolated peripheral neuropathies may follow stretching or compression of nerves while intoxicated with alcohol or drugs. Radial nerve palsy (wrist

drop) often occurs in these circumstances. Patients with foot drop sometimes present to an ED. Both of these conditions should be treated by splintage and referral for investigation.

Acute (transverse) myelitis may look similar to a polyneuritis. It causes a specific sensory level with bilateral leg weakness and bladder and bowel dysfunction.

Multiple sclerosis (MS) is not a peripheral neuropathy but may be mistaken for one as the multiple CNS lesions responsible are scattered in both time and place. MS may present with a vast array of different neurological features including loss of vision, diplopia, spastic weakness of the legs, numbness and parasthesia, sphincter disturbance, painful flexor spasms and cerebellar signs (vertigo, tremor and nystagmus).

For botulism see page 240.

For tetanus see page 239.

For poliomyelitis see page 260.

For myasthenia gravis see page 239.

Guillain–Barré syndrome (acute polyneuritis)

Guillain–Barré syndrome is an ascending polyneuritis of unknown aetiology, which develops over the course of a few days or sometimes several weeks. It is the most common form of acute peripheral neuropathy in the United Kingdom. There may be a history of a preceding infection and then severe backache prior to the development of neurological symptoms and signs as below:

- progressive, symmetrical, ascending weakness, which may include ocular, bulbar and respiratory muscles;
- diminished or absent tendon reflexes;
- variable sensory loss and sometimes pain;
- autonomic disturbances such as tachycardia, cardiac dysrhythmias and labile blood pressure.

Motor involvement (which may be either proximal or distal) usually predominates over sensory loss (often distal). Of the cranial nerves, the facial nerve is the most commonly affected. Measurement of peak expiratory flow rate is useful to assess the degree of respiratory impairment.

Tx

If the condition is clinically suspected, then the patient must be admitted to hospital. Intensive care is appropriate if there is bulbar or respiratory weakness or autonomic signs. Most cases of Guillain–Barré syndrome recover spontaneously over several weeks.

Cholinergic and myasthenic crises

In myasthenia gravis, too high a dose of anti-cholinesterase drugs may make the weakness worse (cholinergic crisis). This is easily mistaken for exacerbation of the primary disease (myasthenic crisis). Differentiation can be achieved by IV injection of edrophonium 2 mg (the 'Tensilon test'), which will induce a transient improvement in myasthenic crisis only.

> This test may precipitate ventilatory failure and so should only be carried out by those who can deal with this eventuality.

Tx

In both conditions, artificial ventilation may be required from the outset. For myasthenic crisis, neostigmine 0.5 mg IM should be given and repeated every 20 min as necessary. For cholinergic crisis, the treatment is pralidoxime 1–2 g by slow IV injection, again repeated every 20 min as required. The muscarinic effects of anticholinesterases must be controlled with IV atropine.

Tetanus

For prophylaxis against tetanus infection in wounds see page 390.
For Clostridium welchii infection (gas gangrene) see page 257.
There were 12 cases of tetanus in the United Kingdom in 2003, with two deaths in the previous year. Infection is caused by contamination of a wound with the spores of the bacillus *Clostridium tetani*. Days or even weeks after infection, local multiplication of the organism occurs with release of its neurotoxin. Even the most trivial of wounds can introduce tetanus into the body, but some wounds carry a particularly high risk of infection. *For factors that help to identify tetanus-prone wounds see Box 21.6 on page 391.* The incubation period of tetanus is between 4 and 21 days (usually about 10 days) and the case fatality rate is nearly 30%. Tetanus is a notifiable disease.

Active immunisation against tetanus was introduced into some areas of the United Kingdom as part of the primary immunisation of infants from the mid-1950s and was adopted nationally from 1961. As a result, tetanus virtually disappeared in children under 15 years old by the 1970s. Until recently, the majority of cases of tetanus in the United Kingdom were in people over 65 years old who had not been previously immunised. Two-thirds of the victims were women who, unlike most older men, had not been vaccinated during military service. (Immunisation against tetanus was provided by the British armed forces from 1938 onwards.) However, in the last few years, men and women seem to be equally at risk from the disease. More recently still, tetanus has been seen in young adults who abuse IV drugs. (In the United States, 20% of tetanus cases are associated with IV drug abuse.) Intramuscular and subcutaneous injection is particularly likely to result in a suitable environment for spore germination as citric acid (which is used to dissolve heroin) may damage muscle tissue. Neonatal tetanus is still a major public health problem in many developing countries but there have been no cases in the United Kingdom for over 30 years. It is usually caused by infection of the umbilical stump due to poor hygiene.

It is important to understand the mechanism of action of tetanus toxin. In the ventral horn of the spinal cord, negative feedback loop neurones (Renshaw cells) limit the activity of the α-motoneurones. Tetanus toxin prevents the release of the inhibitory neurotransmitter glycine from these cells, which allows uncontrolled spasms of skeletal muscle. Strychnine (and brucine) compete with glycine for its receptors on the α-motoneurones and thus cause a very similar clinical picture. Acute dystonic reactions ('occulogyric crises') may also mimic tetanus – *see page 296.*

The clinical features of tetanus can progress slowly over as much as 2 weeks. In the usual order of appearance they are:

- stiff muscles near the wound (or injection site);
- jaw stiffness and trismus ('lock-jaw');
- abdominal rigidity;
- progressive painful muscle spasms (the fixed mocking grin caused by facial muscle tightening is known as the 'risus sardonicus' and extensor spasms of the back, neck and limbs are called opisthotonus);
- dysphagia and respiratory difficulty;
- autonomic dysfunction.

> Consider the diagnosis of tetanus in IV drug abusers presenting with muscle stiffness or muscle spasms.

Tx

Supportive therapy is essential with special attention given to the airway, respiration and autonomic activities. IV benzodiazepines or even general anaesthesia may be required to control spasms. The tetanus bacillus is sensitive to both benzyl penicillin and metronidazole. Immunoglobulin against tetanus toxin (HTIG) 150 iu per kg is given IM in multiple sites. (A range of doses from 30 to 300 iu per kg has been suggested). Tetanus immunoglobulin for IV use is also available on a named patient basis. The dose is 5000–10 000 iu by IV infusion. Surgical debridement of wounds may help to reduce the toxin load. Suspicion of tetanus infection should provoke a discussion with a specialist in infectious diseases. Strychnine poisoning is treated with similar supportive and relaxant therapy.

Wound botulism

This variant of botulism has recently been seen in IV drug abusers, probably as a result of contaminated drugs and citric acid damage to muscle. Unlike the classical food-borne disease (which is caused by the ingestion of preformed toxin), wound botulism occurs when the spores of the anaerobic bacterium *Clostridium botulinum* contaminate a wound, germinate and produce toxin *in vivo*. Botulinum toxin blocks the release of acetyl-choline from the neuromuscular junction and characteristically causes a descending flaccid paralysis:

- blurred or double vision and ptosis;
- dysphonia, dysarthria and dysphagia;
- dizziness and general muscle weakness;
- immobility and respiratory distress.

Patients are afebrile with no sensory loss and no confusion. Autonomic signs include dry mouth, dilated pupils and urinary dysfunction.

Diagnosis is confirmed in a reference laboratory using serum samples and wound swabs. Botulism is fatal in 10% of victims and those who recover are usually debilitated for many months. Botulinum toxin is one of the most poisonous substances known to man. Several countries are known to have attempted weaponisation of the toxin for airborne dispersal leading to inhalation.

Tx

Ventilatory support may be required as may surgical debridement of wounds. *Clostridium botulinum* is sensitive to benzyl penicillin and metronidazole. Botulinum antitoxin should always be given as it is effective in reducing both the severity and duration of symptoms.

Decompression sickness

Decompression sickness or Caisson disease may occur up to 48 h after diving. It is caused by nitrogen (which has been dissolved in the blood under pressure), coming out of solution and forming bubbles in the blood stream and tissues. The patient may present as a collapse without giving a history of recreational diving as many people do not appreciate the potential for delayed onset of symptoms. There is:

- malaise;
- joint pains (the 'bends');
- itching and rashes;
- lymphadenopathy and oedema.

In severe cases there are signs and symptoms of cardiopulmonary, vestibular and CNS involvement such as:

- chest pain;

- dyspnoea;
- coughing and haemoptysis;
- hypertension or hypotension;
- tinnitus or deafness;
- nausea;
- vertigo and nystagmus;
- headache;
- behavioural changes;
- altered consciousness;
- convulsions;
- motor and sensory deficits, including hemiplegia, paraplegia and urinary retention.

Tx

- Give oxygen.
- Commence IV fluid resuscitation.
- Control fits and agitation.
- Discuss the patient with a specialist in diving and hyperbaric medicine. Recompression in a hyperbaric chamber may be required.

Nitrogen narcosis and oxygen toxicity in divers ('Rapture of the deep').

When breathed under pressure (at depths in excess of 100 ft or 30 m), nitrogen has an intoxicating effect. There is light headedness, impairment of judgement and loss of coordination. Hallucinations, coma and death may occur at extreme depths. The narcosis reverses spontaneously on ascent to normal air pressures.

Breathing oxygen at high partial pressures (at depths over 200 ft or 60 m) causes CNS toxicity. Dizziness, nausea, disorientation, visual abnormalities and facial twitching occur; convulsions and coma can prove fatal. Treatment is supportive. Recompression requires careful oxygen monitoring as high inspired concentrations of oxygen may worsen the condition.

Barotrauma from diving

The pressure changes associated with diving may also cause:

- pneumothorax and surgical emphysema;
- air embolism (neurological signs may mimic decompression sickness);

- rupture of the tympanic membrane (pain, bleeding, hearing loss);
- disturbance of the inner ear (nausea, vomiting, vertigo, tinnitus and deafness may also look like decompression sickness);
- pain around the sinuses and in the mouth (from air trapped in cavities beneath fillings or caries);
- GI pain, colic and flatulence.

If the clinical picture suggests a possibility of decompression sickness then the patient must be discussed with a hyperbaric specialist.

Altitude-related illness

Altitude, hypoxia and acclimatisation. Barometric pressure falls logarithmically with increasing altitude. The partial pressure of oxygen (21% of barometric pressure) falls at the same rate. At 19 000 ft (5800 m), these pressures are 50% of their values at sea level, falling to 28% at the summit of Mount Everest. The ambient temperature also drops by 6.5°C with every additional 3300 ft (1000 m) in altitude. The complex physiological changes of acclimatisation include increased minute ventilation, increased sympathetic tone, increased pulmonary vascular resistance and, after several weeks, an increased haematocrit.

Acute mountain sickness. AMS affects around 75% of people who ascend rapidly to heights of more than 10 000 ft (3000 m) above sea level and even troubles 20% of people at just 7500 ft (2300 m). It is usually defined as a headache accompanied by any of the following symptoms: nausea, vomiting, malaise, fatigue, lethargy, anorexia and insomnia. Sleep may be disturbed by periodic breathing or even apnoea. AMS usually resolves within 3 days of arriving at altitude but sometimes leads to life-threatening cerebral or pulmonary oedema. The causes of these altitude-related illnesses are poorly understood. There is some genetic predisposition associated with capillary leakage, fluid retention and stimulation of chemoreceptors in the presence of hypoxaemia. The risk is increased with rapid ascents and failure to acclimatise. All patients will have a low SaO_2. It is said that AMS can be minimised by 'climbing high and sleeping low'.

High altitude cerebral oedema. The most severe manifestation of altitude sickness is acute cerebral oedema, which can be overwhelming if untreated. It is thought to have the same pathophysiology as AMS and may represent the extreme form of the condition. In addition to the usual symptoms of mountain sickness, there is a progressive deterioration in mental status with ataxia and, in some cases, focal neurological deficits. Eventually coma supervenes.

High altitude pulmonary oedema. This is seen in 2–4% of climbers once 14 000 ft (4300 m) is reached and is the most common medical cause of death at altitude. Atmospheric hypoxia is thought to cause pulmonary hypertension, uneven perfusion and capillary leakage. The first symptoms are cough and tachypnoea, followed by increasing dyspnoea and cyanosis.

Tx

Sufferers must be advised to stop and rest immediately before the condition worsens. Oxygen, analgesics and antiemetics should be given and descent arranged. A reduction in altitude of as little as 1500–3000 ft (450–900 m) may be all that is required. Acetazolamide 125–250 mg bd may be given to increase the rate of acclimatisation. High altitude cerebral oedema is treated with dexamethasone 4 mg (by any route) every 6 h and hyperbaric therapy (in a portable unit such as a Gamow bag) if available. Patients with high altitude pulmonary oedema should be given nifedipine 10 mg by mouth 4-hourly and hyperbaric therapy, in addition to standard treatments for the oedema.

Prophylaxis for AMS

Acetazolamide is a sulphonamide that inhibits carbonic anhydrase. It decreases renal bicarbonate reabsorption, causing a mild metabolic acidosis and also decreases the formation of CSF. Acetazolamide 125 mg bd is an effective prophylaxis for AMS, which increases the rate of acclimatisation and reduces the severity of symptoms. Treatment should be started 2 days before ascent and continued for up to 5 days at altitude. The main side effects are diuresis and paraesthesiae. Chemoprophylaxis does not reduce the risk of altitude sickness; gradual ascent and physiological acclimatisation are still essential.

Other risks in climbers

These include hypothermia, frostbite, UV keratitis, exacerbation of pre-existing diseases and of course, trauma.

> British expeditions to peaks higher than 23 000 ft (7000 m) have experienced death rates of 4.3 per 100 climbers.

Cardiovascular and respiratory causes of collapse

For myocardial infarction see page 183.
For pulmonary embolism see pages 197 and 223.
For cardiac dysrhythmias see page 170.
For dyspnoea see chapter 13 on page 205.
For pneumonia see page 218.
For anaphylaxis see page 295.

Shock

Shock is a state of inadequate perfusion of vital tissues. This may be caused by inadequacies in the pump (heart), the delivery system (blood vessels) or the perfusing fluid (blood). There are therefore three basic types of shock:

1 Central shock – pump failure.
2 Hypovolaemic shock – decreased blood volume.
3 Distributive shock – leaky or dilated blood vessels.

The effects of septic, anaphylactic and neurogenic shock are mostly attributable to maldistribution of fluid but there may also be elements of cardiac depression and true hypovolaemia.

For anaphylactic shock see page 295.
For neurogenic shock see page 52.
For hypovolaemic, cardiogenic and septic shock see later.

Hypovolaemic shock

Loss of blood or other body fluid may result in hypovolaemic shock. The classical signs may only

Box 14.9 Blood Loss and Signs of Shock				
Blood loss (percentage of total)	**<15%**	**15–30%**	**30–40%**	**40%**
Blood pressure	Normal	Normal	Decreased	Decreased
Heart rate	Normal	Raised	Rapid	Very rapid
Respiratory rate	Normal	Raised	Rapid	Very rapid

become obvious as sudden decompensation occurs (*see Box 14.9*).

Tx

- Manage the airway and breathing. Give high-concentration oxygen.
- Keep the patient supine.
- Insert two large IV lines. Large (Seldinger-type) peripheral lines are better than central lines. Short thick lines are the best.
- Cross-match blood.
- Give IV fluids in boluses of 10–20 mL per kg for an adult (20 mL per kg for a child).
- Institute full monitoring.
- Look for the cause of the shock (see appropriate section of book for specific treatment).
- Refer to the appropriate speciality, usually surgical.
- Insert a urinary catheter and record the fluid balance.

Cardiogenic shock

Collapse with hypotension may occur secondary to asymptomatic MI or to overt causes of cardiac depression. Cardiogenic shock is 'forward failure' of the heart as opposed to the 'backward failure' of congestive cardiac failure. In the absence of external factors, it is caused by insufficiency in the muscles which power the pump and thus primary electromechanical dissociation (EMD) is the final phase – *see page 157*.

Investigations

There may be ECG changes but these cannot be guaranteed.

Tx

- Ensure the airway and breathing are satisfactory. Give high-concentration oxygen. Intubation and ventilation may become necessary.
- Allow the patient to adopt whatever posture is most comfortable; this will usually be partially sitting up.
- Correct any bradycardia with IV atropine to a rate above 60 bpm, but avoid tachycardia as this impairs coronary perfusion.
- Consider the need for IV fluids. The failing heart needs a high filling pressure, hence left ventricular failure causes pulmonary oedema.
- Institute full monitoring.
- Refer to the ICU.
- Look for the secondary causes of pump (heart) failure. These are identical to the causes of EMD – *see page 157*.
- Insert a central venous line.
- Insert a urinary catheter.
- Request a Chest X-ray, ECG, full blood count and urea and electrolytes.
- Begin inotropic support – an IV infusion of dobutamine or dopamine – *For setting up an IV infusion of dobutamine see Box 14.10.*

Box 14.10 Intravenous Infusion of Dobutamine
- Mix 500 mg of dobutamine in 500 ml of 5% glucose or 0.9% saline to give a solution of 1 mg (1000 μg) per mL.
- This infusion can be given into a peripheral vein in the short term. In contrast, dopamine must always be given into a central vein.
- A reasonable starting dose is 5 μg per kg per min. The infusion rate in millilitres per hour needed to give this dose can be calculated by multiplying the patient's body weight in kilogrammes by 0.3.
e.g. To give 5 μg per kg per min to a 70 kg man:
70 kg × 0.3 = 21 mL per hour of the above mixture

Cardiac tamponade

This causes:
- hypotension;
- raised JVP unless hypovolaemic;
- muffled heart sounds;
- pulsus paradoxus;
- breathlessness.

If the signs suggest a diagnosis of tamponade, then look for an underlying reason for a pericardial effusion or haemorrhage such as:

- MI;
- trauma (*see page 81*);
- neoplasia;
- renal failure.

Tx

In a collapsed patient with a tamponade, attempt pericardiocentesis (*see page 82*). This procedure may buy time but is not a definitive treatment so seek help immediately.

Septicaemia

Septic shock is a common cause of collapse, especially in the elderly and in children. It is often overlooked as:

- the temperature may not be raised;
- the white blood cell count may be normal or low;
- blood cultures may be negative.

The hallmark is impaired tissue perfusion.

Tx

- Give a high-concentration of oxygen.
- Start vigorous fluid resuscitation.
- Take blood for routine tests, serum lactate and blood cultures. (A serum lactate greater than 4 mmol per L (36 mg per dL) denotes very poor tissue perfusion.)
- Monitor ECG, BP and SaO_2.
- Catheterise the bladder and record the fluid balance.
- Look for a source of infection (e.g. chest, abdomen, soft tissue in diabetic, brain, post-splenectomy).
- Start broad spectrum IV antibiotics. Septicaemia is treated with the antibiotics that are appropriate for its most likely source. In the absence of an obvious cause, a broad spectrum antipseudomonal beta-lactam antibacterial should be given (e.g. piperacillin enhanced with tazobactam).

- Refer to the inpatient/ICU team. Low-dose steroids (hydrocortisone 200–300 mg daily or equivalent) are believed to be beneficial for intensive care patients with severe sepsis.

For meningococcal septicaemia in both children and adults see page 336.

Accelerated or very severe hypertension

Accelerated or very severe hypertension (diastolic blood pressure > 140 mmHg) requires urgent treatment in hospital but is not usually an indication for parenteral antihypertensive therapy.

Tx

Oral therapy should be instituted with a beta-blocker (atenolol or labetalol) or a long-acting calcium-channel blocker (modified-release nifedipine or amlodipine). The aim should be to reduce diastolic blood pressure to 100–110 mmHg within the first 24 h. Then, over the next 2 or 3 days, blood pressure can be normalised with additional drugs such as diuretics and ACE inhibitors. Very rapid reduction in blood pressure can reduce organ perfusion leading to cerebral infarction, myocardial ischaemia and renal failure. Parenteral antihypertensive drugs are only rarely necessary; sodium nitroprusside by infusion is the best drug in these exceptional circumstances.

Malignant hypertension refers to the syndrome of:

- severe diastolic hypertension;
- papilloedema;
- retinal exudates and haemorrhages;
- renal failure.

It occurs mainly in men in their third and fourth decades and pursues a rapidly downhill course to death from uraemia within a year unless properly treated.

Hypertensive encephalopathy is a rare condition in which transient neurological symptoms occur in the presence of a very high blood pressure. The underlying acute focal cerebral ischaemia is caused by a mixture of cerebrovascular spasm, oedema and thrombosis. Treatment is as described above for accelerated hypertension.

Myocarditis

Although it can be subclinical, inflammation of the myocardium can lead to debilitating cardiomyopathy. The damage to the muscle tissue is thought to be caused by either toxins or an immunological reaction. A vast array of organisms and diseases have been associated with myocarditis. Enteroviruses (especially *Coxsackie B virus*) are the most common pathogens in the developed world. Diphtheria toxin, HIV infection, Lyme disease (*see page 261*), rheumatoid arthritis and Kawasaki disease (*see page 342*) are less common causes of myocarditis. Ethanol can cause cardiomyopathy and AF. The heart failure that follows Chagas' disease (caused by *Trypanosoma cruzi*), is an enormous problem in Central and South America. Clinical presentations of myocarditis range from a mild flu-like illness to overwhelming congestive cardiac failure. ECG and Chest X-ray changes are variable; echocardiography typically shows a globally dilated left ventricle. ESR, C-reactive protein, CK-MB and troponin may be raised. Treatment is supportive and symptomatic.

Endocarditis

Infective endocarditis is a serious condition with a mortality of 20% or more. Although it is primarily a disease of older people and those with prosthetic heart valves, IV drug abusers have a 30-fold higher incidence of endocarditis than the general population. HIV infection and diabetes are also risk factors. Infected vegetations occur on the endothelium of the heart usually, but not always, on areas of previous abnormality or damage. Left-sided infections are mostly found in patients with acquired valvular heart disease (e.g. rheumatic heart disease) but either side of the heart may be affected in those with congenital heart disease or prosthetic valves. The most common pathogens are *Streptococcus viridans*, *Staphylococcus aureus* and *Staphylococcus epidermis*. Most cases of right-sided endocarditis occur in IV drug abusers as a result of *Staphylococcus aureus* infection of the tricuspid valve.

The symptoms of infective endocarditis are vague and may be the result of valvular emboli.

There is fatigue, weight loss and fever (above 38°C). Nausea, back pain and arthralgia may also occur. Cardiac murmurs are usually pre-existing. Septic emboli cause pulmonary, cerebral or systemic symptoms (e.g. pneumonia, headache, renal or splenic infarcts). Splinter haemorrhages and petechiae are classical signs of the disease.

> Endocarditis should be considered in all patients with malaise and fever of uncertain origin.

Investigations

FBC, ESR, C-reactive protein and blood cultures may all yield useful information. Mild anaemia is often found. Chest X-ray and ECG are usually non-specific. Echocardiography is used to detect predisposing heart disease.

Tx

Initial 'blind' antibiotic therapy is IV flucloxacillin and gentamicin. The flucloxacillin should be replaced with vancomycin and rifampicin if the patient has cardiac prostheses *in situ* or is allergic to penicillins or if MRSA (methicillin-resistant *Staphylococcus aureus*) is thought to be a likely pathogen.

Prophylaxis against infective endocarditis

Surgical procedures and instrumentation may cause a transient bacteraemia, which is sufficient to infect an area of abnormal endothelium. Prophylaxis with antibiotics is thus recommended for patients with congenital or acquired valvular heart disease or with prosthetic valves who are undergoing certain operative procedures. The *British National Formulary* lists both the procedures and the appropriate antibiotics. Surprisingly, drainage of an abscess is not a particularly high risk situation.

Palpitations

Palpitations are a common presentation to an ED. The underlying causes include:
- sinus tachycardia;
- ectopic beats (*see page 180*);
- paroxysmal dysrhythmias (*see Chapter 11*);
- chronic dysrhythmias (*see Chapter 11*).

Sinus tachycardia may result from:

- anxiety or other emotion;
- pyrexia;
- anaemia;
- drugs including excessive caffeine intake;
- hyperthyroidism.

A rapid onset and cessation of palpitations with polyuria in an otherwise normal individual is extremely suggestive of a paroxysmal dysrhythmia.

Investigations

Full blood count, electrolytes, glucose and thyroid function tests should be performed. An ECG is essential to demonstrate:

- the exact rhythm and rate;
- congenital abnormalities of the cardiac conducting tissue;
- unsuspected myocardial ischaemia and infarction.

Tx

For the treatment of patients with a frank cardiac dysrhythmia see Chapter 11.

Patients with an abnormal ECG should be discussed with a physician. Excessive and unexplained sinus tachycardia should also be investigated.

Those with normal physical findings and a normal ECG can be referred to their GP for further assessment.

Metabolic problems

Hypoglycaemia

The symptoms of low blood sugar are the most common presentation of diabetes to an ED. Hypoglycaemia results from:

- too much insulin or oral hypoglycaemic either by accident or intent;
- insufficient food;
- change of routine, for example, site of injection, type of insulin, new syringe size.

Initially, a hypoglycaemic patient is restless and agitated but, if untreated, rapidly becomes unresponsive. There is pallor, profuse sweating and a bounding pulse. Aggression can be such that the patient arrives in police custody and may be thought to be intoxicated. False localising neurological signs are sometimes seen.

Investigations

Venous blood should be taken for measurement of baseline glucose before treatment is instituted. In cases of unexplained hypoglycaemia samples should also be sent for liver function tests, insulin, C-peptide and paracetamol assay.

Tx

Like hypoxia, hypoglycaemia rapidly leads to permanent brain damage. This can be avoided by prompt treatment with IV glucose into a large vein (50 mL of 50% solution for an adult). In a child, the dose is 0.2–0.5 mg per kg of glucose, which should be given as 10% dextrose (i.e. 2–5 mL per kg of 10% dextrose).

Glucagon 1 mg (equal to 1 unit) IM is an alternative treatment if venous access is delayed, although it is rather slow to work. The dose for children is 20 µg per kg.

When the patient has fully recovered, the reasons for the low blood sugar must be explored. The patient should only be allowed home if:

- he or she has been fully awake for a couple of hours and has had some food;
- continuous supervision is available;
- there has been an attempt to prevent a recurrence of the problem;
- follow-up arrangements have been made.

Diabetic ketoacidosis

For DKA in children see page 340.

Most of the cells of the body need insulin to allow them to take up glucose from the blood stream. Ketoacidosis starts when this process is critically interrupted by absolute or relative deficiency in insulin. Two main problems result:

1 The body cells have no glucose to metabolise and so are starving. They burn fat and then produce an excess of the ketoacids.

2 Gross hyperglycaemia causes an osmotic diuresis, decreased tissue perfusion and circulatory

collapse. There is dehydration and gross metabolic upset, failure of all body systems and eventually coma and death.

The patient looks ill and may have a decreased level of consciousness. The skin is dry, not sweaty and there is tachycardia and hypotension. Kussmaul's respiration describes the characteristic deep, sighing breathing.

Tx

Hyperglycaemia is of less importance initially than the hyponatraemic dehydration.
- The airway must be protected and oxygen given.
- Resuscitation should be commenced with normal saline (at least 20 mL per kg in the first hour).
- Full monitoring is essential.
- Plasma sugar and electrolytes, haematocrit and blood gases should be measured.
- Hyperglycaemia is initially treated by rehydration. Soluble insulin is given in a bolus of 6–10 units IV (for an adult). The rate of the subsequent insulin infusion should be governed by the patient's clinical condition and biochemical results (*see Box 14.11*).
- Metabolic acidosis is best treated by restoration of blood volume and renal function. Bicarbonate should not be given.
- Serum potassium may be normal or high initially as a result of haemoconcentration. It will fall rapidly when the hypovolaemia and acidosis are corrected and will follow the glucose into the cells. For this reason, plasma potassium should be measured regularly and replacement initiated early on. (*For potassium therapy see page 254.*)
- Catheterisation allows a careful check on fluid balance.
- A cause for the development of the ketoacidosis must be sought. The condition usually develops over several days and is often precipitated by infection or other coexisting illness. Samples of blood, sputum and urine should be collected for culture and sensitivity. Chest X-ray and ECG should also be requested.
- The patient should be discussed as soon as possible with a physician.

Box 14.11 Insulin Infusion

- Soluble insulin binds to plastic; this can be prevented by mixing the insulin with Haemaccel or a similar modified gelatin solution.
- Fifty units of human soluble insulin added to 50 mL of gelatin solution gives a 1 unit per mL mixture, which is easy to administer via an infusion pump.
- The usual rate for an adult is 2–3 units of insulin per h. A typical variable rate IV insulin regimen ('sliding scale') is shown below:

Blood glucose (mmols per L)	Insulin (units per h)
0–4.0	0.5
4.1–8.0	1
8.1–10.0	2
10.1–14.0	3
14.1–22.0	4
>22.0	6

When restarting subcutaneous insulin, the IV insulin infusion must be continued for 30 min after the administration of the first subcutaneous dose.

It is usually recommended that the long-acting recombinant human insulin analogue, insulin glargine, is continued as a baseline therapy to ensure stabilisation despite the addition of a variable IV infusion.

Hyperosmolar (non-ketotic) diabetic coma

A hyperosmolar state is usually seen in older patients who are not insulin dependent. In fact, most have no history of diabetes although there may have been polyuria and polydipsia for up to 2 weeks before presentation. As there is some insulin available to the body, ketoacidosis is not a feature of this condition. It is precipitated by infection or other illness in just the same way as DKA but drugs, especially diuretics, may also play a part. Hyperosmolar coma has a very high mortality because of coexisting disease and late diagnosis.

There is profound dehydration with depression of consciousness (not necessarily coma) and other neurological signs. There may be symptoms and signs of the precipitating disease.

Investigations

- Blood glucose, urea and electrolytes, haemoglobin, white cell count and haematocrit should be performed together with blood gases. Haemoconcentration and infection are likely findings. Potassium depletion is common. *For potassium therapy see page 254.*

- Serum osmolality is, of course, very high (>350 mmol per L) as a result of hyperglycaemia (>30 mmol per L) and hypernatraemia.
- Investigations for infection and other illness are as detailed above for ketoacidosis.

Tx

This is similar to that for DKA. Vigorous fluid resuscitation is essential. Hypotonic solutions may precipitate cerebral oedema and so should be withheld until monitored parameters have stabilised. Half-normal saline is then used. Insulin requirements are low and so insulin therapy should again await fluid resuscitation.

Patients with hyperosmolar coma are at great risk of thrombo-embolism and so should be given prophylactic subcutaneous or IV heparin.

Hypothermia

Hypothermia is defined as a core temperature below 35°C.

- Mild hypothermia – below 35°C.
- Moderate hypothermia – below 32°C.
- Severe hypothermia – below 30°C.

Core temperature must be measured with a suitably low reading and accurate device.

There are three main types of accidental hypothermia:

1 Acute (immersion) hypothermia. Heat production is overwhelmed by sudden cold stress (immersion, lying injured in snow or drunk on a very cold, wet day).

2 Acute (exhaustion) hypothermia. Cooling only occurs as energy reserves are exhausted (endurance sports, outdoor pursuits and immersion in relatively warm water).

3 Subacute (urban) hypothermia. The victim has been exposed to moderate cold for days, often with several predisposing factors (elderly or other – *see later*).

Up to 3% of medical patients admitted to UK hospitals during winter months have core temperatures below 35°C.

The factors predisposing to hypothermia include the following:

- Relatively large surface area, large head and immature thermoregulatory mechanism in babies and young children.
- Impairment of thermoregulatory mechanisms in old age. This may be potentiated by immobility after a minor accident, poor personal and environmental insulation and inadequate heating in the home.
- Altered behaviour patterns in patients taking drugs or alcohol; alcohol also causes peripheral vasodilatation.
- Direct metabolic effect of certain drugs (e.g. chlorpromazine) and endocrine disorders (e.g. myxoedema).

There are several important haemodynamic changes in hypothermia:

- Profound vasoconstriction occurs. This is accompanied by a diuresis.
- Fluid moves into the extracellular compartment and cells.
- Immersion in water causes hydrostatic compression of the body – an effect similar to vasoconstriction and hence removal from water may cause 'rescue collapse'.
- As the core temperature decreases, the risk of VF increases.

The reversal of these effects during rewarming creates a danger of fluid overload. *For the causes of death in hypothermia see Box 14.12.*

Box 14.12 Causes of Death in Hypothermia

Hypovolaemia and circulatory collapse

Fluid overload leading to cardiac failure and pulmonary or cerebral oedema

Ventricular fibrillation

Hypoxia

Continued cooling and cardiac standstill

Underlying pathology which predisposed patient to hypothermia (e.g. poisoning or CVA)

Hypothermia also induces metabolic upset:
- There is both respiratory and metabolic acidosis. Serum potassium levels rise.
- As the body temperature falls, carbohydrate is progressively replaced by fat as the metabolic fuel.
- Insulin resistance develops but the blood sugar level may be high or low.
- Cortisol levels are uniformly high.
- Pancreatitis may occur.
- Hypothyroidism is only rarely the cause of hypothermia presenting to an ED but cold, elderly patients may look myxoedematous. Consider taking a blood sample for subsequent estimation of thyroid stimulating hormone, T_3 and thyroxine. T_3 (or T_4) must not be given except on the instructions of an endocrinologist – it may precipitate cardiac failure.

Tx

Hypothermia is a reversible condition. Recovery has been reported from core temperatures as low as 13.7°C. Cardiovascular complications may make rewarming hazardous, but if normothermia can be regained patients rarely show any residual stigmata in the CNS or elsewhere. The 'afterdrop' phenomenon – whereby cooling of the patient continues after removal from the cold – is of little clinical significance.
- Seek advice.
- Treat the patient gently – the most common precipitant of VF in hypothermia is mechanical irritation of the body.
- Give oxygen.
- Institute careful monitoring – the key to success.
- Start passive rewarming – *see Box 14.13.*
  Remove clothing, especially if wet.
  Gently dry the skin.
  Wrap the patient in woollen blankets. Space blankets are no better than a comparable sheet of plastic.
  Dry and cover the scalp.
- Establish an IV line, although fluid therapy must be carefully monitored.
- Take blood for baseline Hb, white blood cells, glucose, urea, electrolytes and amylase.

- Obtain an ECG. It may show bradycadia and a characteristic notching of the S wave (usually seen best in V4) referred to as a J wave (present in 80% of patients with severe hypothermia). *See Figure 14.1.*
- Consider coincidental injury. Request radiographs of the chest and skull and any areas that may have been injured. Bruising and swelling are slow to appear in hypothermia and examination

---

Box 14.13 Rewarming in Hypothermia

Rewarming may be of two main types:
1 Passive rewarming. Insulation and other measures to prevent further heat loss.
2 Active rewarming. Heat supplied to the surface or to the core of the body.

Cold is a slow killer but inappropriate warming treatment can be fatal in a matter of minutes. Aim for safe, rather than rapid rewarming.

Active rewarming of the surface of the body
Radiant surface heat can be dangerous because it may:
- reduce vasoconstriction leading to hypotension and collapse and the release of acidotic blood;
- cause burns even at low temperatures if the circulation is sufficiently impaired;
- inhibit shivering and reduce heat production.

However, when applied to the trunk only, radiant heat is useful in patients with mild to moderate hypothermia. A warm bath (40°C) is effective but makes other management difficult. Hot water bottles around the neck, axillae and groins are probably the best compromise.

Active rewarming of the core of the body
This is more effective and logical than surface warming and should be employed in severe hypothermia. Techniques include the following:
- Airway warming. Warm, moist air is supplied from a humidifier. This is effective as the entire cardiac output passes through the lungs. However, the energy which can be supplied is limited (only 10–15 kcal per h) and the main value is to prevent heat loss from the lungs.
- Gastric or peritoneal lavage with warm saline.
- Extracorporeal blood warming. This requires specialised facilities.
- Irrigation of other body cavities and orifices with warm saline. This is usually impractical.

The administration of warm (40°C) IV fluids is attractive but technically difficult to achieve as the high flows and volumes required may lead to fluid overload.

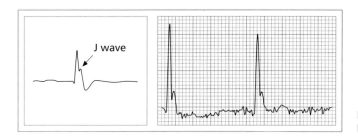

Figure 14.1 J waves on the ECG in hypothermia.

may be deceptively normal. The skin is abnormally susceptible to burns and pressure effects because of its poor blood supply.

• Consider active methods of rewarming – *see Box 14.13* – in elderly patients with a core temperature of less than 32°C and in younger patients with a temperature below 30°C. ICU-level monitoring and facilities for IPPV (intermittent positive pressure ventilation) must be available for these groups. Patients with the slow-onset (subacute) type of hypothermia (invariably the elderly) should probably be rewarmed at a rate no faster than 0.5°C per h to avoid the risk of pulmonary and cerebral oedema.

• Admit the patient to a suitable ward or to the ICU.

Hypothermic patients with no detectable cardiac output

• Diagnosis of arrest (feeling for a central pulse) should take place over about 60 s. The depressed circulation is difficult to assess; inappropriate cardiopulmonary resuscitation may precipitate VF.

• Ventilation and compression for cardiopulmonary resuscitation should then probably follow the same guidelines as in normothermia, although some authorities advocate slower rates. The compliance of the lungs, heart and chest wall is decreased in hypothermia.

• Defibrillation for VF is increasingly ineffective as the core temperature falls – especially below 28°C. Thus it is usually recommended that if there is no response to the initial three shocks, subsequent attempts at defibrillation are delayed until the core temperature rises above 30°C. If the deep

body temperature is less than 25°C, consider opening the chest through the fourth left interspace, assessing cardiac activity directly and, if necessary, performing internal cardiac massage. Warm saline packs can be applied to the heart and internal defibrillation is an option. (*See page 83*).

• Metabolism of drugs is impaired in hypothermia and toxic accumulation of drugs may thus occur. For this reason, it is usually recommended that adrenaline and other drugs are withheld until the patient's core temperature reaches 30°C. At this point, the interval between drug doses is doubled (adrenaline is given every 6–10 mins) until at least 32°C has been reached. Apparently dead patients may be hypothermic but recoverable ('never dead until warm and dead'). The heart can still be working even if this is clinically undetectable. Patients who may have suffered from hypothermia must therefore be rewarmed before assessing viability. This is particularly important in children. However, hypothermia and collapse may be agonal features of a terminal illness. If the prognosis is known to attending relatives discuss the management with them; rewarming is usually inappropriate.

For cardiac arrest see Chapter 11 on page 156.

Hyperpyrexia and hyperthermia

Normal basal metabolism creates a heat load of around 65–90 kcal per h for an adult. This is enough to raise the body temperature by about 1°C per h in the absence of normal thermoregulation. Moderate exercise increases the generation of heat by a factor of five (300–500 kcal per h). A third of basal heat production is the result of cellular membrane ion pumps.

Hyperpyrexia is defined as a core temperature in excess of 41°C. This can result from two main causes:

1 febrile illnesses;

2 hyperthermic conditions.

In a fever, the thermoregulatory set point of the hypothalamus is raised. This usually causes temperatures of between 38 and 41°C, and rarely up to 42°C – a response which may be protective against some infectious diseases. The most effective treatment is antipyretics such as paracetamol, which reset the temperature control mechanism. Cooling measures alone are relatively ineffective and short-lived.

Hyperthermia is a condition in which there is an imbalance between heat production and heat loss. Unlike hypothermia, this is not an inherently benign state. Urgent treatment is required to lower the temperature. Brain damage continues throughout the period of hyperpyrexia.

Causes of hyperthermia include the following:

• The extreme effects of drugs (e.g. levothyroxine and atropine; amphetamines, cocaine, PCP (phencyclidine) and other stimulants).

• Idiosyncratic reactions to drugs (e.g. neuroleptic malignant syndrome and malignant hyperthermia – *see page 297*, Ecstasy and other stimulant drugs – *see pages 280 and 281*).

• Tetanus and other severe tonic–clonic conditions (*see page 239*).

• Excessive exercise, exhaustion and dehydration (heat exhaustion – *see below*).

• Combinations of the above (e.g. febrile illnesses accompanied by convulsions or profound dehydration; stimulant drugs and prolonged dancing with an inadequate fluid intake).

> If the patient's temperature is above 42°C, then hyperthermia is the likely diagnosis rather than fever.

For treatment of hyperthermia see page 270.

Heat exhaustion Heat exhaustion or heat stroke results from a combination of excessive exercise, exhaustion of energy stores and dehydration. Symptoms include headache, malaise, nausea, vomiting, faintness and muscle cramps. Core temperature is usually below 41°C and mental status is unaffected. Treatment is rest, cooling, fluids and glucose. In most cases, the condition runs a benign course and does not lead to a hyperpyrexic emergency.

Addison's disease

Adrenocortical deficiency may be a consequence of autoimmune disease, TB or, most commonly, the cessation of long-term steroid therapy. In the last case, the deficiency may only become obvious several months after the therapy has stopped.

An Addisonian 'crisis' is often precipitated by infection. It presents with hypotension, collapse and vomiting. Pigmentation and weight loss are features of the underlying disease.

Investigations

The plasma potassium and urea are high and the sodium is low (due to aldosterone deficiency). Blood glucose may be normal or low. A plain abdominal radiograph may show calcification in tuberculous adrenal glands and Chest X-ray may also reveal TB.

Tx

• Give high-concentration oxygen.

• Take blood for routine tests and plasma cortisol level.

• Start fluid resuscitation with normal saline.

• Give hydrocortisone 200 mg IV.

• Refer the patient to the general physicians on-call.

Hepatic coma

Acute hepatic failure is usually caused by alcoholic cirrhosis or hepatitis (*see page 304*) but can also be caused by other diseases and drugs. There are three main problems:

1 impaired gluconeogenesis;

2 coagulopathy;

3 failure to breakdown toxic metabolites.

Clinical features include:

• hypoglycaemia;

- hypothermia;
- neurological changes and coma as a result of underlying cerebral oedema or encephalopathy;
- renal failure and metabolic disturbance;
- hypotension and pulmonary oedema;
- bleeding;
- infection;
- jaundice and hepatic fetor.

Paracetamol poisoning – the most common cause of hepatic failure in emergency medicine – may present late with:

- a vague, non-specific history;
- a few days of malaise, anorexia, nausea and vomiting;
- hypoglycaemic coma;
- low levels of paracetamol detectable in the plasma.

> Hepatic coma can be partially reversed by the benzodiazepine antagonist flumazenil; this can be misleading in coma of unknown causation.

Tx

- Oxygen and fluids.
- Treatment of complications (e.g. hypoglycaemia, bleeding).
- Admission.

Renal failure

Shock from any cause may result in a temporary 'prerenal failure' with anuria. Sustained hypotension leads to acute tubular necrosis and, in extreme cases, to acute cortical necrosis also – see Box 14.14.

Acute renal failure is also seen in:

- acute-on-chronic failure – precipitated by renal infection or dehydration;

Box 14.14 Causes of Acute Tubular Necrosis

Sustained hypotension
Massive haemorrhage
Septicaemia, especially Gram-negative
Free circulating haemoglobin or myoglobin – see crush injuries on page 255
Poisoning

- primary renal disease – acute glomerulonephritis or collagen vascular disease;
- hepatorenal syndromes – including Weil's disease – see page 304;
- post-renal obstruction.

Oliguria is the cardinal sign (less than 300 mL in 24 h) since the clinical features of severe uraemia are variable and non-specific:

- *cardiovascular* – hypertension, heart failure, pericarditis;
- *neurological* – lethargy, weakness, confusion and eventually coma;
- *gastrointestinal* – anorexia, nausea, vomiting and hiccoughs;
- *dermatological* – pruritus, pallor, petechiae;
- *haematological* – anaemia, bleeding tendency, immunosuppression.

Other changes seen in acute renal failure are caused by hyperkalaemia and acidosis (see pages 253 and 257).

Investigations

The diagnosis is confirmed by the high blood urea and creatinine. Hyperkalaemia is common. Other investigations that should be performed are:

- full blood count – low platelets;
- blood gases – acidosis;
- Chest X-ray – pulmonary oedema;
- ECG – For ECG changes in hyperkalaemia see Box 14.15;
- blood sugar;
- calcium studies;
- urine microscopy and culture – haematuria, casts and infection.

Box 14.15 ECG Changes in Hyperkalaemia

Tall, peaked (tented) T waves (early change)
Shortened QT interval (early change)
Widened QRS complex
Small or absent P waves
Increased PR interval
Depressed ST segment
Ventricular dysrhythmias (fibrillation and asystole)

NB Tall peaked T waves are higher than they are wide.

Box 14.16 Distinction between Prerenal and Renal Uraemia

In volume depletion or hypoperfusion with a healthy kidney the intact tubules are able to conserve sodium and concentrate the urine by the tubular reabsorption of sodium and water. In contrast, in acute tubular necrosis (renal uraemia) the tubular function is impaired and the urinary sodium concentration rises.

Prerenal problem   Urinary sodium ≤20 mmol per L
Acute tubular necrosis   Urinary sodium ≥40 mmol per L

The urinary sodium concentration is a useful investigation if there is any doubt about whether the oliguria is prerenal and amenable to fluid therapy or a result of acute tubular necrosis – *see Box 14.16.*

Tx

- Record fluid balance carefully.
- Restore intravascular volume in prerenal failure.
- Perform an aseptic catheterisation.
- Treat complications (e.g. left-ventricular failure or hypokalaemia).
- Discuss the patient with a physician and arrange admission.

Nephrotic syndrome. This may present with oedema. There is heavy proteinuria and hypoalbuminaemia. Various types of glomerulonephritis account for 80% of cases in adults while there is usually minimal change glomerulonephritis in children.

Hyperkalaemia

High plasma potassium (above 5.5 mmol per L) may be caused by:
- *release from damaged cells* – burns, crush injury and rhabdomyolysis, transfusion;
- *abnormal movement out of cells* – acidosis, transfusion, hyperkalaemic periodic paralysis;
- *decreased excretion* – renal failure, Addison's disease, drugs such as potassium-sparing diuretics and NSAIDs;
- *poisoning;*
- *excessive intake* – rarely.

The effects of hyperkalaemia are:
- paraesthesia;
- muscle weakness (flaccid paralysis);
- ventricular dysrhythmias (eventually asystole).

Dangerous effects are to be anticipated when the plasma potassium exceeds 6.5 mmol per L.

Investigations

The plasma potassium may be spuriously raised by haemolysis. Blood gases should be taken to check for acidosis in the specimen tube and the plasma potassium should be checked before commencing treatment. There are characteristic ECG changes in hyperkalaemia – *see Box 14.15.*

Tx

Patients with severe symptoms or ECG changes. The first priority is to protect the patient from life-threatening cardiac dysrhythmias by giving:

1 *Calcium.* Under ECG control, give 5 mL of 10% calcium chloride by slow IV injection (10 mL of this solution contains 6.8 mmol of calcium ions). A further 5 mL can be given after 5 min and will have an immediate effect that lasts for up to 1 h. 10–20 mL of 10% calcium gluconate (2.25–4.5 mmol) is an alternative. Calcium stabilises the myocardial cell membrane but does not affect the plasma potassium.

2 *Bicarbonate.* If the patient has a metabolic acidosis (pH < 7.20), give sodium bicarbonate (1 mmol per kg) IV over 5–10 min (*see Box 14.20 on page 257*). This has no direct effect on potassium levels.

Potassium can then be redistributed out of the plasma into the cells by the administration of:

1 *Salbutamol.* Give salbutamol 0.5 mg IV (4 μg per kg in children) or 10 mg by nebuliser (2.5–5.0 mg in children). Patients with known ischaemic heart disease may be safer with inhaled salbutamol. Via β_2-receptors in liver and muscle, salbutamol stimulates the sodium–potassium ATP pump to move potassium into cells. Within 30 min, the plasma potassium begins to fall, (by up to 1.5 mmol per L following IV salbutamol and up to 1.0 mmol per L after the nebulised drug). The effect of salbutamol is additional to that of insulin and reduces unwanted hypoglycaemia.

2 *Insulin.* Give 10 units of soluble insulin in 50 g of glucose IV over 30 min. Insulin stimulates the sodium–potassium ATP pump to increase the intracellular uptake of potassium. This effect is independent of its hypoglycaemic action. Reduction in plasma potassium starts within 15 min and is maintained for 1–2 h; a drop of around 1 mmol per L is to be expected. In children (who increase their insulin production more rapidly than adults) IV glucose 0.5 g per kg may be given alone.

Asymptomatic patients without ECG changes. Monitor the ECG. If renal function is normal, increase potassium excretion with furosemide (frusemide) 0.5 mg per kg orally or IV. Sufficient oral or IV fluid must be given in addition.

For all patients, consider treatment with an ion exchange resin such as sodium (or calcium) polystyrene sulphonate 15 g qds by mouth. Rectal administration is an alternative. Referral to a physician for further investigation is essential; dialysis may be required.

Hypokalaemia

Low plasma potassium (<3.5 mmol per L) results from:
- *abnormal movement into cells* – alkalosis, insulin, hypokalaemic periodic paralysis;
- *excessive loss from the GI tract* – diarrhoea or vomiting;
- *excessive renal loss* – Cushing's disease, diuretics, renal tubular acidosis.

The most common symptoms of hypokalaemia are tiredness and weakness. These may be the only symptoms and examination may be unremarkable. However, there may also be:
- paraesthesia;
- metabolic alkalosis;
- polyuria;
- paralytic ileus.

Investigations

The blood gases should be checked. The ECG may show characteristic changes – *see Box 14.17.*

> **Box 14.17 ECG Changes in Hypokalaemia**
>
> Flattening or inversion of the T wave.
> Depression of the ST segment.
> Prolongation of the QT interval.
> Ventricular dysrhythmias including VF.

Tx

Under ECG control, IV potassium replacement can be commenced in symptomatic or at-risk patients. The rate can be up to 0.5 mmol per kg per h (no more than 30–40 mmol per h for an adult). Many patients with no symptoms and normal ECGs will respond to oral supplements. All patients should be referred to a physician.

Hypercalcaemia

Older people may present with non-specific symptoms that are attributable to hypercalcaemia:
- weakness and lethargy;
- confusion and other mental changes;
- anorexia, nausea and vomiting;
- constipation;
- polyuria and dehydration.

The most common causes are malignancy (lung, breast and kidney) and primary hyperparathyroidism.

Tx

- Monitoring, especially of the ECG.
- Forced saline diuresis.
- IV furosemide (frusemide) 0.5 mg per kg.
- Admission for investigation and specific calcium-reducing therapy (steroids, calcitonin, etc.).

Tetany, hypocalcaemia and hypomagnesaemia

Hypocalcaemia gives rise to the state of increased neuromuscular excitability known as tetany. The features are:
- paraesthesia;
- carpopedal spasm and muscular cramps;
- stridor, caused by laryngospasm;

- other signs of neuromuscular irritability (twitching, hyperreflexia, Trousseau's and Chvostek's signs);
- convulsions.

Tetany most commonly accompanies the calcium changes of hyperventilation (*see page 224*) but may also be seen in hypoparathyroidism and a variety of other diseases. A similar state is seen in hypomagnesaemia – *see below*.

Tx

For hyperventilation syndrome see page 225.
Other patients suffering from tetany should be carefully monitored, given appropriate therapy and discussed with a physician. The initial dose of calcium in hypocalcaemic tetany is 2.25 mmol, which is present in 1 g of calcium gluconate (i.e. 10 mL of calcium gluconate 10% solution). This is given slowly IV and may be doubled if the response is unsatisfactory. It should be followed by an IV infusion of around 9 mmol a day.

> Volume for volume, a solution of calcium chloride contains three times as much ionised calcium as a similar strength solution of calcium gluconate. For example, 10 mL of calcium chloride 10% contains 6.8 mmol of calcium ions; 10 mL of calcium gluconate 10% yields 2.25 mmol of calcium.

Hypomagnesaemia. Magnesium is an essential constituent of many enzyme systems, particularly those involved in energy generation. Its salts are not well absorbed from the GI tract – hence their use as osmotic laxatives. Since magnesium is present in large amounts in the GI secretions, excessive losses in diarrhoea, stoma or fistula fluids are the most common causes of hypomagnesaemia; deficiency may also occur in alcoholics and patients on diuretics.
Hypomagnesaemia often causes secondary hypocalcaemia – with which it may be easily confused (*see before*). Symptomatic patients should be treated with a starting dose of 8 mmol (2 g) of magnesium, diluted to 20 mL with saline and given IV over 15 min.
For serum levels of magnesium see Box 14.18.

> **Box 14.18 Serum Levels of Magnesium**
>
> | | |
> |---|---|
> | Normal range | 0.7–1.1 mmol per L |
> | Therapeutic range | 1.5–2.5 mmol per L |
> | Toxic range | >4 mmol per L |
>
> A bolus dose of 8 mmol of magnesium will approximately double the serum concentration; this will return to normal levels within 20 min.
> Toxic levels of magnesium cause neuromuscular blockade and muscle weakness. Calcium is a specific antagonist and will reverse these effects.

> **Box 14.19 Indications for Magnesium Therapy in Emergency Medicine**
>
> 1 Control of some resistant ventricular dysrhythmias:
> - VT secondary to hypokalaemia
> - VT which is resistant to DC shock
> - Torsades de pointes (*see page 179*)
> - Some tachycardias that are secondary to the effects of drugs including digitalis, anti-arrhythmics and occasionally tricyclics
>
> 2 Treatment of eclamptic fits (*see page 315*)
> 3 Treatment of asthma (*see page 210*)
> 4 Treatment of hypomagnesaemic tetany (*see above*)
>
> The recommended starting dose of IV magnesium varies with the condition being treated. The total dose may be up to 16 mmol, followed by an infusion of 2.5 mmol per h. One gram of magnesium sulphate contains approximately 4 mmol of magnesium ions; a 50% solution contains approximately 2 mmol per mL. Transient flushing – sometimes accompanied by hypotension – is to be expected in almost all patients.

For other indications for treatment with magnesium in emergency medicine see Box 14.19.

Crush injuries and myoglobinuria

Extensive contusion to muscle resulting in rhabdomyolysis and myoglobinuria may occur in several ways:
1 As a consequence of an acute crushing injury (e.g. trapped in a pit or under a lorry) – *see also traumatic asphyxia syndrome on page 81.*
2 From other direct muscle injury for example, deep burns or severe and untreated compartment syndrome.

3 After lying immobile for a long time on a hard surface. This is seen in:

- the elderly or debilitated after a collapse (found on the floor);
- alcohol-intoxicated patients;
- drug abusers;
- those who have been in prolonged coma from an overdose.

4 Following the excessive muscle activity caused by prolonged seizures and some stimulant drugs (e.g. phencyclidine, cocaine and 'ecstasy').

5 In some severe metabolic disorders.

In addition, drugs of the statin class may sometimes cause a dose-related myositis, which in rare cases leads to rhabdomyolysis.

The diagnosis should be suspected in any patient in the above categories. Muscle pain and tenderness may be absent.

The main consequences of the damaged and necrotic muscle are:

- metabolic and volume disturbance;
- acute renal failure from myoglobinuria;
- local tissue destruction;
- compartment syndrome in the limbs (*see page 116*).

Investigations

The urine usually tests positive for blood and the laboratory may find granular casts in it. A raised serum creatinine kinase is also strongly suggestive of the diagnosis of rhabdomyolysis. The serum myoglobin peaks at 4 h and returns to normal within 12 h of injury; because of this rapid clearance, myoglobin in the urine may easily be missed.

Arterial blood gases, plasma electrolytes and calcium studies should also be performed.

Tx

Resuscitation with fluids should be followed by:

- Hartmann's (or saline) infusion to maintain normovolaemia and a steady urine output of over 100 mL per h. Catheterisation is mandatory.
- Careful monitoring of clinical and biochemical parameters.

Hyperkalemia occurs in most cases and may need treatment. Bicarbonate is of use but IV calcium may increase the destruction of the muscle tissue.

Mannitol (0.5–1 g per kg) or furosemide (frusemide) (1–2 mg per kg) is sometimes used to achieve a forced diuresis. Dialysis may be required.

Early amputation of extensively crushed limbs has been advocated to remove the source of toxic metabolites and infection but is of unproven value. In contrast, rapid fluid replacement and electrolyte control will increase the chances of survival.

Necrotising soft tissue infections

There is a large spectrum of clinical conditions in which there is a spreading necrosis of soft tissue ranging from relatively localised pyodermas to fulminating gas gangrene. Anaerobic streptococci, staphylococci and clostridia are the most commonly implicated organisms but many other bacteria are also sometimes involved.

Necrotising fasciitis

Spreading necrosis of the fascial plane is usually polymicrobial in nature with cultures yielding a mixture of anaerobic and aerobic bacteria. Exotoxin-producing anaerobic streptococci are the most common causative organisms at present but 'clostridial cellulitis' was well recognised in the past. Although rare, the condition has a mortality of around 25%. It is more common in males and in people over 60 years old. Victims often have an underlying condition that predisposes to infection such as diabetes or IV drug abuse. Fournier's gangrene of the scrotum (which tracks abdominally via Scarpa's fascia) is an eponymous variant of the same condition.

Necrotising fasciitis can affect any part of the body. It usually follows a trivial injury such as an insect bite or a small abrasion. An initial cellulitis is followed by necrosis of the fascia and subcutaneous tissue with relative sparing of the underlying muscle. Symptoms develop over a period of hours or even days and presentations vary greatly. The patient is pyrexic, tachycardic and unwell with a seemingly disproportionate amount of pain. A diffuse erythema of the whole body (similar to toxic shock syndrome) may occur. The necrosing skin is erythematous and oedematous at first but, as the infection develops, it becomes dusky and haemorrhagic with bullae formation. Overwhelming sepsis can progress rapidly to shock and multi-organ failure.

Gas gangrene (Necrotising myositis)

Fulminating necrosis of muscle occurs when damaged or devitalised tissue becomes contaminated with anaerobic bacteria from soil or the intestines of humans and animals. The Gram-positive anaerobe *Clostridium welchii* (also called *Clostridium perfringens*) is the classical cause of gas gangrene but other clostridial species (e.g. *Clostridium novyi* and *Clostridium septicum*) and anaerobic streptococci are also sometimes implicated. As the bacteria multiply, they produce toxins (such as lecithinase), which digest muscle and subcutaneous tissues. Free gas and an assortment of noxious metabolites are liberated by the destructive processes.

In this situation, Clostridia have a short incubation period; contaminated wounds begin to putrefy around 1–3 days after injury. The surrounding tissues crepitate because of the free gas and emit a foul odour. The patient has a high fever, hypotension and usually a toxic delirium. The condition progresses rapidly to systemic sepsis and organ failure. First World War surgeons noted jaundice as a preterminal feature of gas gangrene.

Investigations

Diagnosis of soft tissue necrosis is almost entirely clinical. However, around 50% of patients with necrotising fasciitis (and many more with gas gangrene) have air in the soft tissues on plain radiography. Almost all patients have an elevated white cell count and urea. In the later stages, there is metabolic acidosis and coagulopathy.

Tx

Resuscitation with IV fluids and administration of broad spectrum IV antibiotics (e.g. co-amoxiclav and metronidazole) is required. Extensive surgical debridement of affected wounds must not be delayed.

> **Box 14.20 Bicarbonate Therapy**
>
> Correction of an acidosis with IV sodium bicarbonate generates CO_2, which must be eliminated via the lungs:
>
> $$HCO_3 + H = H_2O + CO_2$$
>
> Thus adequate ventilation is a prerequisite for treatment.
>
> *Listed below are the two main solutions of bicarbonate:*
> **1** Sodium bicarbonate 8.4% contains 1 mmol of bicarbonate and 1 mmol of sodium per mL. It is thus easy to calculate the required dosage but the concentrated solution is caustic to veins and should be given through a central venous line.
> **2** Sodium bicarbonate 1.26% is isotonic. It contains 150 mmol of bicarbonate and 150 mmol of sodium per L. It is thus similar in composition to normal saline (150 mmol of chloride and 150 mmol of sodium per L). This dilute solution can be given into a peripheral vein and provides fluid in addition to bicarbonate and sodium.

Metabolic acid–base disorders

Metabolic acidosis

In emergency medicine, metabolic acidosis is most commonly a result of hypoxia and increased lactate production. This accompanies poor tissue perfusion or fitting. Other causes of metabolic acidosis include:

- poisoning (e.g. salicylic acid, methanol, carbon monoxide or cyanide);
- renal failure;
- diabetic ketoacidosis;
- rapid saline infusion (dilutional acidaemia).

Correction of hypoxia and restoration of tissue perfusion is the mainstay of emergency treatment. Bicarbonate therapy should be used with caution only in the patient with adequate ventilation (*see Box 14.20*). It is not indicated for diabetic ketoacidosis. *For the use of bicarbonate in tricyclic poisoning see page 277.*

> In a simple metabolic acidosis, the $PaCO_2$ in mmHg will be approximately the same as the last two digits of the arterial pH.

Metabolic alkalosis

For diagnosis and treatment of metabolic alkalosis see Box 14.21.

Box 14.21 Differential Diagnosis of Metabolic Alkalosis

Saline responsive (urinary chloride ≤ 10 mmol per L)

If the urinary chloride concentration is less than 10 mmol per L, the metabolic alkalosis is likely to be responsive to therapy with IV normal saline. The condition is characterised by sodium chloride and volume depletion and so both sodium and chloride are avidly reabsorbed by the kidney. This type of alkalosis usually results from:

- loss of gastric secretions (e.g. vomiting);
- diuretic therapy;
- chloride diarrhoea.

Saline resistant (urinary chloride ≥ 20 mmol per L).

If the urinary chloride concentration exceeds 20 mmol per L, the metabolic alkalosis is probably resistant to simple infusion of saline. The underlying metabolic disturbance is excessive hydrogen ion secretion by the kidney. This occurs in hyperadrenal states and severe hypokalaemia. Chloride excretion remains unaffected. Causes include:

- primary aldosteronism;
- Cushing's disease;
- ACTH-producing tumours;
- steroid therapy;
- severe potassium depletion.

For the rules of compensation in acid–base disorders see Box 14.22. These rules predict the expected compensation that results from a given primary change in acid–base status.

For respiratory causes of acid–base disorders see page 214.

The direction of the pH change (acidosis or alkalosis) indicates the primary disorder; overcompensation does not occur.

Zoonoses and diseases related to travel

Travel to exotic places is now commonplace and so patients with a large variety of tropical and other unusual diseases may present to an ED. In addition, many of the infections described below (especially the zoonoses) have been included because of their potential for 'weaponisation', that is, use in a biowarfare or bioterrorist incident. The UK's Health Protection Agency lists 10 such types of infective organism – *see page 294.*

Meningococcal infection has recently occurred in outbreaks amongst travellers making pilgrimages to holy shrines in the Islamic world.

Malaria

Malaria is commonly misdiagnosed as flu or viral hepatitis. A history of chemoprophylaxis does not exclude the diagnosis as patients may fail to take the right dose for the right period.

Malaria is the world's most important parasitic disease. It is a protozoal infection that is transmitted to man by the bite of an infected female anopheline mosquito. Four species of the parasite are infectious

Box 14.22 Rules of Compensation in Acid–Base Disorders

Primary disturbance	Normal compensatory response
Metabolic acidosis	The $PaCO_2$ (mmHg) is equal to 1.5 times the plasma bicarbonate concentration plus 8 (±2)
Metabolic alkalosis	The $PaCO_2$ (mmHg) is equal to 0.9 times the plasma bicarbonate concentration plus 9 (±2)
Acute respiratory acidosis	For each mmHg rise in $PaCO_2$, the bicarbonate concentration increases by 0.1 mmol per L
Chronic respiratory acidosis	For each mmHg rise in $PaCO_2$, the bicarbonate concentration increases by 0.4 mmol per L
Acute respiratory alkalosis	For each mmHg fall in $PaCO_2$, the bicarbonate concentration decreases by 0.2 mmol per L
Chronic respiratory alkalosis	For each mmHg fall in $PaCO_2$, the bicarbonate concentration decreases by 0.4 mmol per L

to man – *Plasmodium falciparum*, *Plasmodium vivax*, *Plasmodium ovale* and *Plasmodium malariae*. Half of the world's population lives in areas where malaria is endemic; 400 million people contract the disease each year and two million die from it, invariably from *Plasmodium falciparum* malaria.

Even the most fleeting visit to an area where malaria is endemic may result in infection. The time that it takes for an aeroplane to refuel is longer than the time that it takes for a mosquito to bite. *For predisposing factors see Box 14.23.*

The initial features last for 2–3 days – malaise, anorexia, fever and headache. There is then an abrupt onset of rigors and sweating without specific clinical findings. There may also be:
- nausea, vomiting and diarrhoea;
- tachycardia;
- splenomegaly and occasionally splenic rupture;
- jaundice.

The fever may become periodic as the erythrocytic phases of the parasite's life cycle become synchronous; every 48 h or 'tertian' for *Plasmodium vivax* and *Plasmodium ovale* infection and every 72 h or 'quartan' for infection with *Plasmodium malariae*.

The addition of acute neurological findings (disorientation, fits or coma) indicates cerebral malaria, a complication of *Plasmodium falciparum* infection. Blackwater fever, where malaria causes haemoglobinuria and renal failure, is another potentially fatal variant of this infection.

Investigations

The diagnosis is confirmed by microscopic examination of blood films (fresh or EDTA samples if stained within 3 h) but this may require up to six films. Nevertheless, in the vast majority of patients with a final diagnosis of malaria, the first blood film gives a positive result. A negative blood film suggests that the risk of developing an overwhelming disease in the next 24 h is very small because the level of parasitaemia correlates well with the severity of the infection.

Tx

In patients who are very unwell start an IV infusion. Measure the blood sugar and correct any hypoglycaemia. A specialist in infectious diseases should be contacted for advice in all cases. Quinine is still the first-line drug in severe (invariably *Plasmodium falciparum*) infection, although there is increasing evidence that artesunate may be more effective. Quinine is given orally unless the patient is vomiting or is deteriorating rapidly. Admission is usually only required for infection with *Plasmodium falciparum*; other forms of malaria can be treated in the community (with chloroquine). The disease is not contagious and so the patient does not have to be isolated.

Rabies

Any bite from an animal outside of the United Kingdom carries a potential risk of rabies. Within the United Kingdom, bats can transmit EBLV2 (European Bat Lyssavirus type 2), which is closely related to the classical rabies virus. Most cases of rabies occur within a few days of the bite but occasionally symptoms are delayed for weeks or even months. It is said that the more peripheral the wound, the longer the incubation period is likely to be because it takes time for the virus to migrate to the CNS.

> An unprovoked attack may suggest a rabid animal but an animal that is known to be alive and well several days after the bite is unlikely to be rabid.

Rabies flourishes in dirty, contused wounds. The earliest signs are a failure of wound healing and paraesthesia or anaesthesia at the site of the injury. Eventually, florid CNS signs, including hydrophobia, develop. *For features that suggest the development of rabies see Box 14.24.*

> **Box 14.24 Features of an Animal Bite that are Suggestive of Rabies Infection**
>
> Bite occurred outside of the United Kingdom or from a bat within the United Kingdom.
> Animal dead or whereabouts unknown.
> Dirty wound; wound not healing well; paraesthesia.
> Accompanying CNS symptoms or signs.

Tx

- Clean, debride and dress the wound.
- Give antitetanus therapy.
- Discuss the patient with a specialist in infectious diseases. Human diploid cell rabies vaccine should be given as soon as possible.

Poliomyelitis

This highly infectious disease is still prevalent in many parts of the world, although the last 'non-imported' case in the United Kingdom was in 1982. The polio virus is spread by droplet infection and faecal-oral contamination with an incubation period of 3 to 21 days. An initial flu-like illness is followed by a preparalytic phase. This is essentially a meningitis (pyrexia, headache, vomiting and neck stiffness) accompanied by muscle pain and tenderness. Symptoms may subside after 48 h but in susceptible patients (around 1 in 75 adults and 1 in 1000 children) a paralytic phase will ensue as the muscle pain continues and weakness develops. This is a result of the involvement of the anterior horn cells and the onset of an irreversible motor neuropathy. Signs are asymmetrical and may include the brainstem and bladder as well as the limbs.

Tx

Patients must be isolated and discussed with a specialist immediately.

Haemorrhagic fevers

These deadly viral diseases have short incubation periods and are unlikely diagnoses if the patient has been out of an endemic area for more than 3 weeks.

- *Lassa fever:* Nigeria and other West African countries.
- *Marburg fever:* northern Zaire and southern Sudan.
- *Ebola fever:* Zaire.

The haemorrhagic fever starts abruptly as a flu-like illness with malaise, shivering and pyrexia. Other features that quickly develop are:

- severe headache, backache and other myalgia;
- pharyngitis;
- anorexia, nausea and vomiting;
- abdominal pain and diarrhoea (watery stools often containing blood and mucous);
- maculopapular rash;
- chest pain and pleural effusions;
- spontaneous bleeding.

Tx

Seek advice from a consultant specialising in infectious diseases before taking blood samples. Barrier nurse the patient in the interim. Patients are not infectious until they become very ill but transmission may occur through contact with infected body fluids.

Traveller's diarrhoea and vomiting

This has many different infectious causes:

- Viral infections, especially Noro (or Norwalk) virus
- Coliform infections.
- Staphylococcal toxins: abrupt onset of violent symptoms within a few hours of a meal.
- *Bacillus cereus* toxins: diarrhoea 12–24 h after eating recooked rice.
- *Shigella sonnei* and *Shigella shigae*: bacillary dysentery with pyrexia, abdominal pain and bloody diarrhoea.
- *Entamoeba histolytica*: amoebic dysentery (chronic diarrhoea).
- *Salmonella* (including paratyphi A and C): abdominal pain and pyrexia.
- *Salmonella paratyphi* B: paratyphoid fever.

Tx

- Commence rehydration.

- Take blood for full blood count, urea and electrolytes and glucose.
- Send stools for microscopy, including ova, cysts and parasites, and culture.
- Prevent spread of infection – wash hands.

For Scombroid fish poisoning see page 287.
For 'Chinese restaurant syndrome' see page 287.

Other infections in travellers

Cholera

Infection with the causative organism of cholera – *Vibrio cholerae* – causes profound diarrhoea ('rice-water' stools) and the rapid development of life-threatening dehydration. This is accompanied by hyponatraemia and hypokalaemia. Rehydration is essential.

Typhoid fever

Infection with *Salmonella typhi* causes a non-specific fever for the first week of the illness. During the second week more specific signs develop:
- abdominal pain and diarrhoea;
- relative bradycardia, considering the high pyrexia;
- 'rose spots';
- splenomegaly.

Typhoid fever is treated with ciprofloxacin, chloramphenicol or cefotaxime. Infections from India and Southeast Asia may be resistant to antibiotics.

Sandfly fever

This disease is a viral infection, transmitted by the bite of the sandfly. There is sudden onset of:
- pyrexia;
- frontal headache;
- neck stiffness;
- ocular pain;
- muscle pain;
- red face, neck and conjunctivae.

Dengue fever

This is a mosquito-born viral infection with clinical features almost identical to sandfly fever.

Yellow fever

Yellow fever is a dangerous viral infection, which is also transmitted by mosquitoes. Three to six days' incubation is followed by profound illness:
- pyrexia;
- headache, nausea, vomiting and photophobia;
- jaundice;
- hypotension;
- purpura and bleeding.

Plague

Bubonic plague presents with pyrexia, malaise and discharging 'buboes'. These are purulent lymph nodes in the groin or axilla. *Yersinia pestis* is transmitted by flea bites but, if inhaled, causes a very contagious pneumonia (pneumonic plague).

Smallpox

Smallpox starts with an initial febrile episode, followed by severe prostration. The characteristic vesicular rash then develops in a single eruption with a dense distribution on the face and limbs. The palms and soles are particularly badly affected. (Chickenpox begins with a mild prodromal period. The vesicles appear at different times in several crops, mostly on the trunk. The palms and soles are spared and the lesions are relatively superficial.)

For infectious hepatitis see page 304.
For Weil's disease (leptospirosis) see page 304.
For influenza and SARS see pages 221 and 222.

Zoonoses (human infections of animal origin)

Lyme disease

Visits to parks or woods where there may have been deer, or sometimes other animals, may lead to infection by *Borrelia burgdorferi*, a tick-born spirochaete. There is:
- a papule at the site of the bite;
- fever, headache and fatigue;
- polyarthritis and lymphadenopathy.

Lyme disease is on the increase in the United Kingdom.

Brucellosis (Undulant or Mediterranean fever)

Brucellosis is a highly transmissible zoonosis, which is caused by bacteria of the genus *Brucella*. It affects a wide variety of mammals; human infections arise through direct contact with infected animals or their milk, by either ingestion or inhalation. After an incubation period of 5–30 days, there is fever, malaise, headache and joint pains. The disease is rarely fatal but causes debilitation for many weeks. Brucellosis is treated with a combination of doxycycline and rifampicin for at least 6 weeks.

West Nile fever

Despite its name, West Nile virus is endemic in Southern Europe, the United States and Canada. It is transmitted to humans from animals via mosquitoes and causes pyrexia (above 38°C) with encephalitis or meningitis.

Glanders

This zoonosis is caused by the bacterium *Burkholderia mallei* and is primarily a disease of donkeys, mules and horses. Human infection is rare but may be rapidly fatal. Glanders is spread to humans by inhalation or directly into wounds and has an incubation period of 10–14 days before symptoms appear. There is a high fever, malaise and muscle pains. Abscesses of the skin, nasal passages or lungs may be followed by septicaemia. Cases should be isolated.

Melioidosis

The causative organism of melioidosis, *Burkholderia pseudomallei*, is found in the soil and water of tropical regions such as Thailand, India and Northern Australia. It may enter the body through wounds or by inhalation. Features include fever, headache, muscle pains, pneumonia and septicaemia. Untreated severe disease is nearly always fatal. Cases should be isolated.

For Q fever see page 221.
For anthrax see page 402.
For tularaemia see page 402.

Haematological and sexually transmitted diseases

For the indications for transfusion of different blood components see Box 14.25.

Box 14.25 Indications for Transfusion of Blood Components in Emergency Medicine

The codes given are those assigned to the indication by the National Blood Service of the United Kingdom.

Red cell concentrates

R1 Acute blood loss – to maintain circulating blood volume and haemoglobin above 7 g per dL in otherwise fit patients and above 9 g per dL in older patients or those with known cardiovascular disease. Usually only required when there is 30–40% loss of blood volume (1500–2000 mL for an adult).

R7 Anaemia – to maintain the Hb above the symptomatic level (usually around 8 g per dL)

Cryoprecipitate

Dose = 1unit per 5 kg body weight (equivalent to 10 units for an adult)

C1 DIC with bleeding and a fibrinogen level below 1 g per L

C2 Advanced liver disease with bleeding and a fibrinogen level below 1 g per L

C3 Bleeding associated with thrombolytic therapy and hypofibrinogenaemia

C4 Hypofibrinogenaemia (less than 1 g per L) secondary to massive transfusion

C5 Renal or hepatic failure associated with bleeding where DDAVP is ineffective

Fresh frozen plasma

Dose = 12–15mL per kg (equivalent to 4 units for an adult)

F1 Single coagulation factor defeciency where a specific or combined factor concentrate is unavailable (e.g. factor V)

F2 Bleeding due to warfarin

F3 DIC with bleeding and abnormal coagulation results

F5 Massive blood transfusion – coagulation factor defiiciency can be expected after blood loss of 1.5 times blood volume

F6 Liver disease with bleeding

Platelet concentrates

Dose = 15 mL per kg (equivalent to one therapeutic dose for an adult)

P1 Thombocytopenia – to prevent spontaneous bleeding when the platelet count is below 10×10^{-9} per L

P2 Thombocytopenia – to prevent spontaneous bleeding when the platelet count is below 20×10^{-9} per L in the presence of additional risk factors for bleeding such as sepsis

P3 Thombocytopenia – to prevent bleeding associated with invasive procedures (such as central line insertion) when the platelet count is below 50×10^{-9} per L

P4 Massive blood transfusion – the platelet count will usually be less than 50×10^{-9} per litre after replacement of 1.5–2 times the blood volume. Aim to keep the platelet count above 50×10^{-9} per L.

P6 DIC with bleeding and thrombocytopenia

P8 Autoimmune thrombocytopenia with a major haemorrhage

Sickle cell disease

Sickle cell disease is hereditary and occurs predominantly in African and Afro-Caribbean patients. It is also seen to a lesser extent in those from the Middle East, India and Mediterranean countries.

Polymerisation of abnormal haemoglobin-S leads to deformity of the red cells with a consequent increase in blood viscosity and blockage of capillaries. This 'sickling' is usually precipitated by hypoxia, dehydration or infection, although there are many other causes. Induction of anaesthesia can provide just such a stimulus. Attacks start in infancy.

Clinical presentations of sickling include the following 'crises':

- *Severe bone pain* (ischaemic). This may be in the spine.
- *Abdominal pain and vomiting.* Splenic infarction causes pain in the left upper quadrant of the abdomen.
- *Pleuritic chest pain.* Pulmonary infarction.
- *Convulsions and strokes.* Cerebral ischaemia.
- *Visual loss.* Retinal infarction.
- *Infection.* The leading cause of death. NB Loss of splenic function predisposes to pneumococcal infection.
- *Hypotension.* Visceral sequestration of blood; enlarged, tender liver and spleen.
- *Priapism.*
- *Rhabdomyolysis. See page 255.*
- *Haemolytic and anaemic crises.*

Investigations

A full screen should be carried out. Haemoglobin is normally low in patients with sickle cell disease and will be very low in a crisis.

CT brain scan is indicated in the presence of neurological signs.

Prior to general anaesthesia, patients at genetic risk of sickle cell disease need a simple laboratory test to screen for HbS (sickle cell haemoglobin). Application of a tourniquet (e.g. for Bier's block) is contraindicated in sickle cell disease.

Tx

- Give a high-concentration of oxygen.
- Commence rehydration with IV fluids. Blood transfusion dilutes HbS but may increase blood viscosity.
- Give adequate analgesia, usually morphine.
- Arrange admission.

Penicillin prophylaxis against pneumococcal septicaemia is advisable in at-risk children. If in doubt, seek advice from the nearest NHS Sickle Cell and Thalassaemia Counselling Centre.

Acquired haemophilia

Acquired haemophilia is a rare condition caused by an autoimmune depletion of clotting Factor VIII. It is most commonly seen in elderly patients without any underlying disease but also occurs:

- as a feature of autoimmune diseases;
- as a drug reaction;
- in some malignancies and lymphoproliferative disorders;
- in young women up to 12 months post-partum.

The haemophilia may present with a rapid onset of bleeding into the muscles, soft tissues or retroperitoneum or may complicate a situation in which there is already severe bleeding. Sometimes, prolongation of the activated partial thromboplastin time (APTT) is the first sign of abnormal clotting. Diagnosis depends on finding a reduced level of Factor VIII in the plasma together with Factor VIII inhibitors. Acquired haemophilia is treated by intravenous administration of activated recombinant human Factor VIIa (rFVIIa), which directly activates the conversion of Factor X to Factor Xa.

> Children with haemophilia should be given Factor 8 (or 9) concentrate after even very minor injuries.

Low platelets

There are many causes of thrombocytopenia (a platelet count below 150×10^{-9} per L):

1 *Decreased production* (bone-marrow failure due to disease, cytotoxic therapy or irradiation; acute leukaemias; uraemia).

2 *Decreased survival* [usually immunological causation such as idiopathic thrombocytopenic purpura (ITP) or drugs].

3 *Increased consumption* [disseminated intravascular coagulation (DIC); thrombotic thrombocytopenic purpura (TTP); large haemangiomata; some infections].

4 *Sequestration* (hypersplenism and hypothermia).

5 *Excessive loss* (massive haemorrhage and consumption coagulopathy).

6 *Dilution* (massive transfusion of stored blood).

There are also congenital causes of low platelets and conditions where platelets exist in sufficient numbers but are dysfunctional. The diagnosis and specific treatment of all these conditions is beyond the scope of this book. However, severe bleeding and the indications for platelet transfusion are discussed below.

Platelet transfusions are used for the prevention and treatment of bleeding associated with thrombocytopenia or platelet function defects. Serious spontaneous haemorrhage due to thrombocytopenia alone is unlikely to occur at platelet counts above 10×10^{-9} per L. Massive haemorrhage, DIC, bone marrow failure and acute leukaemias are all indications for platelet therapy as is post-transfusion purpura (PTP). In ITP, TTP and heparin-induced thrombocytopenia (HIT) platelets are contraindicated unless there is life-threatening bleeding.

Platelet concentrates from donors of the identical ABO group to the patient should be used. Rhesus-D negative women of child-bearing age should receive Rh-D negative platelets. The initial transfusion should be one adult therapeutic dose over 30 min. This may be expected to increase the patient's platelet level by at least 20×10^{-9} per L. To treat massive bleeding, much larger doses may be required (four bags or more). Small children should be given 10–15 mL per kg of platelet concentrate at a rate of 20–30 mL per kg per h.

Adverse effects from oral anticoagulant drugs

The main adverse effect of drugs such as warfarin and acenocoumarol is haemorrhage. Bruising and bleeding increase significantly with International Normalised Ratios (INRs) greater than 5. (Therapeutic INRs are between 2 and 4.) Vitamin K1 (phytomenadione) can be used to reverse the effects caused by over-anticoagulation, the dose being dependent on the INR result and the presence of bleeding. Oral administration of Vitamin K is nearly as effective as IV administration; it is almost completely absorbed from the gut and the onset of action is not significantly delayed. The solution for injection can be taken by mouth. If given IV, Vitamin K1 should be injected slowly at a rate of 1 mg per min.

INR 6.0–8.0 with minor or no bleeding. Stop oral anticoagulants and recheck the INR every 2 days to ensure that it is falling. Recommence anticoagulants when the INR is below 5. There is no indication for Vitamin K.

INR above 8.0 with minor or no bleeding. Stop oral anticoagulants and recheck the INR every 2 days to ensure that it is falling. Recommence anticoagulants when the INR is below 5. If the patient has risk factors for bleeding (age >70 years, previous history of bleeding including epistaxis), give oral Vitamin K 0.5–2.5 mg stat. Recheck the INR after 24 hours and repeat the Vitamin K if necessary.

Major bleeding. Stop oral anticoagulant drugs. The anticoagulation can be rapidly and effectively reversed with prothrombin complex concentrate 50 units per kg IV and Vitamin K1 5 mg IV stat. Partial reversal can be achieved using fresh frozen plasma 15 mL per kg and Vitamin K1 5 mg IV stat. Complete reversal of anticoagulation with higher doses (6–10 mg) of Vitamin K results in prolonged resistance to oral anticoagulants with the risk of thrombosis. The INR should be rechecked daily.

Box 14.26 Opportunistic Infections in AIDS

Pneumonia, classically caused by *Pneumocystis carinii*

Tuberculosis

Meningitis and encephalitis (headache, fever, fits and coma – toxoplasmosis and sometimes herpes viruses)

Gastrointestinal upset (anorexia, weight loss and diarrhoea – cytomegalovirus, Salmonella or atypical mycobacteria)

Hepatitis

Fungal infections

Skin infections

Acquired Immunodeficiency Syndrome

The causative organism of AIDS – Human Immunodeficiency Virus – is transmitted by:

1 unprotected sexual intercourse with an infected person;

2 injection of infected blood, usually the result of drug abusers sharing equipment;

3 an infected mother to her baby before or during birth or by breast feeding.

Infected blood and other body fluids that are splashed on to body surfaces in the normal course of resuscitation have not been shown to transmit HIV. Current evidence indicates that a significant volume of infected material has to be injected in order to transmit infection.

HIV infection can be encountered in any patient although it is most common in:

• homosexual men;

• IV drug abusers;

• people from sub-Saharan Africa.

HIV is easily neutralised by the common disinfecting agents.

The most common presentation to an ED is with fever and malaise caused by an opportunistic infection (*see Box 14.26*).

Investigations

A full screen should be performed. Chest X-ray shows diffuse interstitial changes in *Pneumocystis* pneumonia. Tuberculosis should also be considered when looking at the Chest X-ray.

Tx

All HIV-positive patients with unexplained fever, neurological signs or any suggestion of significant infection should be admitted for investigation. *Pneumocystis carinii* pneumonia is very suggestive of AIDS and is treated with high dose co-trimoxazole. Tuberculosis is also increasing in the HIV-positive population.

For post-exposure prophylaxis against HIV infection in health care workers see Box 21.11 on page 399.

For TB see page 223.

For pneumonia see page 218.

Syphilis

Syphilis is on the increase in the United Kingdom. Men account for over 90% of the cases, the majority of whom are either homosexual or bisexual. Acquired syphilis is divided into early (primary, secondary and early latent infection) and late (>2 years after infection):

• *Primary syphilis* presents as a painless ulcer usually (but not always) in the anogenital area with regional lymphadenopathy. This ulcer heals in a few weeks and may go unnoticed. The incubation period of the underlying treponemal infection is usually 3–4 weeks (range 9–90 days).

• *Secondary syphilis* causes a widespread, polymorphic rash on the trunk (typically with involvement of the palms and soles as well). There is lymphadenopathy, mucocutaneous ulcers (especially in the mouth), headache and vague malaise.

• *Early latent syphilis* is characterised by positive treponemal serology with no symptoms.

Around one-third of diagnosed patients are found to have primary syphilis, another third secondary syphilis and the remainder early latent syphilis. The incidence of late syphilis (latent, cardiovascular, neurological or gummatous disease) has not increased in the United Kingdom.

Moist primary and secondary syphilitic lesions are highly infectious!

Investigations

Patients from high-risk groups presenting with genital or oral ulceration, non-itchy rashes or lymphadenopathy should be tested for syphilis. The diagnosis is confirmed by positive serology (send 10 mL of clotted blood marked '?syphilis'), although serology may be negative in very early infection.

Tx

Patients with positive serological tests or with suspicious ulcers on their genitalia should be referred urgently to a GU clinic.

For pelvic inflammatory disease (gonococcal or chlamydial infection) see page 310.

Chapter 15

Poisoning

General principles in poisoning

Poisoning may be the result of:

1 accidents;
2 social drug abuse;
3 deliberate self-harm;
4 attempts to harm others.

> Bizarre symptoms and signs or unusual combinations of clinical features should always suggest the possibility of poisoning.

Initial assessment and management

- ABCs as detailed in *Chapter 1*.
- In all cases, approach the patient without condemnation.

If the patient has a reduced level of consciousness or immediately appears unwell:

- protect the airway;
- administer a high concentration of oxygen by mask;
- obtain venous access;
- control fits with IV diazepam;
- connect the patient to monitoring devices – ECG, BP and SaO$_2$. Measurement of core temperature is also important;
- measure the blood glucose;
- request an urgent ECG;
- seek senior/anaesthetic advice.

> Narcotic and sedative drugs may depress the protective reflexes of the airway more than might normally be expected for a given level of consciousness.

Further assessment and management

Ask about

- Nature of substance taken.
- Type of preparation taken.

> Slow-release preparations may cause delayed or protracted poisoning.

- Other substances (e.g. alcohol) also taken. Ask specifically about paracetamol and aspirin. Poisoning with these two drugs is common, dangerous and treatable.
- Route of poisoning (e.g. oral, IV).
- Time taken.
- Intended result of poisoning.
- Previous episodes of poisoning.

> Over half of all self-poisoned patients present less than 4 h after ingestion.

Look for

- Dyspnoea, bronchospasm and pulmonary oedema.
- Tachycardia and hypotension.
- Dysrhythmias and widening of the QRS complex.
- Depressed level of consciousness.
- Agitation, restlessness and hallucinations.

- Pupillary changes.
- Extensor plantar reflexes.
- Lowered or raised core temperature.

Specific actions

- Measure the plasma urea and electrolytes and glucose.
- Measure the blood gases.
- Measure or screen for plasma aspirin and paracetamol levels 4 h after the estimated time of ingestion.
- Obtain a 12-lead ECG.
- Seek specific poisons advice *(for sources see page 270)*.
- Consider the need for gastric decontamination (see later).
- Consider the need for specific supportive measures *(see page 270)*.
- Consider requesting toxicology levels (e.g. lithium, iron, theophylline, methanol, ethylene glycol, digoxin, paraquat and carboxyhaemoglobin).
- Consider the need for specific therapies (see later).

> Most patients should be screened for aspirin and paracetamol 4 h from time of ingestion, irrespective of the history of substances taken.

In patients with a reduced level of consciousness, consider the need to:

- give IV saline (at least 10 mL per kg) unless there is a specific contraindication;
- catheterise the bladder and measure the urine output.

Gastric decontamination

Controversy still surrounds the efficacy of the different modes of gastric decontamination. All methods aim to reduce the absorption of residual toxins from the gastrointestinal tract. The risks must be carefully weighed against the likely benefits. Any form of gastric decontamination is of doubtful value if more than 1 h has passed since the ingestion of poisons, except in specific cases such as:

1 Modified-release preparations of drugs
2 Drugs that possess anticholinergic (antimuscarinic) properties (e.g. tricyclics)
3 Drugs that directly delay gastric emptying (e.g. salicylates)
4 Drugs whose elimination may be increased by active charcoal after they have been absorbed – *see page 269.*

Gastric lavage

Gastric lavage is only effective if the substance ingested is still in the stomach – *see before*. It should be reserved for patients with a depressed level of consciousness or specific indications such as highly toxic drugs. It may be useful to remove large quantities of alcohol in patients with acute poisoning. A general anaesthetic may sometimes be necessary, especially in children. Gastric lavage is contraindicated if:

1 there are not adequate facilities available to protect the airway or deal with any complications that might arise;
2 the substance taken is relatively safe (e.g. benzodiazepines);
3 the substance ingested is safer in the stomach than anywhere else. This applies to the following:

Oily or petroleum-based sustances: Relatively harmless in the stomach, but may cause a life-threatening pneumonitis in the lungs.

Corrosives and caustics: May cause oesophageal perforation, especially with the help of a lavage tube.

Before gastric lavage is performed, the ability of the patient to protect the airway must be assessed.

> An absent gag reflex does not guarantee an unresisted intubation.

Gentle attempted laryngoscopy may be required. In patients whose protective airway reflexes are thought to be relatively intact, (i.e. not deeply unconscious and offering resistance to laryngoscopy or coughing) lavage may be performed without intubation. The patient should be in the recovery position with the suction switched on. Patients in whom the protection of the airway is in doubt should be assessed by an anaesthetist. Many such patients will have depressed airway reflexes but will still need muscle relaxant drugs to facilitate endotracheal intubation.

Box 15.1 Procedure for Gastric Lavage

- Move the patient to the resuscitation area.
- Assess the airway.
- Request anaesthetic help if indicated (significantly depressed consciousness or airway at risk).
- Put the patient in the recovery position on a tiltable trolley. The stomach is easier to drain in the right lateral position.
- Monitor the patient's SaO$_2$ throughout the procedure.
- Have a high-volume suction pump switched on.
- Carefully insert a lubricated lavage tube.
- Syphon the gastric contents into a bucket, checking for tablet material. Gentle pressure over the stomach may facilitate drainage.
- Use litmus paper to ascertain that the tube is in the stomach.
- Lavage the stomach with warm water or saline until the drainage fluid is clear. In small children isotonic dextrose–saline in aliquots of 10 mL per kg should be used.
- Instil activated charcoal if indicated – *see later*.
- Remove the lavage tube.

Gastric lavage is a dangerous procedure that induces hypoxia in many patients.

For the technique of gastric lavage see Box 15.1.

Emesis and whole bowel irrigation

Emesis removes at least as much material from the stomach as gastric lavage. It also has the same contraindications as lavage – *see before*. It is possible to vomit up tablets, which would not fit through the small Murphy's eye of a lavage tube. However, emesis is dangerous in obtunded patients and activated charcoal cannot be subsequently given. For this reason, emesis is no longer routinely recommended in the United Kingdom. For those situations or places where there is no alternative, syrup of ipecacuanha is usually used to induce vomiting (30 mL in an adult and 15 mL in a child). It should be followed by a reasonable volume of fluid and can be repeated after 20 min if necessary.

Whole bowel irrigation is also of doubtful value and has not been shown to improve outcomes.

Milk

Milk is often advocated to assuage the effects of ingested substances, which are:

- irritant;
- of low toxicity;
- dangerous to remove by lavage or emesis.

Activated charcoal

Heating of charcoal with chemical activators increases its surface area to about 1000 m^2 per gram and thus enhances its ability to reversibly absorb small molecules.

Charcoal is extremely dangerous if aspirated; airway protection must therefore be ensured whenever it is used.

Activated charcoal will not absorb:

- iron, lithium and other metallic compounds;
- cyanides;
- strong acids and alkalis;
- alcohols;
- petroleum distillates;
- malathion and DDT.

Repeated administration of charcoal absorbs drugs re-excreted into the bowel via the enterohepatic circulation. It is indicated for:

- theophyllines
- carbamazepine
- phenobarbital
- quinine
- dapsone

and sometimes recommended for:

- tricyclic and related antidepressants
- barbiturates
- salicylates
- sotalol
- phenytoin
- paraquat
- digoxin and other cardiac glycosides
- cyclosporin.

Activated charcoal should be administered in a dose equal to ten times that of the poison to be absorbed. An initial dose of 50–100 g (or 1 g per kg for children) will usually ensure that this ratio is met. Paracetamol and aspirin are taken in gram rather than milligram quantities and so a second dose of charcoal may be needed after a few hours. For repeated dosing 50 g (1 g per kg) should be given every 4 h or smaller doses more frequently. Large doses of charcoal may form concretions in the bowel and so lactulose (or sorbitol) should be given with each repeated dose.

Treatment of respiratory depression

There are four main factors:
1 Airway protection – positioning and suctioning.
2 Airway maintenance – positioning and adjuncts.
3 Support of breathing – assisted ventilation.
4 Reversal of specific opioid-induced respiratory depression – naloxone.

Specific respiratory stimulants (e.g. doxapram) have little place in the treatment of drug-induced respiratory depression.

Treatment of circulatory depression

This involves:
• maintenance of adequate oxygen supply to the heart – see before;
• maintenance of normovolaemia – IV fluids; vasoconstrictors (e.g. ephedrine) are sometimes used in specific treatment situations;
• correction of cardiac dysrhythmias – may need specialist advice to avoid dangerous interactions (e.g. prolongation of the QT interval – *see page 180*);
• correction of bradycardia – atropine initially, may need an adrenaline infusion or cardiac pacing (*see page 170*);
• maintenance of cardiac contractility – inotropes such as dobutamine (*see page 243*). Specialist monitoring is necessary to optimise cardiac output in this situation.

Treatment of hyperthermia

Hyperthermia may result from:
1 stimulant drugs (e.g. amphetamines);
2 excessive exercise and dehydration;
3 idiopathic reactions to drugs (e.g. neuroleptic malignant syndrome – *see page 297* – and malignant hyperthermia);

4 a combination of the above (e.g. 'Ecstasy' and prolonged dancing; amphetamines and convulsions – *see pages 280 and 281*).

Treatment must be promptly instituted to prevent the development of multi-organ failure. Cooling measures include:
• removal of clothing;
• cool sponging and promotion of evaporation with an electric fan;
• placement of ice-packs in the axillae and groins;
• infusion of cooled IV fluids;
• gastric lavage with cool fluids in the unresponsive (intubated) patient;
• administration of oral or rectal paracetamol.

Exotic lavages of cool fluids into the peritoneal and pleural cavities, the colon and the bladder are often advocated but are usually impractical in the ED. Drugs that may be used in some situations by the specialist to promote cooling include:
• chlorpromazine – vasodilator, sedative, hypothermic effect;
• diazepam – muscle relaxant and sedative;
• dantrolene – muscle relaxant. Dantrolene is used for the treatment of malignant hyperthermia and as such is kept in all operating theatres. Its use should usually be discussed with an intensivist. An initial dose of 1 mg per kg is given IV over 10 min, repeated if necessary every 15 min to a maximum of 10 mg per kg in 24 h.

For a discussion of hyperpyrexia and hyperthermia see also pages 250 and 251.

For the treatment of convulsions see page 237.

Many sedative drugs may cause hypothermia – see page 248.

Poisons information services

Specific poisons information may be obtained from:
1 The Internet (TOXBASE, the primary clinical toxicology database of the UK National Poisons Information Service is available on the Internet to registered users).
2 Telephone enquiries to the UK National Poisons Information Service (a single number that directs callers to the local poisons information centre).
3 Textbooks, including the front of the *British National Formulary*.

4 Databases (e.g. tablet identification charts) on CD-ROM.

Poisoning with common medicines

The frequency with which poisoning with a drug occurs usually reflects its availability in a society.

Paracetamol (acetaminophen)

> Paracetamol 150 mg per kg (12 g or 24 standard tablets for an adult) constitutes a significant ingestion of the drug.

Paracetamol is now the most common drug involved in self-poisoning. This reflects its widespread usage and over-the-counter availability. The only early features of poisoning are nausea and vomiting, which usually settle within 24 h. Malaise beyond this time, especially if accompanied by right subcostal pain and tenderness, usually indicates the development of hepatocellular necrosis, the major toxic effect of paracetamol poisoning. There may also sometimes be delayed renal tubular necrosis, usually in association with liver damage. These serious problems occur 3–4 days after ingestion, although patients may sometimes present even later with:

- hypoglycaemia;
- bleeding;
- encephalopathy and cerebral oedema.

The fatal dose of paracetamol may be as low as 10–15 g (20–30 tablets). Fortunately, the specific antidotes, *N*-acetylcysteine and methionine, are very effective if given early enough. Children rarely ingest large quantities of paracetamol and so deaths attributable to this drug before teenage are extremely unusual.

> Patients who present 15 h or longer after ingestion tend to be more severely poisoned and at a greater risk of serious liver damage.

Tx

All patients should have their plasma paracetamol concentration measured as soon as 4 h have passed since the ingestion. (Measurements before 4 h have passed are unreliable because of continuing absorption and distribution.) The plasma salicylate should be simultaneously measured as patients are not always able to differentiate between the two drugs. The need for specific treatment can usually be determined from this single measurement when it is plotted on a reference treatment curve (*see Figure 15.1*). If the time of ingestion is in doubt, the worst case option should be assumed to have occurred. After 15 h, the estimates of risk are less reliable and clinical judgement is more important.

> Be aware of the units used by the laboratory to measure paracetamol concentration. At least two different units are commonly used in the United Kingdom.

The usual antidote is IV *N*-acetylcysteine (NAC) (*see Box 15.2*), but up to 10% of patients treated with this drug may have an allergic response to it (*see Box 15.3*). Oral methionine is an alternative that is widely used in some countries (*see Box 15.4*). Some patients have an increased risk of liver damage following a paracetamol ingestion (*see Box 15.5*). Antidote treatment should be instituted for these patients if their plasma paracetamol concentration is 50% or more of the normal reference treatment value (*see Figure 15.1*).

Patients who have received NAC or methionine will subsequently require measurements of clotting time (INR), glucose, urea, electrolytes and creatinine. Vitamin K should be given if the INR is increased (> 2) with fresh frozen plasma and clotting factors reserved for active bleeding.

Patients with signs of liver damage should be discussed early on with a specialised liver unit. This would include those with:

- INR > 3.0;
- elevated plasma creatinine;
- hypoglycaemia;
- acidosis;
- encephalopathy;
- hypotension (mean arterial pressure < 60 mm Hg);
- pre-existing liver disease.

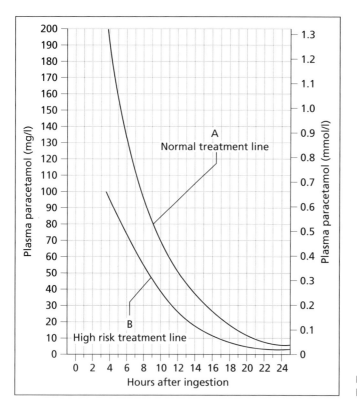

Figure 15.1 Paracetamol treatment lines.

Box 15.2 Treatment with *N*-acetylcysteine

For adults, infuse NAC in three aliquots:
1 150 mg per kg in 200 mL of 5% glucose over 15 min
2 50 mg per kg in 500 ml of 5% glucose over 4 h
3 100 mg per kg in 1000 ml of 5% glucose over 16 h.
For children over 20 kg, use the same dose of NAC in half the volume of 5% glucose. For children under 20 kg, the same doses can be used in a still smaller volume of fluid (e.g. aliquot 1 = 3 mL per kg, aliquot 2 = 7 mL per kg and aliquot 3 = 14 mL per kg).
 Normal saline may be substituted for 5% glucose.

Box 15.3 Adverse Reactions to *N*-acetylcysteine

Reactions usually occur during the first 30 min of treatment and consist of:
• nausea;
• flushing;
• itching, urticaria and other erythematous rashes;
• angioedema;
• bronchospasm;
• hypotension or hypertension (rarely).
Most reactions are mild and will resolve if the infusion is stopped and IV chlorphenamine is given. The infusion can then be restarted at the rate of 50 mg per kg over 4 h. Severe reactions require urgent treatment; methionine can then be given as an alternative.

Severe liver damage following paracetamol poisoning has been defined as a peak plasma alanine aminotransferase (ALT) activity exceeding 1000 iu per L. An aspartate transaminase (AST) level above 1000 iu per L is similarly diagnostic. Most patients who are clinically unwell have ALT and AST levels of several thousand units per litre.

Management of patients who present within 8 h of ingestion

• For patients who present within 1 h of a significant ingestion, give activated charcoal 50 g,

---

Box 15.4 Treatment with Oral Methionine

Oral dose of methionine
2.5 g initially followed by three further doses of 2.5 g every 4 h.
Useful if
- past or present allergic reaction to *N*-acetylcysteine;
- difficulty obtaining, or maintaining, IV access;
- patient refuses other treatment;
- patient is going to take own discharge;
- awaiting plasma paracetamol concentration.
Unsuitable if
- patient is nauseous or vomiting;
- activated charcoal has been given (it will absorb methionine).

Box 15.5 Patients at Special risk of Liver Damage (Treated According to the 'High Risk' Line on the Graph in *Figure 15.1*)

- Has a condition that causes glutathione depletion (i.e. malnourished, failure to thrive, anorexia nervosa, and other eating disorders or cachexic, including HIV infection).
- Is taking enzyme-inducing drugs such as carbamazepine, phenytoin, phenobarbital, primadone, rifampicin or St John's Wort.
- Drinks excessive amounts of alcohol (more than 21 units per week in males and 14 units per week in females).

---

although it is of unproven benefit in this situation.

- Assess whether the patient is at an enhanced risk of severe liver damage (*see Box 15.5*).
- Measure the plasma paracetamol concentration as soon as 4 h or more have elapsed since the ingestion.
- Start treatment with NAC if the plasma paracetamol level is on or above the relevant treatment line (*see Figure 15.1*); (for normal patients, this is 200 mg per L at 4 h and 110 mg per L at 8 h and for high-risk patients 100 mg per L at 4 h and 55 mg per L at 8 h). If the paracetamol concentration is unavailable within 8 h of ingestion and if more than 150 mg per kg (or 12 g) of paracetamol has been taken, then the antidote should be started

anyway and treatment stopped if the result subsequently indicates that it was not required.

- Arrange admission to a medical ward or psychiatric referral as appropriate. INR, ALT and plasma creatinine should be measured before discharging patients who have received NAC. Patients should be advised to return to hospital if vomiting or abdominal pain develop or recur.

Children: Paracetamol poisoning with children's preparations is rarely serious but children poisoned with adult preparations may be at risk of liver damage. Treatment is virtually identical to that for adults. If there is a certainty of an accidental ingestion of a single dose of paracetamol of less than 150 mg per kg (or 75 mg per kg in children at an enhanced risk – see Box 15.5), then measurement of paracetamol levels is unnecessary and the child can be discharged. All children with deliberate self-poisoning, including those who have taken insignificant amounts, should be admitted for child psychiatric assessment – *see page 359.*

Management of patients who present 8–15 h after ingestion

- Measure the plasma paracetamol concentration immediately. Also take blood for INR, plasma creatinine and ALT.
- Start IV NAC whilst waiting for the paracetamol concentration result if a significant amount (> 150 mg per kg or total 12 g) is thought to have been taken. The efficacy of the antidote declines progressively from 8 h after ingestion.
- Assess whether the patient is at special risk of severe liver damage (*see Box 15.5*).
- Continue the antidote only if the paracetamol level is above the relevant treatment line (*see Figure 15.1*) (for normal patients, 110 mg per L at 8 h and 35 mg per L at 15 h; for high-risk patients, 55 mg per L at 8 h and 15 mg per L at 15 h).
- Arrange medical admission or psychiatric referral as appropriate. INR, ALT and plasma creatinine should be measured before discharge in patients who have received a full course of NAC. Patients should be advised to return to hospital if vomiting or abdominal pain develop or recur.

Management of patients who present 15–24 h after ingestion

• Measure the plasma paracetamol concentration together with the INR, ALT, glucose, urea, electrolytes and creatinine.
• Start IV NAC whilst waiting for the paracetamol concentration result in all patients unless convinced that a significant amount (> 150 mg per kg or total 12 g) has not been ingested. Urgent action is required because the efficacy of NAC is limited when more than 15 h have passed since the ingestion.
• Assess whether the patient is at special risk of severe liver damage (*see Box 15.5*).
• Continue the antidote only if the paracetamol level is above the relevant treatment line (*see Figure 15.1*). The prognostic accuracy of these lines after 15 h is uncertain but a plasma paracetamol concentration above the applicable treatment line should be regarded as indicative of a serious risk of severe live damage.
• Arrange admission for patients with abnormal clotting, renal function or liver enzymes or whose paracetamol level exceeds the relevant treatment line.

Patients can be discharged 24 h after paracetamol ingestion if all of the following criteria are met:
• no symptoms;
• normal INR, ALT and creatinine;
• plasma paracetamol concentration less than 10 mg per L;
• normal mental state (confirmed by psychiatric review) and adequate social circumstances.

Management of patients who present more than 24 h after ingestion

• Measure the plasma paracetamol concentration together with the INR, ALT, glucose, urea and electrolytes, creatinine and venous bicarbonate.
• Arrange admission or referral if a significant ingestion is thought to have occurred. All patients with abnormal clotting or liver enzymes or renal function require admission and monitoring and should be discussed with a specialist liver unit.

Management of patients who ingest a significant amount of paracetamol over a period of time, as opposed to a single ingestion

Staggered overdose of paracetamol is particularly difficult to assess and treat.
• Measure the plasma paracetamol concentration, but accept that it is very difficult to interpret.
• These patients should all be considered for treatment with NAC and be discharged only if the INR, ALT and creatinine are normal at 24 h after the last dose of paracetamol.
• In patients who have ingested the paracetamol over less than 12 h, the plasma paracetamol concentration should be measured again 4 h later. If the second level is more than half the first level, then a significant overdose is likely to have occurred.

Aspirin

Aspirin poisoning is now relatively uncommon. The main features of salicylate toxicity are:
• hyperventilation;
• tinnitus and deafness;
• vasodilatation;
• sweating;
• hypoglycaemia (especially in children).
  In severe poisoning, convulsions and coma may occur and complex acid–base disturbances are inevitable. Initial stimulation of the respiratory centre causes a respiratory alkalosis. As more of the drug is absorbed, a metabolic acidosis supervenes. In between these two phases there may be a transitory period with a relatively normal blood gas picture.

Tx

• Plasma salicylate concentration must be measured in all patients in whom analgesic poisoning is suspected. It is usually measured with the plasma paracetamol level 4 h after ingestion. Peak levels however, may not be reached for at least 6 h. Urea and electrolytes, glucose and blood gases must also be measured.

• It is worth attempting to decontaminate the stomach with charcoal for up to 8 h after ingestion as salicylates markedly delay gastric emptying.

> 'It is never too late for salicylate.'

• Repeated doses of charcoal may also be useful.
• Intravenous fluid should be administered.
• Forced alkaline diuresis (with sodium bicarbonate 1.26% – *see page 257*) should be considered in cases of significant poisoning, that is when the plasma salicylate concentration is greater than:
   500 mg per L (3.6 mmol per L) in adults or
   350 mg per L (2.5 mmol per L) in children.
• Haemodialysis may be required if the plasma salicylate concentration is greater than 700 mg per L (5.1 mmol per L) or in the presence of a severe metabolic acidosis.

Ibuprofen, mefenamic acid and other NSAIDs

Ibuprofen is of low toxicity; poisoning with less than 100 mg per kg does not require any treatment. Ingestions in excess of 400 mg per kg will cause symptoms including nausea, vomiting, and epigastric pain. Diarrhoea, GI bleeding, headache and tinnitus may also occur, but more severe toxicity (convulsions, CNS depression and metabolic acidosis) is very uncommon. The half-life of ibuprofen in overdosage is 2–3 h.

Mefenamic acid is the most dangerous NSAID when taken in overdosage. It may cause convulsions.

Tx of ibuprofen and mefenamic acid poisoning

Treatment with activated charcoal is indicated if more than 100 mg per kg of ibuprofen have been taken within the preceding 1 hour (or longer for sustained release preparations). All patients who have ingested in excess of this amount will require observation for at least 4 h and monitoring of plasma electrolytes. A good urine output must be maintained.

Activated charcoal effectively absorbs mefenamic acid and should be considered for all patients, even when only small amounts of the drug have been ingested. Observation and monitoring of plasma electrolytes should be arranged.

Tx of poisoning with other NSAIDS

• Ascertain the time and amount of the ingestion.
• Seek specific information concerning the toxicity and treatment of poisoning with that drug.
• Consider the need for gastric decontamination.
• Consider admission for observation and supportive therapy.

Salbutamol

This beta-2-receptor agonist causes predictable adrenergic side effects:
• tremor;
• tachycardia;
• agitation and headache;
• hypokalaemia.

Tx

• Consider activated charcoal for all patients, especially if a controlled-release preparation has been taken.
• Monitor the heart rate, BP and ECG continuously.
• Measure the urea and electrolytes and glucose.
• Consider specific therapy with a cardioselective beta-blocker. This would probably be contraindicated in patients with a history of bronchospasm.
• Admit for observation and monitoring.

Beta blockers

The effects of poisoning vary considerably according to the specific drug. Sotalol in particular, may cause bizarre dysrhythmias. *(For torsades de pointes and prolongation of the QT interval by sotalol see page 180.)* In overdosage, most beta blockers can cause:
• severe bronchospasm;
• bradycardia, hypotension and syncope;
• heart failure;
• coma and convulsions (especially with propranolol).

Tx

- Apply supportive measures.
- Consider activated charcoal in recent ingestions and for modified-release preparations (repeated doses for sotalol in particular).
- Give nebulised salbutamol for wheezing.
- Administer IV atropine for bradycardia and hypotension (up to 3 mg for an adult and 40 μg per kg for a child).
- Give IV glucagon for hypotension refactory to atropine (boluses of 2 mg, up to a maximum of 10 mg for an adult; 50–150 μg per kg for a child).
- Give IV dobutamine for severe cardiac depression.
- Establish transvenous pacing for intractable bradycardia.

Calcium channel blockers

Poisoning with calcium channel blockers causes nausea, vomiting, dizziness, confusion and coma. Metabolic acidosis and hypoglycaemia can occur. Depending on the exact drug, hypotension may be primarily due to cardiac depression (verapamil and diltiazem) or profound vasodilatation (nifedipine).

Tx

Activated charcoal is effective if given within 1 h of ingestion or after modified-release preparations (when repeated doses may also be considered). IV calcium may be used in severe poisoning – *see page 254*. For symptomatic bradycardias and hypotension, atropine and inotropes are indicated.

Tricyclic and related antidepressants

Poisoning with tricyclic antidepressants (TCAs) is dangerous and common, being implicated in over one-fifth of all fatal ingestions. Dosulepin (dothiepin) is the most common drug involved. Some of the newer cyclic antidepressants – with different ring structures – seem less toxic. Ingested amounts are usually significant as the patient who needs TCAs will often have a mental state compatible with suicide. One in 40 patients who overdoses on tricyclics will die. An ingestion of 35 mg per kg is the median lethal dose for an adult.

The effects of TCAs are largely related to their anticholinergic activity and so include peripheral effects such as:

- blurred vision and dry mouth;
- dilated pupils;
- urinary retention;
- diverse gastrointestinal symptoms;
- tachycardia and dysrhythmias;
and central effects such as:
- agitation and anxiety;
- hyperactivity;
- disorientation and confusion;
- drowsiness and lethargy;
- hallucinations;
- nystagmus, dysarthria, ataxia and movement disorders;
- hyper-reflexia and extensor plantar response;
- hyperthermia or hypothermia:

The most serious signs are probably unrelated to anticholinergic activity:

1 *Coma.* A GCS of 8 or less occurs in about one-third of cases but rarely lasts more than 24 h. Comatose patients are likely to develop complications.

2 *Convulsions.* These are associated with severe toxicity, hypoxia and metabolic acidosis. They occur in up to 20% of patients.

3 *Cardiorespiratory collapse.* Hypotension or cardiac dysrhythmias may occur. The latter are the most common cause of death. Tachycardia (rate > 120 bpm) is worrying, especially with ECG change. Prolongation of the QRS complex > 100 ms suggests cardiotoxicity. A QRS duration of more than 160 ms (four small squares) is associated with a very high risk of life-threatening dysrhythmia.

Tx

This depends very much on the time of ingestion and the condition of the patient. Serious complications occur within 12 h of ingestion. Rapid deterioration may occur. Most patients will require:

- gastric decontamination (worthwhile for up to 8 h after ingestion – little absorption of tricyclics takes place in the stomach). The administration of activated charcoal may be repeated since charcoal prevents absorption in the small intestine.

- a 12-lead ECG;
- referral for monitoring and observation.

Agitation or convulsions should be controlled with IV benzodiazepines.

Patients with a significantly depressed level of consciousness or fitting also require:

- airway protection;
- high-concentration oxygen;
- blood gas analysis;
- monitoring;
- anaesthetic advice and a consideration of the need for paralysis and ventilation (this may need to be accompanied by an infusion of thiopental to control fits);
- ICU admission.

Cardiovascular complications should be treated by alkalinisation (see later). Antidysrhythmic drugs are best avoided in tricyclic poisoning as conduction deficits may make the ECG difficult to interpret. Moreover, some of these drugs will produce a synergistic cardiotoxicity. Torsades de pointes should be treated with magnesium – *see page 179*. Mild hypotension usually responds to IV fluids; for more severe hypotension alkalinisation is appropriate.

Alkali therapy for TCA poisoning

Induction of an alkalosis with IV sodium bicarbonate reduces mortality in TCA poisoning. The mechanism of action is not fully understood but is related to protein-binding of the TCA and the movements of ions into the heart. The benefits of alkalinisation are seen not only in patients who are acidotic; those with a minimal or absent base deficit also show improvement. Suggested indications for bicarbonate in TCA-poisoned patients are:

- systemic acidosis;
- QRS duration of more than 120 ms;
- ventricular dysrhythmia;
- hypotension;
- cardiac arrest.

The aim of therapy is to maintain a pH of between 7.50 and 7.55. The initial dose of bicarbonate can be up to 1–2 mmol per kg; further doses will depend on the clinical picture. Hyperventilation can be used as an adjunct to the bicarbonate to help achieve the desired pH.

For bicarbonate therapy see page 257.

Selective serotonin reuptake inhibitors

Selective serotonin reuptake inhibitor (SSRI) type drugs inhibit the reuptake of serotonin (5-hydroxytryptamine or 5-HT). Some related compounds (SNRIs) also inhibit the reuptake of noradrenaline. These drugs are widely prescribed for the treatment of depression and consequently self-poisoning with them is common. SSRIs in overdose cause:

- sweating and dizziness;
- drowsiness, convulsions and coma;
- tachycardia, hypotension or hypertension. (Prolongation of the duration of the QT and QRS may also occur with consequent ventricular dysrhythmias. Torsades de pointes is a particular risk – *see page 179*);
- serotonin syndrome – *see page 297*.

Tx

Activated charcoal may be given if a significant amount of an SSRI has been ingested within the previous hour. Observation for at least 6 h is indicated. Otherwise, treatment is supportive.

For serotonin syndrome (which may be a feature of poisoning) see page 297.

Theophylline

Large doses of slow-release theophylline preparations may be taken intentionally. They cause:

- severe and intractable vomiting;
- agitation and restlessness;
- dilated pupils;
- tachycardia and tachydysrhythmias;
- convulsions;
- haematemesis;
- hyperglycaemia and hypokalaemia.

Tx

- Consider gastric lavage within 2 h of ingestion and give repeated doses of activated charcoal.
- Administer potassium, anticonvulsants, sedatives and other supportive treatment as indicated.
- Intravenous propranolol may be considered in patients who are not asthmatic to reverse tachycardia, hypokalaemia and hyperglycaemia.
- Large clumps of drug in matrix may require endoscopic removal.

Lithium

Lithium toxicity may occur as a complication of long-term therapy or following a deliberate ingestion. Dehydration and infection may precipitate a crisis by reducing renal excretion of the drug. The symptoms of acute overdosage of lithium may be delayed for 12 h or more. Initially, there is lethargy and restlessness and later the patient may have:

- diarrhoea and vomiting;
- thirst and polyuria;
- ataxia and dysarthria;
- muscle weakness, twitching and tremor;
- convulsions and coma;
- dehydration and hypotension;
- renal failure and electrolyte imbalance.

Tx

The serum lithium should be measured. Therapeutic concentrations are within the range of 0.4–1.0 mmol per L while concentrations in excess of 2.0 mmol per L may be associated with serious toxicity. Forced diuresis is often advocated. Haemodialysis is required in the presence of renal failure. Otherwise, treatment is supportive with special regard to electrolyte imbalance and renal function. Activated charcoal is ineffective.

Phenytoin

The average lethal dose for adults is between 2 and 5 g but there is a marked variation among individuals with respect to the toxic effects of a given serum level of phenytoin. The initial symptoms are nystagmus, ataxia and dysarthria but later on there may be:

- coma;
- fixed pupils;
- hypotension;
- respiratory depression.

Tx

Activated charcoal should be given; repeated doses are sometimes advised. Subsequent treatment is supportive and symptomatic.

Carbamazepine

Overdose may cause:

- tremor and excitation;
- convulsions;
- impairment of consciousness and coma;
- hypotension or sometimes hypertension;
- cardiac dysrhythmias.

Tx

Activated charcoal should be given; repeated doses are indicated, especially if a slow-release preparation has been taken. Subsequent treatment is supportive and symptomatic.

Benzodiazepines and related minor tranquillisers

Self-poisoning with prescribed (or illicit) minor tranquillizers is common but hardly ever fatal. They are often taken in conjunction with alcohol, which leads to a synergistic effect. Benzodiazepines exert their action on specific BZ receptors, which are closely associated with gamma-aminobutyric acid (GABA) receptors. GABA is an inhibitory neurotransmitter that is widely distributed throughout the brain and spinal cord. Potentiation of GABA transmission thus causes a generalised depression of CNS activity and results in:

- a reduced level of consciousness;
- flaccidity;
- ataxia and dysarthria;

Box 15.6 Comparison of Different Benzodiazepines		
Drug	**Half-life (hours)**	**Equivalent dose**
Diazepam	20–50	5 mg
Chlordiazepoxide	6–30	15 mg
Nitrazepam	24	5 mg
Lorazepam	12	0.5 mg
Temazepam	8	10 mg
Oxazepam	6–8	15 mg

- hypotension;
- hypothermia.

Poisoning with non-benzodiazepine hypnotics such as zopiclone, which also act at the benzodiazepine receptor, is similar in both effects and treatment.

Tx

Supportive therapy and observation is usually enough; gastric decontamination is rarely indicated. *For comparative doses and half-lives of benzodiazepines see Box 15.6.*

Flumazenil

This is a specific benzodiazepine antagonist that:
- wears off sooner than most oral ingestions of benzodiazepines;
- may precipitate fitting if tricyclics have also been taken and so should never be used in poisonings with unknown or mixed substances;
- may partially reverse hepatic coma;
- can occasionally be useful as a diagnostic tool. It is given as a bolus of 200 μg (2 mL) by slow IV injection and then repeated doses of 100 μg (1 mL) after 1-min intervals, depending on effect. Infusion of 100–400 μg per h may sometimes be required.

Barbiturates

Barbiturates are now infrequently prescribed and so poisoning with them is much less common than in the past. Findings include:

- depressed level of consciousness;
- respiratory depression;
- hypotension;
- hypothermia;
- palmar and plantar blistering.

Tx

Supportive therapy and admininistration of activated charcoal is appropriate. Repeated doses of charcoal may increase drug elimination, especially of phenobarbital. Forced alkaline diuresis and charcoal haemoperfusion may be necessary.

Phenothiazines and other major tranquillizers

These drugs cause:
- drowsiness and confusion
- hypotension
- hypothermia
- sinus tachycardia and cardiac dysrhythmias, (especially with thioridazine);
- convulsions and coma (with large doses).

There is often less depression of consciousness and respiration than is seen with other sedatives. Extrapyrimidal effects including acute dystonic reactions may occur but are not dose-related. Neuroleptic malignant syndrome is not usually a feature of poisoning – *see page 297.*

Tx

Activated charcoal should be given to all patients who present themselves within 1 h of ingestion of a potentially toxic amount. Otherwise treatment is supportive. Fluids and dobutamine can be used to treat severe hypotension. Convulsions respond to lorazepam. Symptomatic patients should be monitored (including ECG) for at least 4 h.

Poisoning with drugs of abuse

For the Misuse of Drugs Act 1971 and the Misuse of Drugs Regulations 2001 see page 369.
For poisoning with minor tranquillisers see page 278.
For poisoning with barbiturates see page 279.

Narcotic analgesics (opioids)

Opioid poisoning occurs by both oral and parenteral routes. If a combination analgesic has been taken, narcotic effects may accompany paracetamol poisoning (*see page 271*). Signs of acute poisoning with opioids include:

- a depressed level of consciousness;
- respiratory depression (usually the respiratory rate is most affected);
- pinpoint pupils.

Methadone and dextropropoxyphene have particularly long durations of action. The effect of naloxone can be used as a diagnostic test in cases of suspected acute opioid overdose.

Tx

Emergency treatment involves naloxone therapy in variable amounts (and sometimes by IV infusion), support of vital functions and close observation. The initial dose of naloxone for adults is 400–2000 µg IV, repeated at 2–3 min intervals as required. For children 10 µg per kg should be given, increased to 100 µg per kg if the desired improvement is not seen with the first dose. *For a suggested approach to a patient with an overdose of IV narcotics see Box 15.7.*

Withdrawal from opioid drugs is rarely as traumatic as is popularly believed. Most patients should be referred to a specialised treatment and counselling facility. Prescription of substitute opiates is best left to such agencies.

For withdrawal from opioid drugs see page 360.

If a vein cannot be found, naloxone may be given via the endotracheal or intra-osseous routes.

Stimulant drugs

The abuse of stimulant drugs is on the increase. Amfetamine is used as the basis for several more potent variants (e.g. 'Ecstasy' – *see page 281*). Patients present with varying degrees of:

- wakefulness and hyperactivity;
- agitation and confusion;
- paranoia and hallucinations;
- hypertension and dysrhythmias;
- convulsions;
- exhaustion and coma;
- sweating and hyperthermia.

Later on, in extreme cases, gross electrolyte disturbance, rhabdomyolysis, disseminated intravascular coagulation (DIC) and multisystem failure may occur. Sometimes, just one tablet can provoke an idiosyncratic life-threatening hyperthermia.

Tx

This mainly consists of supportive therapy.

- Give oxygen.
- Start vigorous IV rehydration.
- Consider giving activated charcoal in recent ingestions.
- Give sedatives and anticonvulsants (e.g. lorazepam or diazepam) as necessary.
- Summon anaesthetic help early on.
- Measure the core temperature continuously.
- Start active cooling if indicated (*see page 270*).
- Consider the need for paralysis and ventilation and/or ICU care.
- Measure the urea and electrolytes, glucose and blood gases.
- Consider giving bicarbonate for metabolic acidosis.
- Monitor the urine output.
- Consider the use of nifedipine (5–10 mg by mouth) for hypertension and betablockers for

---

Box 15.7 Management of Heroin Overdose

- Attend to the ABCs; assisted ventilation with a bag and mask is often required.
- Draw up two ampoules of naloxone (800 µg) in a 2-mL syringe.
- Insert an IV cannula; this may be difficult. Often only a tiny spidery vein is available. Enter this vein with an orange (25 G) needle attached to the syringe of naloxone.
- Inject the naloxone, ensuring that it is not extravasated.
- Inject a further 800 µg of naloxone IM to sustain the blood levels. This is very important.
- Continue ventilatory support until recovery occurs.
- Once the patient is alert and orientated, discuss the further management options with him or her.

tachycardias. (Do not use betabockers if cocaine may be involved.)

• Consider the need for dantrolene therapy – *see page 270.*

• Consider forced acid diuresis to increase excretion.

The patient with extreme mental disturbance secondary to amphetamines

The patient in a violent, agitated, confusional state may present a challenging problem. The diagnosis is not usually difficult as not many medical conditions look like this. The patient should be restrained and sedated for the safety of both him or herself and others. He or she can then be examined properly. This kind of immediate sedation presents no special legal problems (*see page 373*).

> Do not forget to check the blood sugar – hypoglycaemia is the best mimic of this condition.

Methylenedioxymethamfetamine

Methylenedioxymethamfetamine (MDMA, 'ecstasy') is a semi-synthetic drug that is sold in single tablets containing 30–150 mg of active substance. Effects occur within 1 h and last for 4–6 h after 75 mg and up to 48 h with higher doses. The half-life of MDMA is 7.6 h. *For clinical features that are suggestive of MDMA usage see Box 15.8.* 'Ectasy' gives the user a tremendous feeling of energy and vitality, is mildly hallucinogenic and can engender feelings of peace, love and sensuality.

Box 15.8 Features Suggestive of MDMA Poisoning ('Ecstasy' Usage)

History of ingestion or likely circumstances from user and friends.
Fever, sometimes with absence of perspiration.
Dilated pupils.
Dry mouth and throat.
Tightening of the jaw muscles.
Increased pulse and BP (hypotension in some cases).
New onset of fits or headaches.
Unexplained pains.
Coma or sudden collapse.

Unfortunately, it is much more dangerous than cannabis, its 1960s predecessor. At moderate doses (75–100 mg) it causes:

• mild mental changes as described above;

• variable autonomic upset (dilated pupils, dry mouth, tachycardia and hypertension). These may be influenced by the degree of dehydration;

• an increase in muscle tone, sometimes with myalgia;

• a partial failure of temperature homeostasis. When this is combined with excessive dancing in a hot, dry atmosphere with a low fluid intake, simple heat-stroke type collapse may occur.

At higher doses, panic attacks and even psychosis may appear. Severe and even fatal idiopathic reactions can follow the ingestion of amounts that were previously tolerated. These dramatic, but rare, events seem to be an idiosyncratic reaction related to the neuroleptic malignant syndrome (*see page 297*). There is hyperpyrexia, coma, convulsions and circulatory collapse. Rhabdomyolysis, renal failure and disseminated intravascular coagulation may occur. It must be remembered that similar, unidentified or impure drugs may corrupt the clinical picture described above as may self-induced water intoxication.

Tx

Rehydration and observation is the mainstay of treatment for mild cases. Activated charcoal may be given for recent ingestions. *For severe features, see treatment of poisoning with stimulant drugs on page 280.* 5-HT agonists (e.g. cyproheptadine) may be useful.

Cocaine

Cocaine and its more potent, free base form 'crack' are increasingly abused by smoking, sniffing or injection. The resulting central nervous system stimulation causes:

• agitation and hallucinations;

• dilated pupils;

• tachycardia and hypertension;

• hyperthermia;

- hypertonia and hyper-reflexia;
- convulsions and coma.

There may be a metabolic acidosis and chest pain (caused by coronary vasospasm) often occurs. It may lead to dysrhythmias and even MI.

Tx

- Give supportive therapy (oxygen, rehydration and cooling measures).
- Consider sedation with IV benzodiazepines.
- Treat chest pain with analgesia and nitrates.

Do not use β-blockers as they may cause worsening of the hypertension because of unopposed α-receptor stimulation.

Gamma hydroxybutyrate

Gamma hydroxybutyrate (GHB) is a potent CNS sedative that is easily synthesised and then sold in clubs. Several precursor drugs (such as 1,4-butane-diol or pine needle oil) are metabolised in the body to GHB and so may also be used for the same effect. Gamma hydroxybutyrate may cause a rapid onset of coma and respiratory depression such that 10% of patients presenting to an ED after its ingestion require endotracheal intubation. Concurrent ethanol usage exacerbates its effects. Treatment is largely supportive. One of the hall-marks of GHB intoxication is a rapid recovery to full consciousness following profound coma.

Ketamine and phencyclidine

Ketamine ('Special K') and phencyclidine (PCP) are also encountered as drugs of abuse. They cause a variable depression of consciousness and disso-ciative behaviour. Trance-like staring may occur with hallucinations and agitation. The diagnostic ocular finding is rotatory nystagmus. Treatment is supportive.

Lysergic acid diethylamide

The potent hallucinogen Lysergic acid diethy-lamide (LSD) causes excitement and euphoria

before agitation, tachycardia and vivid visual hallucinations. Extreme dysphoria and bizarre behaviour may require sedation. A similar condi-tion may be seen in people who have eaten bread made with grain (principally rye) contaminated with the fungus *Claviceps purpurea* (which pro-duces ergot alkaloids related to LSD). Outbreaks of collective madness (known in the Middle Ages as 'St Anthony's fire') have occurred in villages and on cruise ships where contaminated bread has been distributed.

Cannabis (marijuana or Indian hemp)

Patients may present to an ED who are intoxicated with tetrahydrocannabinols, the active substances in cannabis resin. They are usually mildly disori-entated; rarely a frank psychosis is seen. No spe-cific therapy is indicated.

Mushroom poisoning

Patients may accidently or deliberately eat poiso-nous fungi.

Death cap mushrooms (Amanita phalloides) are the most dangerous fungi in the British Isles. They con-tain phallotoxins and amatoxins. Several hours after ingestion there is abdominal pain, vomiting and continuous diarrhoea. Renal and hepatic failure may follow in 2–3 days with death within a week.

'Magic mushroooms' contain the hallucinogens psilocybin and psilocin that can cause an organic psychosis. Disturbed patients may require seda-tion with diazepam or lorazepam followed by close observation.

Solvent abuse

This was originally described as glue-sniffing in teenagers; toluene is the usual solvent in glue but benzene and xylene are found in plastic cement. However, the sensations of early anaesthesia can be obtained from most inhalable organic materials and so many products have abuse potential. Lighter fuel (butane) appears to be one of the most dangerous as sudden death may result from a cardiac dysrhyth-mia. Solvent abuse usually causes no symptoms or signs after the initial effects but should always be

considered in young people with bizarre behaviour or collapse. There may sometimes be:
- euphoria and 'drunkenness';
- headache;
- nausea and vomiting;
- dizziness and ataxia;
- fits;
- cardiac dysrhythmias, which are precipitated by a mixture of cardiac irritation, hypoxia and hypercapnia.

Chronic abusers may also have:
- sores around the nose and mouth;
- signs of bone marrow suppression;
- encephalopathy.

Tx

- Give high-concentration oxygen.
- Establish ECG monitoring.
- Obtain blood gas analysis.
- Request a full blood count.
- Refer for observation and follow-up.

> It is often asked why people seek the disordered sensations of cerebral poisoning. The questioner should remember that there are whole industries devoted to providing human beings with strange sensations – the fairground and distilling industries, for example. Every civilisation sets its own standards of acceptable behaviour. The emergency physician must not let these social and legal codes influence management or attitudes to care.

Alcohol (ethanol)

The world's favourite poison is freely available in most societies and is associated with many social problems (*see Chapter 20*). It is frequently taken as a component of self-poisoning. In acute ingestions there may be a combination of signs such as:
- a smell of alcoholic beverage on the breath;
- red, injected conjunctivae;
- loss of inhibition and judgement;
- aggression and excitability;
- ataxia and slurred speech;
- depression of consciousness.

There may also be:
- hypoglycaemia – seen in children and adult patients with poor liver glycogen reserves;
- fluid depletion – in severe poisoning;
- a loss of airway protection – with a risk of aspiration;
- coexisting head injuries – especially subdural haematoma (*see page 46*).

Ethyl alcohol is metabolised in the liver to carbon dioxide and water via acetaldehyde and acetate. This breakdown normally occurs at a constant rate (about 10–15 g per h) irrespective of the amount of alcohol present in the body (zero-order kinetics). Above a level of about 100 mg per dL, liver metabolism is unable to cope and further alcohol intake may cause a very rapid increase in blood concentrations. Similarly, at very high blood levels (probably above 300 mg per dL) alcohol concentration decreases more quickly than can be explained by zero-order kinetics alone.

Tx

Several substances have been shown to hasten the recovery from alcohol intoxication.
- Insulin – speeds up the catabolic process.
- Fructose (laevulose), galactose and sorbitol. These substances may precipitate lactic acidosis, especially in the presence of hypovolaemia.
- Naloxone – inconclusive.
- Intravenous fluids.

The risk is greater than the benefit with all these therapies, except in the case of IV fluids. Isotonic saline should therefore be given (at least 10–20 mL per kg in the first hour if not contraindicated). Further treatment consists of supportive measures and a consideration of other injuries. This frequently necessitates obtaining radiographs of the skull. The blood sugar should be measured routinely in all patients thought to be drunk.

> In a patient with a depressed level of consciousness thought to be caused by alcohol, a CT scan of the brain is indicated if a GCS of 15 is not reached within about 6–8 h of arrival.

Measurement of blood alcohol

Level of consciousness bears little relationship to initial blood alcohol level. However, it is unusual

> **Box 15.9 Management of the Aggressive Drunk**
>
> Observe the patient carefully.
> Inquire about the possibility of trauma from the patient and any bystanders.
> Examine the patient as fully as possible but without risk to yourself. Try especially to feel the head for cuts or swellings.
> Measure the blood sugar.
> Get senior help. Options for further management include:
> • sedate the patient and observe in hospital;
> • let the patient go home with friends or relatives and with verbal and written head injury instructions;
> • let the patient go to a police cell with head injury instructions.

for a blood alcohol concentration below 200 mg per dL to cause depression of consciousness. Coma generally occurs with alcohol levels above 300 mg per dL. Serial measurements of blood alcohol show that the concentration of alcohol in the blood often increases for the first 2 h after presentation. The explanation for this phenomenon is that alcohol is continuing to be absorbed from the gastrointestinal tract at a rate that exceeds its metabolism in the body. Gastric lavage may be useful in unresponsive patients to prevent this continuing absorption of alcohol.

For the management of the aggressive, intoxicated patient see Box 15.9.

For alcohol withdrawal states see page 355.

For medicolegal aspects of alcohol abuse (including driving) see page 370.

Management of poisoning with unknown substance(s)

• Obtain as much history and background information as possible; consider alternative diagnoses.
• Examine the patient and his or her clothing and possessions for further clues. Beware of needles in the pockets.
• Consider trauma or coexistent disease.
• Monitor the patient.
• Check the blood sugar.
• Send off blood for full blood count, urea and electrolytes and aspirin and paracetamol screen.

• Consider the need for ECG and blood gases. Plasma osmolality can be a useful test to establish the presence of extraneous substances in the blood (see page 228).
• Consider the administration of activated charcoal.
• Administer IV fluids and measure urine output.
• Admit for observation.

Poisoning with substances found at home and at work

Iron

Iron poisoning is most common in children under 5 years old and so is usually accidental. The toxicity of iron may be underestimated by both parents and medical staff.

In normal circumstances, iron is absorbed by the mucosal cells of the duodenum and jejunum and transported in the blood bound to transferrin. Following an acute overdose, the intestinal barrier is overwhelmed and the transferrin is saturated. Unbound iron then causes cardiovascular, hepatic, central nervous system and metabolic damage.

Oral iron preparations are ferrous salts and contain differing amounts of elemental iron (e.g. 200 mg of ferrous sulphate contains 60 mg of pure iron). Toxicity is dependent on the amount of elemental iron ingested:
• <30 mg per kg causes mild toxicity;
• >30 mg per kg causes moderate toxicity;
• >60 mg per kg causes severe toxicity;
• >150 mg per kg is potentially lethal.

The early features of iron poisoning, which occur at 1–6 h post-ingestion, result from corrosive damage and haemodynamic effects (vascular dilatation and capillary leakage). There may be:
• nausea and vomiting (vomitus may have a metallic odour);
• abdominal pain and diarrhoea;
• haematemesis and rectal bleeding;
• hypovolaemia, hypoxia, acidosis and collapse.

Drowsiness, coma and convulsions may also occur; signs of gastric and jejunal perforation are a possibility.

A relatively quiescent phase then follows. This lasts for 6–12 h, after which there is either a recovery or a further exacerbation of symptoms. These later effects are mostly the result of intracellular poisoning and include:

- coma and convulsions;
- circulatory collapse and pulmonary oedema;
- profound metabolic acidosis;
- liver failure with hypoglycaemia and coagulopathy;
- renal failure;
- further gastrointestinal haemorrhage.

Delayed sequelae, after at least 2 weeks, include stricture formation, pyloric stenosis and small bowel obstruction.

Investigations

Patients who have ingested less than 30 mg per kg of elemental iron will not require either investigations or active treatment. In those who have taken in excess of this amount:

- an abdominal X-ray should be obtained in order to determine the need for gastrointestinal decontamination and the site to target;
- the serum iron must be measured to determine the need for chelation therapy – see later;
- full blood count, electrolytes and glucose should be requested.

Patients with severe symptoms will also require LFTs, clotting studies, blood gases and ECG. Measurement of total iron-binding capacity (TIBC) is of little value. Raised white cell count and blood sugar are typical findings.

The serum iron should be measured 4 h post-ingestion or immediately before desferrioxamine administration. Levels taken later than 6 h post-ingestion may underestimate the amount of free iron because of tissue uptake. If slow-release tablets have been taken, the serum iron should be rechecked after 4 h. Patients who present late and have low iron levels must be regarded as at high risk of toxicity.

The anticipated effect of the measured serum iron concentration must be interpreted in conjunction with the history and clinical findings:

- Over 20 μmol per L (> 110 μg per dL) – mild toxicity.
- Over 55 μmol per L (>300μg per dL) – moderate toxicity.

- Over 90 μmol per L (>500 μg per dL) – severe toxicity.
- Over 180 μmol per L (>1000 μg per dL) – extreme toxicity.

The advice of a chemical pathologist should be sought as soon as possible.

Tx

Patients who have ingested less than 30 mg per kg of elemental iron do not require either investigations or active treatment.

Tablets that are visible on X-ray must be removed from the stomach by lavage or endoscopy. Iron tablets beyond the pylorus are an indication for whole-bowel irrigation or even surgical removal. Whole-bowel cleansing may be performed with polyethylene glycol electrolyte solution (Klean-Prep). The dose is 15–40 mL per kg per h given orally until the rectal effluent runs clear (maximum 6–8 h). Repeat radiographs must be obtained in all cases requiring decontamination to confirm a satisfactory result.

Dissolved tablets are not radio-opaque. Patients who have ingested a significant amount of iron, which is not visible on X-ray, should be treated with emesis or lavage (with 1% sodium bicarbonate solution, if possible). Activated charcoal is not indicated as it does not bind iron.

Subsequent management depends on clinical findings and serum concentrations of iron. All patients should be rehydrated with care; fluid balance must be recorded. Patients with serum iron levels under 55 μmol per L can be managed at home. Those with serum iron concentrations of 55–90 μmol per L and minimal symptoms should be observed in hospital for 48 h.

Parenteral desferrioxamine chelates free iron and the resulting complex is excreted in the urine, which then turns pink. It should be given to all patients with:

- serum iron concentrations in excess of 90 μmol per L;
- cardiovascular symptoms;
- central nervous system symptoms;
- significant gastrointestinal haemorrhage.

The dose of IV desferrioxamine is 15 mg per kg per h up to a maximum of 80 mg per kg in 24 h.

It may cause hypotension. A successful outcome is heralded by cessation of symptoms, return of normal urine colour and low serum iron (<18 μmol per L). Oral or IM desferrioxamine is no longer recommended.

All patients with significant iron poisoning must be followed up for 6 weeks because of the risk of stricture formation.

Vitamins

These are not harmful in an isolated acute ingestion but the estimated amount taken should be checked against known poisons information. Some compound preparations may contain iron and other substances.

Oral contraceptives

These are not harmful although nausea and vomiting may occur. Female patients should be warned about the slight possibility of withdrawal bleeding.

Methanol and glycols

Substances such as methanol (methyl alcohol or wood alcohol) and ethylene glycol (antifreeze) cause drunkenness in the early stages followed by a severe metabolic acidosis and renal damage. (NB Methylated spirits and surgical spirits contain 95% ethanol).

Tx

Patients who are thought to have ingested this type of poison require IV fluids, arterial blood gas analysis and admission. Fomepizole is a competitive inhibitor of alcohol dehydrogenase, the enzyme that is responsible for the preliminary step in the metabolism of methanol and ethylene glycol to their toxic metabolites. A loading dose of 15 mg per kg should be given, followed by 4 doses of 10 mg per kg at 12 h intervals and then 15 mg per kg every 12 h until the plasma concentration of the poison has reduced to a non-toxic level. All doses are given as a slow IV infusion over 30 min.

The most frequent adverse effects of fomepizole are headache, nausea, dizziness and minor allergic reactions. Ethyl alcohol may be given in an attempt to saturate the alcohol dehydrogenase binding sites if fomepizole is not available. Dialysis may be required in severe cases. Activated charcoal is ineffective.

Household substances

Children may be suspected of ingesting an enormous variety of domestic substances. Most of these are harmless but some are not and so caution is always advisable. Many household substances are caustic or contain petroleum distillates. Thus, in almost all cases, emetics are contraindicated. Treatment consists of milk and the recommendations of a poisons information service.

Cleaning materials

Most are harmless. Two notable exceptions are bleach and dishwasher products for machines. These can burn the mouth and damage the oesophagus. Emesis is therefore contraindicated. Patients should be given milk and observed in hospital.

Turpentine

This can be lethal. Its abbreviated name, "Turps," usually refers to a white spirit substitute that is not very dangerous. Check the bottle.

Cosmetics

These are usually harmless but may contain a large amount of alcohol (*see page 283*). Perfume oil ingestions (which may sometimes be dangerous) should be treated with milk and observation.

Pet foods

Not surprisingly, most pet foods are completely safe to eat.

Mercury

Mercury from a broken thermometer has a very low risk of toxicity.

Plants and garden substances

Earth, faecal material, insects and worms generally present little risk. The possibility of ingesting ova, cysts and parasites is probably quite small.

Berries and seeds are commonly ingested. Some such as laburnum seeds may cause gastrointestinal upset and drowsiness. Deadly nightshade may be mistaken for elderberry and lead to atropine poisoning. If the ingested plant material is presented, it may be identified with the aid of a guide book.

Tx

Most ingestions of this type, including those where the material is unidentified, should be treated by observation for around 6 h.

Paraquat

The industrial liquid (e.g. "Gramoxone") contains 10–20% paraquat and is deadly. Granular preparations for the garden contain only 2.5% paraquat and have caused few deaths. The chemical is highly irritant to the skin, eyes and other membranes. Inhalation of paraquat spray causes a sore throat and epistaxis but not systemic toxicity. Ingestion causes:
- nausea, vomiting and diarrhoea (after a few hours);
- painful ulceration of the lips, tongue and throat (36 h);
- renal failure (48 h);
- dyspnoea (after a few days). There is pulmonary fibrosis with proliferative alveolitis and bronchiolitis.

Tx

- Expert advice should be sought as soon as possible. The Central Toxicology Laboratory at Imperial Chemical Industries Ltd can help with plasma estimations of paraquat in the United Kingdom.
- Activated charcoal should be administered immediately (with an IV antiemetic if required).

Fuller's earth and magnesium sulphate are no longer recommended.
- Oxygen therapy should be avoided in the early stages of treatment since it may exacerbate damage to the lungs. All patients should have blood gas analysis performed.
- Local irritation of mucous membranes, eyes and skin should be treated by irrigation.
- Mannitol (200 mL of 20%) can be given orally as a purgative but is of doubtful value.
- ICU admission must be arranged.

Toxic effects from foods

Scombroid fish

If not completely fresh, fish of the family *Scombridae* (which includes mackerel and tuna) may be decomposed by bacteria such as *Proteus morgani* to form heat-stable substances that are unaffected by cooking. Similar processes may occur in both tinned and fresh fish of other non-scombroid species such as herring. Histamine is produced from histidine and levels are very high in affected fish. However, there are other (as yet unidentified) toxins also involved.

Around 30 min to several hours after eating the fish, the seafood lover experiences widespread erythema and blotchy urticaria of the skin with headache, colic, diarrhoea and vomiting. Bronchospasm, tachycardia and hypotension may also occur. This combination of features is easily mistaken for an allergic reaction or even bacterial food poisoning. The illness is treated with IV antihistamines (both H_1 and H_2 receptor blockers), IV fluids and nebulised bronchodilators. Symptoms resolve within 24 h.

Chinese restaurant syndrome

Monosodium glutamate (MSG) is used as a flavour enhancer in a variety of foods. It is sold as a fine white crystalline powder, which does not have a distinct taste of its own. The mechanism by which MSG adds flavour to other foods is not fully understood. However the human body uses the amino acid glutamate as a neurotransmitter and it may be that MSG stimulates glutamic acid receptors in the tongue to augment meat-like flavours.

Excessive quantities (3 g or more) of MSG cause a toxic reaction in susceptible individuals around one hour after ingestion. There is flushing and parasthesia of the skin with nausea, headache, a sensation of facial pressure and chest discomfort. Bronchospasm may occur in people with asthma. The syndrome is rarely seen nowadays as restaurant cooking practices seem to have changed.

Food poisoning is a notifiable disease throughout the United Kingdom.
For bacterial and viral food poisoning see page 260.
For allergic reactions to foods (and other substances) see page 295.

Envenomation

Exotic pets may inflict exotic bites and stings. In addition, unlucky world travellers may encounter poisonous insects, spiders, snakes, fish, corals, hydroids, anemones, jellyfish and octopi.

Tx

All such wounds must be cleaned thoroughly and then dressed. Tetanus prophylaxis must be ensured. It may occasionally be necessary to give antivenom and it is important that each ED knows where the nearest supply is kept. (The British National Formulary contains up-to-date telephone numbers of regional depots). Twenty-four hour help and advice can be obtained from the following centres in the United Kingdom:
- The Liverpool School of Tropical Medicine
- The Hospital for Tropical Diseases in London.

In the case of travellers, expert local advice is essential for both diagnosis and treatment.
For jellyfish, Weever fish, caterpillar, wasp and bee stings in the British Isles see page 394.

Adder bites

The European Viper or adder (*Vipera berus*) is the only poisonous snake that is native to the British Isles. It is not found in Ireland.

Adder bites are occasionally seen in EDs, especially in the south of England. The viper venom causes three main groups of effects:

1 *Local effects:* pain, swelling and bruising at the site of envenomation with tender enlargement of regional lymph nodes
2 *Early anaphylactoid effects:* angioedema, urticaria, transient hypotension and syncope; diarrhoea and vomiting with colic
3 *Severe systemic toxic effects:* hypotension, ECG abnormalities, coagulopathy, acute renal failure and adult respiratory distress syndrome.

Tx

Anaphylactoid symptoms should be treated with adrenaline (*see page 295*). Systemic effects or persistent and worsening local swelling are indications for treatment with European Viper venom antiserum. The dose for both adults and children is 10 mL (diluted in saline) by IV infusion over 30 min. If there is little improvement, this may be repeated after 1–2 h. The antivenom itself may cause an anaphylactic reaction.

Carbon monoxide

This under-recognised condition hospitalises more than 200 people and causes about 50 deaths every year in the United Kingdom. Carbon monoxide is a colourless, tasteless, non-irritating gas produced by incomplete combustion of any carbon-containing material and so is a sinister and insidious enemy. The main causes of poisoning with carbon monoxide in the United Kingdom are:
1 deliberate self-harm (45%);
2 faulty domestic heating and cooking apparatus (33%);
3 smoke inhalation in fires (20%). (NB Cyanide and other toxic fumes may be released during the combustion of common materials such as polyurethane foam in furniture – *see page 292*).

Think of carbon monoxide poisoning if a patient has:
- a history of smoke inhalation (*see page 146*)
- unexplained neurological symptoms, including headache
- an unexplained metabolic acidosis

and if:
- more than one patient presents from the same site;

- there are known to be animals that are also unwell;
- the patient gets better when away from home;
- the patient comes from a community that uses traditional, ethnic cooking methods
- the patient reports that there are black, sooty marks on the walls around stoves, boilers or fires or that their gas appliances burn with yellow rather than blue flames.

Carbon monoxide causes tissue hypoxia by:

1 binding to haemoglobin and preventing the carriage of oxygen. (Its affinity for haemoglobin is 240 times greater than that of oxygen.);

2 moving the oxyhaemoglobin dissociation curve to the left;

3 binding to cellular proteins essential for oxidation.

Tissues with a high requirement for oxygen, such as nervous tissue and myocardium, are most severely affected. The atmospheric level of carbon monoxide considered to be immediately dangerous is 1500 ppm (0.15%) but exposure to 1000 ppm (0.1%) may result in 50% saturation of haemoglobin with the gas.

Symptoms and signs

Symptoms vary widely and include malaise, headache, nausea and myalgia (*see Box 15.10*). A collection of these vague symptoms may mimic influenza or food poisoning. However, there may also be overt neurological, cardiovascular and biochemical findings such as:

- confusion, coma and psychological changes;
- dysphasia, dyskinesia, paresis and cortical blindness;

- angina, dysrhythmias and left ventricular failure;
- hypotension;
- metabolic acidosis, hypokalaemia and leucocytosis;
- rhabdomyolysis (very rarely).

These problems may persist or reoccur and are not well related to the carboxyhaemoglobin (COHb) level. This is probably because the half-life of carbon monoxide bound to intracellular myoglobin and respiratory enzymes is up to 48 h, as opposed to 5 h (320 min) in the blood as COHb. Binding to mitochondrial cytochrome A3 is thought to be particularly important in the causation of carbon monoxide toxicity. Neurological damage seems to be the result of free radical generation and lipid peroxidation.

Patients with coexisting medical problems (heart disease, respiratory disease and anaemia) and children are usually the worst affected and may experience symptoms at lower levels of COHb. Carbon monoxide has a special affinity for fetal haemoglobin and so babies and pregnant women present a special risk.

The severity of poisoning is related to:

1 the concentration of carbon monoxide inhaled;

2 the length of exposure;

3 the level of activity during the exposure.

Investigations

Investigations may include:

- blood gases – metabolic acidosis with normal oxygen tension;
- ECG – ischaemia;
- fetal cardiotocograph (FCTG) – fetal hypoxia;
- plasma electrolytes, glucose and osmolality – to exclude other causes of poisoning;
- carboxyhaemoglobin levels (*see Box 15.11*).

Box 15.10 Common Symptoms of Carbon Monoxide Poisoning

Symptom	Approximate frequency
Headache	90%
Nausea and vomiting	50%
Vertigo	50%
Alteration in mental state	30%
Subjective weakness	20%

Laboratory measurement of arterial blood gases looks at oxygen dissolved in the plasma rather than oxygen bound to haemoglobin and so the PaO_2 level in CO poisoning may be surprisingly near to normal. Pulse oximeters will also give a false normal value since they cannot differentiate between oxyhaemoglobin and carboxyhaemoglobin.

Box 15.11 The Effects of Increasing Carboxyhaemoglobin Levels

COHb should be less than 5% of total haemoglobin in a non-smoker and less than 10% in a smoker.
COHb > 10% causes mild headache and dyspnoea on vigorous exertion.
COHb > 20% causes severe headache, dyspnoea on mild exertion and sometimes early neurological symptoms and signs.
COHb > 30% causes severe headache, irritability, fatigue, dimness of vision and other neurological symptoms and signs.
COHb > 40% causes severe headache, tachycardia, lethargy, confusion, collapse and sometimes coma.
COHb > 60% causes coma, convulsions and cardiovascular collapse.
COHb > 70% is very rapidly fatal.

Box 15.12 Indications for Hyperbaric Oxygen Therapy in CO Poisoning

Symptoms of poisoning and COHb > 40%.
Last trimester of pregnancy with FCTG changes and COHb > 20%.
Comatose at any time.
Neurological signs after 2 h treatment with high-concentration oxygen.
Severe cardiovascular problems (e.g. continuing myocardial ischaemia on ECG).

Tx

This should include:

• high-concentration oxygen therapy for 120 min, given via an endotracheal tube or tight-fitting mask (The half-life of COHb is reduced to around 1 h (80 min) when breathing 100% oxygen.);
• close observation and monitoring;
• a consideration of the need for hyperbaric oxygen therapy (*see Box 15.12 for indications*). (The half-life of COHb is reduced to 23 min when breathing oxygen at twice atmospheric pressure although there is very little evidence of a beneficial effect from this expensive and inconvenient treatment). The telephone number of the nearest hyperbaric unit should be available in the ED; suitable patients can usually be discussed with an expert at the hyperbaric facility. All unresponsive patients should be intubated and ventilated. Acidosis will resolve with oxygenation and should not be treated with bicarbonate.
For cyanide see page 292.
For noxious fumes, vapours and gases see page 291.
For the diagnosis and management of methaemoglobinaemia see page 291.

Incapacitating sprays and aerosols

Patients may present who have been assaulted with a variety of irritant powder aerosols eg. pepper spray, CS ('tear gas') or CN ('Mace'). There is profound irritation of the eyes, skin and respiratory tract. Water 'activates' the powder and may temporarily increase symptoms but it is usually impractical to avoid irrigation during treatment.

Tx

The effects of these agents are usually self-limiting (within 30 min). Most patients require irrigation to the face and eyes only; a weak alkaline solution (or soap and water) can be used for the skin. Continuing discomfort of the eyes merits examination with fluorescein to exclude chemical damage. Severe dermatitis can be treated with topical steroids. Good ventilation of treatment areas is essential to protect staff and other patients.

Poisoning with harmful agents, which have been released into the environment

Deliberate release of harmful substances

Intentional spread of a chemical or biological agent might occur in a biowarfare or bioterrorist incident anywhere in the world. A deliberate release could be overt and clearly identifiable. In this case, there might be a prior warning or an obvious distribution of a toxic substance by an explosive device. However, covert release is also a possibility, in which circumstances the release would not be apparent until the first cases of disease presented – probably to an ED!

Chemical agents

Chemical warfare has not gone away. With modern aeromedical evacuation patients suffering from its effects may present to distant hospitals. In addition, the threat of terrorist attack has necessitated a knowledge of substances that might be deliberately released into the environment. There are five main types of agents used for such purposes:

1 irritants and asphyxiants such as chlorine, phosgene, ammonia and ammonium nitrate;
2 vesicants (blistering agents) such as mustard gas and the arsenical vesicants;
3 blood agents such as the compounds of cyanide;
4 nerve gases – the G-agents (e.g. tabun, sarin and soman) and the V-agents (e.g. VX);
5 miscellaneous substances (such as ricin).

Tx

All cases should be discussed with a specialist; initially a public health consultant or a poisons unit adviser.
For chlorine, phosgene, ammonia and sulphur dioxide see page 291.
For ammonium nitrate see page 291.
For mustard gas see page 292.
For cyanide see page 292.
For organophosphate and carbamate insecticides and nerve gases see page 293.
For ricin see page 294.
For botulinum toxin see page 240.
For strychnine and brucine see page 239.
For chemical accidents and decontamination see page 297.

> In the United Kingdom, the National Blood Service can supply multi-dose antidote pods containing botulinum antitoxin, cyanide antidote and nerve agent antidotes.

Noxious vapours and gases

Occupational poisoning may occur with gases such as sulphur dioxide, chlorine, ammonia and phosgene. In most cases, there is immediate dyspnoea,

choking, coughing, watering eyes and incapacity. However, pulmonary oedema may develop up to 36 h after a severe exposure.

Tx

Most patients will require inpatient observation. Symptomatic treatment may include:
- oxygen therapy;
- nebulised steroids (e.g. budesonide 2 mg repeated as necessary);
- cough suppressants;
- continuous positive airway pressure (CPAP);
- ventilation with positive end expiratory pressure (PEEP).
- correction of methaemoglobinaemia – *see later.*
For ammonium nitrate (which releases ammonia and other substances) see later.
For carbon monoxide see page 288.
For cyanide see page 292.

Ammonium nitrate

Ammonium nitrate appears as either a colourless, crystalline, solid substance or a white granular powder that is used to make matches, explosives and fertilizers. It is one of the substances that is considered by the Health Protection Agency (UK) to have a high potential for deliberate release. When mixed with other substances, it is highly explosive and can self-ignite to produce ammonia and toxic oxides of nitrogen. Exposure to these fumes causes severe irritation of the eyes, nose, throat and skin; inhalation inflames the respiratory tract and lungs. Absorption may occur through either the skin or lungs and leads to nausea, vomiting, headache and collapse. It may cause methaemoglobinaemia – *see later.* Treatment is symptomatic; nebulised steroids may be of benefit – *see before.*

Methaemoglobinaemia

Exposure to toxic fumes or drugs may oxidise the iron of haem to its ferric (Fe^{3+}) form. The resulting methaemoglobin (met-Hb) cannot carry oxygen. This leads to acute dyspnoea with headache, lethargy, dizziness, nausea and other symptoms of hypoxia. There is a variable degree of cyanosis. Met-Hb causes cyanosis at one-third of the level of deoxygenated haemoglobin (deoxy-Hb) (i.e. 1.5 g per dL of met-Hb causes equivalent cyanosis to 5 g per dL of deoxy-Hb). The presence of met-Hb is suggested by characteristic chocolate-coloured blood but laboratory confirmation of the diagnosis must be obtained. High doses of the local anaesthetic prilocaine may sometimes cause methaemoglobinaemia.

Tx

- Give oxygen.
- Administer IV methylthioninium chloride (methylene blue) 1% at a dose of 1 mg per kg.

Mustard gas

The toxic effect of the vesicant agent mustard gas is primarily due to its alkylating ability. It can penetrate clothing (including leather) and even the 'off-gassing' from casualties may be sufficient to cause symptoms in emergency personnel. There is usually no pain at the time of exposure; symptoms may be delayed for up to 4 to 6 h. Higher environmental concentrations shorten the time for effects to develop but a typical progression is as follows:
- Under 1 hour: Irritation of the eyes, nausea and vomiting are the first signs (if any). Facial erythema may start to appear.
- 2–6 h: There is nausea, fatigue, headache, inflamed eyes, lacrimation, photophobia, rhinorrhoea, sore throat, hoarse voice, erythema of exposed skin (usually face and neck) and tachycardia.
- 8–12 h: The erythema worsens and oedema of the skin develops.
- 12–24 h: There is severe inflammation in areas where there was tight clothing and of the axillae, inner thighs, genitalia, perineum and buttocks. Pendulous blisters appear, which are filled with clear, yellow fluid. Death at this stage is uncommon.
- 48–72 h: This is the stage of maximum blistering. There is intense itching of the skin with an increase in pigmentation. Coughing leads to

expectoration of mucous, pus and necrotic debris from the airways.

Skin changes continue until 7–10 days when healing begins to occur. Recovery is usually complete by 21–28 days.

Treatment is symptomatic and depends on the level of exposure. Patients with minimal symptoms and signs can be discharged after 4–6 h of observation. Those with respiratatory distress may require intensive care.

Cyanide

Cyanide ions block the electron transport chain between the carrier proteins (the mitochondrial cytochromes) and oxygen. This results in a reversible inhibition of oxidative phosphorylation that is the endpoint of cellular respiration. As rapid measurement of blood cyanide levels is not usually available, the diagnosis must be suspected from circumstantial evidence:
- fire brigade suspicion (materials involved, etc.);
- coma/convulsions;
- cardiovascular collapse/dysrhythmias;
- metabolic acidosis/reduced arterio-venous oxygen content difference;
- other signs of inhalation of smoke and fumes (*see page 146*). *For carbon monoxide see page 288*;
- possibility of deliberate release.

Ingestion of cyanide salts may cause delayed poisoning and is an indication for gastric lavage.

Tx

Initial treatment includes administration of 100% oxygen using a non-rebreathing system. Clothing should be removed, skin decontaminated and the eyes irrigated. Cyanide is rapidly detoxified by the human body. Any casualty who is fully conscious and breathing normally more than 5 min after removal from cyanide exposure will recover spontaneously and does not require treatment with an antidote. Blood for cyanide levels (10 mL in a lithium heparin tube) should be taken before antidotes are given as they interfere with the interpretation of cyanide concentrations.

There are several possible antidote regimes for the treatment of severe, life-threatening cyanide poisoning:

1 Combination therapy with sodium nitrite – given IV over 5–20 min (adult dose 300 mg or 10 mL of 3% solution; child 4–10 mg per kg) – and sodium thiosulphate – given IV over 10 min (adult dose 12.5 g or 25 mL of 50% solution; child 400 mg per kg). Sodium nitrite exerts its therapeutic effect by inducing methaemoglobinaemia; methaemoglobin binds cyanide ions. An excess of this process will impair oxygen delivery.

2 Hydroxocobalamin (70 mg per kg by IV infusion; repeated once or twice according to severity of poisoning).

3 If the patient is severely ill (with coma or respiratory depression) and cyanide poisoning is thought most likely to be responsible and sodium nitrite has not been given already, treatment with dicobalt edetate – given IV over 1 min (adult dose 300 mg or 20 mL of 1.5% solution) – followed immediately by 50 mL of 50% glucose IV. This can be repeated once or even twice as necessary. Dicobalt edetate is extremely toxic in the absence of cyanide ions. It can cause laryngeal and pulmonary oedema.

Cholinesterase inhibitors (nerve agents)

This form of poisoning has occurred following the deliberate release of chemical warfare agents and in workers exposed to the related organophosphate and carbamate insecticides. The principle weaponised substances in this group are tabun (GA), sarin (GB), soman (GD), GF and VX. Nerve agents are absorbed through intact skin as well as through the lungs and the gut. Off-gassing from casualties may cause symptoms in emergency personnel. The mechanism of toxicity is inhibition of cholinesterase enzymes (both acetylcholinesterase and pseudocholinesterase) and thus the effects are those of endogenous acetylcholine in massive excess:

1 Muscarinic (parasympathetic) effects: miosis, lacrimation and rhinorrhoea; hypersalivation and sweating; bronchospasm, bronchial hypersecretion and pulmonary oedema; colic and diarrhoea; bradycardia and dysrhythmias

2 Nicotinic (motor and post-ganglionic sympathetic) effects: muscle weakness, fasciculation and flaccid paralysis; hypertension and hyperglycaemia

3 CNS effects: headache, nausea and vomiting; anxiety and restlessness; dizziness, ataxia, confusion, convulsions and coma; central respiratory depression

Death is usually due to respiratory arrest.

Tx

Further absorption must be prevented by emptying the stomach, giving oxygen by mask and removing clothing and washing the skin. Supportive therapy includes oxygen and bronchial suctioning. There are three types of antidote for organophosphorus poisoning:

1 Atropine antagonises the muscarinic effects of acetylcholine (especially hypersecretion and bradycardia). The dose of 2 mg IV (20 μg per kg for a child) can be repeated every 10 min until the pupils dilate and a tachycardia develops.

2 Oximes reactivate inhibited enzyme and thereby decrease the amount of excess acetylcholine. Pralidoxime mesylate (P2S) 30 mg per kg is diluted and given slowly IV over 5–10 min. It improves muscle tone within 30 min and lasts for 4 h. Oximes must be given within 24 h of exposure. Casualties who fail to respond to P2S should be given the second-line cholinesterase reactivator obidoxime (which is also indicated as a first-line drug for tabun (GA) exposure). In the United Kingdom, both drugs are available in multi-dose pods from the National Blood Service.

3 Benzodiazepines are used to control the CNS effects.

The exact treatment depends on the level of exposure and the type of poison. Organophosphates cause an almost irreversible phosphorylation of the active site of the cholinesterase enzymes; carbamates induce a much less stable carbamoylation of the binding sites that may be overcome by atropine alone. Patients with minimal symptoms and signs can be discharged after 4–6 h of observation. Those with respiratatory distress will require intensive care.

Ricin

Ricin, the favourite poison of the old Soviet Secret Service, has recently been linked to terrorist activity. It is a toxalbumin, which is extracted from the beans of the castor oil plant. Accidental poisoning has followed the ingestion of castor oil seeds; as few as 8 seeds have killed an adult. Ricin is particularly toxic if injected, the fatal dose being only 1 μg per kg. Although it is not volatile, it can be effectively spread and inhaled as an aerosol. Ricin inhibits protein synthesis, which rapidly leads to cell death and multi-organ failure. The onset of symptoms and signs may be delayed after absorption via any route. They include:

- fever and widespread mucosal irritation;
- abdominal pain, bloody diarrhoea and vomiting;
- haematuria, proteinuria, raised creatinine and abnormal LFTs;
- pulmonary oedema, pneumonia and ARDS;
- fits and CNS depression.

Tx

Patients should be removed from the source of an aerosol exposure (by personnel with full respiratory and body protection). Their clothing and personal effects should be removed and their skin decontaminated by washing with dilute detergent. Eyes should be irrigated. There is no antidote for ricin and so treatment is supportive. Patients who are still asymptomatic 8 h after ricin ingestion or 24 h after ricin aerosol exposure may be safely discharged.

Biological agents

The Health Protection Agency (UK) considers a number of infectious diseases to have the potential for military or terrorist use. This is either because they are known to have been the subject of attempted weaponisation or because they have characteristics that make deliberate release a dangerous possibility. Such infectious organisms are invariably able to survive for long periods away from their natural host and can usually be distributed as an aerosol for subsequent inhalation by intended victims. Many of these unpleasant infections are zoonoses. The main diseases are:

- Anthrax – *see page 402.*
- Tularaemia – *see page 402.*
- Brucellosis – *see page 262.*
- Q fever – *see page 221.*
- Glanders and melioidosis – *see page 262.*
- Viral haemorrhagic fevers – *see page 260.*
- Plague – *see page 261.*
- Smallpox – *see page 261.*
- Botulism – *see page 240.*

Further considerations in poisoning

Mental state and psychiatric assessment

All patients who have deliberately poisoned themselves should be assessed for suicide risk (*see page 359*). This may entail immediate or delayed psychiatric referral. Most self-poisoned patients need help of some sort and so social and psychological follow-up should be offered (*see page 358*).

Child abuse

Poisoning in childhood is usually the result of accidental ingestion. Public safety measures have highlighted the need for care with the storage of noxious substances. However, there are three circumstances where isolated poisoning in a child may suggest the possibility of child abuse.

1 The ingestion has occurred in an environment of gross neglect. This may also be considered in some episodes of carbon monoxide poisoning following a house fire.

2 The child has been deliberately poisoned, usually as a case of Munchausen's syndrome by proxy – *see page 363.*

3 A crying child has been inappropriately sedated. This is increasingly recognised as the background to some cases of methadone poisoning in childhood. The parents do not intend to harm the child but a disturbed toddler, a bottle of methadone syrup and a rudimentary knowledge of pharmacology may prove to be a disastrous combination. *For the management of suspected child abuse see page 348.*

Chronic poisoning

Heavy metals such as antimony, arsenic, bismuth, gold, mercury and lead are the most usual suspects in chronic poisoning. There have been recent cases of thallium poisoning among political refugees from unstable countries. Suspicion of chronic poisoning merits medical referral for detailed investigation. Antidotes for heavy metals include dimercaprol, penicillamine and sodium calcium edetate.

Forensic aspects

The suspicion of criminal poisoning should provoke a discussion with the police surgeon. Specific urine and blood samples for toxicology may be required. Moreover, there are sometimes coexisting injuries or allegations of sexual interference. Even a detailed history and examination may be carefully dissected in court and so written speculation should be avoided.

Atypical reactions to drugs and other substances

Allergic reactions

> Biphasic reactions, where a second wave of symptoms appears 4–8 h after the initial remission, are seen in a small proportion of patients with anaphylaxis. A single dose of oral prednisolone (1 mg per kg) may be given before discharge to ameliorate such an event, should it occur.

Drugs and foods, especially peanuts, are usually implicated in acute allergic reactions but a collapsed patient will give no history. In the United Kingdom, around one person in 200 (0.5% of the population) is allergic to peanuts. Even minute amounts of peanut allergen can cause very severe reactions.

The presentations of allergy can be divided up according to their immunological basis but for the emergency clinician it is the type and severity of the reaction that is of most significance. Any pattern is possible, combining elements of the following.

Airway (upper airway obstruction)

There is dyspnoea and stridor. This is usually the result of laryngeal oedema but swelling in the mouth or pharynx may also occur.

Tx

- Summon skilled anaesthetic and ENT help.
- Administer adrenaline parenterally *(see Box 15.13)*.
- Consider nebulised adrenaline (5 mg) in less acute cases.
- Give IV hydrocortisone (300 mg) and IV chlorphenamine (10 mg).

Breathing (bronchospasm)

The patient has dyspnoea and wheezing.

Tx

- Request anaesthetic help in severe cases.
- Administer a nebulised bronchodilator (e.g. salbutamol 5 mg).
- Give IV hydrocortisone (300 mg) and IV chlorphenamine (10 mg).
- Consider IV salbutamol or parenteral adrenaline *(see Box 15.13)* in overwhelming reactions.

Circulation (shock)

The circulatory collapse is a result of vasodilatation and maldistribution of fluid. The presence of

---

Box 15.13 Adrenaline for Anaphylaxis

1 in 1000 adrenaline contains 1 mg (1000 μg) per mL. It is usually supplied as a 1 mL (i.e. 1 mg) ampoule.
1 in 10000 adrenaline contains 0.1 mg (100 μg) per mL. It is usually supplied as a 10 mL (i.e. 1 mg) ampoule.
The intravenous dose of adrenaline is 1–3 μg per kg given slowly under ECG control. For an adult this means giving 1 mL (100 μg) aliquots of the 1 in 10,000 solution. The IV (or intra-osseous) route is appropriate in situations that are immediately life-threatening. In less acute situations, the IM route should be used. The IM dose of adrenaline is 5–10 μg per kg.

tachycardia may help to distinguish anaphylaxis from vasovagal syncope.

Tx

- Administer rapid IV fluids (20 mL per kg).
- Give IV hydrocortisone (300 mg) and IV chlorphenamine (10 mg).
- Consider parenteral adrenaline in severe cases (*see Box 15.13*).
- Consider an infusion of IV ephedrine or even IV noradrenaline in prolonged shock.

> Cardiac arrest from acute anaphylaxis is treated in the same way as any other arrest. Intravenous adrenaline will inevitably be given.

Patients who are taking β-blockers appear to have an increased risk of anaphylaxis and may have severe reactions that are difficult to treat. Some effects – especially refractory hypotension – may be lessened by the use of IV glucagon.

Angio-oedema and rashes

Swelling of the face and hands is especially common. The lips and eyelids are often particularly badly affected. In these cases, consideration must be given to the airway. Rashes often occur as an isolated finding. The typical rash is that of urticaria or 'hives'. This is a blotchy, red 'nettle-rash' with raised whitish weals on it. It may persist or reccur for several days or even weeks.

> Diffuse swelling of the face, hands and legs may be due to nephrotic syndrome, rather than allergy.

Tx

- IV or IM antihistamine (e.g. chlorphenamine 10 mg) should be given to all severely affected patients.
- IV or IM hydrocortisone (300 mg) should also be considered in patients with a very severe reaction.
- Supportive and symptomatic treatment should be given as indicated.

- Oral antihistamines are appropriate for continuing treatment or as the sole treatment in minor cases.
- Some patients will benefit from a short course of oral prednisolone.
- Follow-up must be that appropriate for the severity of the allergic reaction–see later.

In all cases, the allergen should be sought and removed as soon as possible. Some clinicians would add an H_2-receptor antagonist (e.g. ranitidine) to the standard antihistamine therapy in severe cases.

Aftercare of allergic reactions

1 Every patient must have a letter for the GP detailing the problem and the treatment.

2 The patient must understand the condition and be aware of the possibility of a further, more serious attack.

3 Patients with potentially serious reactions should be advised to avoid visiting areas where rapid medical help is unavailable – at least until specialist assessment of risk and standby medication has been obtained.

Acute dystonic reactions

Patients presenting with acute dystonic reactions are often misdiagnosed or labelled as hysterical. Young adults and children are most commonly affected. Symptoms vary from isolated problems with swallowing and talking, to generalised spasms of the face, neck and trunk (the occulogyric crisis). Usually, the dystonia is intermittent in severity. It is the reactions affecting only one cranial nerve area that are the most easily mistaken for hysteria. All patients will have recently taken anti-psychotic or anti-emetic drugs (dopamine-receptor antagonists). These may vary from regular depot major tranquillisers to one tablet of metoclopramide. Teenagers may occasionally have abused 'unknown' substances. Anticonvulsants and anti-depressants have also been reported to cause extrapyramidal reactions.

Tx

Symptoms are dramatically relieved by the intravenous injection of a centrally acting anticholinergic (e.g. procyclidine 5–10 mg or benzatropine (benztropine) 1–2 mg). The onset of these drugs, however, usually takes a few minutes and may take longer. Benzodiazepines (e.g. diazepam 10 mg) are also effective. It must be remembered that the antidote is unlikely to last as long as the offending substance. Patients therefore need admission or oral medication to take out.

Occulogyric crises may look very similar to the spasms of both tetanus and strychnine poisoning. *For tetanus (and strychnine poisoning) see page 239.*

Neuroleptic malignant syndrome

This rare, idiosyncratic reaction is most commonly seen soon after starting phenothiazines and related neuroleptic drugs. The relationship between neuroleptic malignant syndrome, serotonin syndrome, severe dystonia and malignant hyperthermia (a life-threatening condition seen during general anaesthesia) is unclear. Typical features of neuroleptic malignant syndrome include:
• muscular rigidity;
• hyperthermia;
• dehydration;
• autonomic instability – pallor, raised BP and tachycardia;
• altered or fluctuating consciousness.

About 10% of patients with this syndrome die, usually as a result of:
• rhabdomyolysis (*see page 255*);
• acute renal failure (*see page 252*);
• pulmonary embolism (*see pages 197 and 223*).

Tx

• Give oxygen.
• Start vigorous rehydration.
• Begin cooling measures (*see page 270*).
• Send blood for electrolytes, glucose, blood gases and creatinine kinase assay.
• Give an antimuscarinic drug to reduce rigidity (e.g. procyclidine 5–10 mg IV).
• Sedate with a benzodiazepine if necessary.
• Consider correcting any acidosis with bicarbonate (*see page 257*).
• Consider arranging admission to HDU or ICU.

Dopamine agonists such as bromocriptine and muscle relaxants such as dantrolene may also have a part to play – *see page 270*. Antipsychotic medication must be stopped.

Serotonin syndrome

Serotonin syndrome is a disorder which is seen infrequently in patients taking selective serotonin reuptake inhibitors (SSRIs). In most cases, it occurs when two or more drugs are taken that interfere with serotonin receptor systems (e.g. SSRI + monoamine oxidase inhibitor or SSRI + tricyclic antidepressant). Symptoms start insidiously within hours of commencing therapy with the second serotinergic drug. The syndrome has also been reported following overdose of SSRIs. There are three main groups of symptoms:
1 Mental changes (seen in 40% of patients) (agitation, confusion, hallucinations, drowsiness and coma)
2 Neuromuscular hyperactivity (seen in 50% of patients) (tremor, shivering and myoclonus)
3 Autonomic instability (seen in 50% of patients) (tachycardia, fever, hypertension or hypotension)

Flushing, diarrhoea and vomiting are also common. In severe cases, fits, hyperthermia, rhabdomyolysis, renal failure and coagulopathies may also develop.

Tx

Most mild cases resolve spontaneously within 24 h. Serotinergic drugs should be stopped and electrolytes and creatinine kinase monitored in all patients. Supportive therapy includes anticonvulsants, IV fluids and cooling measures. There are reported uses of both propranolol and cyproheptadine to control symptoms. Treatment of malignant hyperthermia with dantrolene (*see page 270*) may be required.

For routine treatment of poisoning with SSRIs see page 277.

Contamination and irradiation

Contamination by toxic chemicals

In the United Kingdom there is a national centre called the Focus, which monitors and provides advice on chemical incidents. It is situated at the University of Wales Institute in Cardiff. There is a 24 h emergency hotline.

At the scene

The senior fire officer is responsible for identification of the substance(s) involved and for deciding the level of protection appropriate for personnel and the environment. The fire service will usually carry out immediate decontamination using running water. The patient should be kept warm and removed to a well-ventilated and protected area. Resuscitation may need to precede decontamination, in which case direct skin and mucosal contact with the patient should be avoided.

In the emergency department

The contaminated patient should be taken to a designated area. If volatile substances are involved, the hospital engineers must be alerted to prevent contamination of the air-conditioning systems. Staff should wear protective clothing; gloves and gown are usually sufficient. Further decontamination of the patient may be effected by washing with soap and water or showering for 20 min. A special bath with a collecting tub for contaminated water should be used and movements of the patient in the department must be kept to a minimum. Some substances (e.g. phenol) may cause severe systemic poisoning by skin contact alone.

Contamination by radioactive substances

At the scene

It is the responsibility of the police force to seek advice and to take appropriate measures to secure the scene.

In the emergency department

• The local radiation protection officer should be contacted for advice and to measure the level of radioactive contamination.
• A predetermined and separate entrance and treatment area for isolation and decontamination

should be demarcated. This area must have a shower and water collection facility as detailed above. Floors of treatment and transit areas should be covered with disposable sheeting, as should non-disposable equipment. Air conditioning must be switched off and portable equipment removed.
• Involved staff must wear theatre suits, long plastic aprons, caps, overshoes and two pairs of gloves.
• Patients and staff must not eat, drink or smoke within the designated area.
• There must be a place to decontaminate staff on arrival from the scene and before leaving the designated area. All personnel involved must be checked by the radiation protection adviser and should have a shower before leaving this area.
• Resuscitation is still the first priority but efforts must be made throughout to limit the spread of radioactive particles.
• Levels of radiation should be measured before and after decontamination.
• All clothing, swabs and fluids should be handled carefully and collected in labelled bags and containers.
• Areas of the body unprotected by clothing take priority. Hands and nails should be cleaned with running water and surgical scrub for 5 min. Hair must be washed (with any shampoo) in a similar way; showers should not be taken whilst the hair is contaminated. The face should be cleaned and ears and eyes irrigated. The nose must be blown and the mouth washed out. Vacuum cleaning is sometimes recommended. If radiation monitoring confirms residual contamination of skin, then cleaning should be attempted with 5% potassium permanganate solution for 5 min. The brown staining is removed by the application of 5% sodium bisulphite. This system gives a visual confirmation of coverage and removal.
• Wounds must be covered prior to surface decontamination and later cleaned by direct irrigation.

Irradiation

A patient who has received a toxic dose of ionising radiation alone does not present a contamination threat or need decontamination. Features suggestive of significant penetrating irradiation that may progress to full radiation sickness include:

- a history of loss of consciousness (this suggests a high dose of radiation with a bad prognosis);
- transient erythema after 24 h;
- nausea, diarrhoea and vomiting;
- an early and dramatic fall in the white cell count.

Tx

The development of radiation sickness is a delayed phenomenon and at-risk patients should be referred to the nearest oncology unit after discussion with the local radiation protection adviser. A history of irradiation should not delay immediate resuscitation or surgery. Because of the immuno-suppressive effect of the radiation, all surgery should be carried out as soon as possible and certainly within 36 h of the incident.

It is important to distinguish between patients who have been contaminated by radioactive particles and those who have been irradiated. The former can spread radiation; the latter cannot. Some will be in both categories.

Chapter 16

Abdominal pain

Pain in the abdomen is a common symptom that is managed by surgeons, physicians, gynaecologists, paediatricians and especially by GPs. Patients from all of these domains may present to an ED; they may arrive critically ill and require resuscitation, they may have an acute illness that is best managed by admission or they may present with a problem that can be further investigated on an outpatient basis.

For abdominal injury see page 84.

For abdominal pain in children see pages 341 and 343.

For perineal problems see Chapter 17.

Immediate assessment and management

In the patient who is distressed and in severe pain or otherwise clearly unwell:

- give high-concentration oxygen;
- start an infusion of Hartmann's solution or saline;
- monitor pulse, BP, SaO$_2$ and temperature;
- consider the need for a 12-lead ECG;
- give IV analgesia with an antiemetic;
- pass a urinary catheter if there is a distended bladder or any suggestion of fluid depletion;
- insert a nasogastric tube if there is abdominal distension;
- ask for surgical advice.

> **Box 16.1 Causes of Collapse with Abdominal Pain**
>
> Acute blood loss from the upper gastrointestinal tract (oesophageal varices and peptic ulceration).
> Perforation of a peptic ulcer, sigmoid diverticulum or the appendix.
> Acute pancreatitis.
> Leaking aortic aneurysm.
> Mesenteric infarction.
> Intra-abdominal sepsis with septic shock.
> Ruptured ectopic pregnancy.
> Hypovolaemia from any abdominal cause.
> Diabetic ketoacidosis.
> Cardiorespiratory pathology (e.g. MI or PE).

For causes of collapse with abdominal pain see Box 16.1.

> Leaking abdominal aortic aneurysm is common but the symptoms and signs are often unremarkable. The diagnosis should always be considered in patients who have either collapsed or have trunk pain.

Further assessment

Ask about

- Site and speed of onset of the pain.
- Character and duration of the pain.
- Exacerbating and relieving factors.
- Radiation of the pain.
- Accompanying features such as nausea and vomiting.

- General health, family and past history, drugs and allergies.
- Travel abroad.

Think about the patient's anxieties and why, if there is a long history, the patient chose this moment to present to hospital.

Look for

- Abdominal tenderness and guarding.
- Rebound tenderness.
- Rigidity.
- Bowel sounds.
- Loin tenderness.
- Hernias.
- Perineal signs (*see Boxes 16.2 and 16.3*).
- Chest disease.

> Sudden deterioration in a patient with abdominal symptoms is usually caused by acute blood loss, frequently from the upper gastrointestinal tract or an aortic aneurysm. In the absence of haematemesis, PR examination or the introduction of a nasogastric tube can be diagnostic.

Box 16.2 Rectal Examination

Rectal examination can provide information about:
- perianal pathology
- sphincter tone
- the rectal contents (empty, consistency of stool, presence of blood or melaena)
- the rectal wall (over the age of 50 years carcinoma is increasingly common)
- pelvic masses or tenderness, including the appendix
- the prostate gland.

If the presenting symptoms and signs could not be expected to be associated with any of the abnormalities in this list, then there is no indication to undertake a rectal examination.

Oesophageal pain and bleeding

Haemorrhage from oesophageal varices

This occurs in about one-third of patients with chronic liver disease and has a high mortality. The patient may have ascites and encephalopathy and often has deficient clotting factors.

Box 16.3 Vaginal Examination

This must be acknowledged as a very invasive procedure, particularly in young or nulliparous women. Do not consider undertaking any intimate examination unless you have:
- appropriate training
- an experienced chaperone
- privacy
- the confidence of the patient
- reason to believe that the findings of the examination will influence management.

Before the examination
Explain the need for the procedure and what it will entail (including any potential pain or discomfort).
Give the patient an opportunity to ask questions.
Obtain the patient's permission.
Give the patient privacy to undress and later on to dress; use sheets to protect the patient's dignity.

During the examination
Do not make any irrelevant, personal or ambiguous comments.
Encourage questions and discussion.
Stop if the patient becomes distressed or requests that you terminate the examination.

Tx

See gastrointestinal haemorrhage on page 303.

Oesophageal pain

Oesophagitis is caused by reflux of gastric contents. It is sometimes associated with a hiatus hernia. The patient is often obese and experiences burning retrosternal pain on lying flat and bending down. The pain is relieved by antacids and by sitting up. Severity of symptoms does not correlate well with endoscopic findings.

> Oesophageal spasm is rare and should not be diagnosed in the ED. Myocardial pain is almost identical and is very common.

Investigations

Myocardial infarction should be considered – *see page 183.* A normal ECG does not exclude MI. A trial of antacids and observation may be helpful.

Tx

Patients in whom MI cannot be excluded must be admitted for observation. However if:

- the history is indicative of oesophagitis;
- the examination and ECG are normal; and
- the patient responds to antacid,

then referral can be made to the GP for further care (weight reduction, small regular meals, stopping smoking, antacids and alginates). A course of a proton pump inhibitor (e.g. omeprazole or rabeprazole 20 mg daily for 4 weeks) will give rapid relief of symptoms and promote healing.

Oesophageal pain and bleeding after vomiting

Oesophageal injury may be caused by repeated vomiting, often after excessive alcohol consumption. A small tear of the mucosa may cause bleeding (Mallory–Weiss syndrome – usually seen in chronic alcoholics). Sometimes this is accompanied by diffuse, intense, retrosternal pain, suggestive of a transmural injury. Mediastinitis is then a common sequel and is often fatal.

Investigations

A plain chest X-ray may reveal air in the mediastinum or a foreign body. A Gastrografin swallow should be arranged. Oesophagoscopy is hazardous.

Tx

An IV infusion must be commenced and analgesia prescribed. The patient should be given nil by mouth and then admitted for systemic antibiotics and observation.

Pain in the upper abdomen

Dyspepsia and gastritis

Epigastric pain and tenderness may often be seen in young adults, especially following alcohol ingestion. Some of these cases will settle with minimal therapy while others will subsequently prove to result from peptic ulceration. The non-endoscopic diagnosis of gastritis is thus dependent on the history and on the magnitude and duration of the symptoms and signs.

Tx

The majority of patients with a recent onset of dyspepsia will settle quickly with antacids. However, many GPs will treat undiagnosed dyspepsia in young adults (who have a low risk of gastric malignancy) with a short course of an oral H_2-receptor antagonist. Ranitidine (which can be bought over the counter) is suitable; 150 mg b.d. for a maximum of 14 days should be prescribed. A similar course of a proton pump inhibitor (e.g. omeprazole or rabeprazole 10–20 mg daily) is even more effective. Patients in severe pain will require analgesia and admission for investigation, including barium meal or gastroscopy. The eradication of *Helicobacter pylori* is now thought to be the main aim of long-term therapy.

Peptic ulceration

Dyspeptic pain and tenderness in the epigastrium are the cardinal features of peptic ulceration. Vomiting may also occur, especially with a gastric ulcer. Management depends on the severity and duration of the symptoms and signs – *see before*. The differentiation between gastric and duodenal ulceration is of little clinical importance in the ED. Gastric carcinoma is associated with profound anorexia, weight loss and anaemia.

There are three other serious acute presentations of peptic ulceration, none of which necessarily follow episodes of dyspepsia.

1 Perforation – *For generalised peritonitis secondary to perforation see page 303.*

2 Haemorrhage – *See gastrointestinal haemorrhage on page 303.*

3 Pyloric stenosis – This is usually associated with a chronic ulcer history but there is often no recent pain. It presents with episodic projectile vomiting, unrelated to eating. Examination reveals undernourishment and a succussion splash resulting from the full stomach. Hypochloraemia, hypocalcaemia and metabolic alkalosis are common. Initial management is therefore directed at the

correction of the dehydration and electrolyte disturbance. The stomach is emptied by a wide-bore oral tube prior to endoscopic assessment.

Gastrointestinal haemorrhage

The patient with a gastrointestinal bleed may present with any combination of:

- haematemesis;
- melaena;
- passage of bright red blood per rectum;
- hypotension, shock and collapse;
- sub-acute symptoms (fatigue from anaemia, etc.).

Peptic ulceration is by far the most common cause of serious gastrointestinal haemorrhage (more than half of all cases) but bleeding may also be seen in:

- gastritis and gastric erosions (e.g. following alcohol or NSAIDs);
- oesophagitis;
- Mallory–Weiss syndrome (oesophageal tear after vomiting) – *see page 302*;
- oesophageal varices;
- diverticulitis (copious melaena or bright red blood);
- neoplastic and clotting disorders (variable presentations);
- minor conditions of the rectum (e.g. piles – *see page 322*).

Severe bleeding from the small intestine is rare.

> For patients admitted to hospital with upper GI bleeding, overall mortality rates are around 1 in 7; the majority of deaths occur in older people. *For high risk factors see Box 16.4.*

Tx

- Protect the airway and give oxygen.
- Start immediate volume replacement via two large-bore cannuli. Central venous access may be required.
- Monitor vital functions.
- Discuss the patient with the admitting teams. (Usually both medical and surgical liaison is appropriate).
- Take blood for cross-matching (6 units), clotting screen, full blood count, glucose, urea and electrolytes and LFTs.

> **Box 16.4 Patients Most Likely to Die from Upper GI Bleeding**
>
> Over 60 years old
> Serious concomitant disease
> Systolic BP less than 90 mmHg on admission
> Hb less than 10g per dL on admission
> Evidence of re-bleeding.

- Obtain a chest X-ray and an ECG.
- Catheterise the patient and monitor the urine output.
- Correct clotting abnormalities (vitamin K+/− FFP – *see page 264*). Consider acquired haemophilia – *see page 263*.
- Consider terlipressin (2 mg IV), vasopressin (20 units IV over 15 min), octreotide (a somatostatin analogue given at 50 μg an hour IV) or balloon tamponade in suspected oesophageal variceal bleeding secondary to portal hypertension. (When using a Sengstaken–Blakemore tube, inflation of the gastric balloon alone is usually adequate to control bleeding. The oesophageal balloon may cause damage, especially post-sclerotherapy.)
- Consider an IV infusion of omeprazole (40 mg diluted to 100 mL and given over 20–30 min) in suspected gastroduodenal bleeding.

Endoscopic assessment (which should be performed within 24 h of admission) usually precedes any decision to operate.

Peritonitis

Generalized peritonitis causes:

- severe abdominal pain;
- a rigid (board-like) abdomen;
- hypotension and shock.

It usually occurs secondary to a perforated viscus in:

- peptic ulceration;
- appendicitis;
- diverticulitis;
- neoplastic or inflammatory bowel disease;
- trauma;
- iatrogenic injury.

The pain of perforation begins suddenly. After a few minutes its severity is reduced but the abdomen remains rigid – especially the epigas-trium. The pulse is elevated and the patient is pale and anxious but not initially 'shocked'. Rigidity and pain may decrease after a few hours but bowel sounds remain absent. Symptoms increase again after 6 h as bacterial peritonitis develops. Vomiting may occur. The patient is often elderly or has a recent history of NSAID ingestion.

Investigations

An erect chest X-ray will show gas under the diaphragm in many (but not all) cases.

Tx

Vigorous fluid resuscitation, analgesia and surgi-cal referral. If antibiotics are required, then a cephalosporin and metronidazole are a reasonable first-line choice.

Hepatitis

Hepatitis is caused by:
- viruses with an enteric mode of transmission (hepatitis A and E) – *see later;*
- viruses with a parenteral mode of transmission (hepatitis B, C and D). (*For immunisation against hepatitis B see page 399*);
- Weil's disease (leptospirosis) – *see below;*
- drugs.

Leptospirosis

Leptospirosis or Weil's disease occurs after mucosal contact with water that has been infected by rat's urine. It is sometimes fatal and should always be considered when a pyrexia and abdominal pain is found in:
- sewage workers;
- farmers;
- water board workers;
- people who have been swimming in fresh water;
- people who have been sleeping rough.
The incubation period is about 10 days (range 4–21 days).

Infectious hepatitis (hepatitis A)

This is by far the most common cause of hepatitis. Transmission is by the faecal–oral route and the incubation period is 6 days to 6 weeks. Outbreaks may occur in primary schools and in other insti-tutions. Hepatitis causes a variable degree of:
- anorexia and malaise;
- nausea and vomiting;
- abdominal pain and right upper quadrant tenderness;
- jaundice;
- dark urine and pale stools;
- pyrexia;
- urticaria;
- hepatomegaly and splenomegaly.

Investigations

There is bilirubin and urobilinogen in the urine.

Tx

Admission is required for patients who:
- are significantly jaundiced;
- are clearly very unwell; or
- have an uncertain diagnosis.
   Those with hepatitis A (young, short duration of symptoms and limited signs) can be treated at home and followed-up by the GP. Strict hygiene must be observed with a light diet and no alcohol.

Biliary disease

Acute cholecystitis

Inflammation of the gall-bladder with or without intermittent obstruction at its neck leads to acute cholecystitis. There is:
- constant right upper quadrant pain, referred to the back;
- localised tenderness;
- nausea and vomiting;
- fever and malaise;
- a palpable gall-bladder (sometimes).
   (In more chronic cases, dyspepsia may be the presenting symptom. Pain is worse after a large, fat-laden meal, and heartburn and belching are

common. If these are the only symptoms, then further investigation can be pursued on an outpatient basis.)

Biliary colic

This presents as sudden, colicky, epigastric and right hypochrondrial pain radiating to the back. There is tenderness in the right upper quadrant and vomiting is common. Impaction of the stone may be transient or last for several hours, with the pain disappearing as suddenly as it started. Significant hold-up of a stone in the common bile duct is unusual but will be associated with more prolonged symptoms and the gradual appearance of obstructive jaundice.

Investigations

Early ultrasound examination confirms the diagnosis.

Tx

Analgesia and admission. In the presence of a fever, antibiotics (a cephalosporin or gentamicin) should be prescribed.

Pancreatitis

The main predisposing factors are:
- chronic biliary disease; and
- excess alcohol consumption.

The pain may begin suddenly but is then constant and very severe. It is accompanied by vomiting and may be relieved by sitting forward. The pain differs from that associated with perforation of a peptic ulcer in that it radiates to the back and extends from the epigastrium bilaterally. There is epigastric tenderness and guarding and decreased bowel sounds. Pyrexia is uncommon but tachycardia is usual. In severe cases the BP falls, cyanosis may be present and the patient is brought in as a 'collapse'.

Investigations

- A serum amylase above 1200 iu per mL is considered diagnostic. Lower levels may be caused by

other abdominal conditions or by a myocardial infarction.
- The sodium, potassium and calcium are usually low.
- The plasma white cell count is invariably raised.
- The serum bilirubin may be raised.
- There may be hypoxia and an effusion on chest X-ray.
- ECG may show non-specific abnormalities.

Tx

Initial treatment is nil by mouth, nasogastric aspiration, IV fluids and antibiotics. Analgesia must be given. The patient may need intensive care and laparotomy for peritoneal toilet.

Pain in the central and lower abdomen

Leaking abdominal aortic aneurysm

Leaking aortic aneurysm is most often seen in an older (>55 years) patient who has generalised vascular disease. Symptoms and signs are variable but include:
- back pain (sometimes with a previous episode a few days before);
- generalised abdominal pain with vague tenderness and fullness (pain may radiate to the groin);
- hypotension;
- pallor and sweating;
- sudden collapse.

Classical features are often absent; an expansile, pulsatile mass may not be detected and the femoral pulses may be present and not delayed with respect to the radial. Pain may not be severe.

> Only about 50% of patients with a ruptured aortic aneurysm reach hospital alive. A further 10% are unsuitable for surgery. For the remainder, the operative mortality is between 30 and 60%.

Investigations

Routine blood tests including clotting studies should be ordered. On admission, 60% of patients with a ruptured aortic aneurym have coagulopathy,

40% have low platelets and 30% have impaired renal function.

The ECG usually shows ischaemic changes as 90% of this group of patients have coronary heart disease and the pre-existing coronary ischaemia is worsened by hypotension. (Atherosclerosis of other vascular beds is also common.)

There is no indication for a plain abdominal radiograph. However, if performed in cases where the diagnosis is not yet established, it may show the lumbar vertebrae notched by a chronically expanding aorta and an enlarged, calcified vessel wall.

If there is doubt about the diagnosis, then ultrasound scan of the abdomen will show an aortic mass and free fluid if there is a leaking aneurysm. None of these investigations should delay surgical referral.

Tx

- Give oxygen.
- Start two infusions via large-bore cannuli. Volume replacement in the ED should be carefully controlled; the objective is to maintain adequate cerebral and coronary perfusion without increasing blood loss. Fluids should be given until large pulses are palpable, aiming to keep systolic BP around 70–90 mmHg but no higher.
- Monitor pulse, BP, SaO$_2$ and ECG.
- Call for surgical and anaesthetic help.
- Cross-match 8–10 units of packed red blood cells and order a similar number of units of both fresh frozen plasma and platelets. (Median transfusion requirements are 6–10 units.) Excessive fluids may rupture a leaking aneurysm but anaemia will also be harmful in this low output state. Therefore, transfusion with packed cells should begin as soon as possible. (Haemoglobin should be kept around 10 g per dL and always above 8 g per dL.)
- Send blood for FBC, clotting studies, urea, electrolytes and glucose.
- Obtain an ECG and a chest X-ray.
- Give small increments of IV analgesia as required (but be careful as opiates will reduce vital sympathetic tone).
- Pass a urinary catheter and measure the urine output.

Other intra-abdominal bleeding

- Ruptured ectopic pregnancy – *see page 316*.
- The diseased and enlarged spleen may bleed dramatically after trivial injury or even spontaneously (e.g. during malaria or glandular fever).
- Haemophiliacs and patients on anticoagulant therapy may bleed spontaneously. Consider acquired haemophilia – *see page 263*.

Mesenteric vascular disease

Problems with the blood supply of the bowel are difficult to diagnose clinically and are often only found at laparotomy. These diagnoses should be thought of in older patients (usually over 60 years) with other evidence of cardiovascular disease, who are disproportionately unwell and distressed for their clinical signs.

Mesenteric infarction

This usually involves the superior mesenteric vessels and is approximately equally split between cases of embolism and thrombosis. Symptoms are caused by infected, dying bowel in the abdominal cavity and are compounded by fluid loss into the bowel and perforation.

Once the condition has developed, the patient is hypotensive and looks very ill. The pain is diffuse, severe and poorly localised. There is generalised abdominal tenderness and guarding with shifting dullness. Bowel sounds are decreased and there may be some abdominal distension. Vomiting is an early feature and bloody diarrhoea is passed per rectum. The mortality rate is very high (over 50%).

Mesenteric angina

Recurrent bouts of severe abdominal pain in elderly patients may be a result of ischaemia of the bowel. The pain may be followed by episodes of obstruction or bloody diarrhoea (ischaemic colitis).

Mesenteric venous thrombosis

Venous occlusion gives rise to a similar clinical picture to infarction but is even more insidious in onset and in symptoms and signs.

Investigations

The haemoglobin and amylase are often raised, with a high white cell count. An elevated D-dimer, although not very specific, is a very sensitive indicator of ischaemic bowel. Therefore, a normal D-dimer makes the presence of necrotic bowel extremely unlikely.

Plain radiographs are invariably unremarkable, although 'thumb-printing' of the wall of the bowel is sometimes seen. ECG should be performed to rule out coexisting myocardial ischaemia and to look for a source of emboli. Mesenteric angiography may be used to confirm the diagnosis.

Tx

Comprehensive resuscitation with early fluid replacement and analgesia is essential, together with prompt referral to the admitting surgical team.

Appendicitis

Appendicitis may occur at any age but is most common between the ages of 15 and 30 years and is uncommon under the age of 2 years. The usual features are:

- abdominal pain (the pain is initially periumbilical or epigastric, later radiating to the right iliac fossa);
- localised tenderness;
- nausea and anorexia;
- coated tongue and halitosis;
- mild leucocytosis.

Pyrexia and tachycardia are unusual. The right iliac fossa is usually the most tender and guarded part of the abdomen but symptoms and signs may vary from the classical description:

- *Retrocaecal appendix* – pain may be elicited by right hip extension or be greatest in the right hypochrondrium.
- *Appendix in the pelvis* – rectal examination reveals tenderness high up on the right. There may be diarrhoea.
- *Appendix has become gangrenous or has perforated* – the patient presents with signs of generalised peritonitis (*see page 303*).

> **Box 16.5 The Differential Diagnosis of Acute Appendicitis**
>
> Urinary tract infection.
> Mesenteric adenitis.
> Ovulation pain (Mittelschmerz).
> Salpingitis.
> Ovarian cyst torsion.
> Constipation.
> Pancreatitis.
> Psoas haematoma (in haemophiliacs).
> Perforated Meckel's diverticulum.
> Non-specific abdominal pain.
> Gastrointestinal upset in athlete.

Occasionally, an appendix mass will have developed.

Investigations

As the diagnosis is made on the basis of history and examination, special investigations are not indicated in the ED unless alternative diagnoses are being considered (*see Box 16.5*).

Tx

The patient should be referred for admission. If the appendix is thought to be leaking, then IV metronidazole should be commenced.

Diverticular disease

This usually occurs in patients over the age of 50 years. There are three common acute presentations:

1 Inflammation (diverticulitis) causes periumbilical pain radiating to the left iliac fossa. There is localised tenderness and guarding in the left lower quadrant and a mass may be palpable. The patient may be pyrexial.

2 Perforation may occur without previous symptoms, producing acute peritonitis – *see page 303*.

3 Copious bleeding per rectum may cause profound shock – *see page 303*.

Tx

All three conditions require surgical referral.

Inflammatory bowel disease

Ulcerative colitis

The patient with known ulcerative colitis may present to the ED with a fulminating attack. This is not usually associated with severe abdominal pain. Blood-stained mucusy diarrhoea is the most common feature with fever, tachycardia and hypotension.

Crohn's disease

This may rarely present as undiagnosed abdominal pain to the ED. There is usually a long history of recurrent diarrhoea and colic leading to anaemia and the development of an abdominal mass. The cicatrised small bowel may obstruct or perforate. If the patient presents with acute pain in the right iliac fossa, the previous history of diarrhoea should help to distinguish the condition from appendicitis.

Investigations

Abdominal X-ray may show a dilated colon in ulcerative colitis. Routine blood tests should be requested.

Tx

Intravenous fluid replacement is started and the admitting surgeons contacted.

Intestinal obstruction

The basic causes of intestinal obstruction are:
- *blocked lumen* – food, foreign body, faeces and very rarely a gallstone;
- *thickened wall* – carcinoma, Crohn's disease, tuberculosis;
- *altered geometry* – intussusception, volvulus;
- *external compression* – herniae, inflammatory bands, adhesions;
- *absent peristalsis* – paralytic ileus, mesenteric infarction.

> The early features of intestinal obstruction can be mistaken for mild gastroenteritis. Small-bowel obstruction in the femoral hernia of an obese patient may be overlooked.

Paralytic ileus

This occurs after major abdominal surgery, but is most often seen in the ED in association with retroperitoneal haematomas, spinal and head injuries and electrolyte disturbances.

Small-bowel obstruction

Small-bowel obstruction begins with periumbilical, intermittent, colicky pain. Vomiting is an early feature of jejunal obstruction but is delayed by a few hours in ileal obstruction. The patient usually presents at an early stage of the obstructive process; visible peristalsis may be seen and bowel sounds are increased. Later, the patient becomes dehydrated and oliguric. Central abdominal distension is occasionally evident. After the large bowel has been evacuated there is absolute constipation (no faeces or flatus per rectum).

Large-bowel obstruction

This usually presents as an acute-on-chronic problem. Increasing constipation is the first symptom and abdominal distension is marked before the colicky pains become significant. The caecum becomes enlarged and tender unless the ileocaecal valve is incompetent. Vomiting is a late feature. Dehydration and major electrolyte abnormalities are often present by the time the patient is seen in the ED.

Strangulated bowel

When the blood supply to the obstructed bowel is impaired – for example, by the neck of a hernial sac – strangulation quickly ensues. Pain becomes more generalised and continuous and the tachycardia increases. Rarely, these signs of impending necrosis and perforation are present without early evidence of obstruction if only part of the bowel wall is captured in a hernial sac (Richter's hernia).

Investigations

An abdominal radiograph may show dilated bowel and fluid levels (although there are many causes of fluid levels). Full blood count, urea and electrolytes and glucose may reveal dehydration and metabolic disturbance.

Tx

- Administer IV fluids.
- Insert a nasogastric tube.
- Give analgesia.
- Refer to the surgical team.

For intussusception in children see page 343.

Diarrhoea

For diarrhoea and vomiting in children see page 343.

With diarrhoea, the history is central to the diagnosis. Consider:

- appendicitis – *see page 307*;
- pelvic abscess;
- infective and traveller's diarrhoea – *see page 260*;
- metabolic disturbance;
- recent antibiotic therapy;
- recent surgery; and
- athlete's diarrhoea. (Up to one-third of athletes have a history of gastrointestinal upset. The cause is usually not clearly defined, although gut ischaemia has been implicated.)

Patients who are clearly ill or significantly dehydrated will need admission.

'Renal' colic

Ureteric colic presents as severe and sudden bouts of pain radiating from the loin to the groin. Vomiting and sweating are usual and the patient often strains to pass small quantities of urine. The calculus is frequently held up proximal to the ureteric orifice in the base of the bladder at the trigone. The sensory nerve supply of the latter is identical to that of the external urethral meatus, as they share a common embryological origin. Hence trigonal pain is interpreted as arising from the tip of the external meatus.

> Patients with Munchausen syndrome commonly present with features of renal colic – *see page 362.*

Investigations

Renal colic invariably causes microscopic haematuria. Urine should be tested for blood with reagent sticks and then sent for microscopy and culture. Blood tests should include serum calcium and uric acid levels as well as standard FBC, urea and electrolytes. A plain abdominal radiograph may be requested to show the course of the ureters in the abdomen and pelvis (a 'KUB' X-ray) – 90% of stones are radio-opaque. Early IVU is desirable.

Tx

Analgesia must be given as soon as possible – NSAIDs are effective (e.g. tenoxicam 20 mg IV/IM or diclofenac 75 mg IM). Opiates are an alternative. All patients with renal pain and blood in the urine will require admission for further analgesia and investigation.

Stones elsewhere in the urinary tract

Bladder stones are rare in the United Kingdom. Stones in the renal pelvis are common but usually present to the outpatient clinic or are entirely asymptomatic. (They may cause chronic, dull pain and loin tenderness with intermittent infection or haematuria.)

Urinary tract infection

The symptoms of urinary tract infection (UTI) vary according to the site of infection and the age and sex of the patient. Pyelitis causes unilateral loin pain, tenderness and fever. Cystitis gives dysuria, frequency and urgency with or without haematuria. Both may cause some lower abdominal pain and tenderness. Some patients with urinary tract infection will be generally unwell, with evidence of systemic infection but few localising signs (especially infants and the elderly).

For the investigation and treatment of UTI see page 319.

Acute retention of urine

Acute retention of urine causes severe abdominal pain, which is usually accompanied by a history of inability to pass urine. The enlarged bladder is easily palpable although it may be overlooked in the obese patient. *For causes and treatment see page 320.*

Pain from the testis and epididymus

Pain from the region of the scrotum is usually referred to the lower abdomen. The perineum of all patients with abdominal pain must therefore be examined.
For perineal problems see Chapter 17.

Pelvic inflammatory disease

Inflammation of the pelvic structures is usually caused by chlamydial or gonococcal infection and is therefore a manifestation of sexually transmitted disease in women of child-bearing age. Recurrent or chronic infections may cause ectopic pregnancy and infertility.

The presenting symptom is usually bilateral lower abdominal pain, although unilateral discomfort may be seen. The history may also reveal malaise, nausea, menstrual disturbance and vaginal discharge. Signs include fever, tenderness, guarding and cervical excitation (pain on moving the cervix). There may be tenderness of the uterus and in the fornices.

Investigations

Full blood count, ESR and MSU should be arranged, together with a pregnancy test. High vaginal, urethral and endocervical (chlamydial) swabs are also required but the acquisition of these is usually best left to a specialist. Laparoscopy may be needed to collect definitive specimens for culture.

Tx

The condition is an inflammation and so injection of a NSAID (eg. Tenoxlcam 20 mg IV) can give con-siderable relief. Patients in severe pain or with hard signs should be admitted. Other patients can be followed-up by the GP or in a gynaecology or genitourinary outpatient clinic. A short course of NSAIDs can be given to take out but antibiotics (usually doxycycline for 7 days or erythromycin for 14 days) should only be prescribed after swabs have been taken. Ofloxacin and metronidazole are used for severe infections.

Other gynaecological causes of pain

For bleeding PV see page 315.
For ectopic pregnancy see page 316.
For threatened and incomplete abortion see page 315.
For dysmenorrhoea see page 318.

Rupture of an ovarian cyst causes sudden, lower abdominal pain with localised tenderness.

Torsion of an ovarian cyst causes lower abdominal pain and tenderness that may be recurrent. There may be a mass on abdominal or PV examination.

Endometriosis gives rise to recurrent abdominal pain, which is worse during menstrual bleeding. Other gynaecological symptoms are often present.
For obstetric, gynaecological and perineal problems see Chapter 17.

Non-specific abdominal pain

Some patients have abdominal pain for which no obvious diagnosis can be found. Non-specific abdominal pain should only be diagnosed in an adult under 50 years of age, with minimal symptoms and signs, who settles quickly.

If discharged, the patient should be advised to visit his or her GP within a few days for follow-up.

Non-surgical causes of abdominal pain

Many conditions may present with abdominal pain as a feature. They include the following:
• *Cardiac pain.* Myocardial ischaemia may present as acute upper abdominal pain. Right ventricular

failure, leading to hepatic engorgement, may be associated with right hypochondrial pain.

• *Diaphragmatic irritation.* Pleurisy caused by a chest infection or pulmonary embolus may present with hypochondrial pain, worse on deep inspiration. There is usually referred shoulder tip pain in addition.

• *Pneumonia.* Children with pneumonia may present with abdominal pain – *see page 334.*

• *Alcohol withdrawal – see page 355.*

• *Poisoning.*

• *Diabetes.* Generalised abdominal pain associated with hyperglycaemia precoma.

• *Migraine, epilepsy, lead poisoning and porphyria.* All may present with acute central abdominal pain.

• *Herpes zoster.* Unilateral pain extending round either flank in the distribution of a cutaneous nerve. The herpetic eruption appears 24–48 h after the onset of pain – *see page 203.*

• *Collapsed vertebra.* Usually the result of osteoporosis but may be caused by a secondary neoplastic lesion or tuberculosis. Pain may be generalised and not evidently arising from the spine.

• *Muscle injury.* Rupture of part of the rectus abdominis or avulsion of the origin of the external oblique produces severe abdominal pain. It is exacerbated by attempting to sit up with arms folded over the chest.

• *Sickle cell crisis – see page 263.*

• *Munchausen syndrome – see page 362.*

A patient who has presented with acute abdominal pain should not be discharged unless the diagnosis is confidently recognised as trivial or the patient has been discussed with and assessed by a senior colleague. Arrangements should be made for the patient to be followed-up in a hospital clinic or by the GP.

Chapter 17

Obstetric, gynaecological, genitourinary and perineal problems

Problems in pregnancy

For the abdomen in pregnancy see Figure 17.1.

Precipitant delivery

In the United Kingdom, most pregnant women have planned maternity care and so have made clear arrangements for the delivery of their baby. However, occasionally women arrive at the ED in the second stage of labour (i.e. after the cervix is fully dilated). Delivery of the baby may be imminent and assistance must be given (*see Boxes 17.1 and 17.2 and Figure 17.2*).

Antepartum haemorrhage

This is vaginal bleeding occurring after 24 weeks' gestation and is caused by placental abruption, placenta praevia or other less common lesions. The bleeding of placenta praevia is usually painless and starts around the thirty-second week of gestation as the lower uterine segment is beginning to form. With abruption, severe blood loss

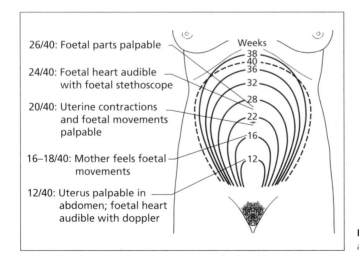

26/40: Foetal parts palpable

24/40: Foetal heart audible with foetal stethoscope

20/40: Uterine contractions and foetal movements palpable

16–18/40: Mother feels foetal movements

12/40: Uterus palpable in abdomen; foetal heart audible with doppler

Weeks
38
40
36
32
28
22
16
12

Figure 17.1 Examination of the abdomen during pregnancy.

Box 17.1 Precipitant Delivery

- Reassure the patient and take her to a private room.
- Summon help (midwife and paediatrician).
- Keep a record of timing throughout.
- Request a delivery pack, turn on the neonatal resuscitation trolley heater and get the Entonox apparatus.
- Try to ascertain the gestational age of the baby and, briefly, the obstetric history of the mother.
- Examine the abdomen to discover the position and number of babies.
- Listen to the foetal heart with a Pinnard's stethoscope. The rate should be over 120 and if it slows with contractions it should recover quickly.
- Allow the patient to adopt any position she chooses.
- Administer Entonox if required.
- If liquor is draining, check the colour. Meconium-staining indicates foetal distress.
- Perform a vaginal examination to assess progress in labour, but NOT if there has been any bleeding because of the risk of placenta praevia. If the cord is prolapsing, push it back into the cervix and hold it there until help arrives. Try to prevent cord compression by the head of the baby.
- If the patient is 'pushing' (i.e. is late in the second stage) look to see if the foetal head, or other presenting part, is visible at the vulva. If it is, put on gown and gloves from the pack and place sterile towels around the delivery area. Cleanse the vulval area.
- Control the descent of the head with the left hand while the right hand supports the perineum with a sterile pad.
- As the head is delivered, encourage the mother to push more gently, while keeping the head flexed. If a breech appears, support the body gently without traction.
- Check for the cord around the baby's neck and free it if necessary.
- Allow the baby's head to turn laterally as the shoulders rotate. With the next contraction the body will be expelled. Deliver it by lifting the baby up and on to the mother's abdomen.
- Tie or clamp the cord in two places at least 10 cm from the umbilicus and cut between the ties.
- *For resuscitation of the baby see Box 17.2.*
- Await spontaneous delivery of the afterbirth.
- Keep the mother warm. If there is excessive bleeding, establish an IV infusion and give an ampoule of an oxytocic (e.g. Syntometrine 1 mL or ergometrine 0.5 mg IM).

Box 17.2 Resuscitation of the Newborn

For the algorithm for life support of the newborn infant see Figure 17.2.
Summon paediatric/anaesthetic help.

The assessment of the newborn infant depends primarily on three factors:

1 colour
2 respiratory effort
3 heart rate.

The Apgar score requires assessment of muscle tone and reflex irritability in addition to these three parameters.

A pink, crying baby needs no active resuscitation. The baby should be dried, wrapped up and given to the mother. Routine suctioning may cause reflex bradycardia and apnoea.

A blue baby who is gasping or apnoeic and has a heart rate above 80 bpm is in a state of primary apnoea. This will often respond to:

- warmth and peripheral stimulation;
- gentle pharyngeal suctioning;
- inflation of the lungs with oxygen using a bag and mask.

A pale, apnoeic, floppy baby with a slow heart rate is in terminal apnoea. He or she needs:

- pharyngeal suctioning (meconium in the mouth indicates the need for inspection of the larynx and, if necessary, tracheal suctioning);
- ventilation with oxygen;
- intubation if there is a skilled operator present (clumsy attempts may result in vagal bradycardia and laryngospasm [endotracheal (ET) tube size = 3 mm after 28 weeks' gestation]);
- cardiac compression if the heart rate is less than 60 bpm (three compressions after each inflation with a compression rate of 120 per min);
- adrenaline via the IV or IO routes (the weight of a full-term neonate is usually about 3.5 kg and the dose of adrenaline = 10–30 μg per kg).

For further details of paediatric resuscitation see Chapter 11 on page 156 and Chapter 18 on page 323.

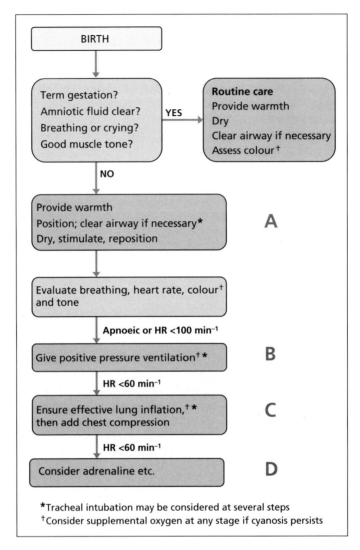

Figure 17.2 Resuscitation Council (UK) Algorithm for life support of the newborn infant.

and shock may occur in the absence of significant external bleeding (concealed haemorrhage). There may be pain and a hard, 'wooden' uterus.

Tx

The patient requires IV fluids, cross-matching of blood and immediate referral to the obstetric service.

> Vaginal examination is contraindicated in antepartum haemorrhage.

Postpartum haemorrhage

Bleeding may occur soon after delivery or later on in the puerperium. It is the later bleeds (secondary postpartum haemorrhage) that may present to the

ED. The causes are retained products of conception and infection.

Tx

Syntometrine (oxytocin 5 units and ergometrine 0.5 mg in 1 mL) IM may contract the uterus and control the bleeding. An IV infusion should be established and blood sent for cross-matching before the patient is referred to the obstetrician.

Eclampsia

Eclampsia occurs in about 1 in 2000 deliveries in the United Kingdom and contributes to around 10% of maternal deaths. Women who are in late pregnancy or postpartum may occasionally present to an ED with eclamptic fits. The signs of pre-eclampsia (hypertension, oedema and proteinuria) may not be immediately apparent.

> In the United Kingdom, high-quality antenatal care has reduced the problems of pre-eclamptic toxaemia to such an extent that 75% of cases of eclampsia now occur in the postpartum period and a similar proportion occurs without pre-existing hypertension.

Tx

- Summon senior anaesthetic and obstetric help.
- Manage the airway and breathing.
- Establish venous access.
- Control the fitting with standard therapy (e.g. lorazepam) followed by IV magnesium sulphate (*see below*).

Magnesium therapy

Magnesium sulphate is now the standard treatment for the control of recurrent eclamptic seizures. An IV injection of 4 g is given over 5–10 min, followed by an IV infusion of 1g per h for at least 24 h. If fits recur then a further 2 g is given IV over 5 min; this dose is increased to 4 g if the patient's weight is over 70 kg. (NB. 1 g of magnesium sulphate is equivalent to approximately 4 mmols of ionised magnesium.) *For more information about magnesium see page 255.*

Major trauma in pregnancy

For the management of major trauma in pregnancy see page 31.

> When patients in late pregnancy are supine, the uterus may compress the inferior vena cava. This impairs the venous return to the heart and causes a profound fall in cardiac output. To avoid this problem, women in the last trimester of pregnancy should be wedged into a left semi-lateral position in the ED.

> Women who may have suffered abdominal trauma and who are Rhesus-D negative will require anti-D immunoglobulin.

Gynaecological problems

For treatment of suspected rape or sexual abuse see page 368.
For guidance about intimate examinations see page 301.

Vaginal bleeding in pregnancy

Vaginal bleeding occurs in up to one-fifth of all pregnant women but in over 50% of cases the pregnancy will continue successfully. After 24 weeks (and effectively after 20 weeks for the purposes of management in the ED) vaginal bleeding is classed as an antepartum haemorrhage (*see page 312*). Before this time it may be:
- a threatened abortion;
- an incomplete abortion;
- a complete abortion;
- other (*see below*).

Loss of the foetus is accompanied by:
- significant pain and tenderness;
- heavy or continuing bleeding;
- the passage of placental material in addition to blood clots;
- an open cervical os;
- the absence of a foetal heart on ultrasound examination.

Investigations

Portable Doppler ultrasound scanners are only useful at gestations of more than 12 weeks, although formal scanning may detect a heart beat at 7 weeks' gestation.

Tx

Patients with the above features of imminent foetal loss require admission for observation. Severe bleeding necessitates IV fluids and, if foetal loss is assured, an oxytocic (e.g. syntometrine 1 mL IM or oxytocin 5 units slowly IV). Pain must be relieved by appropriate analgesia, whatever the course of the pregnancy. Severe pain is sometimes caused by the passage of material through the cervix; great relief can be obtained by the removal of this tissue with sponge-holding forceps via a speculum.

> Loss of a foetus will be an important and sad event for most women; medical care must be accompanied by compassion.

Patients with threatened abortion without symptoms or signs of foetal loss may be referred back to the GP for bed rest at home, although requests for admission from patients must be given serious consideration. If possible, all such patients should be seen in a specialist pregnancy review clinic within 48 h. Early ultrasound scanning is desirable.

The Rhesus-D antibody status of all patients with bleeding in pregnancy after 12 weeks' gestation must be ascertained. It may be recorded on the obstetric cooperation card in later pregnancy.

If antibody status is unknown, then blood should be sent for urgent grouping. Patients who are Rhesus-D negative with a gestation of 12 weeks or more must be protected from developing anti-D antibodies to foetal Rhesus-D positive cells, which may have leaked into the maternal circulation. This is achieved by the administration of anti-D immunoglobulin to destroy any Rhesus-D positive cells before they can sensitise the mother. To be effective, the gammaglobulin must be given within 72 h of the onset of vaginal bleeding. The dose is 250 international units (iu) by deep IM injection for patients with a gestation of less than 20 weeks and and 500 iu for those with a gestation of 20 weeks or more.

Ectopic pregnancy

See Figure 17.3.

There are 1.8 ectopic pregnancies per 1000 total pregnancies in the United Kingdom and it is still one of the most common causes of maternal death. The diagnosis must be considered in any woman of child-bearing age with abdominal or pelvic pain or unexplained collapse. There may be:
• a history of amenorrhoea (perhaps only for a couple of weeks and not by any means essential for the diagnosis);
• vaginal bleeding (follows the pain but may be minimal and is absent in about 25% of cases of tubal pregnancy);

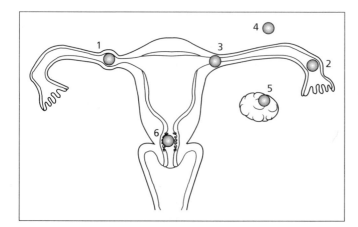

Figure 17.3 Sites for ectopic pregnancies. 1, Fallopian tube – isthmial; 2, Fallopian tube – ampullory; 3, cornual; 4, abdominal; 5, ovarian; 6, cervical.
• UK incidence, 1 in 200 pregnancies, almost all in Fallopian tubes.
• Pregnancy in isthmus of tube ruptures early (4–8 weeks gestation) and causes sudden, acute lower abdominal pain and guarding with shock.
• Pregnancy in ampulla of tube does not cause symptoms until 8–12 weeks gestation. Blood leaking into the peritoneal cavity then causes intermittent pains over several days.

- tenderness in the lower abdomen;
- tenderness in the fornices on vaginal examination;
- sudden onset of severe hypovolaemic shock.

Investigations

The absence of beta human chorionic gonado-trophin (βHCG) in the urine makes the diagnosis of ectopic pregnancy very unlikely as its presence is a highly sensitive test for early pregnancy. Ultrasound scan (preferably a high-resolution transvaginal scan) or even laparoscopy may be needed to con-firm the diagnosis.

Tx

- Establish an IV infusion.
- Cross-match blood.
- Refer the patient to a gynaecologist.

Patients with no abdominal tenderness who are haemodynamically stable may be a seen at an urgent clinic on the following day if local arrange-ments permit this course of action. In the presence of a low serum βHCG concentration (<1000 iu per L), nearly 70% of ectopic pregnancies will resolve without surgical treatment. Medical treat-ment with systemic methotrexate raises this figure to around 80%. However, patients with tubal rupture, a mass >3.5 cm in diameter, free fluid >50 mL or a foetal heart beat on ultrasound scan still require conventional surgical treatment.

Other vaginal bleeding

Women with vaginal bleeding unrelated to preg-nancy should be referred back to their GP for examination and cervical smear. Occasional severe menorrhagia may merit admission. Some reduction in the blood loss during a period can be achieved by taking a short course of oral NSAIDs at the time of the bleeding.

Emergency contraception

Some patients will only present on one occa-sion to one agency in their attempt to get the 'morning-after pill'. This 'window of opportunity' must be grasped by that agency in order to avoid the disaster of an unwanted pregnancy.

> In England and Wales in 2001, one in every 100 young women between the ages of 13 and 16 years became pregnant. Pregnancy in the under-16s is not a planned event and half of these conceptions ended in therapeu-tic abortion.

Two main methods are currently used for emer-gency post-coital contraception:
- hormonal therapy – *see below*;
- immediate insertion of a copper-containing intrauterine contraceptive device (IUCD). (This is more effective than emergency hormonal contra-ception and can be introduced up to 5 days after the earliest predicted ovulation.)

Either of these therapies may be obtained by referral to the GP or a family planning clinic. For those women wishing to be treated in the ED, the hormonal method is the most suitable. It must be started within 72 h of unprotected sexual inter-course (preferably within 12 h) and consists of two 750 μg (0.75 mg) tablets of the synthetic progestogen levonorgestrel to be taken together immediately. This regimen can also be used between 72 and 120 h after unprotected inter-course but this is an unlicensed indication. Emergency contraception with the Yuzpe regime (combined oestrogen and progestogen tablets) is no longer recommended as the progestogen-only system is safer and three times more effective. There is no increased risk of ectopic pregnancy with emergency contraception using progestogens.

Before prescription, a medical and gynaecologi-cal history should be taken to discover the normal menstrual cycle and details of contraceptive usage. There are no absolute contraindications to the use of progestogen-only emergency contracep-tion but caution should be exercised in women with porphyria or severe liver disease.

Women should be given verbal and written information on the following:
- The hormones work by making the lining of the uterus unsuitable for a pregnancy to develop, by delaying the release of an egg from the ovary or by preventing the egg from being fertilised by the

sperm (i.e. by preventing ovulation, fertilisation and implantation).

- There is a failure rate of 1–3% with this method of emergency contraception. Expressed another way, levonorgestrel in the recommended dosage will prevent around 85% of expected pregnancies, if used within 72 h of unprotected intercourse. (The overall risk of pregnancy following one act of unprotected sexual intercourse at any time during the menstrual cycle is about 2–4%. However, around the time of ovulation (days 10 to 17) this figure climbs to 20–30%).
- The next period may come earlier or later than usual and may be unusually light or heavy. A pregnancy test is required if proper menstruation has not occurred within 3 weeks.
- The main side effects of the tablets are nausea and occasionally vomiting. If vomiting occurs within 3 h of taking the pills, another dose must be taken as soon as possible.
- If the method fails and pregnancy ensues, there is no evidence that the hormones may harm the foetus.
- A barrier method of contraception should be used until the start of the next period.
- All women should attend the GP or family planning clinic as soon as possible to get definitive contraceptive advice.

Dysmenorrhoea

This complaint should be dealt with sympathetically even if definitive treatment cannot be offered. Other causes of abdominal pain must be excluded before the patient is referred back to their GP. NSAIDs may give great relief, both as drugs to take out and as a parenteral therapy in the ED.

Pelvic inflammatory disease

For PID see page 310.

Mid-cycle pain

Ovulation may sometimes be associated with pain and slight vaginal bleeding. This is called Mittelschmerz and can be followed up by the GP.

Vaginal discharge

A slight discharge is normal in women of reproductive age. It may be increased by the oral contraceptive pill. Candidiasis causes an irritant creamy discharge.

Tx

Suspected thrush may be treated by a short course of pessaries (e.g. miconazole). The partner will also need treatment to prevent reinfection.

Other patients should be referred to their GP for vaginal examination, swabs and cervical smear.

Vaginal foreign bodies

Women may present with retained vaginal foreign bodies; most commonly tampons or contraceptive sheaths. The posterior fornix is the site where such objects are often lodged.

Tx

The foreign body should be visualised with the aid of a Cusco's speculum and removed with sponge-holding forceps. A digital examination must also be performed if the object is not found. It is worth noting that occasional cases of missed intravesical foreign body have been described.

Women who have had a retained vaginal foreign body for some days may be at risk of toxic shock syndrome (*see page 345*). An unpleasant discharge may be treated with a short course of antiseptic pessaries (e.g. Betadine pessaries one bd for 5 days).

Labial abscess

An abscess may form in the Bartholin's gland, which is situated in the posterior third of the labia majora. The whole labia is swollen, inflamed and extremely tender. The patient must be referred to the gynaecologist on call for drainage and marsupialisation.

Breast abscesses and lumps

A combination of lactation and staphylococcal infection may lead to a breast abscess. The patient needs admission as the tender, red lump in the breast must be drained under general anaesthesia; anything less is inappropriate. Suppression of lactation may be required.

Breast lumps should be examined and the findings discussed with the patient. Referral should then be made to the GP who can arrange appropriate treatment, usually a surgical opinion and excision-biopsy.

Genitourinary problems

Urinary tract infection

Urinary tract infection (UTI) is more common in women than in men; when it occurs in men there is often an underlying anatomical or pathological abnormality. Recurrent episodes of infection, especially in children, are an indication for radiological investigation. Infection of the lower urinary tract is characterised by the classical symptoms of dysuria, frequency and urgency. Haematuria and proteinuria may be present but physical signs are usually minimal. Suprapubic pain and tenderness are sometimes seen. A patient with pyelitis or pyelonephritis is usually systemically unwell with pyrexia, loin pain, rigors and tenderness over the affected kidney.

> In children and the elderly, UTI may cause general malaise with non-specific features such as pyrexia, vomiting, abdominal pain and confusion.

Tx

- Test the urine for glucose to exclude diabetes.
- Send a MSU (midstream specimen of urine) to the laboratory with the results forwarded to the GP.
- Commence antibiotic therapy – see later.
- Advise the patient to drink an increased amount of fluids.
- Refer the patient to see their GP after 3 days for follow-up when the MSU result is available.

But note the following:

- Patients with features of pyelitis or pyelonephritis require admission under a general surgeon.
- Children with UTI should be followed-up in the paediatric clinic. Investigations may reveal ureteric reflux or congenital abnormality.

- In men, UTI is often secondary to venereal infection and so genitourinary clinic follow-up should be arranged.

Antibiotics for UTI

The most common organism found in urinary tract infection is *Escherichia coli*. Other causative bacteria include Gram-negative bacilli of the *Proteus* and *Klebsiella* genera and enterococci. *Staphylococcus saprophyticus* is a common cause of UTI in sexually active young women. The sensitivity patterns of coliforms are changing – around half are resistant to ampicillin/amoxicillin and nearly a third are resistant to trimethoprim. Therefore, a 3–5 day course of cefalexin (cephalexin) or cefadroxil is a good first choice in uncomplicated cystitis; nitrofurantoin, nalidixic acid or trimethoprim are alternatives. Females above 50 years of age and male patients are more difficult to treat and may require a longer course (7 days) of co-amoxiclav or a combination that includes ciprofloxacin (for *Pseudomonas aeruginosa*). Ascending infections of the urinary tract (pyelitis or pyelonephritis) should be treated with a quinolone or a broad spectrum cephalosporin for 14 days.

Haematuria in the absence of signs of infection

Patients with mild haematuria may be referred back to their GP. Macroscopic, painless haematuria should be discussed with a member of the surgical team. Severe haematuria merits admission.

Prostatitis

Bacterial infection of the prostate gland can occur with *Escherichia coli* and *Streptococcus faecalis*. The patient has:

1 the features of prostatism – frequency, hesitancy and poor stream – possibly leading to retention;
2 pyrexia, leucocytosis and a very tender prostate gland on rectal examination.

Tx

The patient should be referred to the on-call surgical team. Acute prostatitis is treated with either ciprofloxacin or trimethoprim for 28 days.

Testicular swelling and pain

A male patient under 25 years of age with testicular pain must be assumed to have a torsion until proved otherwise.

The pain of a *testicular torsion* is unilateral and usually, but not always, sudden in onset. It may radiate to the lower abdomen. There may have been previous episodes of the same pain. The testis is swollen and tender with a small hydrocoele.

Epididymo-orchitis may be seen in older males after a urinary tract infection. The testis and cord are painful, tender and swollen and the patient is pyrexial. Orchitis may also occur as a feature of mumps – *see page 420.*

Investigations

An ultrasound scan of the scrotum can distinguish testicular swelling from paratesticular lesions and demonstrate free fluid and tumours.

Tx

Patients with testicular pain or swelling should be seen by the surgeon on call.

Suspected venereal disease

Ulcers, warts or herpetic lesions of the genitalia may present to the ED. They should be assumed to be highly infectious. Referral should be made to the local genitourinary clinic.

Penile discharge is also invariably a symptom of venereal disease. It may be accompanied by dysuria. Referral should again be made to the genitourinary clinic.

Post-coital bleeding

Post-coital bleeding may occur in both sexes. Women with this symptom should be referred back to their GP for speculum examination and cervical smear. Men are usually found to have torn the frenulum of the foreskin. A small blood vessel may be bleeding profusely. It should be cauterised with silver nitrate.

Retention of urine

Acute retention of urine causes extreme distress. There is lower abdominal pain and an inability to micturate, although the patient may be unaware of the latter problem if obtunded. Usually, the enlarged bladder is obvious but it may be overlooked in the obese patient, especially if there is retention with overflow (i.e. a large volume remains in the bladder after voiding a small amount of urine).

In male patients, retention is most often caused by obstruction of the urethra by an enlarged prostate gland but a variety of other conditions may also cause it, including:
- pain around the pelvis and perineum;
- drugs (e.g. anticholinergics, antihypertensives and antihistamines);
- neurological problems.

Tx

Treatment consists of careful, aseptic catheterisation and controlled drainage of urine. Most patients should then be admitted for investigation.

Catheter problems

Elderly male patients commonly present with blocked catheters. The catheter should be changed for a suitable long-term replacement and free drainage of urine confirmed. It is essential that arrangements are made with the district nursing team for follow-up and advice about future catheter care.

Balanitis

Infection of the prepuce and glans may occur, especially in boys with an unretractable foreskin.

Tx

Severe infection or difficulty with micturition merits referral. Other patients need:
- a urine test for glucose to exclude diabetes;
- a local swab to be sent to the laboratory;

- a consideration of the possibility of infection with *Candida* or *Trichomonas* – ask about symptoms in the partner;
- cleaning of the infected area and advice on hygiene, especially in the elderly; and
- referral to the GP.

Some patients will go on to require circumcision.

Paraphimosis

Retraction of a tight foreskin can impair the venous return from the glans causing distal engorgement and extreme swelling.

Tx

Reduction may be attempted in the ED. Analgesia and lubrication is obtained by the application of lidocaine gel. The thumb is placed on the prepuce and gentle but increasing pressure applied as the foreskin is drawn over it with the index and middle fingers. If this is unsuccessful, the patient should be referred to a general surgeon. Reduction under anaesthetic may be required and occasionally, in adults, a dorsal slit is needed.

'Fracture' of the penis

Trauma to the erect penis during intercourse may sometimes rupture one of the engorged corpora cavernosa. This is known as a 'fracture' of the penis. The patient presents with a history of increasing perineal discomfort and bruising after intercourse. The penis, scrotum and suprapubic area is found to be very swollen and bruised without any other external sign of injury. Patients with this condition should be referred immediately to a urologist for exploration of the damaged area. If left untreated, impotency can result.

Iatrogenic priapism

This problem is sometimes seen in patients who are under the care of a clinic that treats aspects of sexual dysfunction. Intracavernosal injections of papaverine (up to 120 mg) may be used by a patient as often as twice weekly to obtain an erection, which should subside spontaneously within 3 h. If this does not occur, the prolonged erection (priapism) becomes uncomfortable and distressing.

Tx

Discuss the patient with a urologist or the doctor who prescribed the injections before contemplating treatment. If priapism is long-standing, surgical evacuation of blood clots may be necessary. In cases of a shorter duration, decompression may be achieved by the following technique:
- Draw up 5 mg of the α-agonist phenylephrine into a syringe, diluted with saline to 10 mL.
- Insert a 19 G butterfly needle into either corpus cavernosum.
- Withdraw 20–40 mL of blood using a syringe. This will usually relieve the pain.
- Inject 1 mg of the phenylephrine solution (via the same needle) while monitoring the patient's blood pressure. If there is no hypertension, inject a further 4 mg (to a total of 5 mg).
- Massage the penis gently. This may be painful.
- If there is little improvement, repeat the above procedure after 1 hour.
- Observe the patient for an hour after the last treatment.
- Advise no further intracavernosal injections until the patient has consulted the doctor who prescribed the treatment.

Perineal problems

Perianal abscess

Abscesses arising from the glands of the anal canal present as extremely painful swellings around the anus. Deeper infection in the ischiorectal fossa may cause a more diffuse swelling of the buttock. The patient should be referred to the surgical team for drainage under general anaesthesia. It is totally inappropriate to attempt incision under local anaesthesia in the ED.

Pilonidal abscess

This presents as a tender, red swelling in the upper part of the natal cleft. The underlying pilonidal sinus may not be visible. Inpatient care is necessary for this condition.

Gluteal abscesses may extend deep into the buttock and are also generally best treated in theatre.

Foreign bodies in the rectum

Rectal foreign bodies may be difficult to remove because of spasm of the sphincters. Removal under general anaesthesia is often needed.

Rectal bleeding

The loss of a significant amount of blood from the rectum should be treated in the same manner as any other bleeding, that is, resuscitation, cross-matching of blood and immediate specialist referral. *See page 303.*

Lesser amounts of bleeding, in an apparently well patient, can be referred back to the GP for investigation and referral as appropriate.

Haemorrhoids

Haemorrhoids or piles are enlarged cushions of anal mucosa accompanied by varicosities of the neighbouring (superior haemorrhoidal) veins. They may cause:
- bright red blood with and after the motions;
- pain on defaecation and consequent constipation;
- perianal irritation;
- a prolapse of mucosal tissue (on straining – second-degree piles; or constant – third-degree piles).

Tx

If the bleeding has stopped and abdominal and rectal examination is unremarkable, then further investigation can be undertaken by the GP. Extreme pain such as that caused by a strangulated pile or suppurative, ulcerated lesions should be referred to the duty surgeon.

Thrombosed external pile

This is a perianal haematoma caused by the rupture of a tributary of the inferior haemorrhoidal vein. There is pain and a dark blue swelling at the anal margin. If it discharges or begins to resolve spontaneously then no further treatment is needed. If not, incision may be required either in the ED under local anaesthetic or in some cases by a surgeon in theatre.

Anal fissure

A tear at the anal margin may cause severe pain with defaecation. It may be associated with a tag of anal epithelium known as a sentinel pile. Multiple fissures are a feature of Crohn's disease. Treatment is the province of a general surgeon.

Perianal irritation

Pruritis ani is the predominant symptom of a perianal dermatitis. A build-up of moisture and small particles of faeces reduces the efficacy of the normal skin barrier in a manner similar to that which causes nappy rash. Scratching and secondary bacterial infection then compound the damage.

Tx

- The perianal skin must be kept clean and dry.
- Scratching and chemical irritants should be avoided.
- After every bowel action, the area must be cleaned by bathing or by using shower jets, a bidet or medicated wipes. Strong soap and abrasive methods of cleaning are not suitable.
- The area should be gently dried after cleaning with a soft towel or a hairdryer.
- Talcum powder, ointments and creams should not be used.

Chapter 18

Children's problems in the emergency department

Patients under 16 years of age account for about 25–30% of the attendances at a typical ED in the United Kingdom. Experiences of hospitals gained in childhood may influence patients throughout their lives.

Assessment of the ill or injured child: the differences between adults and children

The principles of paediatric assessment are identical to those applicable to an adult. Problems arise because of the following.

The size of children

The variable age and hence size of children affects physiological measurements, drug doses and equipment sizes. An expected adult weight range might be 45–90 kg: that is a two-fold difference. Children may easily vary from 3 to 60 kg: a 20-fold range. A factor of two is often disregarded – most adults are given a standard dose of drugs and assumed to have similar physiological parameters. A 20-fold difference is impossible to ignore; treatment must be tailored to the size of the child.

The age of a child is usually known but the weight is more difficult to ascertain. Because of this it is important to be able to estimate a child's weight from a knowledge of his or her age. *For a method of estimating a child's weight from his or her age see Box 18.1.*

The causes of illness in children

The conditions with which children present are different. They do not generally suffer from the degenerative diseases of adult life but have more problems with infective conditions.

The causes of cardiac arrest in children

Children usually die from hypoxia, secondary to respiratory distress or depression, or from hypovolaemia (fluid loss or maldistribution). These lead to cardiac asystole, which has a very poor prognosis. Therefore, it is vital to recognise and reverse these conditions before terminal bradycardia supervenes. Coronary artery disease and thus ventricular fibrillation is very uncommon in children.

Box 18.1 The Weight of a Child

Average birth weight of a full-term infant = 3.5 kg.
Weight at age 5 months = double the birth weight.
Weight at age 12 months = triple the birth weight.
Between the ages of 1 and 10 years the approximate weight of a child in kilograms can be calculated by the following formula:
(Age in years + 4) × 2 = weight in kg.

The anatomy and physiology of children

Children differ from adults in their body proportions. They also have a more elastic skeleton. This leads to a different pattern of injury and an airway that can be more difficult to manage. Because of the elastic chest wall, children are far less likely to have rib fractures, although they may have severe underlying damage to the lung, liver or spleen (*see also Chapter 6*).

The fast metabolism and low reserves of children explain why they get ill, hypoxic, hypoglycaemic and hypothermic very quickly. However, their general health and high capacity for repair make for a speedy recovery.

The psychology of children

The interaction with the assessor is as variable as the age of the child. Only practice can teach the subtle parts of this relationship but those with children of their own have a distinct advantage.

Immediate assessment and management

For the principles of immediate assessment see Chapter 1.
For cardiac arrest protocols for children see Chapter 11.
For resuscitation of the newborn infant see page 313.

> The skills required for the resuscitation of infants and children are best learned on a paediatric life support course such as APLS (Advanced Life Support Group, Manchester) or PALS (Resuscitation Council UK, London).

A – Airway

Checking for responsiveness

The presence of a response is usually immediately obvious. If it is not then gentle shaking may establish verbal communication with an older child. The young child will respond by eye movement, cry or body posture – the mother will know.

> Always consider the possibility of an inhaled foreign body in children who are unresponsive or dyspnoeic.

The child's airway

Children are particularly prone to airway obstruction because of the following:
- The airway has a small diameter. Its narrowest point is at the subglottis, rather than at the cords as in an adult.
- The tongue and pharyngeal soft tissues are relatively bulky.
- The voice box (larynx) is more of a voice bag with a large, floppy epiglottis and pliable cords. It lies more anteriorly than in an adult.
- In the submucosa of the airway there is a large amount of lymphoid tissue that can enlarge.
- The airway reflexes are particularly sensitive.
- Toddlers put things in their mouths.
- There is a high incidence of upper respiratory tract infection in children, including several infections that target the airway.
- Children under the age of 6 months are compulsory nose breathers. Nasal obstruction is thus critical in this age group.

For choking protocols see page 205.
For management of other laryngotracheal obstruction in children see page 330.

> Do not examine the throat with any instrument in children with stridor or suspected partial airway obstruction. Doing so may convert the problem to complete obstruction.

Maintenance and protection of the airway

The need for aids to maintain the airway is assessed on the same criteria in the child as in the adult. However, if a child's airway is maintainable by simple manoeuvres, an oropharyngeal (Guedel) airway is best avoided. This is because retching is easily induced in children and may be followed by laryngospasm or aspiration.

For assessment of artificial airway and endotracheal tube sizes see Box 18.2.

Box 18.2 Artificial Airway and Endotracheal Tube Sizes

Oropharyngeal airway size = approximately the distance from the centre of the lips to the angle of the jaw.
Nasopharyngeal airway size = approximately the distance from the tip of the nose to the tragus of the ear.
Endotracheal tube size
- Internal diameter in mm = (age/4) + 4
(neonate 3–3.5 mm tube).
- Oral tube length in cm = (age/2) + 12.
- Nasal tube length in cm = (age/2) + 15.

Box 18.3 Normal Respiratory Rates and Pulse Rates in Children (Per Minute)

Age	Respiratory rate	Heart rate
Under 1 year	30–40	110–160
1–5 years	25–30	95–140
5–12 years	20–25	80–120
Over 12 years	15–20	60–100

NB: The heart rate is roughly four times the respiratory rate at all ages.

The presence or absence of the gag reflex gives no useful information. Testing for it in children may easily induce retching or laryngospasm and create a certain airway problem.

Endotracheal intubation of infants

The large, floppy epiglottis of the infant prevents a standard intubation technique whereby the tip of the laryngoscope is positioned in the vallecula – the angle between the base of the tongue and the anterior surface of the epiglottis. Instead, the epiglottis must be lifted forward by a laryngoscope, which is placed posterior to it.

For this reason, paediatric laryngoscopes have relatively straight blades (e.g. Seward, Soper, Robertshaw, Miller or Wisconsin blades). The Robertshaw laryngoscope, which has characteristics of both typical adult and paediatric designs, is probably the easiest to use. After the age of about 18 months, a standard adult technique can be adopted, although many anaesthetists prefer to use a straight blade for children up to the age of 5 years.

B – Breathing

The oxygen saturation shown by the pulse oximeter should be close to 100% in a normal healthy child breathing air.

For the normal respiratory rates in children see Box 18.3.
Very slow respiratory rates in children suggest imminent respiratory arrest or poisoning with narcotic drugs (e.g. methadone).

Oxygen therapy

Almost all ill or injured children will benefit from high-concentration oxygen therapy. There is no need to assess risk as in adults with chronic lung disease. Only a small group of infants with duct-dependent congenital heart disease need controlled oxygen therapy.

It is usually counterproductive to make an unwilling child wear an oxygen mask.

Therapy with brochodilators

All wheezy children should be given nebulised bronchodilators, whether they are known to be asthmatic or not. Ask the parents how much of this type of drug they have already had and look for agitation, tachycardia and tremor – the signs of overdosage. Remember, however, that these may also be signs of hypoxia.

Artificial ventilation

Ventilation is indicated as an emergency procedure for respiratory insufficiency in a child in the same way as in an adult. *For a method of estimating appropriate ventilator settings see Box 18.4.*

Box 18.4 Suggested Ventilator Settings

Tidal volume = 10 mL per kg.
Minute volume = 100 mL per kg.

C – Circulation

Checking for a central pulse

The brachial or femoral pulses should be used in infants rather than the carotid pulse. The absence of a central pulse or a rate of less than 60 bpm in infants indicates the need to follow procedures for cardiorespiratory arrest (*see page 156*).

> In a child with ventricular fibrillation and no obvious precipitating factors, consider poisoning with tricyclic antidepressants.

For cardiac arrest and dysrhythmia protocols see Chapter 11 on page 156.

Cardiovascular parameters

- For normal heart rates – *see Box 18.3*.
- Blood pressure varies with age. It can be difficult to measure in young, moving children. A useful formula is:
Expected systolic BP in mmHg = 80 + (age in years × 2).
- Blood volume is approximately 80 mL per kg.
   The ECG is rarely as helpful in making a diagnosis in children as in adults. The exception is, of course, dysrhythmias. A cardiac monitor does, however, provide constant information about the heart rate.

Important signs of circulatory disturbance in children

- Purpura (meningococcal disease).
- Dehydration – a dry non-elastic skin or sunken eyes. In infants a floppy anterior fontanelle is a useful, if late, sign of severe fluid loss. Diarrhoea and vomiting can quickly dehydrate a small child.
- Wet nappies confirm urine output in young children. As usual, the mother will know their normal state.

Access to the circulation

The need for and site of this should be assessed carefully. There is nothing worse than looking for veins on a screaming child who is covered with bruises from previous attempts by someone else. Remember the possibility of intra-osseous infusion and venous cut-down (*see Box 18.5*).

> **Box 18.5 Intra-osseous Cannulation**
>
> This is recommended in children if IV access cannot be achieved rapidly. It is a safe technique and so every ED should have the equipment and expertise. The intra-osseous route can be used for both volume resuscitation and drug therapy.
> - Mark the anteromedial tibia 2–3 cm below the tibial tuberosity or the anterolateral femur about 3 cm above the lateral femoral condyle.
> - Prepare the skin and insert local anaesthetic in a conscious child.
> - Make a small cut in the skin.
> - Insert the special intra-osseous needle with the trochar at 90° to skin. A gentle twisting motion results in penetration of the cortex. The needle should then be fixed in the bone.
> - Remove the trochar and use a 5-mL syringe to aspirate and confirm the cannula's position. Blood samples may be taken.
> - Connect an extension tube and three-way tap.
> - Fix the needle in position.
> - Give drugs or fluid in boluses from a syringe. A standard drip will not run adequately.

Fluid replacement

- Bolus fluid therapy = 20 mL per kg, repeated as necessary after further assessment. (This is reduced to 10 mL per kg for children with trauma in hospital and 5 mL per kg for children with trauma in the pre-hospital setting.)
- Maintenance fluid therapy:
   4 mL per kg per hour for the first 10 kg;
   2 mL per kg per hour for the next 10 kg; and
   1 mL per kg per hour for subsequent weight.
For example, a 25-kg child needs:
   (4 mL per kg × 10 kg) + (2 mL per kg × 10 kg) + (1 mL per kg × 5 kg) = (40) + (20) + (5) mL per hour = 65 mL per hour.

> As a routine maintenance fluid, children should be given glucose 5% with sodium chloride 0.45%.

• The palm and adducted fingers of a child's hand is approximately equal to 1% of their body surface area and can be used to make a quick estimate of the fluid replacement required for a burn (*see page 149*).

D – Disability

> Always consider hypoglycaemia as a cause for a reduced level of consciousness in children.

Level of consciousness

AVPU scoring (*see page 7*) is as useful for children as for adults. The standard, adult GCS is suitable for children of school age but special variants of the GCS are more appropriate in children under 4 years old – *see Box 18.6*. Even sleepy children should be fairly easy to rouse.

Box 18.6 The Children's Coma Scale	
Response elicited	**Score**
Best eye response	
Open spontaneously	4
Open to speech	3
Open to pain	2
No response	1
Best motor response	
Moves normally and spontaneously or obeys commands	6
Localises pain	5
Withdraws in response to pain	4
Flexes abnormally to pain (decorticate movements)	3
Extends abnormally to pain (decerebrate movements)	2
No response	1
Best verbal response	
Smiles, follows sounds and objects, interacts	5
Cries consolably or interacts inappropriately	4
Cries with inconsistent relief or moans	3
Cries inconsolably or is irritable	2
No response	1

Other signs

• Agitation or an odd cry or affect may be the first signs of cerebral irritation.
• Children may be flaccid or show abnormal posturing.
• Limb movements may be unequal – sometimes this is congenital but it is best never to assume so.

E – Exposure and environment

Comfort, warmth and the proximity of the mother or other carer are extremely important to children. Attention to these details early on can radically change the well-being and demeanour (and hence ease of assessment) of a child. Clothing may have to be removed to facilitate assessment. However, it must be remembered that children easily become cold and embarrassed.

> In a child, cold limbs usually indicate a cold trunk and head.

F – Fits

For anticonvulsant therapy and cooling measures for children see page 338.
In the apyrexic fitting child consider:
• hypoglycaemia;
• meningitis;
• poisoning;
• causes of cerebral oedema.

G – Glucose

Children are like fast-burning little engines and become short of oxygen and fuel very quickly. Their fuel is glucose and they have relatively low glycogen reserves.

All diabetic children will be on insulin; oral hypoglycaemic drugs are generally only used in adults. This does not mean, of course, that a child cannot take someone else's drugs and become hypoglycaemic.

Hypoglycaemia should be corrected with 2–5 mL per kg of 10% dextrose solution (0.2–0.5 mg per kg of glucose) through a large vein. Glucagon

(20 µg per kg) is an alternative if venous access is delayed.

H – History

The initial AMPLE history (*see page 9*) should be obtained from the child or from the carers.
For additional features of the history in children see later.

I – Immediate needs of the child

Some immediate needs will have been assessed as part of the 'environment'. These include the provision of warmth, the removal of wet clothing and the need to ensure psychological support from the mother or other carer. A position of comfort is also mandatory; it may be life-saving in conditions such as epiglottitis. As usual the relief of suffering is of paramount importance.

Assess
- *The need for analgesia.* Exact localisation of pain is difficult in very young children but careful observation and discussion with the mother often helps considerably. Analgesia can turn an unmanageable situation into a calm one. It also reassures the carers. It is far better to give analgesia freely to children who may be in pain than to withhold it on the spurious grounds that it alters conscious level or masks pupillary or abdominal signs.
- *The need for limb splintage.* Simple limb support with troughs and pillows can be very helpful in children with limb injuries. Distal circulation should be assessed before and after positioning limbs in the same way in children as in adults.
- *The tolerance of cervical and other spinal splintage.* Conscious children often do not tolerate this sort of restraint very well. If a collar is distressing a child significantly, it is better to remove it. The mother's hands and pillows can be more acceptable substitutes. A child who is struggling to remove a collar is actually moving his or her neck more than a child with no splint who is lying still. The indications for spinal immobilisation are the same in children as in adults although young children are less accurate in localising the pain of spinal injury.

Ask yourself
Does this child need:
- drugs to relieve pain? (*See Boxes 18.7 and 18.8.*)
- splintage?
- freedom from splintage?

Further assessment of the child

This will be greatly facilitated by a gentle approach and a tailored environment.

Additional features in a paediatric history

Maternal health and pregnancy

The health of the mother may affect the development of the fetus. Maternal infections (e.g. rubella) may lead to a damaged baby.

Box 18.7 Narcotic Analgesics for Children

Children over 12 months old

Morphine injection	0.1–0.2 mg per kg
Fentanyl injection	Increments of 0.5 µg per kg
Pethidine injection	1–2 mg per kg
Diamorphine intranasal spray	0.1 mg per kg
Morphine elixir	0.2–0.4 mg per kg
Codeine elixir	1–1.5 mg per kg

The above doses of morphine should be halved for children under the age of 12 months.
Children under 3 months old are especially sensitive to opioids and so should be given one-quarter of the usual paediatric dose.
Codeine is best avoided in infants.

Box 18.8 Antipyretic Analgesics for Children

Paracetamol suspension
10–15 mg per kg every 4–6 h. Paracetamol may also be given rectally as a suppository (Loading dose = 15–20 mg per kg).
Ibuprofen suspension
5 mg per kg up to four times a day.

Birth problems

A difficult birth (caesarean section or forceps delivery) may later manifest itself as developmental problems or fits. Was the child on the special care baby unit? If so, then the perinatal period was not as smooth as it might have been.

Siblings

The health of brothers and sisters may give useful information concerning a child's illness.

Development

The continuing rapid development of a child distinguishes it from the adult. Questions should be asked about relationships, behaviour, play, school, sports and activities.

Immunisations

Children in the United Kingdom benefit from the existence of a planned programme of immunisations (*see Box 18.18*). The immunisations actually received should always be ascertained.

Communication with a child

Children vary widely in their ability to communicate. A neonate may make signals that are only understood by its mother whereas teenagers use the same level of communication as adults. The type and level of language used is also influenced by the child's intelligence and environment. Consequently, communicating with a child is a difficult art, which comes more naturally to some than to others.

Questions must be pitched at the right level and the responses of the child constantly reassessed. It is obviously a mistake to phrase a question in language that a small child cannot understand. However, it is equally inappropriate to patronise an older child.

A child's account of events can be extremely accurate. It should not be assumed that an adult's story of events is any more credible than an older child's.

Language problems

Children from ethnic communities may be multilingual and revert to their domestic tongue in a crisis. Gentle rephrasing of questions may reassure them and encourage dialogue but sometimes the help of a translator is required.

The needs of the parents

Children usually have someone in close proximity to look after them. Sometimes the worries of these carers predominate over the symptoms of the child. Requirements vary from simple reassurance to medical interventions. The satisfactory treatment of the child often depends on the support of those closest to him or her; the child's mental state may be inseparable from that of the mother. Parental anxiety or difficulty coping is a good reason for admitting a child to hospital.

Continuing assessment

Assessment must continue during initial treatment and transportation. Children may change their physiological status very rapidly. It is particularly important to assess the effect of any interventions.

Monitoring must be appropriate to the child's condition and should not replace careful observation. It needs to be considered in terms of: (1) usefulness of information obtained; and (2) acceptability to the child.

In a conscious child, this probably means that:
- pulse oximetry is better than
- ECG monitoring, which is better than
- BP monitoring.

Consideration of other children in the vicinity

In many situations, such as severe infections, fires, poisoning and abuse, other children may have been exposed to the same agents as the patient. In such cases it is appropriate to assess the risk to these children also.

Respiratory problems

See also Chapter 13.

Respiratory disorders are responsible for around a third of all paediatric admissions to hospital in the United Kingdom.

Stridor

For foreign body obstruction see page 205.
For angio-oedema see page 295.

Stridor is a harsh respiratory noise, which is loudest in inspiration and usually indicates obstruction of the extrathoracic airways. It can be caused by:

- epiglottitis (supraglottitis);
- laryngotracheobronchitis (croup);
- bacterial tracheitis;
- foreign body obstruction;
- angio-oedema;
- thermal, chemical or other damage to the airways;
- other rarer causes of obstruction (e.g. diphtheria, quinsy, glandular fever).

Accompanying features, including the degree of respiratory distress, depend on the cause of the stridor. They may include:

- hoarseness or inability to speak;
- coughing;
- drooling;
- sternal and subcostal recession (this is a good indicator of the degree of obstruction whereas the intensity of the stridor is not);
- tachypnoea and tachycardia;
- indicators of hypoxia such as cyanosis, agitation or drowsiness.

> Do not put anything, including a spatula or a thermometer, in the mouth of a child with stridor – it may precipitate complete respiratory obstruction.

Differences between epiglottitis and croup

Despite its name, the swelling of epiglottitis usually involves more than just the bright red, cherry-like epiglottis. It is, in fact, a complete 'top of the larynx-itis'. This is different from the 'bottom of the laryngitis' caused by croup. Spasmodic or recurrent croup is a variant form of the disease, which is more common in atopic children and is thought to have an allergic component. *For the differences between the two most common infectious causes of stridor see Box 18.9.*

XR

There is no place for radiographs in the management of stridor.

TX

- Leave the child in the position of comfort, usually sitting up and possibly on the mother's knee.

Box 18.9 Differences between Epiglottitis and Croup

	Epiglottitis	Croup
Age of child	1–6 years	6 months–5 years
Onset of symptoms	Hours	Days
Runny nose	No	Yes
Cough	Slight	Characteristic barking
Speech	Difficult	Hoarse
Stridor	Soft	Harsh
Able to drink	No	Yes
Drooling	Yes	No
Pyrexia	$> 38.5°C$	$< 38.5°C$
Appearance	Pale and toxic	Variable
Respiratory distress	Severe	Variable
Site affected	Supraglottis	Lower larynx and trachea
Causative organism	*Haemophilus influenzae* B	Parainfluenza and other viruses
Decreased incidence (since HiB vaccine)	Yes – now rare in the UK	No – still common
Need for observation	Yes	Yes
Need for intubation	Yes	Sometimes (5%)
Need for antibiotics	Yes	No
Helped by steroids	No	Yes

- Avoid interventions that may precipitate crying; oxygen may sometimes be tolerated but attempts at IV access will not.
- Ask for paediatric help.

If respiratory distress accompanies the stridor, then:
- summon skilled senior help immediately, including an anaesthetist and an ENT surgeon (a consultant anaesthetist is the most appropriate grade);
- notify theatre of the situation.

Gaseous induction of anaesthesia, with a volatile agent such as halothane in oxygen, followed by gentle laryngoscopy is the only appropriate treatment in the distressed child who is still breathing. Intubation should, of course, be attempted if respiratory arrest occurs.

As a holding measure, 5 mg nebulised adrenaline may be life-saving (5 ml of 1 in 1000 adrenaline nebulised in oxygen) with ECG monitoring. For children under 10, 0.5 mL per kg of a 1 in 1000 solution of adrenaline is appropriate. The benefit of the adrenaline only lasts for 30 min and so, in suspected Croup, it should be followed immediately by nebulised or oral steroids – *see later*.

Croup

A croup score is used in some hospitals to describe the clinical severity of the illness. It is calculated by scoring five features:
1 inspiratory stridor;
2 cough;
3 retractions;
4 dyspnoea;
5 colour.

Two alternative steroid treatments have been shown to lead to marked clinical improvement in croup. Either of the following should be administered as soon as the diagnosis is suspected:
- nebulised budesonide 2 mg (4 mL) stat or 1 mg (2 mL) repeated after 30 min;
- oral dexamethasone (0.15 mg per kg).
Oral prednisolone (1 mg per kg) is also used by some units.

Bacterial tracheitis

Infection of the airway with staphylococci, streptococci or *Haemophilus influenzae* may cause bacterial tracheitis (pseudomembranous croup). The trachea contains copious purulent secretions with mucosal oedema and necrosis, features that can lead to severe airway obstruction. An affected child is unwell and toxic with a high pyrexia and stridulous breathing. Intensive care should be arranged immediately; three-quarters of such children require intubation. Antibiotic therapy should be a combination of cefotaxime and flucloxacillin.

Asthma in children*

For asthma in adults and older children see page 210.
An acute attack of asthma is one of the commonest reasons for admission to a paediatric ward in the United Kingdom although admissions for asthma have been declining rapidly over the last 5 years. Throughout Western Europe, around 13% of children and over 8% of adults suffer from asthma. These figures confirm that childhood asthma often remits in adult life. Persistence into adulthood is more likely with:
1 Co-existent atopy
2 Female gender
3 Severe and frequent exacerbations of asthma in childhood
4 Smoking in adulthood.
The first severe episode of asthma usually occurs at around 18 months of age. Attacks are often precipitated by a viral infection; in older children exercise and emotional upset may be the triggers. Asthma is an allergic bronchitis and is not primarily an infectious condition. The inflammatory process causes smooth muscle irritability, oedema and sputum retention resulting in obstruction of the intrathoracic airways. The clinical signs of this obstructive process are:
1 increased work of breathing – wheezing, tachypnoea, recession and use of accessory muscles;
2 reduced efficacy of breathing – poor air entry and hyperexpansion;

---

* This section is mostly concerned with asthma in young children.

3 failure of gas exchange – tachycardia, agitation and eventually drowsiness and cyanosis.

Clinical signs correlate poorly with the severity of airways obstruction; some very ill children do not appear to be distressed.

Severe attacks are characterised by:

• child too breathless to talk or too breathless to feed (cannot complete sentences in one breath);

• respiratory rate > 50 per min in children aged 2–5 years or > 30 per min in children aged over 5 years (usually with marked recession and use of accessory muscles);

• pulse rate > 130 per min in children aged 2–5 years or > 120 per min in children aged over 5 years;

• SaO_2 < 92% on air, but any reduction in SaO_2 from the normal of 97% or above must be given serious consideration.

Life-threatening features include:

• fatigue or exhaustion;

• agitation, drowsiness, confusion or a depressed level of consciousness;

• cyanosis;

• a silent chest;

• poor respiratory efforts;

• bradycardia or hypotension (Bradycardia is often a preterminal sign.);

• SaO_2 < 85% on air.

It is very useful to know what has happened during previous attacks:

• Oral steroids? How many times? For how long?

• Admission? How many times? For how long?

• ICU admission? How many times? For how long?

Investigations

Measurement of peak expiratory flow rate (PEF) can usually be performed on children over 5 years old provided they are not too breathless or too distressed to cooperate. *For predicted peak expiratory flow rates in children see Figure 18.1.* Investigations including chest X-ray are not generally indicated in recurrent attacks of asthma, unless there is a possible history of foreign body inhalation or severe systemic upset. Close observation and pulse oximetry are more important. The aim should be to keep the SaO_2 above 92%.

Tx

• *Nebulised salbutamol 5 mg or terbutaline 10 mg* in 100% oxygen (salbutamol 2.5 mg or terbutaline 5 mg if the child is less than 5 years old). The oxygen flow rate should be around 5 L per min to produce small particles without excess loss of drug from around the face mask. In children with mild to moderate asthma and an SaO_2 above 92% in air, there are some advantages in using a pressurised aerosol via a spacer device (+/− a facemask) to administer the beta-2 agonist. Ten puffs are given, one at a time, and inhaled sequentially.

• *Soluble prednisolone* 1 mg per kg orally (up to a maximum of 40 mg). Children who are already receiving maintenance steroid tablets should be given prednisolone 2 mg per kg (up to a maximum of 60 mg). If the child is unable to swallow liquids or is vomiting, give IV hydrocortisone 4 mg per kg. This should be repeated every 6 h or followed by a continuous infusion of hydrocortisone 1 mg per kg per h.

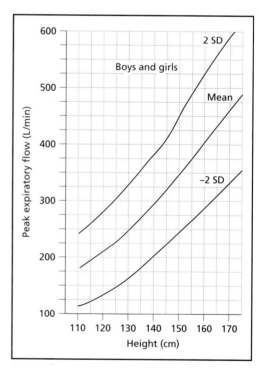

Figure 18.1 Predicted peak expiratory flow rates in children.

With life-threatening features or in a deteriorating situation get senior help, including an anaesthetist or PICU consultant, so that intubation and ventilation can be performed if the child does not improve. (Induction of anaesthesia is usually performed with the bronchodilating agents ketamine or halothane.) Children whose SaO_2 remains below 92% on air after initial treatment should also be considered for PICU referral. Then consider adding:

- *Nebulised ipratropium bromide* 250 μg (125 μg if the child is less than 2 years old). This may be repeated after every 20–30 min for children who are responding poorly to beta-2 agonists.
- *Continuous nebulised beta-2 agonists.*
- *IV salbutamol* 15 μg per kg given over 10 min. This is an alternative to repeated salbutamol or terbutaline nebulisers for children over 2 years old. It is followed by a salbutamol infusion at a rate of 1–5 μg per kg per min. ECG and electrolytes must be monitored to detect dysrhythmias and hypokalaemia.
- *Magnesium sulphate* 25–40 mg per kg given IV over 20 min (maximum dose 2 g; single dose only). *For further information on magnesium see page 255.*
- *Aminophylline* 5 mg per kg given IV over 20 min under ECG control, followed by a maintenance infusion of 1 mg per kg per hour in 5% dextrose. The infusion rate is reduced to 800 μg per kg per h for children between the ages of 10 and 16 years and to 500–700 μg per kg per h for adults. The initial loading dose should not be given to patients who are already receiving oral theophyllines.

Signs of clinical improvement include:

1 improved activity levels or responsiveness; urge to eat, drink or play;

2 falling pulse rate;

3 rising peak flow rate.

Potential discharge

Even if a child responds very well to therapy, discharge from hospital needs careful consideration. No child should be discharged unless his or her SaO_2 is more than 94% on air and the PEF is more than 75% of the predicted value. All children with features of severe asthma must be admitted. If the asthma attack was bad enough to come to an ED, then the child almost certainly requires the following:

- A period of observation (e.g. 4 h) in either a ward or a special area in an ED.
- Oral (soluble) prednisolone for 3–5 days (for infants 1–2 mg per kg per day in either one morning or two divided doses and for children age 1–5 years 20 mg per day).
- Follow-up in a paediatric clinic for reassessment and a review of his or her current therapy.

For more details about the discharge of a patient with asthma see also page 213.

Acute asthma in children under 2 years old

Attacks of wheezing in children under 2 years old are usually due to viral infection. The differential diagnosis includes bronchiolitis, pneumonia, aspiration pneumonitis, cystic fibrosis, tracheomalacia and other congenital conditions. Prematurity and low birth weight are risk factors for recurrent wheezing. A trial of bronchodilator therapy should be considered although children under 18 months old often respond poorly to beta-2 agonists. Metered dose inhalers coupled to spacer devices fitted with face masks may be more effective than nebulisers in this age group. Nebulised ipratropium bromide (125 μg) may lead to some improvement in the clinical picture. Early use of steroid tablets in the ED has been shown to reduce both admission rates and the duration of hospitalisation. Soluble prednisolone 10 mg for 3 days is the recommended regimen. Many children with recurrent episodes of viral-induced wheezing in infancy do not go on to develop chronic atopic asthma and so do not require regular prophylactic medication. The parents of these children should be advised about the relationship between exposure to cigarette smoke and the wheezy illnesses of childhood.

Bronchiolitis

Bronchiolitis is the commonest serious respiratory infection of childhood, affecting 10% of all children at some time. It is a disease of infants; 90% of attacks occur in children under 9 months old and it is rare over the age of 2 years. Bronchiolitis is usually caused by respiratory syncytial virus and may occur in epidemics, invariably in the winter. Initial fever and upper respiratory tract symptoms progress to dry coughing and signs of dyspnoea:

- poor feeding;
- tachypnoea (up to 100 breaths per min) with rib recession;
- hyperinflated lungs and thus easily palpable liver;
- fine inspiratory crepitations and expiratory wheezes;
- mild hypoxia on pulse oximetry;
- tachycardia.

Some infants with severe bronchiolitis (around 2%) will require ventilation, usually because of exhaustion. Signs of imminent deterioration include:

- pallor;
- extreme tachypnoea (>60 breaths per min);
- exhaustion;
- apnoeic spells;
- significant hypoxia.

Some babies can be predicted to have a stormier course including those with a history of:

- heart disease;
- failure to thrive;
- prematurity.

XR

Chest X-ray may show hyperinflated lungs and, in about one-third of infants, areas of segmental collapse or consolidation.

TX

Almost all babies will require admission for observation, monitoring and therapy with humidified oxygen. The disease usually settles over 10–14 days. Traditional bronchodilators and antibiotics are rarely helpful. Steroids, nebulised adrenaline and nebulised antiviral agents (ribavirin) are sometimes used but their role in bronchiolitis is still uncertain.

Pneumonia

Children with congenital abnormalities or chronic illnesses are at a high risk of pneumonia. Fever and cough may be accompanied by non-specific symptoms such as lethargy and abdominal pain.

XR

Chest X-ray may show minimal changes, consolidation or widespread bronchopneumonia.

TX

Most children will require admission for assessment. A wide spectrum of pathogens may cause pneumonia in children and so the choice of antibiotic depends on the clinical features and the age of the child. IV cefotaxime or oral amoxicillin or erythromycin are reasonable first prescriptions, depending on the severity of the illness. (*For doses see Box 18.10.*) Children with cystic fibrosis may present with complicated chest infections, which require specialist advice from the outset.

For pneumonia in older children and adults see page 218.

Other major problems

Bacterial meningitis

Bacterial meningitis occurs all year round although it usually peaks in winter months. Unfortunately, early diagnosis can be difficult and so the possibility of meningitis must always be considered in any patient with an unexplained illness or fever. Symptoms and signs in older children and adults include:

- severe headache;
- nausea and vomiting;
- fever;
- back or joint pains;
- drowsiness or confusion;
- photophobia;
- neck stiffness (often absent!).

Infants may have relatively non-specific signs such as:

Box 18.10 Doses of Common Antibiotics for Children

	1–5 years	Under 12 years	Adult
Oral			
Amoxicillin	125 mg tds	125–250 mg tds	250–500 mg tds
Erythromycin	125 mg qds	250 mg qds	250–500 mg qds
Trimethoprim	50 mg bd	100 mg bd	200 mg bd
Flucloxacillin	125 mg qds	125–250 mg qds	250–500 mg qds
Parenteral			
Cefotaxime	50–80 mg per kg tds	1–2 g tds	1–2 g tds
Benzyl penicillin	300 mg (0.5 megaunit) qds	600 mg (1 megaunit) qds	1200 mg (2 megaunit) qds

- drowsiness and irritability;
- poor feeding;
- distress on handling;
- vomiting or diarrhoea;
- high-pitched or moaning cry;
- tense or bulging fontanelle;
- apnoiec or cyanotic attacks;
- fever;
- neck stiffness.

In meningococcal infection photophobia and neck stiffness are relatively uncommon features; the most common symptoms are fever, malaise and drowsiness – *see page 336.*

Tx

- Give oxygen.
- Gain IV access. Shock must be treated but in its absence fluids should be given sparingly.
- Obtain routine blood specimens and blood cultures if possible.
- Control fits (*see page 339*).
- Check for and treat hypoglycaemia (*see page 327*).
- Start antibiotics. Cefotaxime is used as a first-line monotherapy for meningitis in an IV dose of 80 mg per kg (maximum dose = 2 g). It is effective against the meningococcus, the pneumococcus and *Haemophilus influenza*. About 10% of penicillin-sensitive patients will also be allergic to cephalosporins but, depending on the history, in this infection the risk may be worth taking. For those children (or adults) who have had a previous anaphylactic reaction to penicillin, chloramphenicol should be given IV in a dose of 12.5–25 mg per kg. To cover Listeria infection, IV ampicillin 2 g qds may be added for adults over 55 years old.
- Consider giving dexamethasone 0.15 mg per kg qds for 4 days (started with the first dose of antibiotics), especially where pneumococcal meningitis is suspected. (It may help to prevent deafnesss.)
- Refer the patient to in-patient physicians for further investigation and treatment. Consider the need for a CT scan of the brain to exclude other diagnoses. *For the contraindications to lumbar puncture see Box 18.11.*

Viral meningitis

Many different viruses may cause a meningitis. The clinical picture is very similar to a bacterial infection although the severity of the illness is usually much less. Until the diagnosis is confirmed by lumbar puncture, the treatment is identical to that for bacterial meningitis.

Encephalitis

Coxsackie viruses, other enteroviruses, arboviruses and Herpes simplex virus may all infect the brain. Drowsiness, lethargy and confusion are the commonest symptoms, usually with very few hard signs. Lumbar puncture may be helpful; CT scan is usually normal. The treatment is similar to that for suspected bacterial meningitis but with the addition of drugs directed against Herpes simplex. Aciclovir (acyclovir) 10 mg per kg is given by IV infusion every 8 h for 10 days (calculated on ideal body weight in obese patients).

Box 18.11 Contraindications to Lumbar Puncture

GCS less than 13
Papilloedema
Slow pulse, raised BP and irregular breathing (Cushing's triad)
Impaired brain stem reflexes
Abnormal posturing
Dilated pupils
Prolonged or focal seizure
Focal neurological signs
Widespread purpuric rash
Coagulopathy
Shock
Severe hypertension

Meningococcal disease

Meningococcal disease is the commonest cause of death from infectious disease in the United Kingdom; the mortality in diagnosed cases is still 10%. The disease is on the increase and is most commonly seen in young children. However, in recent years, there has been a marked rise in incidence in young people aged 15 to 24 and the case fatality rate in this age group is twice as high as that in children under 5. Meningococcal group B disease is responsible for over 80% of cases with group C (since the introduction of the MenC vaccine) accounting for less than 10% of infections. There may be a history of travel to Saudi Arabia or sub-Saharan Africa or contact with Islamic pilgrims.

Endotoxin released by meningococci is responsible for many of the features of the infection. In the bloodstream, it triggers an intense inflammatory response, which causes vascular endothelium to become 'leaky'. Plasma then moves into interstitial spaces. Circulating endotoxin also activates the coagulation cascade and may cause disseminated intravascular coagulation (DIC). Together with cytokines, it depresses myocardial contractility. In the brain, endotoxin damages the blood brain barrier leading to cerebral oedema. It causes microvascular thrombosis in the meninges and brain with a consequent reduction in cerebral perfusion.

Meningococcal disease can present as either meningitis, septicaemia or both with a great variety of clinical features. A sudden onset of fever and malaise is characteristic. Alternatively, initially trivial symptoms may suddenly become more serious. In meningococcal meningitis, photophobia and neck stiffness are relatively unusual features; the commonest symptoms are fever, malaise and drowsiness. Headache, vomiting and irritability are also often seen. Raised intracranial pressure (ICP) may lead to confusion, fits, abnormal posturing and florid neurological signs. Septicaemia can be very difficult to diagnose at first and patients can look relatively well and alert. Fever, malaise and weakness may be accompanied by myalgia, arthralgia and isolated limb pain. Rigors are common. Abdominal pain, diarrhoea and vomiting may occur; faecal incontinence has been described. As the infection takes hold, septicaemia manifests itself as shock with a vasculitic skin rash. A rapid increase in the distribution of the purpura is often associated with circulatory failure. Extensive purpura ('purpura fulminans') are indicative of coagulopathy.

The characteristic purpuric skin rash can be found in over 70% of cases of meningococcal septicaemia if a careful examination is made. However, the rash is macular and blanching in the early stages of the disease in 30% of cases.

For common mistakes in the diagnosis and treatment of meningococcal disease see Box 18.12.

Tx

- Call for senior help (including paediatrics and anaesthesia or PICU).
- Give oxygen (10–12 L per min by mask).
- Monitor and record continuously the heart rate, BP, temperature, respiratory rate, SaO$_2$, capillary refill time, GCS, pupillary size/reactions and the spread of any rash.
- Start antibiotics – IV cefotaxime 80 mg per kg or IV ceftriaxone 80 mg per kg (maximum dose of either cephalosporin = 2 g). (For those children or adults who have had a previous anaphylactic reaction to penicillin, chloramphenicol should be given in a dose of 12.5–25 mg per kg IV.)

Box 18.12 Common Mistakes in the Diagnosis and Treatment of Meningococcal Disease

1 *Expecting patients always to look very ill.* (They soon do!) In the early stages of meningococcal disease, patients may look relatively well and alert. Their mental state may remain unchanged until very late.

2 *Expecting the signs of meningitis in all cases.* The bacterium would be better named the septococcus rather than the meningococcus! Symptoms of meningitis (neck stiffness and photophobia) are absent in pure septicaemia and in young children (especially those under 2 years old) with meningitis. Teenagers may be aggressive and combative rather than drowsy.

3 *Expecting the rash to develop early and be purpuric and non-blanching in all patients.* It appears late and is blanching in 30% of cases of septicaemia – then early pinprick spots appear. The rash may be scanty, atypical or absent in pure meningitis. It is more difficult to see on darker skins – look at the soles, palms, palate and conjunctivae.

4 *Failing to recognise the significance of common symptoms and signs.* Sudden onset of fever and malaise is typical. Rigors, weakness and muscle pains are common.

5 *Failing to recognise the significance of uncommon symptoms and signs.* Isolated severe limb pain may occur in early septicaemia. In meningitis, ophthalmoplegia (new squint) is a sign of raised intracranial pressure caused by herniation of the brain through the tentorial opening.

6 *Failing to recognise features that predict a poor prognosis (and the need for urgent action) at the time of presentation.* These features include depressed level of consciousness, absence of meningism, shock, rapidly progressive purpuric rash, coagulopathy, low white cell count and thrombocytopenia.

7 *Failing to anticipate and then treat pulmonary oedema promptly and effectively.* The oedema is caused by leakage from the adjacent capillaries and the treatment is intubation, ventilation and PEEP to increase oxygenation – not diuretics.

8 *Failing to treat impending shock aggressively.* Up to 60 mL per kg of fluid may be required in the first hour together with inotropic support of the circulation. The same problem that causes the shock – capillary leakage – may also cause pulmonary oedema. The fluid should be continued and the oedema treated as stated in the previous point. Most deaths result from shock and multiorgan failure; only a few are caused by raised ICP.

9 *Failing to get PICU help early on.* PICU advice and invasive monitoring are essential as soon as possible.

- Begin resuscitation with IV fluids (*see page 326*). Excess fluids should not be given if there is a possibility of raised ICP.
- Obtain routine blood specimens and blood cultures. If possible, also take blood for clotting studies, calcium, magnesium, phosphate, venous blood gases, meningococcal PCR and blood grouping. (Low platelets, low WCC, raised urea and creatinine, coagulopathy and a base deficit greater than minus 5 mmol per L suggest a poor prognosis.)
- Check for and treat hypoglycaemia (*see page 327*).
- Control fits (*see page 338*).
- Give IV dexamethasone (0.4 mg per kg stat and then bd for two days) to children with clinical features of meningitis or raised ICP.

All children with raised ICP will require intubation and ventilation to control the $PaCO_2$ (at around 4 to 4.5 kPa). They should be nursed with a 30° head-up tilt and mannitol 0.25 g per kg and furosemide (frusemide) 1 mg per kg should be given IV to reduce ICP. A urinary catheter will be required to monitor fluid balance. Lumbar puncture and insertion of internal jugular lines should be avoided. (*For contraindications to lumbar puncture see Box 18.11*).

Septicaemic children are very likely to require early intubation and ventilation with inotropic support. Boluses of colloid (10–20 mL per kg) should be given and a urinary catheter inserted. A urinary output of at least 1ml per kg per hour is the aim. Patients who do not respond to peripheral inotropes (dopamine or dobutamine at 10–20 μg per kg per min) will require a central infusion of adrenaline (0.1 μg per kg per min). There will be gross systemic and metabolic disturbance. Therefore, it is essential to anticipate, monitor and correct if required:

- *Worsening shock* (fluids and inotropes; *see previously*)
- *Pulmonary oedema* (ventilation with PEEP – positive end expiratory pressure)
- *Raised ICP* (*see before*)
- *Hypoglycaemia* (5 mL per kg of 10% glucose)
- *Raised urea and creatinine* (secondary to inadequate renal perfusion – treat the shock and monitor the urinary output)

- *Acidosis* (1 mmol per kg of sodium bicarbonate if pH < 7.2)
- *Hypokalaemia* (0.25 mmol per kg of potassium chloride over 30 min with ECG monitoring)
- *Hypomagnesaemia* (0.2 mL per kg of 50% magnesium sulphate over 30 min if serum magnesium <0.75 mmol per L)
- *Hypocalcaemia* (0.1 mL per kg of 10% calcium chloride over 30 min if ionised calcium < 1.0 mmol per L)
- *Hypophosphataemia*
- *Anaemia, neutropenia and thrombocytopaenia*
- *Coagulopathy* (FFP 10 mL per kg)

Prevention of transmission of the meningococcus

The meningococcus is carried in the nasopharynx of many healthy children and adults without causing any disease. Some people, however, may develop invasive disease within a few days of colonisation. Illness only occurs in the first few days following this colonisation and not during established carriage. The incubation period is generally 3–4 days with a range of 2–10 days.

Most cases of meningitis in this country are sporadic but when a case occurs the risk for other members of the immediate family is increased by up to 1000-fold. The risk factors for transmission are physical intimacy and prolonged close contact. The people most at risk are those who within the 7 days prior to the onset of a patient's symptoms have:
- slept under the same roof as the patient;
- been 'kissing contacts' (friends and close relatives likely to have had mouth-to-mouth contact).

Childminders should be dealt with as part of the family unit but school contact or other community contact is not generally an indication for prophylaxis.

Health care staff only require prophylaxis when they have given a patient with meningococcal disease mouth-to-mouth resuscitation during the acute stage of the illness.

Chemoprophylaxis with rifampicin is given to eliminate nasopharyngeal carriage so as to reduce the likelihood of transmission in the community –

see Box 18.13. It is a misconception that rifampicin is given primarily to protect the recipient of the drug. The responsibility for tracing other contacts lies with the department of public health medicine.

For adults, a single dose of ciprofloxacin (500 mg) is an effective alternative to rifampicin as a prophylaxis against meningococcal infection. A single IM dose of ceftriaxone is also sometimes used (125 mg for patients under 12 years old and 250 mg for those over 12 years).

Box 18.13 Rifampicin Dosage for Prophylaxis against Meningococcal Infection

Children 0–11 months	5 mg per kg bd × 2 days
Children over 12 months and adults	10 mg per kg bd × 2 days

(to a maximum dosage of 600 mg per dose or 1200 mg per day)

Prevention of transmission of *Haemophilus influenzae* B

Invasive disease caused by this infection is most common in children under 4 years of age and has a peak incidence between the ages of 3 and 12 months inclusive. The introduction of the HiB vaccine as part of the routine immunisations of childhood has resulted in a dramatic reduction in *Haemophilus influenzae* B infection. Prophylaxis with rifampicin (but at a higher dosage than in meningococcal disease) is only indicated for members of households where there is a child under 4 years who is not immunised. Children in this category also require immediate HiB immunisation.

Fits

Around 7% of children have had a fit by the age of 3 years but only 0.5% of school age children have epilepsy. In the neonatal period birth injury, hypoglycaemia and hypocalcaemia are common causes of convulsions while intracranial infection, encephalopathy and poisoning occur at all ages. Children with congenital abnormalities often present with fits.

Febrile convulsions occur in about 3% of children between the ages of 5 months and 5 years. They are thought to be caused by a viraemia and are often recurrent. The child may present with prolonged fitting or there may have been a short period of clonic or tonic activity. Sometimes there is a story of an apparently well child suddenly becoming limp and falling to the floor. A history of stiffness, cyanosis, drooling or of the eyes rolling upwards is extremely suggestive of a childhood fit. Children with known epilepsy are more likely to have a fit during a pyrexia.

Investigations

The blood glucose should be checked in all cases at the bedside and the SaO_2 monitored. Children with atypical convulsions may need toxicological, septic and metabolic screening together with a CT scan of the brain.

Tx

The fitting child must be protected from harm and IV access obtained. Anticonvulsant therapy should follow the following progression:

1 Lorazepam 0.1 mg per kg by slow IV injection (or by the intra-osseus route). Diazepam emulsion 0.25 mg per kg IV/IO is an alternative. This can be repeated after a few minutes if the fitting continues. Rectal diazepam (0.5 mg per kg) or buccal midazolam (0.5 mg per kg) can be given if IV access is delayed – see Box 18.14. Midazolam 0.1 mg per kg IV has a shorter duration of action than other IV benzodiazepines.

2 Paraldehyde 0.4 ml per kg per rectum (0.3 mL per kg for infants) diluted 50:50 with olive oil or saline. (The diluted solution is thus given in a dose

of 0.8 mL per kg.) Paraldehyde must be given immediately if drawn up in a plastic syringe as it quickly degrades the plastic.

3 Phenytoin 18 mg per kg IV (or IO) over 30 min with ECG monitoring. This should not be given to any infants or to children who are already on phenytoin. Instead, they should have phenobarbital 15–20 mg per kg IV (or IO) over 10 min.

4 Thiopental (4 mg per kg given IV or IO by an anaesthetist), usually with accompanying rapid sequence intubation and ventilation.

If cerebral oedema or intracerebral infection are suspected, then consider the need for:

- Intubation and ventilation to maintain a $PaCO_2$ of around 4.5 kPa.
- Nursing with a 30° head-up tilt to facilitate cerebral venous drainage.
- Dexamethasone 0.4–0.5 mg per kg IV (especially for oedema around a space-occupying lesion).
- Mannitol 0.25–0.5 mg per kg by IV infusion over 15 min, repeated as required to reduce cerebral swelling.
- Cefotaxime and acyclovir IV for undiagnosed infection.

After the fitting has stopped, children with febrile convulsions should be cooled and given paracetamol or ibuprofen. Cooling measures will have only a transitory effect whereas antipyretic drugs 'reset' the hypothalamic temperature control mechanisms.

All children who have had prolonged or recurrent seizures should be admitted. Others may go home provided that:

- recovery is complete and sustained;
- there is a definite diagnosis (known epilepsy or febrile illness in an appropriate age group);
- the parents agree to the discharge;
- the home circumstances are satisfactory;
- there are adequate arrangements for follow-up.

Some hospitals have a policy of admitting all children with a first febrile convulsion. In known epileptics, blood for anticonvulsant levels should be taken before discharge.

Diabetic ketoacidosis in children

This may be seen in both known and new diabetics and is the commonest cause of death in children

Box 18.14 Rectal Dose of Diazepan	
Age	**Dose (mg)**
Over 1 year	5
Over 3 years	7.5
Over 5 years	10
Over 12 years	20
Adult	30

with diabetes. Most deaths occur as a result of cerebral oedema, hypokalaemia or aspiration pneumonia. There may be a history of increasing polyuria, polydipsia and weight loss, although more usually a concurrent infection precipitates the diabetic crisis. Abdominal pain and vomiting are common symptoms. The metabolic derangement may lead to coma, respiratory disturbance and ileus. Dehydration may be so profound as to cause shock.

Investigations

The clinical condition of the child is the best guide to severity. However, biochemical markers of severe diabetic ketoacidosis (DKA) include:
- pH < 7.2;
- glucose > 16 mmol per L;
- ketones > 2 mmol per L.

Tx

Diabetic ketoacidosis has a mortality rate of 9% in children. The cause of death is cerebral oedema in 50% of cases. To minimise the risk of this, metabolic abnormalities must be corrected slowly.
- Protect the airway and give high-concentration oxygen.
- Monitor vital functions.
- Gain IV access and take blood samples (electrolytes, glucose, blood gases, full blood count and blood cultures).
- If clinically shocked resuscitate with 10 mL per kg plasma, repeated as necessary up to 30 mL per kg. Normal saline is an alternative.
- Weigh the child and keep an exact record of fluid balance. Catheterisation may be required.
- Discuss the child with a paediatrician as soon as possible; intensive care should be arranged.
- Commence a normal (0.9%) saline infusion with added potassium (20 mmol per L) – see Box 18.15.
- Start an infusion of soluble insulin at a rate of 0.1 units per kg per h.

Bicarbonate should be avoided unless the pH is less than 7.0. Acute gastric dilatation is common in DKA and so a nasogastric tube is often required, especially if the child is comatose or vomiting.

> **Box 18.15 Fluids for a Child with DKA**
>
> Twenty-four hour fluid requirement
> = maintenance fluids + deficit.
> Fluid deficit in litres = dehydration (%) × body weight in kg.
> Deficit should be calculated assuming a maximum of 10% dehydration but ignoring any plasma that has been given.

Once the blood sugar has fallen below 10 mmol per L, the IV infusion should be changed to 0.45% saline in 5% glucose with 20 mmol potassium in each 500 mL. The insulin infusion can often then be reduced to 0.05 units per kg per h. If the blood sugar falls to less than 4 mmol per L, the insulin infusion should not be stopped because the insulin is needed to switch off ketone production. Instead, 10% glucose (2 mL per kg) should be given.

NB: Children who are less than 5% dehydrated (dry mucous membranes and reduced skin turgor only) will often tolerate oral rehydration and subcutaneous insulin.

For recognition and treatment of cerebral oedema, see Box 18.16.

Congenital abnormalities

Children with congenital abnormalities may present frequently with fits, chest infections and general illness. Their parents are under enormous

> **Box 18.16 Recognition and Treatment of Cerebral Oedema**
>
> In DKA, cerebral oedema usually occurs in the first 24 h after starting rehydration. There is headache, restlessness and drowsiness followed by bradycardia, hypertension, convulsions and coma.
> - Administer oxygen
> - Exclude hypoglycaemia
> - Nurse the patient with head elevated
> - Give mannitol 1 g per kg over 20 min (5 mL per kg of 20% solution)
> - Restrict fluids to 2/3 maintenance only
> - Discuss the need for intubation and hyperventilation (to reduce PCO_2) with an intensivist
> - Arrange a CT scan of the brain
> - Repeat the dose of mannitol after 2 h if no improvement

strain and so admission should always be considered as an option. Background information from the GP may be useful.

Common complaints

For mumps see page 420.
For herpes simplex stomatitis see page 401.

Upper respiratory tract infections and earache

Young children may have upper respiratory problems up to 10 times a year. Such infections may precipitate asthma attacks or lead to more serious chest infections. Symptoms of upper respiratory tract infection (URTI) include the following:

• *Cough and/or runny nose.* The most common signs of infection. The barking cough of croup is important to recognise as it may accompany stridor. Whooping cough is very distressing; severe coughing empties the lungs and is followed by an inspiratory 'whoop'. The problem may persist for weeks.

• *Sore throat.* This is caused by pharyngitis or enlarged lymph nodes in the neck.

• *Earache.* Young children may pull at their ears if they have earache. Otitis media is a frequent accompaniment of URTI in children.

• *Abdominal pain.* This is caused by mesenteric adenitis and is common. There are usually no localising signs. Specific tenderness may be difficult to distinguish from appendicitis or urinary tract infection.

• *Non-specific symptoms.* Pyrexia, poor feeding, malaise, crying and vomiting.

Tx

Reassurance, fluids and paracetamol are the mainstays of treatment. The former is greatly enhanced if preceded by a thorough examination. Unilateral red eardrums are suggestive of bacterial infection and should be treated with antibiotics (amoxicillin or erythromycin – *see Box 18.10*). Some children with URTIs will need admission for a large variety of reasons.

The risk of sudden infant death syndrome

A high proportion of infants who die from sudden infant death syndrome (SIDS) will have had a minor infection in the previous few days. To minimise this risk the following advice should be given, without necessarily discussing the possibility of SIDS.

• The infant should be positioned on his or her back, or perhaps on the side if there are increased secretions or a risk of vomiting.

• The bedding should not be capable of causing restriction of movement or overheating.

• It is probably wise to have infants sleeping within range of hearing.

Rashes

> The rash in meningococcal disease is classically purpuric but may be macular in the initial stages.

The common exanthemas (rashes) of childhood may baffle the staff of an ED. However, their recognition is important for prognosis, detection of severe illness and sometimes for credibility. The main types are the following.

• *Purpuric.* A non-blanching red or purple rash is caused by extravasation of blood. The septicaemia of meningococcal disease is the most serious cause – *see page 336*. It also occurs in vasculitis (Henoch–Schönlein purpura) and platelet deficiency (idiopathic thrombocytopenic purpura, leukaemia or drugs). All children with purpura must be seen by a paediatrician.

• *Urticarial.* Blotchy, raised, itchy, red and hot. There is diffuse erythema and sometimes swelling of the face and hands. Areas may look like nettle-stings, which are also caused by histamine release – *see page 296*. Itchy scratch marks with either little else to see or some urticaria are usually caused by scabies infection – *see page 404*.

• *Vesicular.* Small, itchy, fluid-filled vesicles that develop at different rates are typical of chickenpox. Later, they become pustular and, if badly infected, should be treated with flucloxacillin.

(*For the differences between chickenpox and smallpox see page 261*). Vesicles may also be seen in:

– herpes simplex (perioral and on the fingers) (*see page 401*);

– impetigo (*see page 401*);

– hand, foot and mouth disease (which starts as painful red dots);

– insect bites (often on the legs).

A single, dark, pus-filled vesicle is often found at the centre of a streptococcal cellulitis.

• *Morbilliform.* The maculopapular rash of measles is diffuse, irregular and usually bright red. It is accompanied by an URTI, swollen watery eyes (conjunctivitis) and Koplick's spots (white dots on the buccal surface of the cheeks). Allergy may sometimes cause a similar rash, which is unaccompanied by the high pyrexia of measles.

• *Pink and papular.* A large variety of viral infections may cause a diffuse maculopapular rash accompanied by upper respiratory symptoms including:

– Rubella – which is accompanied by post-auricular and occipital lymphadenopathy;

– Fourth disease (roseola infantum or exanthem subitum) – discrete pink macules on the trunk;

– Fifth disease (erythema infectiosum or slapped cheek syndrome) – a parvovirus infection, which begins with erythema of the cheeks and circumoral pallor.

> The diagnosis of Kawasaki disease should be considered in any child with a febrile erythematous illness that persists longer than 4 or 5 days – see later.

Kawasaki disease

Kawasaki disease is an acute febrile illness of unknown aetiology. Although uncommon, it is included in this section because of its non-specific features. Eighty per cent of cases occur in children under 5 years old, sometimes in small epidemics. There is an underlying vasculitis. The diagnosis is usually only confirmed if at least 5 of the following clinical features are present:

• fever;

• reddening of the oropharyngeal mucosa including the tongue;

• dry, fissured lips;

• conjunctivitis;

• peeling fingers or toes;

• erythema of the hands and feet, which become swollen and indurated (oedema and pain in the extremities may be the predominant symptom);

• a morbilliform, maculopapular or urticarial rash on the trunk and limbs (within 5 days of the onset of the fever);

• enlarged cervical lymph nodes (in over half of patients);

• arthralgia;

• thrombocytosis.

During the illness, the coronary arteries can become dilated. This may result in the development of coronary aneurysms and delayed but sudden death.

Tx

All patients in whom the diagnosis of Kawasaki disease is a possibility must be referred to a paediatrician immediately. The administration of oral aspirin and IV human immunoglobulin can protect the coronary arteries from damage, but only if given within 10 days of the onset of the illness.

Urinary tract infection

Infections of the urinary tract in children are associated with vesicoureteric reflux and with obstructive lesions. There may be an obvious urinary problem (dysuria, frequency, urgency, haematuria, enuresis or incontinence) or non-specific symptoms such as:

• pyrexia;

• vomiting;

• abdominal or renal pain.

Recurrent infections may lead to renal damage and chronic renal failure.

Tx

A clean urine specimen for culture must be sent to the laboratory before antibiotic treatment is started (e.g. trimethoprim, *see Box 18.10*). All children with UTIs must be referred to a paediatrician via the GP for investigation of the urinary tract (micturating cystogram and renal imaging).

Diarrhoea and vomiting

> Children often vomit after minor injuries and during the course of many illnesses.

The main dangers of gastroenteritis are dehydration and electrolyte imbalance. Infants are particularly susceptible to dehydration because of their very high turnover of water relative to their size. An infant's normal daily intake of 120–150 mL per kg represents up to 15% of his or her body weight. Gastoenteritis in an infant is thus similar in effect to cholera in an adult! *For the signs of dehydration see Box 18.17.*

> Dehydration may be underestimated in hypernatraemia or in plump children.

Box 18.17 Signs of Dehydration

Percentage of body weight lost	Signs
Under 5%	Generally well: dry membranes, slight oliguria
5–10%	Unwell: apathetic, sunken eyes and fontanelle, reduced skin elasticity, tachypnoea, oliguria
Over 10%	Shocked: tachycardia and vasoconstriction
Over 15%	Moribund

Tx

Most children can be managed at home with oral rehydration fluids (although clear liquids do not affect the frequency, amount or duration of loose stools). Vomiting may be reduced by giving fluids frequently and in small amounts. After 24 h, milk or a light diet can be reintroduced, although sometimes lactose intolerance will prolong diarrhoea.

Admission to hospital is required for children who are more than 5% dehydrated or whose parents are having difficulty in dealing with the problem. The type of fluid replacement will depend on the severity of the condition. In severe cases, the plasma electrolytes should be measured; hypoglycaemia may occur.

Intussusception

Although not a common illness, this cause of intestinal obstruction is included in this section because of its often non-specific presentation. Intussusception usually affects children between the ages of 3 months and 3 years and is most common in the first year of life. It occurs when the terminal ileum and ileocaecal valve invaginate into the caecum and ascending colon. The classic triad of intermittent colicky abdominal pain, vomiting and red currant jelly stools is seen in less than 10% of children with intussusception. Lethargy and malaise are the commonest signs. There may be a palpable mass in the right hypochondrium.

Investigations

Red currant jelly stool is rare but the faeces usually test positive for blood. Ultrasound scan is the diagnostic study of choice; barium or air enema is a treatment.

Tx

All children with suspected intussusception should be referred immediately to a surgeon. IV fluids are usually required.

Three months' colic

This is a condition that affects babies in the first few months of life. Spasms of severe crying and drawing up of the legs suggest a painful colic. Stools or flatus may be passed.

Tx

No specific therapy has been shown to help. Paracetamol elixir and tummy rubbing are useful placebos. Admission should be considered for distressed parents, as discussed before.

Infants crying and parents not coping

Crying infants may be brought to the ED by their distraught parents. A thorough history and examination must be conducted, both to exclude serious illness or trauma and to reassure the parents. No tests are better than careful observation and taking the temperature.

> Occasionally, a hair or a thread that has spontaneously become wrapped around a digit is found to be the cause of the child's distress.

Tx

If no abnormality is discovered, then professional reassurance may be all that is needed. The GP should be notified. Some areas have the facility for late night visits by a health visitor.

Parents who feel that that they cannot cope with crying or minor illness must be taken seriously. The child should be admitted for care and assessment. A crying child causes enormous stress and may even in some cases provoke physical abuse.

Threadworms

Infestation with threadworms causes perianal irritation at night. This is the time when the mature female worm crawls out of the bowel to lay her eggs around the anus. Scratching transfers the eggs to the fingers, from where they find their way (via food, clothing and linen) back to the bowel. The small, white worms may easily be seen at the time of the symptoms.

Tx

A single dose of 100 mg of mebendazole will kill threadworms. All close contacts should be treated. The dosage may be repeated after 2–3 weeks to prevent reinfection. Mebendazole is not suitable for children under the age of 2 years or for pregnant or lactating women.

Hygienic precautions are necessary to prevent both reinfection and spread:
- hand-washing;
- daily bathing and washing around the bottom;
- wearing pyjamas in bed;
- having a personal towel;
- changing clothes and bed-linen frequently.

Injuries and accidents

Refer to the relevant sections in the appropriate chapters.
For the limping child see page 95.
For the child who is not moving an arm see page 124.
For burns see Chapter 10.
For swallowed foreign bodies see page 415.
For foreign bodies in the ears and nose see page 413.
For minor injuries see Chapter 21.
For finger tip injuries see page 138.
For impetigo see page 401.
For poisoning see Chapter 15.

Poisoning

See Chapter 15.
Bizarre symptoms and signs and unexplained combinations of findings suggest poisoning. Younger children may ingest substances accidentally; older children may experiment with drugs. Either may have been given inappropriate medication by an adult. The most common non-specific signs are:
- confusion, agitation and drowsiness;
- tachycardia;
- dilated pupils;
- evidence at the scene (which is of enormous help to hospital staff).

Gastric decontamination is rarely required in children. Charcoal is now available in relatively palatable syrup suspensions. Milk is a simple treatment for many ingestions.

Osteochondritis

There are several conditions in which there is an abnormality of bone in an area of growth. Children with one of these diseases may present to the ED with pain and reduced movements, often exacerbated by a minor injury. There is often slight swelling around the affected area.

These osteochondritides are most commonly seen in the lower limb:

- head of the femur – Perthes' disease (*see page 95*);
- lower pole of the patella – Sindig–Laarson's disease (*see page 104*);
- tibial tuberosity – Osgood–Schlatter's disease (*see page 104*);
- posterior calcaneum – Sever's disease;
- navicular bone – Köhler's disease (*see page 112*);
- head of a metatarsal bone (usually the second metatarsus) – Freiberg's disease.

XR

The affected area may be deformed or fragmented. It is thought that a deficiency in the blood supply of the growing bone leads to aseptic necrosis.

Tx

Symptoms usually resolve with time. Rest from sports should be advised and an appointment at the orthopaedic clinic should be given.

Epiphyseal injuries

Injuries to the epiphyses are specific to childhood and adolescence. The epiphyseal plate is a weak area of the bone and so is often damaged. Bilateral or unilateral growth retardation may then occur. The Salter–Harris classification describes 5 types of epiphyseal injury of which type II is the most common – *see Fig. 18.2 on page 346.*

For wrist injuries in children see page 130.
For elbow injuries in children (and a description of the growing elbow) see page 123.
For ankle injuries in children see page 107.

Immunisation in childhood

It is every child's right to be protected against infectious diseases. No child should be denied immunisation without serious thought as to the consequences, both for the individual child and for the community.

Department of Health (1996).

> One in 10 children with meningococcal group C infection dies.
> One in 20 children with Haemophilus Influenzae B meningitis dies.
> One in 500 infants with pertussis dies.

For an ED, good practice in the area of immunisation is essential. No child should be given a single anti-tetanus vaccine. If protection against tetanus is needed, this should be given together with the other vaccines indicated for that age group (*see Box 18.18*). Unimmunised children should either

Box 18.18 UK Immunisation Schedule for Children		
Age	**Target of immunisation**	**Name of vaccine**
2, 3 and 4 months	Diphtheria, tetanus, pertussis, polio and *H. Influenzae* B	DTaP/IPV/Hib (5 in 1)
	Meningococcus Group C	MenC
13 months	Measles, mumps and rubella	MMR
3.5 to 5 years	Diphtheria, tetanus, pertussis and polio	DTaP/IPV
	Measles, mumps and rubella	MMR
10 to 14 years	Tuberculosis	Tuberculin test then BCG if required
13 to 18 years	Diphtheria, tetanus and polio	Td/IPV

Note: Td = tetanus vaccine combined with low-dose diphtheria vaccine. Low-dose (adult) diphtheria vaccine (d) should always be given after the age of 10 years rather than standard full-strength (paediatric) diphtheria vaccine (D). In older patients, use of the D vaccine results in a high number of both localised and generalised reactions.
Pneumococcal vaccination for all children is due to start in 2006. Hepatitis B immunisation for children may soon become routine in the United Kingdom.

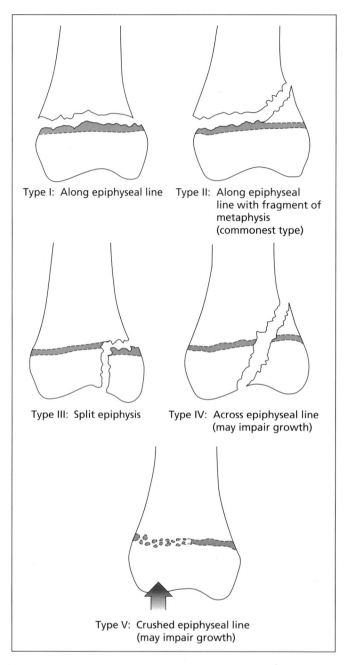

Type I: Along epiphyseal line

Type II: Along epiphyseal line with fragment of metaphysis (commonest type)

Type III: Split epiphysis

Type IV: Across epiphyseal line (may impair growth)

Type V: Crushed epiphyseal line (may impair growth)

Figure 18.2 The Salter–Harris classifications of epiphyseal injuries.

be immunised opportunistically or else referred to the GP and health visitor for follow-up.

Toxic shock syndrome

At any one time, around 3% of the population harbour a toxin-producing strain of *Staphylococcus*

aureus on their skin. Infection of burns or other wounds with these pathogenic bacteria may lead to a life-threatening toxaemia. This toxic shock syndrome is characterised by:

- malaise, anorexia and lethargy;
- dizziness or faintness;

- pyrexia (usually above 39°C);
- myalgia;
- vomiting or diarrhoea;
- a rash (often erythematous or maculopapular);
- peripheral shutdown and frank shock.

Burns information cards should advise parents of the possible dangers of these symptoms in their children. This syndrome may also be seen in women whose vaginal tampons have become infected.

Tx

Resuscitation should be commenced immediately with oxygen and fluids. Anti-staphylococcal therapy must be instituted as soon as possible and purulent lesions should be drained. In severe cases, steroids have been used to limit the endogenous inflammatory response.

Sedation and analgesia for children undergoing procedures in the emergency department

Midazolam elixir

This is an effective tranquilliser for minor procedures in children. The usual dose is 0.5 mg per kg. The onset of sedation occurs within about 20 min and the peak effect may be reached a few minutes later. Recovery is rapid – within less than 2 h – but even so, the parents of all children who have been sedated should have written aftercare instructions to take home (*see page 385*). Some children (around 10%) who have been given midazolam in the above dosage will become hyperexcited. As with all benzodiazepines, the effects of midazolam can be reversed with flumazenil (*see page 279*).

> Sedative drugs used in isolation do not provide analgesia.

Local anaesthetic agents

These must be used with care in children as the maximum safe dose is easily exceeded – *see Box 18.19.*

> **Box 18.19 Maximum Doses of Local Anaesthetic Agents**
>
> | | |
> |---|---|
> | Bupivacaine | 2 mg per kg |
> | Lidocaine | 3 mg per kg |
> | Prilocaine | 4 mg per kg |

Morphine elixir

This can be used to alleviate the pain of a procedure where local anaesthesia is not practicable, such as changing a dressing on a large burn. The dose is 0.2–0.4 mg per kg for a child over 12 months old. The elixir must be given at least 60 min before the procedure to give adequate time for it to work.

Parenteral doses of narcotic analgesics

These can sometimes be useful in instances where a combination of sedation and analgesia is desirable and oral therapy is not suitable – *for dosages see Box 18.7.*

Gaseous analgesia and sedation

Analgesic gas from a premixed nitrous oxide/oxygen cylinder (e.g. Entonox) should be administered via a demand valve with a low opening pressure. An excellent sedative effect may be obtained with a continuous flow apparatus such as the Quantiflex machine. *See page 19.*

Ketamine

Ketamine given IM in a dose of 2 mg per kg creates a unique analgesic, dissociative and sedative effect. Although it is very safe, it should only be used by practitioners experienced in sedative techniques. *See page 19.*

Local anaesthetic creams

Topical local anaesthetic preparations are available. Mixtures such as Emla and Ametop are suitable for procedures on intact skin such as venepuncture and splinter removal. Cocaine and adrenaline cream is used to provide analgesia for suturing in some departments.

Diversional therapies

These are a long-established psychological means of helping with difficult situations. Elaborate coloured pattern and bubble generators are now available as well as traditional diversions such as music and stories. Some departments employ a play specialist who can advise on this aspect of care.

Rewards such as balloons, badges and bravery certificates can help to soften the trauma of an unpleasant experience. Raisins and sweets – sugar-free of course – are also used in some departments. As Mary Poppins said in 1910, 'a spoonful of sugar helps the medicine go down'.

Child abuse

Five main types of child abuse are now recognised:
1 emotional abuse;
2 neglect;
3 sexual abuse;
4 physical abuse (non-accidental injury, NAI);
5 organised abuse.

The above list is in approximate order of prevalence, although the exact ranking is unknown.

> Inclusion of a child's name in the Child Protection Register is a useful finding in a case of suspected abuse but does not influence the initial management.

Physical abuse

Child abuse occurs in every culture and is perpetrated by all social classes and by both sexes. Nevertheless, certain factors are associated with abuse and include:
• parents abused as children (learned behaviour);
• parents with alcohol or other drug problems (alcohol is a factor in most violence);
• frequent address changes (without a permanent address a family has almost nothing);
• undesirable and stressful living conditions or other social circumstances (of course).

The stress of looking after very young children also increases the risk and so:

• one-third of NAI occurs under 6 months of age;
• one-third of NAI occurs between 6 months and 3 years of age;
• one-third of NAI occurs over 3 years of age.

A crying baby is an enormous strain and is the provocation for some cases of methadone poisoning.

> Diagnosis of abuse is a complex problem. False accusations may cause great distress. In suspicious circumstances, experienced advice should be obtained before a full examination is undertaken.

There are patterns of physical signs for some types of abuse but the history and the context in which the events occurred are the most important first indicators to alert the health worker. Some features of a history of injury that should raise a suspicion of abuse are the following.
• Inappropriate delay in seeking help and advice after a significant injury.
• History of previous frequent accidents.
• The history of the accident is not a likely mechanism for that injury.
• Vague or absent history of an accident.
• Different carers give different explanations for the same injury.
• The history keeps changing.
• The child gives a different history.
• The child is supposed to have sustained the injury in a way that is inconsistent with his or her development, (e.g. fell over before the child has started walking).
• The adults with the child are either unconcerned or hostile during questioning. Their attention is focused on their own needs throughout.

The following list of signs of child abuse is by no means comprehensive.
• Unexplained head, facial, chest or limb injuries, especially in children who are not able to walk and thus fall. (Few children walk under the age of 11 months.)
• Multiple bruising.
• Symmetrical bruising.
• Linear bruising, especially to the buttocks or back.
• Bruising around the eye, especially if bilateral.
• Bruising around the ears, especially if bilateral.

- Other facial bruising including in or around the mouth.
- Facial petechiae/subconjunctival haemorrhages.
- Tears of the frenulum of the upper lip.
- Grasp marks or fingertip bruising especially to the face, arms or chest.
- Unusual cuts and bruises. Outline imprints of hands, sticks, cords, shoes, belts and teeth may be present.
- Marks to the neck.
- Marks to the genitalia.
- A tender, red scalp (hair-pulling).
- Unusual burns, e.g. those of a glove or stocking distribution or to the perineum or cigarette-type.
- Injuries of different ages.
- Multiple old scars.
- Any fractures in children under 12 months old.
- Coexisting signs of neglect.

> Look for the child's name on the Child Protection Register (*see page 380*).

For intracerebral injury in the shaken baby see page 43.

> All children in whom the diagnosis of abuse is suspected should be fully examined from top to toe by an experienced doctor. The investigation and management of a case of possible deliberate harm to a child must be approached in the same systematic and rigorous manner as the investigation and management of any other potentially fatal disease.

Xʀ

There are also typical radiographic findings of abuse, which are more common in younger children.
- Old unsuspected fractures.
- Fractures at different stages of healing.
- Rib fractures (posterior rib fractures are particularly specific for abuse).
- Skull fractures in children who cannot walk (especially if multiple, depressed or in areas other than the parietal bones) – *see page 43*.
- Spiral fractures of long bones (twisting injuries).

Box 18.20 Radiographic Healing of Fractures

Periosteal new bone formation	10–14 days
Loss of fracture line definition	14–21 days
Soft callus formation	14–21 days
Hard callus visible	Over 21 days

- Injuries to the metaphyses of long bones (twisting injuries). These are very specific for abuse.
- Periosteal injuries (twisting forces again).

A skeletal survey – to look for occult injuries – is usually only indicated in children under 2 years of age. Dating of a fracture is a job for a radiologist (*see Box 18.20*).

Tx

There will be a local protocol for the management of suspected abuse. The child should always be discussed with a senior member of the ED or paediatric staff. The duty social worker for child protection must also be notified of the concern as soon as possible. This should be followed up in writing within 48 h.

The child must be examined from head to toe and all findings measured and carefully documented (*see page 365*). Injuries should be treated and referred to other departments as appropriate. Specialised investigations in cases of abuse (e.g. clotting screen, platelets, LFTs and calcium studies) are usually obtained by the paediatric staff at a later date.

The reasons for admission to hospital are the same as for non-abused children (unless admission is used as a method to prevent the child from leaving a place of safety). The Child Protection Unit now places most abused children in the care of the extended family or foster parents.

For the legal aspects of child protection, including emergency powers, see page 380.

Neglect and emotional abuse

Only gross forms of neglect can be recognised in an ED. Some of the characteristics are:
- short in stature and underweight for age;

- cold, mottled, discoloured extremities;
- poor skin condition (especially in the nappy area);
- dry, sparse hair;
- wasting;
- diarrhoea;
- voracious appetite;
- flat affect and unresponsiveness;
- lack of energy and failure to play.

Emotional abuse is even more subtle than physical neglect.

Tx

As for other forms of abuse, these children should be discussed with a social worker and a senior paediatrician.

Sexual abuse

Before the age of 16, at least one in 10 girls and one in 15 boys will have been sexually assaulted. The peak incidence of first assault is at about 8 years of age.

Sexual abuse of children can again occur in all socio-economic, cultural and religious groups and is associated with:
- acute perineal injury;
- chronic perineal damage;
- genitourinary infection;
- sexually precocious behaviour;
- sexualised drawings and play;
- regressive patterns of behaviour;
- eating and sleep disorders;
- psychosomatic symptoms;
- withdrawal and depression;
- self-harm;
- promiscuity;
- running away from home.

Profound anal dilatation can occur after failed cardiopulmonary resuscitation in children.

The most common victim is a girl of school age, the offender is usually male and disclosure to an adult is the most frequent way in which the abuse comes to light. A surprising number of patients who present with self-harm will later give a history of sexual abuse.

Tx

All suspected cases should be referred for consideration of the need for child protection as described before. Examination of acute injuries should be deferred to a specialist police surgeon as forensic evidence must be collected.

Sudden infant death syndrome

One baby in every 1400 live births dies suddenly and unexpectedly for no obvious reason. This sudden infant death syndrome is the most common cause of death in the United Kingdom in infants over 1 month of age. The diagnosis does not include all cot deaths as some infants die suddenly from well-understood causes.
- SIDS is more common among boys and with babies of low birth weight.
- It has a peak incidence at 2–5 months of age.
- It is more common in the winter months.
- Most deaths from SIDS seem to occur during sleep.
- Half of all babies who die from SIDS have had a recent URTI (*see page 341*).

Tx

Always bring an infant or young child into the resuscitation room and assess the situation properly, however cold or apparently dead. Children can withstand long periods of hypoxia and still recover. Parents often follow the ambulance not knowing the fate of their child. They need to know that the action taken was immediate and appropriate. Parents should have constant access to their child – even during resuscitation. A nurse should act as a communicator.

The principles of care of bereaved relatives are described on *page 169*. After a child's death the following procedure should apply:
- A senior member of the medical staff should break the news. The baby's name should be used in conversation.

- The parents should be encouraged to sit with or hold their child in a quiet room – for as long as they want.
- They should be asked if they would like a photograph of the child or a lock of hair or a handprint.
- The parents should be given the Foundation for the Study of Infant Deaths (FSID) leaflet, *Information for parents following the unexpected death of their baby*, and also FSID local contact numbers.
- Contact should be made with other family members, the hospital chaplain and a translator if necessary.
- The coroner's officer must be informed. Postmortem examination is not always required by the coroner in cases of SIDS. The purpose of the coroner's procedures should be explained to the parents.
- The GP and the health visitor should be informed. They must ensure that the local health authority deletes the child's name from the immunisation register, etc. Suppression of lactation may be required.
- A senior paediatrician should be involved in the follow-up.
- Transport home should be offered to the relatives.
- The need for continued support should be recognised; a bereavement counsellor is invaluable in this respect.

Infant death can be a very difficult situation for many doctors and nurses who may have children who are the same age as the deceased. Staff support should always be available.

Chapter 19

The disturbed patient

People come to an ED to get medical help. Mental distress is as valid a reason for seeking that help as any physical problem.

One person in seven has a diagnosable neurotic disorder, mainly depression and anxiety, and one person in 250 has a functional psychosis.

Behaviour is influenced by the interplay between the environment and the psyche and is modified by drugs. A disturbed patient may be suffering from a psychiatric condition, an organic brain lesion, a personality disorder or an emotional upset. *See Box 19.1* for common acute presentations of mental disturbance. The task of the ED is to:

- identify those patients who need immediate therapy;
- support the coping strategies of the patient;
- liaise with the appropriate agency for further care.

Initial assessment and management of the disturbed patient

Ask about

- Presenting complaints as described by the patient and those accompanying him or her.
- The history of the presenting complaints and any accompanying problems.
- Current drug therapy and other management and support.
- Previous psychiatric history: symptoms, duration, diagnoses, admissions and any treatment received.
- Coincidental physical illnesses.

Look for

- Abnormal appearance or behaviour.
- Disorientation or altered conscious level.
- Lack of attention or concentration.
- Poor memory.
- Unusual form or content of speech.
- Depressed or elevated mood.
- Disordered thought content.
- Abnormal beliefs: delusions, misinterpretations and overvalued ideas.

Box 19.1 The Presentation of Mental Disorders to the Emergency Department

Acute psychiatric disturbance (patient with little insight brought to ED by relatives, social workers or the police).

Psychological symptoms (patient usually self-referred with depression, anxiety).

Exacerbation of symptoms or loss of control in known psychiatric disease (patient usually has good insight and self-refers; may request admission).

Personality disorder (self-referred patient with no apparent insight; often manipulative).

Self-harm.

Alcohol and drug abuse.

Acute emotional upset.

- Hallucinations (visual or auditory) and disorders of perception.
- Obsessions and compulsions.
- The level of insight that the patient has into his or her problems.

These are the main features of the mental state examination. Concise notes may be augmented by verbatim quotes of the patient's responses to questioning. A brief but comprehensive physical examination is also important to exclude organic causes of disturbance (*see later*). This must include:

- temperature;
- heart rate;
- palpation of the scalp;
- blood sugar;
- gross neurological signs (walking and talking).

Therapeutic manoeuvres include:

- correction of organic problems (e.g. hypoxia and hypoglycaemia);
- sedation (oral lorazepam 2 mg initially and then IV benzodiazepines +/− IV major tranquillizers);
- referral to a psychiatrist or other agency.

Distinction must be made between:

- responses to adverse life events that may appear logical to the patient, however bizarre to the doctor;
- major psychiatric disease, which may be distinguished by the history or examination;
- other medical conditions, which masquerade as psychiatric illness (e.g. head injury, hypoglycaemia, infection, drug disturbance, epilepsy and cerebrovascular disease).

Interaction with the disturbed patient

The image portrayed by staff is very important. The patient is extremely vulnerable and sees doctors and nurses as being in a position of power. Occasionally, this will provoke an aggressive response. It is important, therefore, not only that actions cannot be interpreted as threatening but also that staff are never put in a position of vulnerability themselves. Staff should avoid being judgemental and must be sensitive to a patient's affect. They need to be aware of the potential for manipulative behaviour but must not react to it in a critical manner.

> Promises should only be made if they can be visibly kept; unfulfilled promises increase distrust and the risk of further aggression.

The aim is to support the patient at a time of crisis and to identify appropriate agencies that can provide sustained care. The latter can include the patient's relatives and friends and the patient's own resources. Medication and admission – rarely against the patient's will – may be necessary but physical restraint can only be justified as a prelude to a specific therapy (e.g. holding down a patient while an injection of glucagon or IV glucose is administered).

The patient's behaviour must be responded to appropriately. For example, if a patient is rude or abusive this must not be a cue for clever retaliation. Neither must it be ignored. The situation should be briefly summarised and an explanation that such behaviour is unacceptable must be given. Surprisingly, this sometimes works but, if it does not, lengthy interrogation must be avoided and an early decision made to seek further help from the duty psychiatrist.

Throughout care in the ED it is essential to reassure the patient constantly about the intended course of action and to keep the patient up to date with events.

Confusion and psychotic behaviour

Acute confusional states

Confusion, disorientation and clouding of consciousness may be caused by a wide range of underlying conditions.

- Hypoxia may present as a toxic confusional state and a psychosis of rapid onset with disorientation, hallucination and delusions. There will be a clouding of consciousness and impairment of recent memory. These sudden alterations in cerebration are very frightening and sufficient to cause aggression in many patients.
- Hypoglycaemia may cause considerable violence and aggression.

- Infection, particularly of the central nervous system, can also cause an acute confusional state. Elderly patients with any infection (e.g. chest or urinary tract) can present in such a way that the underlying medical condition is completely masked.
- Drug intoxication (*see later and Chapter 15*).
- Gross metabolic disturbance, including that found with hepatic and renal failure.
- Organic brain lesions may occasionally present in this way.
- Postictal states.
- Cerebrovascular accidents.
- Myocardial infarction may present with acute confusion in the elderly.

Tx

It is often impossible to assess fully or manage a confused and distressed patient. Adequate sedation makes further therapy possible. Intravenous lorazepam or midazolam are effective and have a rapid onset of action but careful observation and monitoring are necessary. Hypoglycaemia is one of the few situations where rapid diagnosis and specific therapy obviate the need for sedation. The use of depressant drugs has been criticised in hypoxaemia as it may decrease respiratory effort. However, in situations of extreme restlessness, judicious sedation decreases oxygen requirements and makes possible the administration of high-concentration oxygen by mask.

Once the patient is reasonably calm, attention should be directed to discovering and treating the primary pathology. A full physical examination should be carried out and the patient's temperature measured accurately. In elderly patients, an ECG and a chest X-ray should be obtained together with FBC and blood chemistry. In this same group of patients, a troponin level – taken 12 h after the onset of symptoms – may reveal an unsuspected myocardial infarction (*see page 183*). Agitation can be greatly reduced if any accompanying pain is relieved and so analgesia is often helpful. Splintage of injuries and drainage of a full bladder may have a similar effect.

If rapid tranquillisation is considered necessary, prior to formal diagnosis and where there is uncertainty about previous medical history (including history of cardiovascular disease, unknown prescribed medications and a possibility of current drug or alcohol intoxication), lorazepam is the drug of choice. Where there is a confirmed history of previous significant antipsychotic exposure (and response), haloperidol may be given in addition.

Drug-induced psychiatric syndromes

Prescribed drugs

Mental disturbance caused by prescribed drugs is particularly common in the elderly but may occur with central nervous system depressant drugs, beta-blockers, digoxin and cimetidine at all ages. Symptoms include fluctuating clouding of consciousness and restlessness with paranoid delusions and visual hallucinations in severe cases. Although usually a result of overdosage, these reactions may sometimes occur because of intolerance to the normal dose or after withdrawal of the drug.

Recreational drugs

Patients may retain full consciousness but experience paranoid delusions and visual hallucinations after ingestion of cocaine, amphetamines, lysergic acid diethylamide (LSD) and psychotropic fungi. Fear and restlessness lead to disruptive and aggressive behaviour. The condition can be distinguished from schizophrenia by the history and often by the extreme nature of the patient's behaviour.

For treatment of specific poisonings, see Chapter 15.

Psychoses

A psychosis is defined as a significant mental illness that robs the patient of insight and distorts appreciation of the environment. It follows that a psychotic patient cannot be held responsible for his or her actions.

Schizophrenia is now no longer thought to be a single condition. The name embraces a heterogeneous group of clinical syndromes in which hallucinations, delusions and thought disorder are present. The intensity of these symptoms is constantly changing and they may be modified or abolished by drugs. Mood and behaviour are similarly fluctuant.

Patients with both schizophrenia and mania may present acutely to the ED with obvious psychotic behaviour. The distinction between the two conditions can be difficult at times but is not initially important since pharmacological control of symptoms is similar in both conditions.

More commonly, a patient with a known history of schizophrenia comes to the ED with an exacerbation of usually well-controlled symptoms. Loss of therapeutic control may be precipitated by:
- pressure of outside events;
- moving area of residence away from long-term support;
- omitting depot therapy;
- absence of usual support (friends, relatives or care workers).

Tx

Psychotic behaviour may necessitate the administration of neuroleptic drugs (e.g. haloperidol 5–10 mg IV or IM), although oral lorazepam 2 mg and/or oral haloperidol 5 mg may be tried initially. These patients will subsequently require expert care from psychiatrists. In less acute cases, community psychiatric nurses can be a useful source of information and advice.

> It is important to distinguish patients with psychoses from those with neurotic conditions. Patients with neuroses are likely to be less disturbed and more amenable to therapy and advice from the non-specialist.

Medical conditions in psychiatric patients

Up to 50% of psychiatric patients have a medical condition and, in some cases, this may exacerbate psychiatric symptoms. In particular, patients with a diagnosis of schizophrenia have an increased

incidence of:
- cardiovascular disease;
- endocrine diseases;
- infections;
- nutritional problems.

There is a corresponding increase in mortality from these conditions and thus medical symptoms in psychiatric patients should always be investigated appropriately.

Alcohol-related problems

Acute intoxication with alcohol

The patient who smells of alcohol may appear merely drunk and disorderly but never assume that this is the only pathology. A coexistent head injury or hypoglycaemia may look identical to the effects of alcohol. Diagnosis of alcohol intoxication must always be made by exclusion – never by neglect.

Alcohol absorption from the gastrointestinal tract will continue for some time after last ingestion. In comatose patients, blood levels continue to rise for about 2 h after presentation. The patient may appear to be becoming quieter and more cooperative when he or she is in fact becoming more intoxicated. Respiratory depression and inhalation of vomitus can occur quite suddenly.

For the signs of intoxication with alcohol and for the treatment of acute alcohol poisoning see page 283.

Alcohol withdrawal states

Alcohol withdrawal is not synonymous with delirium tremens. There are in fact several possible presentations that can follow the cessation of drinking in patients who are physically dependent on ethanol.

Acute withdrawal syndrome

This occurs within 6–12 h of abstinence and presents as:
- agitation and restlessness (sometimes extreme);
- tremulousness;
- sweating;

- tachycardia;
- anorexia, nausea and retching;
- upper abdominal pain (but beware of pancreatitis or ulcer).

Tx

Most of the symptoms respond well to IV diazepam. Enormous doses may be needed; the correct dose is apparent by the relief it affords. Upper abdominal symptoms may be helped by antacids. The patient should be admitted for a reducing dose of oral chlordiazepoxide accompanied by IV fluids and multivitamins (e.g. Pabrinex 1 pair of ampoules IV daily for 5 days).

A lower risk group (i.e. those without signs of weight loss or malnutrition) can be given thiamine 50 mg tds by mouth and vitamin B compound strong two tablets tds. The thiamine can be discontinued once the chlordiazepoxide detoxification regime is complete but the high dose vitamin B should be continued indefinitely.

Generalised convulsions

Fits may be recurrent and require short-term treatment as well as a long-term management strategy. Concurrent head injury must be excluded as a cause. Patients with withdrawal seizures should be prescribed carbamazepine 200 mg tds throughout the period of withdrawal. The drug can be reduced and stopped over 3 to 5 days when the detoxification is complete. If the patient is already taking an anticonvulsant drug such as phenytoin, there is no need to prescribe additional carbamazepine.

Acute alcohol hallucinosis

This is a distinct condition in which auditory hallucinations occur without sensorial clouding. It merits discussion with a psychiatrist. Intravenous haloperidol (5–10 mg) may be helpful.

Delirium tremens

This occurs after 24–72 h of abstinence and is recognised by:

- agitation and restlessness;
- tremulousness;
- fever and tachycardia;
- delirium (acute confusional psychosis with bizarre visual hallucinations often concerning animals or insects);
- fits.

Tx

Delirium tremens has a high mortality and so intensive monitoring and observation is mandatory. The patient will need adequate sedation and supportive therapy.

Alcoholism

Alcoholism is a descriptive rather than a diagnostic term. The alcoholic continues to drink despite obvious harm to self and family. Addiction is a more specific description indicating tolerance, craving and withdrawal symptoms attributable to the drug. Every alcohol addict is an alcoholic but not every alcoholic is an addict. Many simply binge drink, wreak havoc with their lives for a brief period and then return to 'normality'. This, of course, is very disruptive to home and family.

Signs of chronic alcohol abuse include:
- poor nutritional status;
- raised gamma glutamyl transpeptidase;
- macrocytosis in the absence of folate or B_{12} deficiency;
- multiple rib fractures at various stages of healing on chest X-ray (pulmonary TB may also be present);
- atrial fibrillation.

A slow downward spiral often leads to the loss of driving licence, job and home and then to residence in a hostel or on the streets.

Requests for detoxification are often made to ED staff. Unfortunately, there are very few acute facilities available for people requiring this sort of help and those that are require a completely sober individual. This is difficult to achieve as sobriety is usually accompanied by any one of the withdrawal states detailed above. The best policy is probably to provide the patient with a short course of sedative drugs (e.g. chlordiazepoxide

20 mg qds for 3 days) to hold off the worst of the withdrawal symptoms and to arrange a clinic appointment as soon as possible.

> Treatment of alcohol dependence is more effective if it is started early on in the downward spiral. Changes in funding for 'alcohol' services in the United Kingdom reflect a growing recognition that this help must be accessible by patients presenting to both primary and emergency care facilities.

Complications of chronic alcohol abuse

Many health problems accompany chronic alcohol abuse.

Wernicke–Korsakoff syndrome

The common causation of these two eponymous conditions has led to the description of one syndrome with two extreme forms:

1 Korsakoff's psychosis – Severe loss of short-term memory causes the patient to invent his or her immediate past (confabulation). The patient may also be confused and disorientated.

2 Wernicke's encephalopathy – There is ophthalmoplegia, ataxia and peripheral neuropathy. In extreme cases hypothermia, hypotension and coma may also be seen.

The syndrome is often precipitated in alcohol-dependent patients by the stress of an intercurrent illness. It may be very difficult to diagnose. There is an underlying imbalance between the brain's energy requirements and CNS B vitamin availability. Consequent failure of the citric acid cycle can lead to irreversible brain damage. Oral thiamine has little effect. To restore CNS vitamin levels, parenteral vitamins should be given two or three times a day (e.g. Pabrinex 2 pairs of ampoules IV tds for 2 days).

Suicide and parasuicide

Suicide and parasuicide have an increased incidence in alcoholics. Therefore, possible ingestion of other drugs should always be considered.

Injury

Alcoholics are more prone to injury and very much more susceptible to assault than most people. A full physical examination is essential. Loss of reflex protective mechanisms when drunk contributes to the increased incidence of subdural haematoma as a complication of head injury in alcohol abusers (*see page 46*).

Detection of alcohol abuse

Excessive alcohol intake is common throughout the world (*for UK figures see pages 13 and 370*). Its detection and control is a major global health problem. Patients may present to emergency services with a large variety of medical and traumatic complaints, which are related to underlying alcohol abuse.

> The maximum recommended weekly intake of alcohol is 21 units for men and 14 units for women – with at least one or two alcohol-free days. (*For definition of a unit see page 370.*)

The CAGE questions were designed as a quick and effective screen for use by health workers – *see Box 19.2*. CAGE is an acronym made from the first letters of the key word in each question. More than one affirmative answer indicates problem drinking.

If this is found to be the case, then the patient should be advised to reduce his or her consumption of alcohol and the relevant information communicated in writing to the patient's GP. Contrary to popular belief, confronting a patient with the evidence of their alcohol problem may limit further damaging behaviour.

> **Box 19.2 The CAGE Questions**
>
> **1** Do you feel that you should Cut down on your drinking?
> **2** Does anyone Annoy you or get on your nerves by telling you to cut down your drinking?
> **3** Do you feel bad or Guilty about your drinking?
> **4** Do you have a drink first thing in the morning to steady your nerves or get rid of a hangover? (Eye-opener)

Depressed mood and self-harm

Depression

About one in seven people experience some of the symptoms of depression in any one year and a substantially greater number will experience an episode of a depressive disorder at some time during their lives. The problem is underdiagnosed and undertreated and so:

- enquire about depressed mood in anyone who seems 'low';
- enquire about suicidal thoughts in anyone who may be depressed.

> Questioning about suicidal intent will not encourage a patient to attempt self-harm.

Severe depression is usually accompanied by disturbance of eating, sleeping and working. Relationships are strained and retardation of all normal activities may be profound. The risk of suicide is paradoxically at its greatest during the early stages of recovery from depression.

Tx

If suicidal thoughts are present or if there are profound somatic symptoms, psychiatric advice should be sought. Otherwise depression should be treated by the GP with antidepressants at full therapeutic dose. Supervision of a depressed person by a close relative or friend is essential for both their safety and their mental well-being.

Suicide

Suicide has been called the ultimate act of the individual and, indeed, to attempt to take one's own life is to have lost all faith in the help offered by society and its members. The highest rates are in men aged 35–44 years and men over 85 years old. Some professions carry an abnormally high risk of suicide: doctors, pharmacists, vets, nurses and farmers. In the United Kingdom, the incidence of suicide is increasing in men under 24 years old and in young Asian women.

Most suicides have informed somebody of their intention before death.

Self-harm

Self-harm accounts for around 1.5% of all ED attendances in the United Kingdom and is one of the top five causes of acute medical admission. Patients may harm themselves by either poisoning or physical injury, the latter usually taking the form of cuts to the forearms or neck. In extreme cases it is obvious that there was a genuine attempt to commit suicide but often the intent of the patient is unclear. However, in the 12 months after attending an ED, about 1 in 6 patients will harm themselves again and nearly 1% will die by suicide. It is therefore very important to distinguish between the different psychological states, which underlie the self-harming behaviour:

- depression and attempted suicide;
- psychosis and attempted suicide;
- emotional upset and impulsive self-harm (parasuicide);
- psychopathic behaviour;
- sexual or other experimentation and unintentional self-harm.

> Around 40% of patients who poison themselves express a wish to die.

Tx

The poisoning or injury must be treated appropriately and sensitively. Psychosocial assessment should take place in parallel to the physical treatment rather than waiting for its completion. In many hospitals, all patients who have harmed themselves are examined by a psychiatrist. This may follow admission for medical treatment or direct referral from the ED. If this is not the case, then the risk of suicide or further self-harm must be assessed before discharge (see Box 19.3). The key psychological characteristics associated with risk are depression, hopelessness and continuing suicidal intent. All discharged patients must be accompanied home and should be followed-up by their GP.

> Patients who harm themselves have a 100 fold increased risk of suicide in the following year.

Box 19.3 Assessment of Suicide Risk

Certain features of the social and medical history coupled with aspects of the presentation suggest serious
intention to commit suicide.

High-risk individuals
Elderly. (All self-harm in people over 65 should be taken
   as evidence of suicidal intent.)
Male.
Widowed.
Recently bereaved.
Living alone with little support.
Unemployed.
There are special risk factors in women:
- three or more children under the age of 5 years;
- lack of either a close, caring relationship or a job.

High-risk backgrounds
Chronic disabling physical illness.
Previous psychiatric illness or suicide attempt.
Chronic pain.
History of alcohol or other drug abuse.
Family history of mental illness, suicide or alcoholism.

Serious circumstances
Overdose or injury performed in isolated circumstances.
Active precautions taken to avoid detection.
Self-harm timed to reduce likelihood of detection.
Did not confide in a potential helper.
Left a suicide note.
Modified a will or insurance, etc.

Suicidal thoughts
Wanted, and still wants, to die. (Asking about this will
   not increase the risk of a repeat attempt.)
Has had these thoughts and planned suicide for at least
   24 h.
Thought that the method used would succeed in killing
   him or her.
Is sorry that he or she has recovered.
Has intense feelings of hopelessness and worthlessness.

Deliberate self-harm in young people under the age of 16 years

Self-harm is common in teenagers with as many as
1 in 10 affected. It is seven times more common in
girls than in boys. There may be self-poisoning or
various types of physical injury. The commonest
trigger is an argument with a parent or close friend.
As in adults, self-harm in adolescents may reflect
a variety of different underlying mental states

and patients give many different reasons for hurt-
ing themselves. Unfortunately from a diagnostic
perspective, the younger the child the less likely it is
that the severity of the act that they perform reflects
the actual seriousness of the urge to harm themselves. In all such cases, consideration needs to be
given to the child's mental state, care and protection and parental management. Thus it is the policy
of the British Paediatric Association and the Royal
College of Psychiatrists that all young people under
16 years old who harm themselves should receive a
specialist assessment by an appropriately trained
person, usually a child psychiatrist. This generally
entails temporary admission to a paediatric ward.

In the United Kingdom in 2005, 1 in 10 children has a
recognised mental disorder, ranging from depression to
autism. This prevalence of psychological disease doubles
in children whose parents are both unemployed.

Special situations

*For compulsory admission and treatment see page 374
and Box 20.5 on page 375.*

People with learning disabilities

Approximately 3% of the population have a learning disability (defined as an IQ of less than 70).
People with all levels of learning disability live in
the community, in their family homes and in supported accomodation. Many lead independent
lives in their own homes. They develop similar
physical and mental health problems to non-dis-
abled people, although they have a higher prevalence of epilepsy, head injury and difficulties with
hearing and speech. Their presentations may be
atypical because of difficulties in communication.
Common presenting problems to the ED include
physical injuries, medical illness, self-harm and
alcohol misuse. Mental illness may manifest itself
as a change in the person's usual pattern of behaviour. These patients should be treated as adults
with a normal capacity for making decisions about
their health, although simple language may need
to be used. Family and carers may sometimes need
to be involved but only with the patient's consent.

Personality disorders

People with a wide range of unusual or, in the statistical sense, abnormal personality types are seen in an ED. They may demonstate features of histrionic, inadequate, sociopathic, psychopathic and other personalities.

Brief assessment of a patient presenting with unreasonable behaviour tempts the busy doctor to attribute symptoms to long-term personality disorders and to make judgemental decisions. However, even patients who are known psychopaths can develop new treatable conditions.

Tx

As with any patient, a careful assessment should be made at each attendance. The advice of a psychiatrist, even by telephone, can be very useful as many of these patients and their patterns of behaviour are well-known to the mental health services. If it is concluded that the patient's presentation to the ED is exclusively caused by a personality disorder then there is no therapy to be offered, although attempts should be made to ensure that community support is available and that appropriate agencies know of the patient's hospital attendance. Good records are essential to help at future presentations and to adjudicate in any dispute.

Neuroses

Patients with specific neuroses may present to an ED. They usually have some insight into their problems and so referral can be made to an appropriate agency, be it a psychiatrist, GP or psychologist.
For depressive states see page 358.

Requests for drugs

Patients sometimes present to an ED with requests for psychotropic drugs. Generally speaking, it is inappropriate for such prescriptions to be dispensed by doctors who do not have on-going care of a patient. However, there are no absolutes in medicine and every request should be listened to and dealt with according to the clinical situation.

Never feel pressurised into prescribing.

It is helpful to remember that most patients who stop taking heroin do not experience major withdrawal symptoms. 'Cold turkey' is very unusual. According to many ex-users, the discomfort experienced during opiate withdrawal is no worse than a bad dose of flu and is certainly not akin to the life-threatening states caused by cessation of alcohol intake. However, staying away from recreational drugs in the long-term is much more difficult than just stopping for a limited period.
For withdrawal from opiates see later.
For alcohol withdrawal states see page 355.

Withdrawal from opioid drugs (narcotic analgesics)

Why do people take heroin? Most users experience a pleasant, relaxing effect with a sensation of deep inner warmth and complete detachment from all of life's problems.

Patients with a physical dependence to opioids commonly present to an ED with psychiatric problems, drug overdose, alcohol intoxication, DVT or infections secondary to drug injection. They may require admission to an observation area or ward. Symptoms and signs of withdrawal usually occur 6–12 h after the last dose of heroin or 18–48 h after a dose of methadone. There is:
- anxiety, restlessness, irritability, insomnia, cravings, dysphoria;
- lacrimation, rhinorrhoea, sneezing, yawning;
- muscle cramps, sweating, piloerection ('gooseflesh');
- nausea, diarrhoea, vomiting;
- tachycardia, raised BP, dilated pupils.

The state of opioid withdrawal is unpleasant but not dangerous. However, failure to manage it effectively may limit the patient's compliance with other treatment or lead to self-discharge. Symptoms gradually decrease spontaneously over 5–10 days.

Tx

The initial level of treatment depends on the clinical features but it is important to reassure the patient that any worsening of their symptoms will trigger a review of the therapy. Oral methadone mixture (1 mg per mL) is usually prescribed. Buprenorphine is sometimes given as an alternative and, in an emergency, dihydrocodeine is reasonably effective. Benzodiazepines will also alleviate most of the symptoms of opiate withdrawal. The dose of methadone is 30 mg immediately followed by 10 mg every 4 h if signs of withdrawal recur (total daily dose up to 60–80 mg). Equivalent doses of methadone are:

Oral methadone 2 mg = injectable methadone 2 mg = injectable diamorphine 1 mg. (Street heroin is not equivalent to medical diamorphine and so an empirical approach is necessary.)

Lofexidine (an alpha-adrenergic agonist) is prescribed by specialists to control the symptoms of opiate withdrawal. The dose is 0.2–0.4 mg every 6 h. Naltrexone, a long-acting opioid antagonist, is used to prevent relapse in former addicts.

Patients who regularly abuse drugs should be referred to the community drug team. If already on a registered drug programme, their key worker should be contacted. It is important to consider the welfare of any children who may be in the care of people who abuse drugs.

For child protection issues see page 348.

For acute poisoning with opioids (narcotics) see page 280.

Withdrawal from other drugs

Patients with a physical addiction to sedatives and tranquillisers may display symptoms similar to alcohol withdrawal; these drugs should not be stopped abruptly. People who regularly use stimulant drugs such as amphetamines or cocaine will not usually suffer from a withdrawal state although they may become quite depressed.

For alcohol withdrawal states see page 355.

Violent behaviour

Disturbed or violent behaviour may be provoked by environmental, organisational, situational or attitudinal factors. Some aspects of a person's past life are associated with an increased risk of violent behaviour:

- history of violent behaviour or of cruelty towards animals;
- relatives and carers reporting previous extreme anger or violence;
- previous expressions of intent to harm others;
- previous use of weapons;
- previous dangerous impulsive acts (including reckless driving);
- denial of previous violent or dangerous actions;
- evidence of 'rootlessness' or social exclusion;
- evidence of recent stressful events;
- history of misuse of drugs or alcohol;
- loss of a parent before the age of 8 years in association with any of the factors above;
- history of bed-wetting in association with any of the factors above.

Certain behaviours indicate that a person's discontent may be escalating towards violence:
- restlessness and pacing around the floor;
- increased volume of speech and erratic movements;
- refusal to communicate;
- prolonged eye contact;
- tense and angry facial expressions;
- delusions or hallucinations with a violent content;
- verbal threats or gestures.

Members of staff must realise that they are responsible for avoiding provocation in potentially violent situations. It is not reasonable to expect a person exhibiting angry behaviour to simply 'calm down'. ED staff must learn to monitor and control their own verbal and non-verbal behaviour such as body posture and eye contact. In addition, they must be able to defuse a difficult situation.

De-escalation techniques include:
- adopting a non-threatening but safe posture;
- allowing greater personal space than normal;
- relocating to a safer enviroment if at all possible;
- asking for weapons to be placed in a neutral location rather than just handed over;
- paying attention to non-verbal clues;
- attempting to establish a rapport and emphasising cooperation;
- offering and negotiating realistic options and avoiding threats;

- asking open questions and inquiring about the reasons for the person's anger;
- showing concern and attentiveness through both verbal and non-verbal responses;
- listening carefully and showing empathy;
- acknowledging any grievances, concerns or frustrations and not being patronising or minimising these concerns.

Protection of ED staff from violent people

It is the duty of all staff to ensure that they and their colleagues are not placed at unreasonable risk of injury during the course of their duties. For this reason, the police should be involved early on in any potentially violent situation. Many hospitals now have their own security personnel who can attend at short notice.

Most people who express aggression are completely responsible for their own actions. In the eyes of the law, intoxication with alcohol or drugs is no justification for unreasonable behaviour. The exceptions to this generalisation are functional psychoses and organic confusional states, which are not the direct result of the person's own actions. In schizophrenia, for example, auditory hallucinations and paranoid delusions may induce aggression as a defence mechanism. Thus, before an individual is removed from the ED, these conditions must be excluded. In a person who is not intoxicated this is usually fairly easy. However, it must be remembered that staff have a duty of care even to aggressive and 'unpleasant' patients.

Angry relatives

Dissatisfied or frankly aggressive relatives or friends of patients are not uncommon in an ED. There are several frequently met reasons for this:
- inappropriate reaction to the stress of sudden illness or bereavement;
- guilt and redirection of blame;
- unrealistic expectations of a resource-limited system;
- misunderstanding of the situation (a failure of communication);

- unexplained delays at any stage;
- understandable reaction to a failure of care.

The departmental staff must reply calmly, politely, clearly and firmly to all expressions of anger (*see page 361*). If resolution cannot easily be achieved then the case must be referred to a senior member of staff. There is a clear procedure to be followed for all formal complaints, which will usually be directed through a central office of the hospital (*see page 382*).

> Do not be frightened of saying that you are sorry. You can express regret that the patient is upset without implying that you are to blame.

Distressed relatives

For sudden bereavement see page 169.
For cot death see page 350.

In exceptional circumstances it may be appropriate to give distressed relatives a short course (3–5 days) of night sedation. If this is prescribed, the GP should be informed.

Munchausen syndrome (Factitious disorders)

Patients affected by this behavioural disorder display a recurrent need to adopt the sick role. Effectively, this means feigning illness to get attention, analgesia or admission to hospital. The underlying psychology of this behaviour is unclear but there is obviously a secondary gain to the patient. Presumably, Munchausen syndrome is an acute form of the well-known disorder whereby an unrequited need for caring attention leads some healthy people to behave as chronic invalids. Vicarious forms of Munchausen syndrome (Munchausen syndrome by proxy) may be expressed as symptoms attributed to close relatives, especially children (*see page 363*).

The diagnosis of Munchausen syndrome should be made by exclusion (and in retrospect if necessary) by an experienced emergency physician. It must be distinguished from:
- psychopathic behaviour, including some self-harm;
- hypochondriasis;

- hysterical behaviour;
- exaggeration of real symptoms;
- genuine and unexaggerated illness.

Features associated with Munchausen syndrome include:

- apparently complex social background, no relatives;
- stranger to the district, 'passing through';
- numerous previous hospital admissions elsewhere, usually undisclosed;
- classical, textbook symptoms and signs, usually of painful conditions (e.g. renal colic);
- scars from previous surgery;
- negative tests contrasting with positive history (beware of extraneous blood in urine specimens);
- specific requests for opiate analgesia.

Tx

If the diagnosis is strongly suspected, the case should be discussed with senior medical and nursing staff. Additional evidence may be obtainable. All departments should have a Munchausen file in which letters about such patients from other hospitals are kept. The validity of distant addresses can be checked by the police.

The patient should be confronted; the response may clinch the diagnosis. The hospital management and/or department of public health should be sent details of the attendance together with a description of the patient and the presenting features; they will contact other hospitals. Wasting hospital time is illegal under UK law and the patient can be charged in court.

> It is better to give morphine misguidedly to a few patients with Munchausen syndrome than to withhold it inappropriately from one patient with genuine pain. The doctor is not a detective; if there is a suspicion of genuine distress then analgesia should be given.

Munchausen syndrome by proxy

This syndrome – which is more correctly called 'factitious illness by proxy' – occurs when a carer feigns illness in a child. The gain to the adults involved is presumably similar to that which would be obtained if they were the patient themselves. The factitious illness may be directly produced (induced illness), imitated with false signs or fabricated with misleading stories of colourful symptoms. This is an unusual form of child abuse and should be treated as such (*see page 348*).

Post-traumatic stress disorder

There are three main groups of people who may need psychosocial care after traumatic events:
1 Survivors/injured victims.
2 People who have participated in events as rescuers, emergency staff etc.
3 The families of those who have died or been injured.
Adults, children and people from various ethnic groups may all have differing needs. Most people involved will have a normal emotional reaction with features of grief and distress; some may appear dazed and confused by events. The use of standardised individual or group 'debriefing' should be avoided as it is of no proven benefit and may do harm.

Some people will have features of acute stress soon after the traumatic event. Typical early symptoms include fear, anxiety, anger, guilt, sadness, feelings of helplessness and distressing thoughts and dreams. Physical symptoms such as fatigue, muscle aches, tension headaches and dry mouth may also occur. Features may be accentuated by the presence of co-existing conditions such as depression or substance abuse and anxiety, panic or phobic disorders. A few individuals may appear unaffected at first, only to experience problems hours or days later. For most people, symptoms subside without intervention. 'Psychological first aid' consists of:
- information about possible symptoms that may be experienced;
- education for the individual and their family about the reasons for their altered attitude, mood and behaviour (including advice to avoid telling the sufferer to 'snap out of it');
- advice to avoid using alcohol, tobacco or drugs to cope with anxiety;
- practical and social support as required.

The use of antidepressant drugs for adults in this early phase may be helpful if signs of depression are present.

All individuals with on-going or worsening symptoms should be assessed if:
- symptoms have lasted longer than one month;
- symptoms are complicated by other mental health problems;
- the person has suicidal thoughts;
- the person is unable to cope with normal activities;
- there is marked hyperarousal.

Post-traumatic stress disorder (PTSD) is usually only diagnosed after a month of persistent symptoms. It is treated with cognitive behaviour therapy by trained staff and this is associated with good long-term outcomes – *see later*. Prolonged use of anxiolytic drugs should be avoided although they may be helpful for adults in the first 2 weeks after a traumatic event to alleviate panic attacks or sleep disturbance. Antidepressant therapy may be required for many months in some patients.

For victim support see pages 368 and 369.

Counselling

The constant recollection of distressing thoughts reinforces a negative perception of problems and further lowers mood. Counselling aims to break this cycle.
- cognitive behavioural counselling helps a patient to focus on positive rather than negative thoughts;
- psychodynamic counselling takes an historical view of human mental processes and analyses the effect of past events on present thinking;
- supportive counselling encourages the patient to focus on current daily problems rather than dwelling on traumatic events.

For bereavement counselling see page 169.

Chapter 20

Medicolegal aspects of emergency medicine

The information given in this chapter applies to the United Kingdom. In other parts of the world, the social and legal framework may lead to differences in some aspects of the practice and principles of medicine.

Clinical forensic medicine

Description of injuries

Many descriptions of injury are intended for either lay people, the police or the legal profession. Medical terminology is unlikely to be familiar to them. It is therefore inappropriate to use the language of medicine in documents that are not medical records. A pair of erythematous haematomata on the pretibial area thus becomes two red lumps on the shin. Nevertheless, this simplification of terminology must not compromise accuracy. In both medical records and non-medical documents the description of a wound must include:

1 site – described in everyday language;
2 side – left or right;
3 shape – circular, V-shaped, etc.;
4 size – measured with a ruler;
5 structures which are also involved – such as nerves, tendon and bone, including X-ray findings;
6 sutures – number inserted in the skin.

Drawings or photographs can be very helpful. Some idea of the age of a wound is also desirable, although with older injuries this can take a considerable amount of experience. Opinions as to causation should only be expressed if requested and only then if the doctor's experience makes this reasonable.

Types of wounds

According to the Offences Against the Person Act (1861), to wound is to destroy or damage, however superficially, a bodily surface, be it skin or mucous membrane. For the purposes of medicolegal description, there are five main types of wound.

1 *Bruises.* These are also known as contusions or ecchymoses. Blunt force applied to the body surface causes rupturing of small blood vessels and allows blood to escape into the surrounding tissues. This is dependent on the pressure in the vessels and thus post-mortem wounds are not associated with significant bruising. Petechial and subconjunctival haemorrhages are particular types of bruising that may be caused by direct trauma or by indirect force (e.g. strangulation).

Bruises change in both colour and size with time. They are initially red/blue or purple/black and gradually become green/yellow over a few days. Older bruises have a blurred, fading edge. Tracking of blood along a tissue plane may result in bruising at a site well removed from the original injury.

2 *Abrasions.* An abrasion or graze involves only the outer layers of the skin. Unlike a bruise, it

always indicates the exact point of impact. Direction may also be apparent as may dirt from the source of trauma.

3 *Lacerations*. Whenever blunt force splits the whole thickness of the skin, the wound is called a laceration. Such wounds may be inflicted with sticks or bottles or sustained in falls. The characteristic features are ragged, abraded, contused edges and irregular division of the tissue planes.

4 *Incised wounds*. Sharp cutting objects make even wounds with straight, unbruised edges. An incised wound is longer than its depth.

5 *Stab wounds*. A stab wound is different from an incision because its depth is greater than its length. The shape and edges of the wound depend on the object used. A puncture wound is a very small stab wound. The external dimensions of a stab wound are a very poor guide as to the size of the weapon (e.g. knife blade). This is because:

• the weapon may be tapered and not introduced to the full extent of its width;

• the weapon may not have been used perpendicularly to the skin surface;

• the skin contracts after the blade is withdrawn.

Areas of transient redness should also be noted. Erythema may be caused by pressure or by a blow. There may be accompanying swelling or tenderness. Such injuries might include the red finger marks on a slapped face or the tender, red scalp that results from hair-pulling. Fading occurs within a matter of hours.

Specific mechanisms of injury may give rise to a defined type of wound, such as a burn. Burns are distinct patterns of damage that result from thermal or chemical injury – *for types of burns see Chapter 10* and *for child abuse see page 348*. Gunshot injuries are usually self-evident, although the type of gun used can be more difficult to determine. Bite wounds also have characteristic patterns. Most wounds, however, can result from a variety of different mechanisms and so their causation is a matter of judgement.

> All clothing from a wounded patient should be preserved in a sealed, labelled bag for the attention of the investigating police officers.

Gunshot wounds

Airguns

Airguns propel a small, blunt pellet that does not tend to penetrate very far, although it may severely damage the eyeball or even cause a pneumothorax.

Shotguns

Shotguns fire a large number of lead pellets. The wound that they create depends upon the distance from the gun, as a result of the fanning out of the shot. At up to 1 m the entry wound will appear as a single hole less than 3 cm in diameter. At such close range widespread tissue damage and skin burns will occur. Exit wounds are uncommon. At 2 m the shot is already beginning to disperse while at 6 m the shot will be spread over a diameter of about 15 cm. At 12 m the pellets are scattered over an area with a diameter of around 30 cm. These are only rough guides and should not be ventured as a definitive ballistics opinion in court.

Other firearms

Other firearms cause damage proportional to the amount of energy that their bullets transfer to the tissues. Handguns usually fire a large bullet at a relatively low velocity and so result in localised damage to the structures directly in the path of the missile. Military rifles have a high muzzle velocity and cause extensive damage. The high-energy transfer from the bullet to the surrounding tissues causes a large cavity to be formed along the track, which finishes in a large exit wound. Also the missile itself may roll and shatter in the tissues.

For Taser injuries see page 374.

Asphyxia

Attempted suffocation and strangulation both may cause a picture similar to traumatic asphyxia syndrome (*see page 81*). Signs of compression of the face or the neck may be present as may the marks of a violent struggle. Hanging causes death through a mixture of asphyxia, cerebral ischaemia and spinal disruption. *For drowning see page 30.* The asphyxia resulting from a bag over the head, seen in children and sexual asphyxia, usually causes death by hypoxia and subsequent bradycardia.

Violent crime

Contrary to popular belief, most of the victims of violent crime who present to an ED are young men and not elderly women (*see Box 20.1*). They are assaulted in a bar or a club or in the street and are often intoxicated, whereas 75% of the attacks on women occur in the home of either the victim or the assailant.

> Only about half of all violent crimes are reported to the police, with men much less likely to report than women. Fifty per cent of victims suffer 80% of all recorded crimes and an unfortunate 4% suffer over half of these.

Injuries to the face, head and hands are the most common unless weapons are used in the assault. There may be long-term psychological and psychosomatic effects including:
- depression;
- loss of confidence, fear and anxiety;
- irritability, decreased concentration and mood changes;
- lethargy, sleep and appetite disturbances;
- headaches, nausea and muscle tension;
- behavioural changes (e.g. withdrawal or increased alcohol consumption).

In some cases, the problems may be so severe and prolonged as to merit a diagnosis of post-traumatic stress disorder (PTSD) – *see page 363*. This diagnosis would not normally be made unless

Box 20.1 Risk Factors for Violent Crime

Male sex
Age 16–29 years
Low income
Single
Member of ethnic minority group
Alcohol intoxication

symptoms persisted for at least 1 month and caused impairment of normal life functions.

Domestic violence

More than 25% of all violent crime reported to the police is domestic violence of men against women, making it the second most common violent crime in the United Kingdom. It is thought to account for around 1% of all emergency department (ED) attendances. Up to one in four women will be physically assaulted by a partner during their lifetime and around one in ten will suffer an attack each year. It is estimated that a woman in an abusive relationship will suffer over 30 physical assaults before disclosing the abuse – usually when asked directly. Patterns of presentation with sufficient sensitivity to identify victims of domestic violence are few but facial bruising should always alert suspicion. Deliberate self-harm and pregnancy are associated with all types of abuse.

- Severe, repeated violence occurs in at least 5% of all long-term relationships in Britain. It affects women of all cultures, religions, ages and social groups.
- Over 45% of all murdered women are killed by their male partners; this amounts to one or two women per week in the United Kingdom. Women who leave their abusers are at a 75% greater risk of being killed than those who stay.
- Nearly half of all assaults against women are committed by a partner or former partner, compared with 4% of assaults against men.

Abuse may be:
- psychological – shouting, swearing, humiliation or enforced isolation from family and friends;
- economic – withholding of money and transport;
- sexual;
- physical.

Physical injury is the most likely form of domestic violence to present to an ED. Possible signs of it are:
- delayed presentation of injuries;
- injuries that are inconsistent with the mechanism described in the history;
- multiple injuries, especially when symmetrically distributed or of differing ages;
- injuries such as bites, burns, scalds or bruises;

- injuries on areas of the body that are normally clothed;
- injuries to the face, neck, breasts, genitals or pregnant abdomen;
- perforated eardrums or detached retinas;
- evidence of rape or other sexual assault;
- pelvic pain;
- multiple somatic complaints;
- psychiatric illness;
- drug abuse.

> Domestic violence may occur in same sex relationships and may be perpetrated by women against men.

Tx

Injuries should be treated appropriately and social services contacted for advice and shelter if necessary. Specialist helplines to various organisations are now available. A friend or relative of the victim should be enlisted for support and inquiries made about the current safety of any children in the family. (The risks of violence to children growing up in an abusive household are substantial. Such children are much more likely than most to be listed on the child protection register. Concerns about the welfare of children should lead to immediate contact with local child protection services.) The police can only be involved with the consent of the injured party.

> Failure by victims of domestic violence to involve outside help is common. This may frustrate staff who believe that immediate action is required. However, research has shown that information provided in EDs may be used at a later date when the patient finally feels that the time is right.

Rape and sexual assault

Around 17% of women and 3% of men in the United Kingdom state that they have been subjected to non-consensual sexual experiences as adults. Approximately two-thirds of assaults of this type are committed by someone known to the victim. The experience of sexual violence can be life threatening and degrading. Not surprisingly, psychological upset and a specific form of PTSD (rape

trauma syndrome) are common sequelae. Not all patients who have been sexually assaulted have visible genital (or oral) injuries although around 50% have other physical injuries. Examination should be left to the police surgeon as forensic evidence will need to be collected in a way that does not contaminate it or render it invalid as evidence. Locard's principle states that 'every contact leaves a trace'. This includes ED staff!

Tx

There should be early involvement of social services; there may be a dedicated rape crisis centre. Specialist police officers are allocated to this type of investigation.

The police surgeon will also consider the need for emergency contraception (*see page 317*) and the exclusion or treatment of sexually transmitted diseases.

Drug-assisted sexual assault

Alcohol (self-administered or in laced drinks) is by far the most common drug to be associated with sexual assault. However, gamma hydroxybutyrate (GHB), ketamine, flunitrazepam and zopiclone have all been reported as being used to facilitate sexual assault. Patients drugged and assaulted in this way present a very difficult problem as they will have an impaired memory of events and may just feel that 'something wrong happened'.

Child abuse

For the types of and signs of child abuse see page 348. For child protection procedures see page 380.

Abuse of the elderly

Physical abuse of the elderly is surprisingly common; neglect and emotional abuse is even more common. The recent increase in the number of small, privately run nursing homes has done nothing to decrease the problem. Signs may be minimal or similar to those of other forms of domestic violence (*see page 367*). As soon as the diagnosis is suspected, advice should be sought from social workers and senior geriatricians.

Victim support and counselling

Details of local victim support schemes and the witness support service in the Crown Court can be found in the telephone directory, although the police will usually negotiate contact if asked. Victim Support (a registered UK charity) can help with:

- practical matters such as insurance and compensation;
- personal and emotional support;
- liaison with the police and other agencies;
- explanation of the criminal justice system;
- witness support.

People suffering from PTSD or depression should be referred to psychiatric services. Counselling is often advised (*see page 364*).

Alcohol and other drugs / fitness to drive

Misuse of drugs

The Misuse of Drugs Act 1971 prohibits certain activities in relation to 'Controlled Drugs', in particular their manufacture, supply and possession. The penalties applicable to offences which contravene the Act, are graded according to the harmfulness attributable to a drug when it is misused. For this purpose, the controlled drugs are divided into three classes called A, B and C – *see Box 20.2*. The Misuse of Drugs Regulations 2001 define the classes of person who are authorised to supply and possess controlled drugs while acting in a professional capacity and lay down the conditions under which their activities may be carried out. In these regulations, drugs are divided into five schedules, each with its own specific legal requirements – *see Box 20.2*.

The Misuse of Drugs (Supply to Addicts) Regulations 1997 instruct that only those medical practitioners who hold a special licence from the Home Office may prescribe, administer or supply diamorphine, dipipanone or cocaine in the treatment of drug addiction. This does not apply to the prescription of these drugs to known addicts for the relief of pain from organic disease or injury.

Box 20.2 The Misuse of Drugs Act 1971 and The Misuse of Drugs Regulations 2001

The main offences under the Misuse of Drugs Act 1971 are as follows:

Section 4 (2) Production of a controlled drug (i.e. Schedule 1, 2 and 3 drugs)

Section 4 (3) Supplying or offering to supply a controlled drug

Section 5 (2) Having possession of a controlled drug without a prescription or other authority

Section 5 (3) Having possession of a controlled drug with intent to supply it to another person

Section 6 (2) Cultivation of a cannabis plant

Section 8 Being the occupier or manager of premises and knowingly permitting or suffering:

- the production or attempted production of controlled drugs;
- the supply, attempt to supply or offer to supply a controlled drug to another person;
- the preparation of opium for smoking;
- the smoking of cannabis, cannabis resin or prepared opium.

The penalties applicable to these offences are graded according to the harmfulness of a drug when it is misused. For this purpose, the controlled drugs are divided into three classes:

Class A includes: Cocaine, LSD, diamorphine, morphine, pethidine, methadone, opium, MDMA, phencyclidine and class B substances when prepared for injection.

Class B includes: Codeine, amphetamines and barbiturates.

Class C includes: Buprenorphine, cannabis, cannabis resin, most benzodiazepines, zolpidem, anabolic steroids and some hormones.

The Misuse of Drugs Regulations 2001 define the classes of person who are authorised to supply and possess controlled drugs in a professional capacity and lay down the conditions under which professional activities may be carried out. In these regulations, drugs are divided into five schedules, each with its own specific legal requirements:

Schedule 1 includes: Cannabis, LSD and other drugs, which are not used medicinally.

Schedule 2 includes: Diamorphine, morphine, pethidine, cocaine, amfetamine and secobarbital.

Schedule 3 includes: Buprenorphine, most barbiturates and temazepam.

Schedule 4 includes: Benzodiazepines (except temazepam), zolpidem, anabolic steroids and some hormones.

Schedule 5 includes: Those preparations that (because of their strength) are exempt from virtually all controlled drug requirements.

Neither does it apply to methadone or dihydrocodeine. *For requests for drugs in the ED and drug withdrawal see page 360.*

In England, health professionals are expected to report cases of drug misuse to their regional drug misuse centre as part of the National Drugs Treatment Monitoring System (NDTMS). Wales and Scotland have a similar national reporting system. All three countries require notification of misuse of all types of drugs including opiates, benzodiazepines and CNS stimulants. In Northern Ireland, the Misuse of Drugs (Notification of and Supply to Addicts) (Northern Ireland) Regulations 1973 require doctors to send particulars of persons whom they consider to be addicted to controlled drugs to the Department of Health and Social Services.

For the Misuse of Drugs Act 1971 and the Misuse of Drugs Regulations 2001, see Box 20.2 on page 369.

Alcohol and trauma

Ethyl alcohol is probably the most dangerous substance in the world. It is freely available in many societies and, unlike other psychotropic drugs, it is dispensed by a barman rather than by a pharmacist. It is so frequently involved in the causation of accidents that no discussion of the work of an ED would be complete without it. In the United Kingdom, one-tenth of all road accidents that result in injury are a result of the effects of excess alcohol in the blood and almost all other injuries have a significant association with alcohol usage (*see Figure 20.1*). *For the detection and treatment of alcohol abuse see pages 355–357.*

For the treatment of alcohol poisoning see page 283.

> Nearly a quarter of all ED attendances are alcohol-related. Over a quarter of all male hospital inpatients have a current or previous alcohol problem.

Measurement of alcohol in the human body

Units of alcohol

A unit of alcohol has become the standard measure by which public health information on alcohol

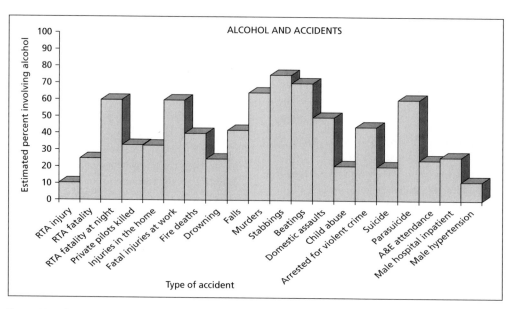

Figure 20.1 The involvement of alcohol in trauma.

consumption is expressed. It is defined as 10 mL by volume (=8 g by weight) of pure alcohol – roughly the alcohol content of a standard measure of 25 mL of many spirits. Half a pint of beer (3% strength) or a glass of wine (125 mL of 8% alcohol) is also roughly equivalent to one unit. Within the first hour, a unit of alcohol increases the blood level by approximately 15 mg per dL in an average man.

Elimination of alcohol

In a healthy person, about 90% of ingested alcohol is cleared from the blood by the liver. This occurs at a steady rate of about 15 mg per dL per h.

Laboratory units of alcohol

Several units of blood alcohol measurement are in use worldwide including milligrams per litre and millimoles per litre. The unit used in UK legal practice, although not necessarily in hospital laboratories, is milligrams per decilitre (i.e. mg per dL or mg% – 1 dL is 100 mL). *See also Box 20.3.*

Conventionally, breath alcohol levels are converted to equivalent blood alcohol levels by multiplying by a factor of 2300. The comparison is not strictly accurate as alcohol concentration in the breath rises faster and falls earlier than it does in venous blood.

Requests for specimens for analysis from patients in hospital

The Police Reform Act (2002), provided new powers concerning the taking of blood specimens from patients involved in road traffic accidents to test for levels of alcohol or drugs. As before, while a person is in hospital (as a patient!), he or she is not required to provide a specimen for breath or laboratory testing unless the medical practitioner in immediate charge of the case has consented. (It must be remembered, however, that there are very few med-ical circumstances that preclude sampling.) If there is no clinical objection, then a person from whom a police constable requires a blood sample and who (without reasonable excuse) refuses to consent, commits an offence. Under the previous legislation, it was a statutory requirement to obtain consent for blood sampling from the person concerned. Therefore, when a patient lacked capacity to consent (usually because of a depressed level of consciousness), a specimen could not be obtained. This led to people escaping prosecution for very serious offences, such as causing death by careless driving while under the influence of alcohol.

The provisions of the Police Reform Act aimed to eliminate this inequity between those with capacity to consent and those without it. A police constable may now request that a blood sample be taken from a patient who, for medical reasons, is incapable of giving consent. This request would normally be made to a police surgeon but, in exceptional situations, may be made to another medical practitioner who is not directly involved in the clinical care of the patient. If the doctor considers it appropriate to take the specimen, then the police constable will provide a special kit to be used for this purpose. The location of all forensic specimens is required by law to be recorded at all times – 'the chain of custody'. As soon as possible, the police will inform the patient that a blood sample has been taken and obtain his (or her) consent for it to be analysed. In this case, failure to give permission for analysis may render the person liable to prosecution.

Driving and other drugs

Many drugs may impair the ability of a patient to drive or to operate machinery. Drowsiness and impaired psychomotor performance are the most common drug-related effects to interfere with driving but postural hypotension, fatigue, hypoglycaemia and impaired vision may also occur. Drivers taking minor tranquillisers or tricyclic antidepressants are 2–5 times more likely to be involved in an accident than untreated controls. The early stages of treatment are associated with the highest risk and the effects of centrally acting drugs are often potentiated by alcohol.

Because of these risks, patients must always be warned whenever their treatment could alter their ability to drive or perform other activities safely. A recommended list of advice is given in *Box 20.12 on page 385.*

> Frequent users of cannabis are 10 times more likely to be injured or to cause injury to others in motor vehicle accidents than other road users.

For the Misuse of Drugs Act 1971 and the Misuse of Drugs Regulations 2001 see Box 20.2 on page 369.

Driving and medical conditions

Medical conditions in drivers contribute to about 1% of the road accidents in the United Kingdom which result in injury or death *(see Box 20.4).*

There are two sets of medical criteria for fitness to drive; one for an ordinary licence and another for a vocational licence [i.e. for a passenger carrying vehicle (PCV) or for a large goods vehicle (LGV)]. Licence holders have a statutory obligation to notify the licensing authority as soon as they become aware that they have any condition that might affect safe driving, unless the condition is not expected to last more than 3 months. Failure to notify is a legal offence.

> The General Medical Council advises that a doctor should notify the licensing authority when a patient is placing themselves or others in danger by continuing to drive. This does not constitute a breach of confidentiality.

The Road Traffic Act (1988), Section 92 lists prescribed disabilities that bar the sufferer from driving. They are:

A epilepsy;

B severe mental handicap;

C liability to sudden attacks of disabling giddiness or fainting (from any cause);

Box 20.4 Most Common Causes of Collapse at the Wheel

- Fits
- Unspecified blackouts
- Hypoglycaemia
- Myocardial infarction
- Strokes

D disorder of the heart requiring a pacemaker;

E inability to meet the eyesight requirements (the number-plate test).

In practice, a person with any of these conditions can drive once they have satisfied the licensing authority that they do not present any significant risk. The rules for vocational drivers are more stringent. Vocational licence holders are responsible for more than twice as many accidents that result in serious injury or death as ordinary car drivers, even when the statistics are corrected for mileage.

For the purposes of the ED, patients should be advised to (temporarily) refrain from driving whenever there is a possibility of a condition being diagnosed that could make driving or other complex tasks dangerous to themselves or others. Such problems may include:

- fits;
- blackouts other than simple faints;
- dizziness and vertigo;
- head injury;
- sudden cardiac dysrhythmias;
- myocardial infarction;
- CVAs (cerebrovascular accidents) and TIAs (transient ischaemic attacks);
- application of an eye pad in the ED *(see page 406)*;
- decreased ability to use a limb (e.g. forearm in plaster);
- post-sedation or strong analgesia *(see page 385)*.

Driving, or other prohibited activities, should only be recommended when:

- the condition has resolved completely;
- the diagnosis has been ruled out after specialist investigation;
- the condition has been controlled and a symptom-free period has elapsed.

In the United Kingdom, the Medical Advisory Branch of the Driver and Vehicle Licensing Authority in Swansea supplies written and verbal advice for doctors on all aspects of fitness to drive.

Payment for emergency treatment of patients involved in road traffic accidents

The Road Traffic (NHS Charges) Act of 1999 allows hospitals to recover some of their costs for treating the victims of motor vehicle accidents from the insurers of the drivers involved. The value of this system to any particular hospital usually depends on the efficacy of local data collection systems.

Legal issues

Consent

In the competent adult, treatment can only be given if the patient gives consent. Any physical contact or treatment without this consent may be construed as trespass or battery. These legal torts do not require harm to have resulted to the patient. Consent may be given verbally, in writing, by gestures or by actions. A signature on a consent form does not by itself prove that consent was valid. In addition, the following points should be noted:

• Valid consent or refusal is dependent on a patient's ability (capacity) to make decisions, namely to:

1 understand and remember information;

2 believe this information;

3 evaluate this information.

Capacity to give meaningful consent or make a valid refusal is a legal concept and not a medical one. However, the law presupposes that all registered medical practitioners are qualified to make an assessment of capacity. It also assumes that all adults have the capacity to consent or refuse unless proven otherwise.

> Conscious adults without serious mental dysfunction are always regarded by the law as capable of giving consent.

For children see page 379.

For patients with mental illness see page 352.

• A patient may be competent to make some health care decisions, even if they are not competent to make others.

• Consent is only valid if the patient understood what he or she was consenting to (i.e. gave informed consent). However, a doctor must only provide that information about a procedure and its attendant risks that a reasonable group of doctors would disclose in the same circumstances. The concepts of the 'reasonable man' and 'the responsible body of medical opinion' pervade this type of law. Compliance with the latter tenet forms the basis of the so-called Bolam test.

• The patient's right to self-determination takes precedence over the physician's duty to preserve life. A competent adult has the right to refuse any treatment or investigation even if it puts his or her life or health at risk. The patient has no obligation to justify this decision with valid and rational argument. The only exception to this rule is where treatment is for a mental disorder and the patient is detained under the Mental Health Act (1983) – and most such patients will lack the capacity to make decisions.

• A competent pregnant woman may refuse any treatment, even if this would be detrimental to the foetus.

• No one can give consent on behalf of an incompetent adult. However, such patients may still be treated provided that the proposed treatment is in their 'best interests'. 'Best interests' extend wider than best medical interests to include such factors as previous wishes and beliefs and general well being. People close to the patient may be able to provide valuable information on some of these factors. Where a patient has never been competent, relatives, carers and friends may be best placed to advise on the patient's needs and preferences.

• An incompetent patient who has indicated in the past (while competent) that they would refuse treatment in certain circumstances ('an advance refusal') must not be treated should those circumstances arise.

• Consent obtained by deceit or with unreasonable pressure is invalid.

• Consent may be withdrawn at any time.

Treatment under common law

A patient who is incapable of giving consent (e.g. in cardiac arrest or coma) may be treated under common law. This means that so long as staff only perform those procedures, which are reasonable to protect life and limb, then they are not liable to be sued for assault. Furthermore, to do less than this would be to neglect their duty of care. The law requires that all decisions must be made in accordance with the patient's best interests. Section 62 of the Mental Health Act (1983) codifies in statute this long-accepted practice.

Emergency treatment

The emergency treatment of physical and psychiatric problems in a fully conscious patient who cannot or will not give informed consent is an extremely difficult area. Treatment cannot be given without a patient's consent unless, by virtue of an abnormal mental state, he or she is incompetent to give or withhold consent. The difficulty is in deciding, in the acute situation, which patients are competent in the eyes of the law and which are not. In general, patients with frank psychotic symptoms can be detained and sedated under common law (see above). Others are likely to be competent, even if depressed or agitated. The help of relatives and psychiatric specialists should be enlisted as soon as possible. Detailed records are essential.

Blood transfusion for Jehovah's Witnesses

There are 140 000 Jehovah's Witnesses in the United Kingdom and Ireland; their faith does not allow them to accept the transfusion of blood or its primary components. Administration of blood in the face of a refusal by an informed and rational patient is obviously unlawful. Similarly, if written evidence in the form of a signed and witnessed advance directive exists, this should be acted upon. Such directive cards are commonly carried by Jehovah's Witnesses and usually state that the physician is released from liability if harm results from failure to transfuse. In the absence of verbal or written instructions from the patient, clinical judgement should take precedence over the opinion of relatives or friends.

The children of Jehovah's Witnesses may be denied blood transfusion by their parents. If the well being of a child is at risk, a court order (a specific issue order) may be applied for to provide legal sanction for an isolated treatment. However, in an emergency, blood should be given to a child as soon as it is needed to save life.

Compulsory detention for assessment or treatment

Part I of the Mental Health Act (1983 England and Wales and 1984 Scotland) defines mental disorder as:

1 mental illness;
2 mental impairment (learning disability);
3 psychopathic disorder;
4 any other disorder or disability of mind.

In Part II, civil detention orders are specified (*see Box 20.5*). The indication for these orders is that the patient is suffering from a mental disorder of a nature or degree that warrants detention of the patient in hospital in the interests of his or her own health or safety or with a view to the protection of others.

In the ED, the sequence of orders would usually be:

- Section 4 (emergency admission order) or
- Section 136 (police admission order) *(For further information see page 376.)*

changed as soon as possible to

- Section 2 (assessment order)

converted later in hospital to

- Section 3 (treatment order).

The patient in police custody

The fact that a patient is in police custody does not affect the duty of care that a doctor has towards him or her. Neither should reasonable constraints on his or her freedom prevent an adequate examination.

Handcuffs may cause a circumferential reddening of the wrists. Occasionally, abrasions and even anaesthesia in the distribution of the superficial radial nerve may be seen.

The decision of 'fitness to be detained' is one for a police surgeon to make as is the similar examination for 'fitness to be interviewed'.

The police surgeon should also be involved as soon as possible in any case that looks as if it might have a complicated forensic element.

Taser injuries. 'Tasers' are hand-held electrical devices, which can be used to incapacitate dangerous offenders. They belong to a group of new non-lethal weapons designed as an alternative to

Box 20.5 Orders (Sections) of the Mental Health Act (1983 England and Wales) with Corresponding Provisions for Scotland and Northern Ireland

Section 2
- Admission for assessment followed by treatment.
- Duration up to 28 days.
- Application by nearest relative or approved social worker.
- Medical recommendation by two doctors (one Section 12 approved).

Section 3
- Admission for treatment.
- Duration up to 6 months.
- Application by nearest relative or approved social worker.
- Medical recommendation by two doctors (one Section 12 approved).

Section 4
- Admission for assessment in cases of emergency.
- Duration up to 72 h.
- Application by nearest relative or approved social worker.
- Medical recommendation by one doctor (preferably acquainted with patient) (must state that admission under Section 2 will involve undesirable delay).

Section 5 (2)
- Detention of patient already in hospital for any form of inpatient treatment.
- Duration up to 72 h.
- Invoked by doctor in charge of the case or one nominated deputy.

Section 5 (4)
- Nurse's holding power applicable to any patient already receiving treatment for a mental disorder.
- Duration up to 6 h while a doctor is found.
- Invoked by nurses of a prescribed class (RMN and RMNH).

Section 136
- Police admission order that allows a police officer to remove a person apparently suffering from a mental disorder from a public place to a designated place of safety (usually a police station or a local hospital ED) for assessment by a doctor and a social worker.
- Duration up to 72 h.
- Invoked by any police officer.

Section 135
- Under this order, and with a magistrate's warrant, a police officer, accompanied by a doctor and a social worker, may enter the residence of a person they believe to be suffering from a mental disorder to take them to a place of safety.
- Duration up to 72 h.
- Warrant must be obtained to use this order.

Corresponding provisions of the relevant legislation in Scotland and Northern Ireland
The following information is given as guidance only

Mental Health Act 1983 (England and Wales)	Mental Health (Scotland) Act 1984	Mental Health Act (Northern Ireland) Order 1986
Section 2	Section 26	Article 4
Section 3	Section 18	Article 12
Section 4	Section 24	Article 6
Section 5(2)	Section 25	Articles 7 & 7A
Section 136	Section 118	Place of Safety provisions

firearms in critical situations. The Taser fires two barbed probes into its target, which are attached to the 'gun' by a pair of thin wires. A high-voltage current is then immediately discharged down these wires, causing painful and overwhelming muscle contractions in the victim. The 'Advanced Tasers' used by most police forces rely on 'electro-muscular disruption' technology, which uses higher energies than older 'stun guns'. A signal powered at 18 to 26 W completely overides the CNS to cause an uncontrollable spasm of skeletal muscle that even large and determined subjects cannot resist. Similar weapons have been used for over 20 years in the United States without significant harmful effects. However, they may be used against individuals suffering from drug intoxication, psychiatric illness or extreme agitation. Consequently, it is recommended that all recipients of a Taser discharge should have a routine medical examination as soon as possible after the shock. Cardiovascular stability should be ascertained. The electrodes with their tiny barbs are easily removed by direct traction.

Patients detained under a Police Admission Order – Section 136 of the Mental Health Act (1983). Police officers frequently bring disturbed people to an ED (if it is a designated place of safety) under Section 136 of the Mental Health Act (1983). This police admission order can be invoked by any police officer and has a maximum duration of 72 h (*see Box 20.5*). The stated purpose of the order is to allow police officers to remove a person who is apparently suffering from a mental disorder from a public place to a safe area where the person can be assessed by a registered medical practitioner and an approved social worker. The Code of Practice (which is not actually legally binding) says that the doctor examining the patient should, wherever possible, be approved under Section 12 of the Mental Health Act. Where the examination is conducted by a doctor who is not approved by Section 12, the reasons for this should be recorded. Social workers are understandably reluctant to see a patient who the doctor does not recommend for detention. However, the Code of Practice states that the patient should not normally be discharged unless both professional assessments have been carried out. It then, rather

confusingly, goes on to say: 'Where the doctor, having examined the individual, concludes that he or she is not mentally disordered within the meaning of the Act, then that individual can no longer be detained under the section and should be immediately discharged from detention'.

In our society, bizarre behaviour in a public place is not always a sign of mental illness. Many patients have 'calmed down' by the time they arrive at the ED. Such patients can be assessed and discharged by a responsible doctor after discussion with the accompanying police officers. Other patients will need to remain in the department while awaiting a detailed assessment by a psychiatrist (preferably Section 12 approved!). In extreme cases, the police officers must be asked to maintain their Section 136-empowered forcible detention until the psychiatrist has concluded his assessment and perhaps even arranged to detain the patient further under Section 2 of the Mental Health Act.

The violent and uncontrollable patient in police custody. Occasionally, a patient who is obviously dangerously disturbed and violent may be brought in by the police (usually without any Section 136 paperwork!). The most common causes are:

• drug intoxication (usually amphetamines or other stimulant drugs);
• hypoglycaemia;
• post-ictal confusion;
• head injury;
• gross psychiatric disturbance.

There is a duty to protect the hospital staff, police and other patients in the ED. The patient is inevitably handcuffed and is best temporarily left so, while the above are excluded. Sedation is often necessary; the quickest and safest way of achieving this is with an intravenous benzodiazepine (e.g. lorazepam or midazolam). The usual rules regarding the administration of sedating drugs must be applied (*see page 17*). Once the patient is calmer, a more detailed assessment can be performed in relative safety.

Release of information to the police

Most information requested by the police relates to injuries sustained by victims of assaults. It is

Box 20.6 Personal and Sensitive Information

Personal information	Sensitive information
Names or initials	Sexuality
Date of birth	Ethnicity
Gender	Physical or mental health conditions
Address or postcode	Religious or similar beliefs
Occupation	Political opinions or memberships
Identity numbers (e.g. NHS or National Insurance numbers)	Offences committed or court proceedings

Under the Data Protection Act (1998) and the NHS Caldicott guidance, there is a duty to keep personal and sensitive information on patients (and staff) confidential and secure.

provided on a standard form with the patient's written consent (*for 'Statements by professional witnesses' see page 379*). However, police officers sometimes request information about patients who are suspects rather than victims (e.g. 'Did a young man attend with a hand injury last night?'). The vast majority of circumstances require the disclosure of personal rather than sensitive or clinical information *(see Box 20.6)*. Clinical information should almost never be divulged without the informed written consent of the patient. The laws that control the release of information to the police in England and Wales and the situations in which they apply are described below:

Legal duty to disclose, even without consent

Terrorism. Under the provisions of the Prevention of Terrorism Act (1989) and the Terrorism Act (2000), there is a statutory duty to immediately inform the police if any information is gained either personally or professionally about suspected terrorist activity.

Motor vehicle offences. Section 172 of the Road Traffic Act (1988) makes it a statutory duty to provide the police, on request, with the names and addresses of drivers who are allegedly guilty of offences under this act. Clinical information should not be given.

Court orders. Where the courts have made an order, the required information must be disclosed unless the decision is challenged at a higher court.

Legal power to disclose, but must consider implications of gaining consent

Serious crimes. Since the introduction of the Police and Criminal Evidence (PACE) Act (1984), the judicial system has accepted that Section 116 and Schedule 5 (parts I and II) of the act, which describe offences that are always considered serious, can be used as suitable guidelines for the release of non-clinical information – without the need to obtain the consent of the patient. These crimes are known as serious arrestable offences and are defined by PACE, Section 116 (*see Box 20.7*). If offences of this type have been committed, then the appropriate non-clinical information can be released by a consultant or his or her deputy at the request of a police officer of the rank of inspector or above. The request is usually made in writing on an agreed form of inquiry.

Aggregated data. The Crime and Disorder Act (1998), recognises that information may sometimes be required in the form of aggregated data (e.g. statistics) for the detection, prevention or reduction of crime. Such information may be required on an individual for the purposes of strategic cross-organisational planning to reduce crime or disorder in which that person is involved.

Child protection. Under Section 47 of the Children Act (1989), a local authority must make all necessary enquiries (either directly or through

377

Box 20.7 Serious Arrestable Offences (PACE, Section 116)

An arrestable offence is 'serious' if its commission (or threatened commission) has led to or is intended or likely to lead to the consequences listed below:
- Serious harm to the security of the state or to public order.
- Serious interference with the administration of justice or with the investigation of an offence.
- The death of any person (including by dangerous driving).
- Serious injury to any person, which includes any disease or any impairment of a person's physical or mental state.
- Substantial financial gain to any person.
- Serious financial loss to any person. Loss is defined as 'serious' for the purposes of this section if, having regard to all the circumstances, it is serious for the person who suffers it.

the police) to safeguard or promote a child's welfare. In such a situation, information should be released without the consent of either parent or child (and without an obligation to inform them) unless 'to do so would be unreasonable in the circumstances of the case'. If you suspect that a child is being abused, then you have a legal power to disclose information to social services (under 'vital interest' conditions of the Data Protection Act) or to the police (under PACE Act).

Information where gaining consent may be prejudicial to an investigation. The police may also seek personal information under an exemption of the Data Protection Act (1998). A Section 29(3) Crime Exemption allows information to be provided by an organisation about an individual without their consent. This is used when the police believe that the seeking of consent would prejudice their inquiries regarding either (a) the prevention or detection of crime or (b) the apprehension or prosecution of offenders. The police should produce a Section 29(3) form requesting the required information, signed by the police inspector who has decided to serve the exemption.

Information to protect vital interests. A similar clause of the Data Protection Act (1998) – Schedule 2(4) and/or Schedule 3(3) (Vital Interests Disclosure) – allows police officers to seek personal information without consent in order to 'protect the vital interests of the data subject or another person'. To release data under this Schedule, an appropriate form signed by a police officer of the rank of inspector or above must again be produced.

Injuries from firearms. Gun-related crimes have a devastating impact on the communities where they occur. Current guidance from the UK General Medical Council (developed in conjunction with the Association of Chief Police Officers) requires the staff of UK EDs to contact the police when a person attends with a gunshot wound. The patient's identity need not be disclosed, although their consent should be sought for both their name and other information to be provided. Without this consent, information should only be given to the police where it is judged that disclosure is necessary to prevent serious harm occurring or to prevent, detect or prosecute a serious crime. This can be seen as a public health measure to protect staff, the police and the public and to limit the likelihood of further injuries.

The Freedom of Information Act

The Freedom of Information Act (2000) gives everyone in the United Kingdom greater rights of access to the information held by public authorities such as NHS Trusts. Requests can be made by anyone (e.g. members of the public, the media and pressure groups) to access information such as reports, policies, guidelines, correspondence, e-mails and minutes of meetings. The Act applies to all public bodies and specifies that the request must be met within 20 working days. There are 23 exemptions from the Act, which may restrict the release of some types of information. Personal and sensitive information (*see Box 20.6*) is still covered by the provisions of the Data Protection Act (1998).

Statements by professional witnesses

All doctors who work in UK EDs will receive regular requests from the police for written statements regarding patients they have seen. These police statements should be carefully and legibly written using the case notes and should follow the format as shown in *Box 20.8. See also the section on clinical forensic medicine at the beginning of this chapter.*

The witness statement form must be signed and dated in the space provided at the top of the form and after the last handwritten word on the statement.

Box 20.8 Statement by a Professional Witness

I am Dr (Name). My qualifications are (Qualifications) and my GMC registration number is (Number). I am employed as a (Grade of doctor) in the Accident and Emergency Department of (Name of hospital). On (Date of incident) I was on duty when I examined [Name of Patient, Date of Birth, Do Not Give Address (1)] who attended the hospital (or was brought to the hospital by ambulance) at (Time of registration using 24-h clock).

(Name of patient) alleged [Brief history and details of incident as reported to doctor (2)].

On examination there were [Clinical findings in layman's terms (3)].

These injuries were treated with [Details of treatment (4)].

He or she was referred to (Details of any referral or follow-up). He or she was discharged from the hospital at (Time of departure using 24-h clock).

The relevant medical records can be produced to the court if required, labelled exhibit (Your initials – 1).

Notes on the above

1 *No address.* To protect the victim from possible intimidation when the statement is made available to the defence.

2 *Details of incident.* The history is part of the complete medical examination and so is more than hearsay evidence. A brief description such as 'hit on the head with a baseball bat' will suffice. Do not be tempted to expand this or other sections in relation to either causation or outcome. This statement is the evidence of a professional witness not the opinion of an expert witness.

3 *Clinical findings. See page 365.*

4 *Treatment.* Including number of stitches, etc.

Going to court

Most doctors and nurse practitioners who work in an ED will have to go to court at some time to give evidence as a professional witness. This is different from appearing as an expert witness. The professional witness must give an accurate account of his or her findings and actions but is not expected to be the ultimate authority on the subject. He or she should be:

- punctual, smartly dressed and courteous;
- well informed and willing to answer all questions without evasion;
- in possession of copies of the relevant notes (however, these notes can only be consulted in court with the permission of the bench);
- honest about the limitations of his or her own knowledge of the subject;
- able to describe the work of his or her profession in a way that everyone can understand.

> Attendance at court is not the same as going to an MRCP examination. The aim is to inform rather than to impress.

Rather more is expected of the expert witness. Both the defence and the prosecution may call their own expert but sometimes the judge will now request only one expert to give advice.

Different levels of court may be attended such as Magistrate's and Crown Courts in England and Sheriff's and High Courts in Scotland. The types of alleged crime that end up in each court again vary with the two legal systems.

Responsibilities to children

Consent and confidentiality for patients under the age of 16 years

The Children Act of 1989, changed the way that the law dealt with children by emphasising for the first time that the interests of the child must be paramount. For doctors, the biggest change was to the issues of consent and confidentiality as paraphrased below:

- Any competent young person, regardless of age, can independently seek medical advice and give valid consent to medical treatment.

- Competency is understood in terms of the patient's ability to understand the choices and their consequences, including the nature, purpose and possible risk of any treatment or non-treatment. Clearly, the more serious the procedure proposed, the more important it is that the doctor is sure that the child has a complete grasp of the situation.
- Parental consent to that treatment is not necessary, although it is obviously preferable for young people to have their parents' support for important and potentially life-changing decisions. It is the doctor's duty to discuss the value of this parental support with a young patient. However, if a competent child has consented to treatment, then a parent cannot over-ride that consent.
- Legally, a parent (or legal guardian) can give consent for treatment even if a competent child refuses – a situation that is best avoided. A refusal can also be overridden by a decision of the High Court.
- The duty of confidentiality owed to a person under the age of 16 years is as great as that owed to any other person. Regardless of whether or not the requested treatment is given, the confidentiality of the consultation should still be respected, unless there are convincing reasons to the contrary.
- When young people consult a doctor other than their usual GP, they are unlikely to refuse a request for details to be passed on to their GP, providing that the chain of confidentiality is maintained.

The legal framework for the above was established in the 1985 House of Lords' ruling in the Gillick case. This was particularly concerned with contraceptive advice but in general allowed for a person under the age of 16 years to submit to examination and treatment without a parent being informed, provided that was the wish of the child.

These guidelines are obviously applicable to teenagers but, for younger children, consent for examination and treatment should still be obtained from a person with parental responsibility. It should also be obtained from the child if he or she is of sufficient understanding to make an informed decision. Lawyers generally believe that in a normal child this would be at 10 years of age or more.

For blood transfusion in the children of Jehovah's Witnesses see page 374.

Child protection procedures

The Area Child Protection Committee

The Area Child Protection Committee (ACPC) is a forum that has representation from many different agencies and takes an overview of child protection issues in the area in which it has jurisdiction. The local social services department will usually have a specialist Child Protection Unit, from amongst whose senior staff the conference coordinators are selected. A child protection conference will be convened in the case of all children where there is reason to believe that there may be a need to coordinate a protection plan for their welfare.

The Child Protection Register

The Child Protection Register (CPR) is often colloquially called the 'at-risk' register. Its compilation and maintenance is the responsibility of the Area Child Protection Committee via the social services department. The NSPCC also usually have a copy. Computerised access from departments of emergency medicine is becoming much more commonplace.

Before a child is registered, the child protection conference must decide that there has been, or is a likelihood of significant harm leading to the need for a child protection plan. The cause of this harm must be established as far as is possible. If the risk can be applied to other children living in the same household, then it may justify their registration also.

Removal from the register is considered at review conferences usually held at least every 6 months. Reasons for deregistration include the following:

- the original factors that led to registration no longer apply;
- the child and family have moved permanently to another area and the child's name is included on the new area's register;

• the child has reached 18 years of age or has married.

The Emergency Protection Order

The Emergency Protection Order (EPO) (Children Act 1989, sections 44 and 45) replaced the Place of Safety Order. It may be made for a maximum of 8 days and extended for up to a further 7 days. Any person may apply for this order but applications are usually made by employees of either a social services department or the NSPCC. The court will only make the order if there is reasonable cause to believe that the child is likely to suffer significant harm if:

• he or she is not removed to another place;
• his or her removal from a safe place (e.g. a hospital) is not prevented;
• inquiries being made are frustrated by access to the child being unreasonably refused.

The Police Protection Order

The Police Protection Order (PPO) (Children Act 1989, section 46) gives a police officer the power to take a child 'into police protection' for up to 72 h if he or she believes that the child is at risk. This useful order can be used to prevent the removal of a child from the ED – at much shorter notice than the EPO.

Death

Reporting of death

About three-quarters of the 580 000 deaths in England and Wales each year are certified by a doctor and the remainder by a coroner. The local coroner must be informed if death is associated with any of the following:

• suspicion of homicide;
• suspicion of suicide;
• recent violence or other trauma;
• any accident (road traffic, domestic or industrial);
• drugs, poisons or alcohol;
• abortion;
• infancy;
• self-neglect or neglect by others;
• death in police custody or in prison;

• recent surgical procedure;
• allegation of medical negligence;
• industrial or occupational disease.

In such cases, a death certificate should not be issued without the coroner's permission. The coroner, or more usually a police officer acting on his or her behalf, must also be informed of any sudden death or in cases where the cause of death is uncertain. This includes most patients who are brought to hospital dead or who arrive in cardiac arrest and are not able to be resuscitated. A death from AIDS or of an HIV-positive individual does not need referral to the coroner unless there are other grounds for concern as detailed above.

In Scotland, the procurator fiscal fulfils the office of the coroner, the main difference being that he or she is less likely to request a post-mortem examination than his or her English counterpart.

> If in doubt, discuss the patient with the coroner.

Clinical diagnosis of death

For most purposes, death is signalled by the irreversible failure of respiration, circulation and innervation. Diagnosis of death in an apparently lifeless patient should thus depend on:

• absence of respiratory movements or breath sounds;
• absence of central pulses or heart sounds;
• absence of the protective reflexes of the eye (e.g. the corneal reflex);
• absence of the pupillary response to light.

It may sometimes but not necessarily include an ECG examination and inspection of the fundi. A state of near-death simulated by hypothermia, cold-water drowning or sedative poisoning must be excluded.

Rigor mortis is usually fully established 12 h after death, lasts about 12 h and then wears off over the next 12 h.

Brainstem death

Sometimes a patient may be brought to an ED with a functioning circulation but no other apparent signs of life. The criteria necessary for the diagnosis of brainstem death were laid down in a statement issued by the Conference of Medical Royal Colleges and their Faculties in the United Kingdom on 11 October 1976.

Loss of brainstem function is diagnosed by:
1 coma;
2 no spontaneous respiration;
3 no abnormal postures or epileptic jerking;
4 no brainstem reflexes.

Essential preconditions to testing

Before a diagnosis of brainstem death can be considered all of the following must coexist:
1 the patient is deeply comatose;
2 the patient is maintained on a ventilator because spontaneous respiration had previously become inadequate or had ceased;
3 there is no doubt that the patient's condition is caused by irremediable, structural brain damage.

Necessary exclusions

Before proceeding to testing, the following must be ruled out:
1 coma secondary to drugs, hypothermia or metabolic disorder;
2 respiratory failure and unresponsiveness secondary to neuromuscular blocking agents. Spinal reflexes should still be present.

Testing for absent brainstem function

Seizures and abnormal posturing (decorticate or decerebrate) imply that there is a passage of nervous impulses through the brainstem, which therefore has live neurons in it.

The oculocephalic reflex ('doll's eye phenomenon') is a brainstem reflex not mentioned in the UK code. If positive, the brainstem is still alive. There is often confusion about what is a positive reflex. Any deviation of the eyes with head movements is positive. In a dead patient, the eyes (obviously) always move in a fixed way with the head.

The brainstem findings used to confirm death in the UK code are:
• no pupillary response to light;
• no corneal reflex;
• no vestibulo-ocular reflexes;

• no motor responses within the distribution of the cranial nerves in response to adequate stimulation of any somatic area;
• no gag reflex or reflex response to bronchial stimulation by a suction catheter passed down the trachea;
• apnoea over a 10-min period during which the patient is oxygenated by diffusion and attains a $PaCO_2$ level of at least 50 mm Hg. Failure of the respiratory centre is the ultimate sign of loss of brainstem function.

Tests should be carried out by an experienced clinician, usually in the presence of another doctor. Retesting is performed after an interval of 2–3 h for the purposes of ensuring that:
• there is no observer error;
• there is no change in signs.

The decision to remove life support is a difficult one to make in an ED unless gross cerebral disruption is visible. A patient maintained on a ventilator whose brainstem is dead will inevitably develop asystole within a matter of hours.

Organ donation

Because it takes several hours to confirm brainstem death and because the patient must be stabilised on a ventilator first, organ donation does not often involve the ED directly. ICU staff may introduce the subject to the relatives at an early stage. The coroner must be informed. Donation of corneas is a different matter and, if this is a possibility, the duty ophthalmologist should be contacted. Eyes may be removed for up to 15 h after death. *See Box 20.9.*

Box 20.9 Suitable Patient for Organ Donation

Age 5–65 years (flexible).
Brainstem dead on a ventilator (early contact with the transplant team should be made once the first brainstem death test has been performed).
No major sepsis.
No malignancy except primary brain tumour.

Complaints

Any effective organisation that serves the public must have a well-structured system for dealing with complaints. Problems, which are dealt with in a rapid, efficient and courteous manner, will often resolve satisfactorily. The current NHS complaints system aims to achieve this by using several levels of response.

Local resolution

Verbal discussion of the problem usually follows a direct approach to a member of the clinical or reception staff at the time of treatment. A senior member of the medical or nursing staff should be involved from the outset.

Written complaints, which should be made within 6 months of the problem revealing itself, are forwarded to the hospital complaints manager who then gathers information from the relevant clinical staff. The chief executive subsequently replies in writing.

Independent review

Patients who are dissatisfied with the results of local resolution can apply for an independent review. A local convener may then set up a panel of three people who will investigate the complaint and prepare a report. This document will have conclusions and recommendations, which the chief executive will then respond to.

Investigation by the Health Service Commissioner

The next level of the system is a complaint to the Health Service Commissioner or Ombudsman. The Ombudsman is independent of the NHS and acts as a final arbiter of both complaints and complaints procedures.

The most common areas of complaint to a department of emergency medicine are:
• waiting times;
• attitude of staff;
• communication and information given;
• aspects of clinical care, such as failure to X-ray.
Staff dealing with a complaining patient or relative should consider the following guidelines in an attempt to defuse the situation.

• Do not be confrontational or defensive.
• Listen attentively and sympathetically.
• Do not be afraid of saying that you are sorry. You can empathise with a patient's distress without admitting liability or error (e.g. 'I am sorry that you are not happy with your treatment').
• Ask questions and obtain the full facts about the perceived problems.
• Do not attempt to justify; explain if appropriate.
• Agree a course of action and ensure that it is carried out quickly and efficiently and moreover that it is seen to be carried out.
• Provide written information about the NHS complaints system if the complainant wishes to take the matter further.
The content and conclusion of the discussion should be recorded in the patient's case notes.

Notifiable diseases

In the United Kingdom, the occurrence of certain infectious diseases must be notified, by law, to the medical officer responsible for environmental health (the consultant in public health medicine with responsibility for communicable diseases). All types of these infections must be notified, whatever the causative organism. This statutory obligation applies on suspicion alone. Legal action may be taken by an infected person if the index case has not been notified. In England and Wales, these notifiable diseases are designated by the Public Health (Control of Disease) Act 1984 and the Public Health (Infectious Diseases) Regulations 1988. There are some differences in Scotland and Northern Ireland where the notifiable diseases are listed in the Public Health (Notification of Infectious Diseases) (Scotland) Regulations 1988 and Schedule 1 of the Public Health Act (Northern Ireland) 1967 respectively. *For a list of notifiable diseases in the United Kingdom see Box 20.10.* HIV infection / AIDS is not a statutorily notifiable disease in the United Kingdom. There is, however, a voluntary confidential reporting scheme (with a special form) to the Public Health Laboratory Service Communicable Disease Surveillance Centre.

Box 20.10 Notifiable Diseases in the United Kingdom

Acute encephalitis* (England, Wales and Northern Ireland only)

Acute poliomyelitis

Anthrax

Chickenpox* (Scotland and Northern Ireland only)

Cholera

Diphtheria

Dysentery (amoebic or bacillary)

Erysipelas* (Scotland only)

Food poisoning

Gastro-enteritis in children under the age of two years* (Northern Ireland only)

Legionellosis (Scotland and Northern Ireland only)

Leprosy* (England and Wales only)

Leptospirosis*

Malaria*

Measles*

Membranous croup* (Scotland only)

Meningitis (Not in Scotland unless meningococcal)

Meningococcal septicaemia

Mumps*

Ophthalmia neonatorum* (England and Wales only)

Paratyphoid fever

Plague

Puerperal fever* (Scotland only)

Rabies

Relapsing fever*

Rubella*

Scarlet fever*

Smallpox

Tetanus

Tuberculosis

Typhoid fever

Typhus

Viral haemorrhagic fever

Viral hepatitis*

Whooping cough *

Yellow fever

An initial telephone call should be followed by written notification, except in the case of those diseases asterisked* where writing alone is adequate.

Box 20.11 Form Med 3

Closed statements – has return to work date
The note is for less than 2 weeks from the day of examination. It should indicate the earliest day on which the patient is likely to be fit for work.

Open statements – no return to work date
If a doctor is unable to issue a closed statement as above, then an open statement may be issued by entering a period during which the absence from work is likely to continue. This period may not be for more than 6 months from the date of issue unless the patient has been certified as unfit to work for the previous 6 months. When a patient who has been given an open statement recovers, he or she must be given a closed statement as above to terminate the spell of incapacity and allow a return to work.

• The statement must be based on an examination of the patient and issued no later than the day after this examination.

• The 'remarks' space of the statement can be used for any additional background information, which may be relevant.

• Only one statement can be issued for one period of absence. If this is lost, it can be replaced by another marked 'duplicate'.

allows for 7 days' absence before a doctor's note is required. The relevant forms are:

1 Form SC1 for people who are self-employed or unemployed. It is usually available in the ED.

2 Form SC2 for people who work for an employer. It is obtained from the place of work.

Medical certificates (doctor's statements) should be issued to patients who will clearly be away from work for a longer period without seeing another doctor.

• Form Med 3 is the usual doctor's statement. It should be issued by the doctor who, at the time, has clinical responsibility for the patient. The rules governing its use are described in *Box 20.11*.

• Form Med 5 is the doctor's special statement. It should be used when Form Med 3 is not appropriate:

1 The patient requires a statement for a past period during which he or she saw the doctor but no statement was issued.

2 The doctor wishes to advise a patient whom he or she has not examined to refrain from

Discharge of patients from an ED

Sick notes

Most patients who attend an ED will only require a few days away from work. Self-certification work for up to 1 month on the basis of a written report which is not more than a month old from another doctor.

Conditions for safe discharge

To send a patient home you must be sure of the following.

1 The patient does not have a life-threatening condition.

2 The symptoms can be adequately controlled in the environment in which the patient lives.

3 Any further investigation or treatment that the patient may need can be reasonably carried out at or arranged from home.

4 The patient has access to further help, and carers, should it be necessary.

5 You have communicated your plan for present and future management to both the patient and any others necessary for this care (e.g. relatives, GP, health visitor, district nurse, social worker, etc.).

Patients who have received sedative or narcotic drugs in the ED

Many patients receive drugs likely to cause sedation as part of their treatment in the ED. For both practical and medicolegal reasons, these patients need to be given verbal and written warnings about the possible residual effects of these drugs. *Box 20.12* summarises this information as it

should appear on a card for the patient to take home.

Box 20.12 Instructions about the Care of a Patient who has Received Sedative Medicines in the ED

Your relative/child/friend has received sedative medicines or injections in the Accident and Emergency Department. These drugs may cause:

- drowsiness;
- unsteadiness and loss of balance;
- poor coordination and clumsiness.

Some of these effects may last for up to 24 h. Because of this, a person who has received sedatives should:

- be accompanied home;
- be escorted when going upstairs;
- take care when using the toilet or bathroom.

They must NOT:

- be left alone in the house until fully recovered (e.g. overnight);
- drive or go cycling;
- go out walking alone;
- use machinery or go into situations where poor balance or coordination could be dangerous;
- drink alcohol;
- sign any legally binding documents.

However, they can:

- eat and drink light meals;
- sit around the house;
- take painkillers and regular medicines.

If you have any worries or problems with this patient, then telephone the Accident and Emergency Department helpline.

Chapter 21

Small wounds and localised infections

Small wounds

Small does not mean trivial. The wound may be:
- the only visible manifestation of a significant deep injury;
- simple yet serious if not treated promptly or properly;
- capable of leaving a considerable amount of disfigurement or loss of function;
- of no consequence in the doctor's eyes but worrying to the patient.

> Inadequately treated small wounds cause much distress for patients, a lot of worry for doctors and a considerable amount of work for lawyers.

Assessment of wounds

Certain features of a wound are associated with a high risk of complications. The following must always be considered.
- *Mechanism of injury* – excessive force, high speed, retained glass, dangerous weapon.
- *Site of injury* – trunk, perineum, neck, near a joint, over a neurovascular bundle.
- *Time of injury* – wounds more than 6 h old are more likely to get infected.
- *Place of injury* – field or garden injuries carry a greater risk of contamination with tetanus and gas-forming organisms.

> A butcher's knife may be contaminated with many organisms from animal carcasses. When boning a carcass and holding the knife with both hands it is possible to receive a deep, penetrating and highly contaminated wound.

Also ask about
- allergies to drugs including antibiotics;
- previous injuries if the patient is a child. Always consider child abuse (*see page 348*);
- current medication, as some drugs may affect local treatment (e.g. anticoagulants);
- implants, for example, arthroplasties and heart valves. There is a risk of infection at the site of the implant and so these patients must receive a short course of prophylactic antibiotics (*see later*).

Look for
- site, extent and character of the wound;
- evidence of contamination, non-viable tissue or foreign bodies;
- involvement of deep structures. Assess distal neurovascular and tendon function and record the findings.

Bleeding is exacerbated by alcohol, anticoagulants, partial (rather than complete) tears of vessels and continued interference with wounds. If there is a potential for significant bleeding, IV access should be established.

Pain may be extreme with some small injuries. Less painful and more serious injuries may have been inflicted in the same incident and can easily be missed. Local anaesthetic may be needed prior to further investigation; sensory loss must be recorded first.

Anaesthesia for wounds

All wounds must be explored and cleaned before closure is contemplated. This usually requires anaesthesia as does the subsequent closure. A general anaesthetic will be required when the areas involved are multiple or large, or belong to children or anxious adults (*see Boxes 21.1 and 21.2*).

Cleaning and exploration of wounds

Wound cleaning must be extensive and thorough. Particulate matter and contamination must be mechanically removed. This can be achieved by high-pressure irrigation or by scrubbing with a sterile nail or toothbrush and an antiseptic solution. Hydrogen peroxide is not recommended nowadays. Dirt left in a wound may cause infection or be taken up by inflammatory cells to produce a permanent tattoo effect.

Exploration of a wound is essential to identify:
- the depth and extent of damage;
- structures exposed or damaged;
- foreign bodies.

An appreciation of the direction and force of the injuring agent will facilitate exploration.

Resection of tissue

- Use a scalpel to remove dead tissue and trim the edges of old wounds.
- Be very cautious in the face, scalp, foot and hand. Skin is at a premium here. Always ask for help with complex wounds in these areas.

Box 21.1 Local Infiltration

For maximum doses of local anaesthetics see page 347.
- Use lidocaine, always without adrenaline.

  2% is suitable for nerve blocks. In a digital ring block this reduces the volume required and hence the risk of vascular compression.

  1% is appropriate for general use.

  0.5% should be used when large areas of tissue are involved and more than 10 mL of anaesthetic are required.
- Clean the wound edge with an antiseptic solution. If local anaesthetic is injected before the antiseptic has dried then the patient will be given a painful subcutaneous injection of both.
- Always trim hair for at least 2 cm around the wound, prior to injecting local anaesthetic. The aim is to expose the wounds fully and to prevent hair from interfering with the sutures. Scissors are usually adequate. A razor is sometimes necessary. Never shave the eyebrows.
- Using a short 23 G needle, inject a small amount of lidocaine under the wound edge, either through the wound edge if the wound is fresh and socially clean or through the skin if the wound is grossly contaminated or contused (safer but more painful).
- Once this small area is anaesthetised inject through it to raise a weal a little further on. Wait and then repeat. In this way, the patient feels only the first injection.

Box 21.2 Ring Block

This is effective for procedures involving distal wounds of the finger. There is a risk of damage to, or spasm of, the digital arteries and it must not be used if there is a history of Raynaud's disease or other upper limb circulatory problems.
- Use only plain lidocaine (2% for an adult). Adrenaline added to the lidocaine will produce irreversible spasm of the digital arteries and loss of the finger.
- Clean the base of the finger with antiseptic solution.
- Insert a 23 G needle into the dorsolateral border of the base of the finger. The tip of the needle should end up near the bone on the palmar side of the finger. Aspirate and if blood is seen withdraw the needle and start again.
- Inject no more than 2 mL of solution and much less in a child. The more fluid that is introduced the greater is the risk of vascular damage. Repeat on the opposite side of the finger.
- Wait for at least 5 min for full anaesthesia of the finger.
- If digital artery spasm occurs stop the procedure. Massage the base of the finger where the anaesthetic has been injected and instruct the patient to move the finger vigorously. These manoeuvres should dissipate the fluid and release the spasm.

The risk of digital artery spasm is increased if digital tourniquets are used. Most procedures on fingers in the ED do not require them.

Radiographs for foreign bodies

Foreign bodies are often surprisingly difficult to locate. The X-ray request card must indicate that a foreign body is being sought so that the radiographer can adjust the exposure accordingly. Glass is usually radio-opaque. Some thin metals (e.g. razor blades) can be surprisingly difficult to visualise on the film. Conversely, small fragments, obvious on X-ray, can be very difficult to find and remove. Occasionally, less damage is done by leaving them *in situ*. This decision must be made after consultation with a senior colleague.

> All wounds involving glass must have radiographs to exclude retained fragments.

Closure of wounds

- *Primary.* For most recent incised wounds.
- *Delayed primary.* After 3–10 days, for crush injuries.
- *Secondary* (i.e. by natural processes). When operative closure is impossible and granulation and epithelialisation is encouraged.

   Monofilament synthetic sutures are more difficult to handle than silk but are resistant to infection tracking up the thread and will give a better cosmetic result. Polyglycolic acid and catgut sutures evoke a pronounced tissue response as a necessary part of their autodestruction and are unsuitable for skin closure in an ED. For most wounds 4–0 G sutures are used, with finer gauges for cosmetically sensitive areas. Catgut may be used to close subcutaneous spaces.

- Plan sutures strategically – do not just start at one end.
- Use interrupted sutures – not continuous or subcuticular as these cause increased risk of infection tracking along the suture.

> Suturing skills cannot be learned from a book.

   Tissue glue, adhesive strips and skin staples are alternative methods of closure with several advantages:

- less traumatic for children;
- sometimes less scarring but only if good apposition is achieved;
- sometimes cheaper;
- sometimes quicker to apply.

However, wounds closed with these methods still require thorough cleaning, possibly under local anaesthesia.

> Tissue glue is applied to the carefully opposed skin surfaces and not to the open wound.

Skin loss

When closing defects in the skin, excessive tension should be avoided at all costs. If there is extensive skin loss or any loss on the face or hand, seek advice. Small skin defects elsewhere may be closed by undermining. This is achieved using a scalpel about 3 mm below the skin in the horizontal plane. A tissue plane may then be opened up using blunt scissors.

Aftercare of wounds

Dressings may not be required (e.g. on the face) or may be of simple non-adherent type. Splintage should be minimal but may be necessary if a wound is over the extensor aspect of a joint.

   Removal time for sutures varies with the site: 3–4 days on the face, up to 14 days in lower limbs or over joints but usually about 7 days for most other parts of the body. Earlier replacement with adhesive strips may avoid permanent puncture-mark scars. Sutures may be removed in the GP clinic provided that adequate documentation accompanies the patient.

   Postoperative analgesia depends on the patient's needs. Efficacy, suitability of formulation and cost should all be considered (*see page 328*).

Resuturing wounds

Patients returning with wounds which have broken down should have a senior opinion. Such wounds must be cleaned and dressed until ready for resuture. Anything more than local infection requires oral antibiotics. Facial wounds need a specialised opinion and wounds in children may need reclosure under general anaesthetic. The possibility of a retained foreign body should always be considered.

Skin grafts

These can be full thickness (Wolfe) or partial thickness (Thiersch); only the latter is generally used in EDs. The objective is to transplant the tops of the dermal papillae from the donor site, leaving the bases and skin appendages as a partial thickness defect. This will heal by secondary intention. The donor skin must be applied directly to a clean, granulating wound. It will be nourished initially by direct tissue perfusion and then later by new capillary buds. The technique may not be suitable for patients on steroids with very thin, friable skin – *see Box 21.3*.

Reimplantation of body parts

Successful reimplantation of amputated body parts is possible using microsurgical techniques. Clean injuries without contamination or contusion have the best chances of success. Suitable structures for reimplantation include:
- the whole or part of a finger (with amputations proximal to the distal interphalangeal joint only);
- the penis;
- ears;
- large pieces of scalp;
- hands, feet and more extensive parts of a limb.

Patients with these injuries should be discussed as soon as possible with the nearest plastic surgery unit. The amputated part should be wrapped in saline-soaked gauze and then put in a plastic bag in a container full of crushed ice. The body tissue must not come into direct contact with the ice.

Prevention of wound infection

This is achieved in most cases by:
- cleaning the wound;
- excising necrotic tissue;
- closing the wound as appropriate;
- dressing the wound carefully;
- using antibiotics when indicated (*see Box 21.4*);
- anticipating the presence of spore-forming organisms (*see later*).

Patient compliance in after-care is essential.
The most common wound contaminants are bacteria from the skin and so flucloxacillin or

---

Box 21.3 Skin Grafting

A clean theatre with a good light is essential. Aseptic theatre technique must be followed, with the operator using gown and gloves. Infection is the most common cause of graft failure. Antibiotics should not be used routinely.

Anaesthesia. This may be general or local. The latter is often preferable. Lidocaine 0.5% or 1% is infiltrated subcutaneously around donor and graft sites.

Donor site. The donor site should be discussed with the patient. Upper arm and inner thigh are usually appropriate.

Graft site. The graft site should be clean and granulating. Avascular eschar should be removed. Clinical evidence of infection precludes operation. Any doubt should be resolved by prior bacteriological investigation.

Technique of removing graft. A small graft knife designed to take a razor blade is appropriate for most cases (a Silva knife). The thickness of the graft is determined by the distance between the blade and the underlying roller. The donor site is dressed with paraffin gauze, a non-adherent dressing and crepe.

Application of graft. The graft is reversed on to paraffin gauze which is then trimmed to the graft size to provide support. Postage stamp sized grafts are ideal, the defect being covered by a number of grafts with minimal overlapping. Any subsequent haematoma formation then lifts and devitalises only one small area and most of the graft survives. Apposition of graft and granulating bed is maintained by suturing the edges and tying in antiseptic-impregnated cotton wool (*see Figure 21.1*).

Follow-up. The outer dressing of the grafted area is removed after 2–3 days to check for infection. Smell and exudate warrant further investigation. In the absence of either, the top dressing is replaced and neither wound disturbed for 10–14 days. Fiddling with the dressings greatly increases pain at the donor site and the risk of failure of the graft.

When the dressings and sutures are removed the graft should not be cleaned vigorously but merely examined and then covered with a non-adherent dressing. Small defects usually close quickly by secondary intention. The graft will take months to stabilize. Initially, it will need constant protection by a dressing. Later, a hand cream should be applied. The split skin will not sweat or produce grease and tends to dry out and break down easily. The patient should be advised to protect it while sunbathing for at least a year.

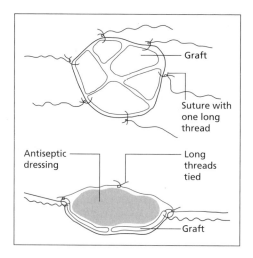

Figure 21.1 Application of a split skin graft.

erythromycin is adequate cover. In bites, however, a wider spectrum of organisms is involved and so co-amoxiclav or erythromycin should be prescribed.

Spore-forming organisms are more likely to contaminate wounds incurred on sports fields or in gardens and also injuries of the lower limb. They will flourish in areas of hypoxia, for example, deep, penetrating and contused wounds. Primary prevention involves scrubbing all wounds under effective anaesthesia and surgically removing all necrotic tissue. Contused wounds should not be closed. All foreign material must be removed.

Gas gangrene can be prevented if wounds are managed as outlined above. Long-acting penicillins are no substitute for adequate wound toilet.

Prevention of tetanus

For the diagnosis and treatment of tetanus see page 239.
For the routine UK immunisation schedule for children see Box 18.18 on page 345.
For a summary of tetanus prophylaxis see Box 21.5.
There were 12 cases of tetanus in the United Kingdom in 2003, although prophylaxis against tetanus is cheap and safe. Infection is caused by contamination of a wound with the spores of the bacillus *Clostridium tetani*. Days or even weeks after infection, local multiplication of the organism

---

Box 21.4 Indications for Antibiotics in Wound-care

Antibiotics are indicated for wounds which:
● are already showing signs of infection when seen;
● are more than 12 h old and in need of primary closure;
● have a definite history of contamination with problem organisms (e.g. human and cat bites);
● are possibly contaminated with deep areas that are not amenable to cleaning (e.g. some puncture wounds);
● have exposed or damaged deep structures (e.g. bone in compound fractures, tendon or nerve).

Box 21.5 Tetanus Prophylaxis

Patient immunisation status	Tetanus-prone wound	Other wound
Has had five or more doses of vaccine during lifetime	Nothing required (HTIG if very high risk of contamination)	Nothing required
Has had complete course of three doses or booster dose within the last 10 years	Nothing required (HTIG if very high risk of contamination)	Nothing required
Has had three-dose course of vaccine or single booster more than 10 years ago	Booster dose + consider HTIG if wound contaminated	Booster dose
Has not ever had complete course of vaccine or immune status unknown	Complete course of vaccine + HTIG if wound contaminated	Complete course of vaccine

Box 21.6 Tetanus-Prone Wounds

Wounds that are particularly tetanus-prone include those which:
- are more than 6 h old at presentation;
- are deeper than they are long (stab or puncture wounds);
- contain devitalised tissue;
- are possibly contaminated with soil or manure;
- show clinical evidence of sepsis.

occurs with release of its neurotoxin – *see page 239.* Until recently, most cases of tetanus in the United Kingdom were in people over 65 years old who had not been previously immunised. In the last few years, tetanus has also been seen in young adults who abuse IV drugs. Even the most trivial of wounds can introduce tetanus into the body but some wounds carry a particularly high risk. *For - factors that identify tetanus-prone wounds see Box 21.6.*

Active immunisation against tetanus was introduced into some areas of the United Kingdom as part of the primary immunisation of infants from the mid-1950s and was adopted nationally from 1961. It was provided by the British armed forces (mostly to men!) from 1938 onwards. Knowledge of these dates and the age of the patient will help to determine the likelihood of previous immunisation.

With diphtheria on the increase in Eastern Europe, single antigen tetanus vaccine (T) has been replaced by the combined tetanus and low-dose diphtheria vaccine for adults and adolescents (Td) for all routine uses. Td replaced single tetanus as the standard booster for UK school-leavers in 1994. For both diphtheria and tetanus, a total of five doses of vaccine are considered to give life-long immunity. These may have been given either as the primary three-dose course in childhood followed by school entry and school leaving doses or as a primary course at any time followed by a booster dose 10 years later and a second booster 10 years after that. Polio vaccine is usually also included in the booster doses.

Unscheduled booster doses are therefore indicated only:

1 Following a tetanus-prone wound (*see Box 21.6*) where the patient has not received a full five-dose course and is due a further dose.

2 Following a tetanus-prone wound (*see Box 21.6*) where the patient's immunisation status is unknown (e.g. elderly patients and immigrants to the United Kingdom).

3 For travellers to areas where medical attention may not be accessible, should a tetanus-prone injury occur, and whose last dose was more than 10 years previously.

Tetanus toxoid vaccine confers active immunity. It stimulates the production of antibodies, which may take several weeks to reach a peak. Therefore, in the case of contaminated wounds, patients receiving Td vaccine in the first two categories above should also be given passive immunisation with human tetanus immunoglobulin (HTIG) – *see later.* The two injections should be given into separate areas. Patients with impaired immunity may not respond to active immunisation and may therefore also need HTIG.

Patients with doubtful or unknown immune status to tetanus and diphtheria require a full primary course of Td vaccine (three doses at 1-month intervals). Notification should be sent to the patient's GP to this effect. Two further booster doses at 10-year intervals will also be required to confer life-long immunity.

Td vaccine is given by deep subcutaneous or intramuscular (IM) injection. Local reactions such as pain, redness and swelling around the injection site may occur and persist for several days. Acute allergic reactions (anaphylaxis or urticaria) are uncommon; peripheral neuropathy is a rare but recognised side effect. Vague post-vaccination symptoms such as headache, pyrexia, lethargy, malaise and myalgia may also occur occasionally. Persistent nodules at the injection site may arise after shallow injections.

The contraindications to Td vaccine are:

1 Coincidental acute febrile illness – unless there is a tetanus-prone wound. Minor infections without fever or systemic upset should not postpone immunisation.

2 Severe reactions (e.g. anaphylaxis or peripheral neuropathy) after a previous dose.

HIV-positive status is not a contraindication to immunisation.

Human tetanus immunoglobulin

Human tetanus immunoglobulin (HTIG) gives passive immunity. It is a preparation of human antibodies, which is not associated with significant side effects or allergy, unlike the previously used horse serum. The dose is 250 iu by deep IM injection. This may be increased to 500 iu if more than 24 h have elapsed or if there is a risk of heavy contamination or after large burns.

Tetanus and diphtheria immunisation for children

The administration of an unscheduled tetanus and diphtheria vaccination to a child may cause great difficulty with the correct timing of other immunisations. For this reason, concurrent administration of the other recommended vaccinations for that age group or referral to the child's health visitor is usually the better practice.
For the routine UK immunisation schedule for children see Box 18.18 on page 345.

Wound botulism

This related Clostridial infection has recently re-emerged in the United Kingdom.
For the diagnosis and treatment of wound botulism see page 240.

Protection from infection of patients with prosthetic heart valves and arthroplasties

A significant number of patients who attend an ED will have some sort of implant *in situ* and many of them will have a wound or an illness that may result in a bacteraemia. Even a transient passage of pathogens through the blood stream may be enough to infect the area around an implant and so these patients must be protected with a short course of prophylactic antibiotics. The

British National Formulary should be consulted as to the exact choice of drugs for each situation.

Specific types of wounds

For forensic aspects of wounds see page 365.
For chest wounds see page 76.
For neck wounds see page 64.
For abdominal wounds see page 85.
For facial wounds see page 70.
For scalp wounds see page 39.
For wrist wounds see page 127.
For serious hand injuries see page 136.
For burns see page 146.

Abrasions

Motorcyclists and children may present with dirty abrasions.

Tx

The basic care is as for any wound. However, the ingrained dirt must be removed to prevent infection and to avoid the development of a permanent 'tattoo'. Scrubbing with a swab or a small brush may be necessary. Analgesia for this purpose can be obtained by:
- application of local anaesthetic gel;
- infiltration of local anaesthetic;
- general anaesthesia.

Crush wounds

Where there is an element of crush or bursting in the mechanism of injury there is widespread damage to tissues. Extracellular fluid accumulates and the tissues continue to swell for 24–48 h.

Tx

The wound should be cleaned, explored and then dressed.

> If crush wounds are closed immediately, interstitial pressure will rise, resulting in tissue necrosis and infection.

The patient must be reviewed on the following day. Severe crush injuries require admission for elevation and observation. Decompression may sometimes be needed, especially if the crush has damaged deep tissues without tearing the skin or if there is a deep, closed compartment.

For compartment syndrome see page 116.

Degloving injuries

When skin is traumatically removed from limbs in this way it is tempting to simply replace and suture it. However, the injured skin is always contused and often dead. The risks of necrosis and sloughing are very great. A patient with a degloving injury must be referred for inpatient surgical management.

Roller injuries

These have features of both degloving and crush injuries. The injury may seem trivial at first but widespread tissue necrosis can occur. Admission, elevation and careful observation are essential. Vascular compromise is suggested by:

- failure to blanch on pressure;
- failure of capillary refill;
- paraesthesia.

Flap wounds

Flaps are caused by initial contact at the apex of the wound and then a tearing of the skin towards the base. Contusion of the skin flap is inevitable. Narrow, distally based flaps have a poor blood supply.

Tx

If the flap has a wide base or is thick with obviously viable tissues, it may be sutured in the normal way. If not, consider defatting the flap and replacing it as a skin graft with a pressure dressing. The skin of children is very elastic and a V-shaped cut may appear to have lost tissue or have a narrow base as a result of contraction. The skin flap should be stretched back to its normal position without undue tension before viability and skin loss are assessed.

Stab wounds

Stab wounds are defined as wounds that are deeper than they are long. As such they have an invisible deep part. The risk of severe damage relates to the anatomical site of the injury, but particular areas of concern are:

- the chest – back or front (*see page 76*);
- the neck (*see page 64*);
- the abdomen (*see page 85*);
- near joints;
- near large limb vessels.

> The presence of distal pulses does not exclude vascular damage. Swelling is always worrying.

Xʀ

Radiographs are used to show air shadows:

- pneumothorax and surgical emphysema on chest X-ray with chest wounds;
- air under the diaphragm on chest X-ray following an abdominal injury;
- surgical emphysema on the lateral soft-tissue view of the neck after a neck wound;
- air in a joint showing synovial penetration after a wound to a limb.

Tx

Stab wounds must be assessed by an experienced doctor. Uncomplicated injuries are best treated by cleaning and simple dressing; immediate closure tends to trap any haematoma that forms. All patients with this type of injury should be either admitted for observation or reviewed on the following day.

For legal aspects of stab wounds see Chapter 20.

Gunshot wounds

Gunshot wounds have a twofold potential for damage:

1 direct injury to structures along the track;

2 damage to neighbouring structures from dissipated kinetic energy. This depends on the type of weapon involved. High-velocity weapons fire bullets that transfer a large amount of energy to the

surrounding tissues. Damage is greatest to solid organs in closed spaces. Bone splinters may cause secondary damage. Vascular injury can be overt and extensive or confined to the endothelium (with intact pulses); delayed thrombosis may result.

XR

As for stab wounds above.

Tx

All patients with gunshot wounds require:
- resuscitation;
- assessment;
- admission and observation;

Most need surgical exploration of the bullet track to remove necrotic tissue and clothing fragments. *For legal aspects of gunshot wounds see Chapter 20.*

Bites in the British Isles

Bite wounds account for up to 2% of all attendances at an ED. Dog bites are the most common and bites from humans and other primates usually are the worst.

Tx

Teeth produce dirty, contused wounds, which must be cleaned thoroughly; this can be difficult with deep puncture wounds. Once cleaned and irrigated, bites are often considered for delayed closure. However, gaping wounds should always be approximated with adhesive strips or loose sutures (not tissue glue). On the face, the excellent blood supply usually prevents infection and this rule can be ignored – especially as the cosmetic results of delayed closure are poor.

Shallow dog bites do not need antibiotics at first presentation. Patients with cat bites, human bites or deep puncture wounds should be given a short course of co-amoxiclav (or erythromycin or metronidazole if allergic to penicillins) to protect against anaerobic infections. All patients must be covered for tetanus (*see page 390*).

> Human bites may carry a risk of hepatitis B transmission. *For prophylaxis against blood-borne viruses see page 397.*

For envenomation (especially adder bites) see page 288.

For rabies see page 259.

Stings in the British Isles

Wasp and bee stings. The stings from almost all *Hymenoptera* arthropods cause local pain, redness and swelling but rarely result in severe problems. Exceptions are anaphylactic reactions and intra-oral swellings, both of which need appropriate treatment (*see pages 295 and 418*). (It is said that up to 0.5% of the population is hypersensitive to either bee or wasp venom.) Unlike wasps, bees leave their stings imbedded in the skin and these should be removed with splinter forceps. The acid bee venom may then be neutralised by the application of bicarbonate, while vinegar may help to soothe the caustic wasp sting. The inflammation from all stings can be treated with local applications of calamine lotion, antihistamine cream or hydrocortisone 1% cream.

Caterpillar stings. The Brown Tail moth, *Euproctis chrysorrhoea*, is common throughout central and southern Europe, including the south of England and is found in all types of habitat. The hairs of its caterpillars may cause an extremely painful rash if touched. (This ordinary-looking caterpillar is brownish grey with red spots along its back and is not particularly hairy.) Hydrocortisone cream may ease the pain.

Weever fish stings. The Lesser Weever fish, *Trachinus vipera*, is found in shallow sandy water around the shores of the British Isles; the Greater Weever fish, *Trachinus draco*, is caught by anglers in deeper water. The dorsal and gill cover spines of both fish may give a very painful sting. The venom can be denatured by immersing the injured part in very hot (but not more than 45°C) water.

Jellyfish stings. The Portuguese Man-of-War jellyfish, *Physalia physalis*, has friable and venomous tentacles as do several other jellyfish found in British waters. Adherent tentacles should be removed with forceps and then a strong solution of sodium bicarbonate applied to the injured area. The stings from other British species of jellyfish (e.g. the Lion's mane jellyfish, *Cyanea capillata*) are also treated with alkaline solutions unlike tropical species (such as the Box jellyfish, *Chironex fleckeri*, of Australasia) for which vinegar is an essential first-aid remedy.

Bites and stings from exotic creatures

Exotic pets may inflict exotic bites and stings on their keepers. In addition, world travellers may encounter poisonous insects, spiders, snakes, fish, corals, hydroids, anemones, jellyfish and octopi.

Tx

All such wounds must be cleaned thoroughly and then dressed. Tetanus prophylaxis must be ensured. It may occasionally be necessary to give antivenom and it is important that each ED knows where the nearest supply is kept. (The *British National Formulary* contains up-to-date telephone numbers of regional depots.) In the United Kingdom 24 hour help and advice can be obtained from the following centres:

1 The Liverpool School of Tropical Medicine;
2 The Hospital for Tropical Diseases in London.

In the case of travellers, expert local advice is essential for both diagnosis and treatment.

For non-venomous injuries from the spines of sea urchins and other marine creatures see page 397.
For envenomation (especially adder bites) see page 288. For rabies see page 259.

High-pressure injection injuries

High-pressure hoses containing air, water, oil and paint are used in many industries. Skin penetration occurs easily and leaves minimal superficial injury but causes significant damage to deep structures. Initially, the injury appears trivial but within 24 h swelling, paraesthesia and loss of function occurs. Tissue necrosis follows and damage is often widespread.

Tx

All of these injuries must be referred for inpatient treatment at the time that they are first seen. Laying open of the track and removal of injected particulate matter is often required. Tetanus prophylaxis is essential. *See also page 138.*

Pretibial injuries

Pretibial lacerations are common in elderly female patients and often follow comparatively minor trauma. The area has a poor blood supply and little deep tissue to support the skin. Despite this, most pretibial wounds heal well, albeit slowly. More problems can be anticipated with:

- distally based flaps;
- very contused flaps;
- very elderly patients;
- patients with very thin skin or those on steroids.

Tx

Most pretibial lacerations should not be sutured – the stitches tear the thin skin. Adhesive strips are ideal but must not be applied until the wound has been adequately cleaned, usually under local anaesthesia. Tension should be avoided when laying back the skin. Blood clots must be removed and the flap laid closely on to a clean bed. A secure non-adherent pressure dressing can then be applied.

The patient should be encouraged to continue ankle movements but to elevate the foot when at rest. Initial follow-up should be arranged for a couple of days post-injury and then as appropriate. Admission for bed rest may be required for frail patients with extensive wounds. In extreme cases, plastic surgical advice may be needed.

Pretibial haematomata

Following injury, patients occasionally present with a large tender, pretibial haematoma.

Tx

Waiting for this swelling to resolve taxes the patience of both the doctor and the sufferer.

A better outcome may be achieved by draining the blood clot through a surgical incision. Needle aspiration is unlikely to succeed. The mode of anaesthesia for the procedure depends on the patient and the size of the haematoma. Observation in clinic over a few days will help to determine the best form of treatment.

Puncture wounds of the feet

Puncture wounds of the feet are common and are often caused by nails, needles and glass. There is usually a tender but unremarkable wound on the sole.

Xʀ

Radiographs are indicated for any suspicion of foreign body and with all glass wounds. A retained fragment is common with wounds from a needle and with glass but not when a nail is involved. A skin marker, applied to the skin at the site of entry, will greatly help with localisation on X-ray.

Tx

The wound must be cleaned, an antiseptic dressing applied and antitetanus prophylaxis given if indicated. The patient should be instructed to return if there are any signs of infection.

> Retained foreign bodies can be very difficult to locate, even if they appear superficial on X-ray.

Foreign bodies must be removed in a suitable environment – usually an operating theatre – by an experienced doctor working in good conditions (fine instruments, a bloodless field and adequate anaesthesia).

Patients returning with obvious infection must be seen by a senior member of staff. Antibiotics, further consideration of the possibility of foreign bodies and follow-up are indicated. Infections in puncture wounds can be very difficult to treat. Exploration of the track and IV antibiotics may be required in some cases.

> *Pseudomonas* likes to live in the damp environment of training shoes and similar footwear.

Nails through hands or feet

It is quite common for a patient to present with a nail protruding from a finger or a foot. The patient should be asked if the nail is from a nail-gun. The nail fired from this tool has two copper barbs on it, which impede withdrawal. Sensation must be assessed before local anaesthesia is administered and then movements assessed after the nail is removed.

Xʀ

Initial radiographs can be helpful if there is difficulty removing the nail. Otherwise they should be obtained after removal to look for bony damage.

Tx

The nail should be removed under local anaesthesia and the wound protected with an antiseptic dressing. If there is bony damage, antibiotic cover is indicated (flucloxacillin or erythromycin).

Foreign bodies in the feet or hands

The removal of a foreign body from the palm of the hand or the sole of the foot can be particularly difficult despite often appearing to be easy. It may require:
- a bloodless field and hence a tourniquet;
- good anaesthesia, usually general;
- skill and experience;
- adequate equipment – a metal detector may be helpful.

Management should be discussed with a senior colleague; inpatient care may be required.

Some foreign bodies can be removed in the ED. These will be:
- superficial;
- easily palpable;
- recently implanted;
- discussed with a senior member of staff.

Other foreign bodies

Other foreign bodies (e.g. airgun pellets) need localisation and then a similar consideration given to the mode of removal.

Sea urchin spines

Patients may present with sea urchin spines imbedded in their hands or feet; usually acquired while swimming in the Mediterranean Sea. The dark brown spines are very friable and so are difficult to remove intact. Softening the skin with salicylic acid 2% ointment, applied overnight, may facilitate the process. Analgesia can be achieved with local anaesthetic cream before attempting to remove the larger pieces with a hypodermic needle. Smaller pieces may be scrubbed out with a toothbrush but most of the remaining debris usually ends up being left *in situ*. Fortunately, with appropriate dressings and analgesia, the injury settles down very quickly.

Other spine-bearing marine creatures including stingrays, scorpionfish, stonefish, weeverfish, catfish and crown-of-thorns starfish may inflict painful puncture wounds on the unwary. The pain is usually very marked in the case of venomous species. Expert local advice is essential for both diagnosis and treatment.
For stings from weeverfish spines see page 394.
For envenomation see page 288.

Subungual collections

Subungual haematomas can be drained by trephining (*see page 144*). This procedure does not introduce infection and thus antibiotics are not required for an associated fracture. Collections of pus under the nail are usually treated by removing the nail under a ring block.

Fish hooks

Fish hooks can be removed under local anaesthesia (ring block or infiltration of lidocaine). The barbed end of the hook should be pushed forwards through the anaesthetised skin and the hook cut in two with K-wire cutters. It can then be withdrawn easily.

Splinters under the nail

Splinters under the nail should be removed under ring block. Attempts may be made with splinter forceps initially but it is often necessary to trim back or remove the nail. Thorns can cause serious infection including tetanus and must be removed.

Oil-based veterinary vaccines

Accidental self-inoculation leads to intense local pain. The wound may appear trivial but can lead to widespread necrosis. Inpatient referral is essential. Debridement is usually necessary.

Blood and body fluid exposure incidents ('needlestick injuries')

Both hospital staff and members of the public may present after a needlestick injury or other body fluid exposure incident. Hepatitis B, hepatitis C and HIV are the major blood-borne viruses (BBVs) but several other pathogens (*see page 15*) may also be transmitted by this route. Exposure incidents include:
1 piercing of the skin by any contaminated sharp objects;
2 splashes into the eyes with body fluids;
3 contamination of broken skin by body fluids;
4 significant human bites;
5 ingestion by mouth of body fluids.
An assessment of risk must be made. People at a high risk of having (and thus transmitting) BBVs are listed in *Box 21.7*. However, all patients in an ED should be regarded as potential sources of BBVs as some apparently benign groups contain a high number of hepatitis B carriers (e.g. elderly ex-servicemen). Around a third of IV drug abusers in the United Kingdom carry hepatitis C but HIV prevalence in this group is still less than 1%. The features of an injury or other incident that increase the risk of transmission of BBVs are listed in *Box 21.8*. The estimated risks of seroconversion are shown in *Box 21.9*. The HIV risk with an unknown source is generally minimal and so patients can be reassured. Hepatitis B is the major problem as transmission can occur with much smaller quantities of blood and with older blood.

Tx

Skin punctures should be encouraged to bleed freely. If the eyes are involved, they should be

Box 21.7 High Risk Sources for Transmission of BBVs

Known carriers of BBVs.
Close family contacts or sexual partners of known carriers of BBVs.
Children of mothers who are known carriers of BBVs.
Homosexual or bisexual people (especially men).
Intravenous drug abusers.
Recent residents of sub-Saharan Africa (and Egypt for HCV).
Inmates of custodial institutions.
Residents of enclosed units for the mentally subnormal, including staff.
Health care workers and trainees (especially from developing countries).
Morticians, embalmers and tattooists.
Patients on long-term renal dialysis.
Patients with chronic liver infection.
Haemophiliacs or others receiving regular blood products and any relatives responsible for the administration of these products.
Patients with jaundice under investigation.

Box 21.8 High Risk Exposure Incidents for Transmission of BBVs

Percutaneous rather than mucocutaneous exposure (puncture wound rather than splash)
Exposure to blood rather than blood-stained fluid or any other body fluid
Injury from hollow-bore rather than solid needle (wider gauge = worse)
Injury from hollow-bore needle that has directly entered a blood vessel
Visible blood on the injuring device
Deep wound rather than shallow abrasion
No protective equipment used
Immediate washing and/or bleeding not performed
Highly infected source (HBV e-antigen detectable, HCV RNA detectable, HIV high viral load)
Source terminally ill
Source infected with more than one blood-borne virus.
Exposed person not immunised

Box 21.9 Estimated Risks of Seroconversion after Blood Exposure

Source infection	Route	Risk
HIV	mucocutaneous	<0.1%
HIV	percutaneous	0.3%
HCV (detectable RNA)	percutaneous	0.5–1.8%
HBV (e-antigen +ve)	percutaneous	30% (for non-immune individual)

Counselling can be arranged in special situations. In all cases, the patient's GP and occupational health department must be notified of the type and date of the injury, the action taken and any further action or follow-up required.

Unknown source of needle

Send 10 mL of unclotted blood from the patient to the Public Health Laboratory Service for storage and possible later testing. (In the unlikely event of seroconversion, this sample can be used to prove that the disease was occupationally acquired.) Ensure protection against hepatitis B – *see later and Box 21.10* – but assume the source of the needle to be low risk for this and other BBVs.

Known source of blood or body fluid

Take 10 mL of unclotted blood from the patient and the same from the person who was the source of the blood or body fluid. Send both samples together to the Public Health Laboratory Service for storage and possible later testing. (In the unlikely event of seroconversion, these samples can be used to prove that the disease was occupationally acquired.) Ensure protection against hepatitis B – *see later and Box 21.10*. All cases that involve a known HIV-positive source, must be discussed with a consultant virologist who may recommend prophylaxis with zidovudine and other antiretroviral drugs – *see Box 21.11*. Treatment with these drugs – ideally started within 2 h of

irrigated with water. Wounds must be cleaned and dressed and prophylaxis against tetanus ensured. The patient should be informed of the general risks from BBVs, the risk from this particular incident and the benefits of the proposed treatment.

Box 21.10 Post-exposure Prophylaxis Against Hepatitis B Infection

● If vaccinated within the last 5 years with a known level of antibodies (100 units or more) no further action need be taken.
● If more than 5 years have elapsed since vaccination or if the antibody level is low (between 10 and 100 units) give a booster dose of hepatitis B vaccine.
● If the antibody status is unknown following a previous course of vaccine, then give a booster dose of hepatitis B vaccine. Assess the risk of the source and the exposure (see Boxes 21.7 and 21.8) and if high, give hepatitis B immunoglobulin (HBIG) in addition.
● If the patient has not been vaccinated against hepatitis B, then start an accelerated course of hepatitis B vaccine. Assess the risk of the source and the exposure (see Boxes 21.7 and 21.8) and if high, give HBIG in addition.

Box 21.11 Post-exposure Prophylaxis Against HIV Infection

The risk of HIV transmission through occupational exposure in health care workers is approximately 0.3% from a percutaneous injury and less than 0.1% after mucous membrane exposure. Prophylaxis with drugs reduces the risk of infection by over 70%. Triple therapy with anti-retroviral agents is usually offered to health care workers following high risk exposure to body fluids from a HIV-positive source:

1 Zidovudine (AZT) 250 mg bd or 200 mg tds
2 Lamivudine 150 mg bd
3 Nelfinavir 1250 mg bd or Indinavir 800 mg tds
These drugs are continued for 28 days and are not without side-effects. Zidovudine and lamivudine are nucleo-side reverse transcriptase inhibitors. Nelfinavir and indinavir are protease inhibitors.

exposure – reduces the transmission rate of HIV by over 70%.

Hepatitis B vaccination

The usual course is three doses of 1 ml (20 μg), the second 1 month and the third 6 months after the first dose. For children (birth up to 12 years) this is reduced to three doses of 0.5 mL (10 μg). The deltoid muscle is the preferred site of injection in adults while the anterolateral thigh is used in children. The buttock must not be used as vaccine

efficacy may be reduced. An accelerated course of hepatitis B vaccine is the preferred schedule for emergency usage; one dose is given immediately and then two more doses with an interval of 1 month between each injection. *For the indications for hepatitis B vaccination in an individual patient see Box 21.10.*

Hepatitis B immunoglobulin

Hepatitis B immunoglobulin (HBIG) is usually obtained from the nearest Public Health Laboratory. It must be given as soon as possible after the incident for maximum effect and certainly within 48 h. The dose of HBIG varies with age:

● age 0–4 years: 200 iu (2 mL);
● age 5–9 years: 300 iu (3 mL);
● adults and children aged 10 and above: 500 iu (5 mL).

The large volume of HBIG should be given by deep intramuscular injection into the upper outer quadrant of the buttock. Concurrent hepatitis B vaccine should be given into a separate site (e.g. the deltoid area of the upper arm). *For the indications for HBIG in an individual patient see Box 21.10.*

Hepatitis B immunisation should be considered for all IV drug injectors who attend an ED.

Localised infections and inflammations

Hot red joints

Patients may present to an ED with a single acutely inflamed joint. This may be caused by:

● septic arthritis including gonococcal arthritis;
● crystal arthropathy (e.g. gout or pseudogout – *see page 400*);
● a bursitis in the area of the joint (*see pages 103 and 127 and Bunions on page 400*);
● a connective tissue disorder (rarely).

Septic arthritis

This is most likely to occur following:

● trauma, often minor;
● soft-tissue infection;

● osteomyelitis;

● a non-septic joint inflammation.

The most common joints to become infected are the interphalangeal joints and the knee. The joint is held in flexion and all movements are restricted by intense pain.

XR

Loss of joint space may be seen in septic arthritis. It is apparent early on in small joints. However, a normal radiograph does not exclude infection.

TX

If there is doubt then the patient should be assumed to have a septic arthritis until proved otherwise. Diagnostic joint aspiration is not recommended in the ED. Admission must be arranged under the care of either the orthopaedic or the rheumatology departments, as seems most appropriate from the likely underlying pathology.

Acute gout

The first metatarsophalangeal joint is the most common site for acute gout although the knee may sometimes be primarily affected. The patient presents with severe local pain and a red, swollen joint. There is extreme tenderness such that even the weight of the bedclothes can be unbearable. A pyrexia often accompanies the inflammation. Other causes of a painful joint must be excluded.

TX

A wool and crepe bandage is required to protect the joint, together with non-weight-bearing crutches. The inflamed area must be rested and elevated. A makeshift 'cage' to protect a painful foot at night can be made by cutting a hole out of a large cardboard box. Initial analgesia and anti-inflammatory activity is provided by NSAIDs. A first parenteral dose can be very beneficial.

The patient should be referred back to the GP in order that he or she can:

● assess progress;

● measure serum urate;

● exclude precipitating causes (full blood count and ESR indicated);

● consider allopurinol therapy.

Bunions

Hallux valgus with varus deformity of the first metatarsal bone causes prominence and osteoarthrosis of the first (big toe) metatarsophalangeal joint. An enlarged bursa develops on its medial aspect – this is termed a bunion. The patient may present to the ED with an acute exacerbation of this chronic condition.

TX

An infected bunion should be treated with oral antibiotics (e.g. flucloxacillin) and the patient advised to consult the GP about an orthopaedic referral.

Osteomyelitis

This diagnosis should always be considered when there is spontaneous or unresolving bony pain. The distal phalanges of the hands and the feet are the most common sites of osteomyelitis in ED patients. There is usually a history of a minor injury but then pain, swelling and redness persist beyond the expected time of resolution. An accompanying septic arthritis is common.

> Bone tumours may masquerade as bone or joint infection.

XR

After 10–14 days, radiographs show absorption of the underlying bone, giving a characteristic moth-eaten appearance. The neighbouring joint space may be lost if infection has spread to the joint.

TX

All patients with suspected osteomyelitis must be referred to the orthopaedic department immediately.

Cellulitis

Infection of the skin may arise around a wound or without any obvious port of entry. The patient is usually tired and anorexic with a raised temperature; slight nausea is common. The skin is red, swollen and hot but the degree of pain is variable. A cause should be sought but is usually not found.

Tx

Antipyretic analgesics and antibiotics should be prescribed. The infection may be streptococcal or staphylococcal and so a combination of flucloxacillin and penicillin V (phenoxymethylpenicillin) is appropriate. (The penicillin V is probably unnecessary as flucloxacillin has good activity against streptococci). Erythromycin can be given to patients who are allergic to penicillins. Admission for observation and IV therapy is necessary for extensive or progressing infections. Lesser cases can be treated with oral antibiotics at home but should be reviewed within 24–48 h. The limits of the infection should be marked on the skin with a pen so that changes are obvious at review.

Athlete's foot

This is a fungal infection, which gives rise to an itchy whitish area between the toes, usually in the space between the middle and the ring toes. It may be the cause of an ascending cellulitis and should always be looked for. It is treated with a topical cream such as clotrimazole.

Impetigo

A localised staphylococcal infection of the skin may cause an area of weeping inflammation with a yellow crust. This is impetigo and is a highly infectious condition. It is most commonly seen in children in the area around the mouth but may spread to other parts of the patient or to relatives and medical staff.

Tx

All patients should be advised of measures to contain the spread by:
• frequent and appropriate hand washing;
• avoidance of contact with the infected area;
• using own towel and cutlery, etc.
An anti-staphylococcal cream should be prescribed (e.g. mupirocin or fusidic acid). Severe cases or those with systemic upset will need oral flucloxacillin.

Herpes simplex infections

Herpes simplex may cause painful yellow blisters with surrounding inflammation on the fingers or face. There is often accompanying malaise, pyrexia and enlargement of related lymph nodes. Treatment is symptomatic – hygiene, dressings, analgesia and flucloxacillin for superadded infection. However, extensive gingivo-stomatitis in distressed children may necessitate admission.

Large abscesses

A great variety of large abscesses is inevitably seen in patients presenting to an ED. Amongst the commonest types are:
• axillary
• breast – *see page 318.*
• perianal – *see page 321.*
• pilonidal – *see page 321.*
• gluteal – *see page 322.*
• labial – *see page 318.*
These painful and distressing conditions should be treated under general anaesthesia in the privacy of an operating theatre.

Boils (furuncles)

A boil is an abscess arising from a hair follicle. The problem may be multiple or recurrent.

Tx

Small abscesses in appropriate sites in adults may be drained in the ED under local anaesthesia. Others need inpatient care.

Most abscesses should be drained with an incision along the lines of cleavage of the skin. In the limbs, a longitudinal incision is more appropriate to avoid damage to nerves, vessels and tendons. A surprising amount of lidocaine may be needed to achieve adequate anaesthesia for this procedure. The cavity should then be cleaned out and a ribbon coated with antiseptic inserted. This stops any bleeding and allows free drainage. (The cavity should not be packed too tightly as this impairs both drainage and healing.) A dressing should be applied over the whole area.

The patient will require oral analgesics to take out. The wound should be reviewed on the following day and the dressing changed.

Infected sebaceous cysts

Sebaceous cysts may become infected and painful. The resulting tender, red lump may be distinguished from a boil by:
1 the history of a pre-existing swelling;
2 the site (cysts are common in certain areas such as the back and the neck);
3 the presence of a central punctum (only sometimes visible);
4 the contents of the swelling (white, cheesy material).

Tx

In the early stages of infection, the inflamed cyst may respond to antibiotics (e.g. co-fluampicil). However, incision and drainage are often necessary and management is then identical to that detailed above for a boil. Sometimes an infected sebaceous cyst will disappear after discharging its contents but often the wall will need surgical removal at a later date.

Carbuncles

A carbuncle is a deep multiloculated infection of the skin, which involves a group of hair follicles. It has several openings each of which discharges pus. The patient is often a middle-aged male and the most common site is the back of the neck. The infection is painful and slow to settle; it may become chronic or recurrent.

Tx

The area should be cleaned and then pus extruded. Debridement or deroofing under local anaesthesia may be necessary. The patient will need oral antibiotics (e.g. flucloxacillin) and analgesia to take out. The carbuncle must be reviewed and frequent dressing changes arranged; this may be undertaken at the local health centre.

Skin lesions acquired from animals (zoonoses)

Orf begins as painless vesicles, which progress to red nodules with sunken centres containing pus.

The lesions then gradually discolour, crust and heal. No specific treatment is required. The causative virus is acquired from sheep and goats.

Cutaneous anthrax starts as a small vesicle, which becomes purulent. A painless skin lesion then develops at the site with a black eschar and a considerable amount of surrounding oedema and induration. Anthrax can be an occupational disease of people who work with large herbivorous mammals or their hide products but has also been spread by terrorist action. If inhaled, the spores of *Bacillus anthracis* cause a haemorrhagic pneumonia and septicaemia. Anthrax is a notifiable disease.

Tularaemia presents as pyrexia and indurated skin ulcers with lymphadenopathy. It is transmitted to humans by close contact with rabbits. Tularaemia is not endemic in the United Kingdom but occurs in Scandinavia, Eastern Europe and the United States. If inhaled, *Francisella tularensis* may cause a plague-like pneumonia.

Other skin lesions

Patients with an enormous variety of other skin lesions present to an ED over the years. Their detailed description is beyond the scope of this book. However, three lesions cause confusion more often than most:
1 *Erythema nodosum.* The characteristic fiery red, infiltrated lesions of erythema nodosum are seen on the knees, shins and forearms. They are very tender with an ill-defined border. Bruising may occur. Erythema nodosum is sometimes mistaken for an allergic reaction; larger patches may look like cellulitis. The condition is a reactive vasculitis to systemic diseases, infections and drugs. A recent streptococcal illness is by far the most common precipitant.
2 *Acute psoriasis.* A shower of small round patches of psoriasis (guttate psoriasis) may appear shortly after an infection (usually streptococcal in nature). It is most common in children. The rash settles slowly over several weeks and is often mistaken for a reaction to antibiotics.
3 *Lichen planus.* This dermatosis of uncertain aetiology is encountered far more frequently in MRCP

examinations than in reality. Shiny pink papules appear on the wrists, shins and lumbosacral area, often with involvement of the mucous membranes. Itching is a variable feature. The rash can look non-specific with an atypical distribution and so often gives rise to confusion. Treatment is aimed at controlling the itching with steroid creams and calamine lotion.

For the common rashes of childhood see page 341.

Paronychial infections

Infections around the nail folds of the fingers are a common cause of presentation to an ED.

Tx

Occasionally, the infection can be treated with antibiotics (e.g. flucloxacillin). More usually an abscess has formed, which requires drainage rather than antibiotics. The finger should be ring-blocked and a longitudinal incision made into the abscess such that the cut extends across the nail fold (*see Figure 21.2*). An antiseptic dressing is then applied and changed on the following day.

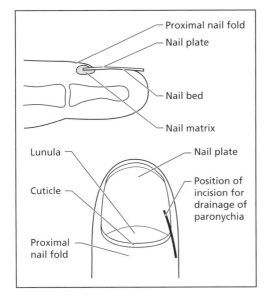

Figure 21.2 Direction of incision for paronychia. Divide the nail fold (but not the nail!).

Ingrowing toenails

This paronychial infection of the big toe commonly presents to an ED. The area alongside the distal toenail is red and tender. There may be a yellow exudate and, in chronic cases, tissue granulation.

Tx

Local policy varies according to the availability of chiropody services. A chiropodist will usually perform a wedge resection of the side of the nail and give advice on foot care. Recurrent cases should have the germinal matrix of the nail destroyed with phenol.

In the absence of a chiropodist, severe infection is best treated by removal of the entire nail under ring block. The patient then requires an antiseptic dressing, crutches and analgesia. He or she must be told to rest and elevate the foot. The dressing should be changed on the following day.

Frostbite

Cold injury is most likely to affect peripheral exposed parts such as fingers and toes and is not only seen in extreme climates. The frostbitten area is initially pale and extremely painful but, if exposure continues, the pain subsides. On rewarming, there is erythema, oedema and blistering and eventually a line of demarcation will appear at the junction with the undamaged tissue.

Tx

Analgesia should be given (together with IV fluids if more than fingers or toes are involved). Rapid rewarming of acute cases is achieved by total immersion of the affected part in warm water. The degree of permanent damage cannot be assessed when first seen and so admission for observation may be indicated.

Trench foot

This is a similar condition where tissue damage and maceration results from prolonged contact with cold, wet, muddy footwear. Treatment follows the same principles.

Wanderer's foot

No discussion of foot problems in a textbook of emergency medicine would be complete without a mention of this condition. The patient presents with macerated soles of the feet that are causing pain while walking. The shoes and socks are usually in poor condition and extremely smelly. There may be a history of homelessness and prolonged walking.

Tx

The feet should be washed and then soaked in antiseptic for an hour. Blisters should be slit open and any obvious infection treated. Crutches may be needed. Definitive treatment necessitates a place to stay so as to rest and bathe. New footwear may be required.
For homelessness see page 12.

Scabies

Infestation by the scabies mite causes intense itching, which is worse at night. Other close contacts may be affected.

If it itches, think of scabies.

At first, the mites affect only the areas where they burrow – between the fingers, wrists, genitalia, buttocks, axillae, waistline and the soles of the feet in children. Small linear tracks of papules may be the only evidence. Later, a sensitivity reaction to the mite causes a widespread papular eruption.

Tx

Malathion 0.5% aqueous lotion is applied to all areas of the body including the head and the face. It is left to dry naturally and then washed off after 24 h. Only one application is necessary provided that all areas are covered (e.g. the web spaces and under the finger nails). This will eradicate scabies in around 75% of cases. For those with persistent symptoms, a second application after 1 week is recommended. Permethrin 5% cream is a more expensive – and possibly more effective – alternative. It is applied to the whole body, washed off after 8–12 h and then reapplied after a week. The whole family and any close contacts must be treated, whether or not they have a rash; the GP should be asked to coordinate this. An oral sedative antihistamine may be required at night to control the itching.

Chapter 22

Ophthalmic, ENT and facial conditions

Injuries to the eye

Ophthalmic problems account for over 5% of all ED attendances.

Assessment of intra-ocular damage

- Obtain an accurate history.
- Ask about vision.
- Test the visual acuity (*see Box 22.1*).

Box 22.1 How to Test Visual Acuity

- Place a Snellen letter chart 6 m in front of the patient (or equivalent distance using a mirror).
- Test each eye separately with patient wearing normal spectacles.
- The number adjacent to each line of print on the chart is the denominator and the distance from the eye to print in metres is the numerator in the acuity equation.
- The largest print on the top line is usually '60' and the smallest print on the bottom line is usually '5'.
- A patient with normal acuity can read down to line 6 and is said to have 6/6 vision.
- If the patient cannot read the top line (i.e. acuity worse than 6/60) repeat the test at 3 m. Ability to read the top line is now described as 3/60 vision.

The bigger the fraction, the better the vision, i.e. 6/6 is good normal vision and 6/60 is poor reduced vision. Additional information can be obtained by asking the patient to look at the chart through a pinhole. Looking through a small hole improves vision in patients with a refractive or corneal abnormality but worsens vision in those with macular problems.

- Examine the eye with a pen torch looking for redness, discharge and other gross abnormalities. Look also for asymmetry and irregularity of the pupils.
- Note the pupillary response to direct light. Switch on the light after it has been placed in front of the eye. This is more likely to detect a small pupillary response than the more usual method of moving a light across the front of the eye.
- Test the cross-pupil reflex. When the damaged eye is illuminated, absence of pupil constriction in the opposite eye indicates interruption of the visual pathway.
- Assess ocular movements and visual fields, noting any diplopia. Eyelid movements must also be noted.

In the presence of blepharospasm (inability to open the eyes), further examination may require the application of local anaesthetic eye-drops, e.g. tetracaine (amethocaine) 1% or oxybuprocaine 0.4%.

- Evert the eyelids to allow examination of the fornices.
- Instil orange-coloured fluorescein drops to highlight any corneal damage – the injured epithelium appears green. A blue light makes a shallow pool of fluorescein much more easily visible.
- Examine the eye systematically from front to back using a slit-lamp and an ophthalmoscope. This may sometimes necessitate the administration of a short-acting mydriatic (a drug that dilates the pupil) such as tropicamide.

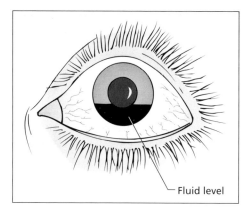

Figure 22.1 Hyphaema – blood in the anterior chamber.

The anterior chamber may contain blood, which collects inferiorly in the erect patient to produce a fluid level. This haemorrhage is called a hyphaema (*see Figure 22.1*). Damage to the lens or pupillary muscle will result in irregularities in the shape of the iris and disorganised or absent constriction to light. A laceration through the cornea will allow aqueous humour, muscle and even part of the lens to herniate anteriorly. Vitreous humour may be opacified by bleeding and the fundus thereby totally obscured.

> Whenever local anaesthetic has been applied to the conjunctival sac in the ED, it is advisable to pad the eye for protection for a few hours.

Corneal abrasions

Corneal abrasions may result from a scratch or other injury to the eye. Sometimes they follow prolonged rubbing of an irritating eye.
- The eye is red, injected, painful and watering.
- There is often pronounced blepharospasm (spasm of the eyelids).
- There may be a sensation of a foreign body.

Tx

A foreign body must be excluded, especially a subtarsal one (*see page 407*). The patient then requires the following:
- Dilatation of the pupil of the affected eye with a medium-duration mydriatic (e.g. cyclopentolate).

> **Box 22.2 Padding an Eye**
> - A single pad will not keep an eye closed.
> - To double pad, fold one pad in half and place it over the closed eyelids. Then place a second, flat pad over the first and secure it in place with three pieces of tape.
> - The patient should then be advised not to drive. Monocular vision impairs judgement of speed and distance; it may also invalidate motor insurance. Patients who intend to drive must be instructed on how to apply eye pads once at home.
> - Bilateral eye padding should be left until at home for all patients.
> - Patients require spare pads and tape to take away.

- Antibiotic ointment or viscous drops (e.g. fucidic acid) – three times a day for 3 days is sufficient and also easy to remember. The first dose should be instilled in the ED.
- A firm eyepad overnight (*see Box 22.2*).
- Instructions not to drive or operate machinery.
- Either a review appointment or instructions to return if there is not a marked improvement within 24 h.

Most abrasions heal spontaneously within 2 days. Remember to check tetanus immunisation status.

> Never give a patient local anaesthetic drops for outpatient use. They impede epithelial healing and invite additional injury. Similarly, NSAID drops or ointment are very effective at relieving pain but have the same effect on the corneal epithelium as oral NSAIDs have on the gastric mucosa.

Contact lens abrasions

Contact lense wearers may present with bilateral, large, shallow abrasions. There is often a history of prolonged use of hard lenses in a hot, dry, smoky atmosphere such as a night club.

Tx

This is similar to the treatment for any other abrasion but is complicated by the fact that the lesions affect both eyes. Bilateral pads leave the patient without vision and can be deferred until safely home. Glasses should be used instead of contact lenses for at least a week. The patient should be advised to get a supply of artificial tear drops to lubricate the eyes whenever they are in similar circumstances to those in which the problem occurred.

Subtarsal foreign body

Foreign material may lodge in the conjunctival sac. There is an anatomical trap under the upper eyelid. The signs are those of corneal damage.
• The eye is red, injected and watering.
• There is pain and blepharospasm.
• There is a marked foreign body sensation.
• There is increased discomfort on blinking (but small children may keep their eyes tightly shut for relief).
• Linear scratches to the superior cornea are extremely suggestive of a subtarsal foreign body.

Tx

Evert the eyelid, remove any foreign material, swab the tarsal conjunctiva and then treat as for a corneal abrasion. Local anaesthesia should be avoided if possible as the pain and foreign body sensation are dramatically relieved by the removal of the offending particles – a useful confirmation of the diagnosis.

Superficial foreign bodies imbedded in the eye

Fragments may fly into the eye while working (e.g. grinding) or may be blown in by the wind.
• The patient complains of a red, painful, watering eye.
• There is marked blepharospasm. (It may be necessary to instil local anaesthetic drops before the eyelids can even be opened satisfactorily.)
• The eye is injected and vision may be slightly blurred.
 Always consider the possibility of deeper damage with higher velocity injuries (*see page 408*).

Tx

Superficial fragments may be removed from the anaesthetised cornea using a cotton bud or a hypodermic needle. The resulting corneal ulcer should then be treated in the same way as a corneal abrasion.

Rust rings: Metallic, ferrous, foreign bodies produce rust rings if left in the cornea for more than a few hours. If the rust is not removed completely, the patient should be reviewed at the eye clinic after 48 h when the softened area of damage will easily 'shell out'.

'Arc' eye

This occurs in a welder, skier or ultraviolet sunbather with inadequate eye protection. The condition is caused by corneal absorption of ultraviolet light. Problems usually start several hours after exposure.
• Both eyes may be affected.
• The eyes are painful, weeping and red.
• There is usually blepharospasm and a sensation of a foreign body.
• Fluoroscein may reveal multiple tiny corneal erosions.

Tx

Symptoms can be relieved by the instillation of local anaesthetic and dilatation of the pupil. The patient is then given topical antibiotics and an eye pad. The condition should settle within 48 h.

Chemical splashes

Chemicals may cause inflammation of the conjunctiva or even a corneal burn. Patients present with an irritant or painful, watery, red eye. Alkalis may cause a penetrating eye injury.

Tx

Irrigate the eye with copious amounts of saline. This is best achieved by emptying a 500-mL bag into the conjunctival sac through a standard giving-set or by using a purpose-built irrigator. Ensure that both fornices are thoroughly washed and remove any lime or other fragments.

Fluorescein drops will help reveal the extent of the damage. Antibiotic ointment should then be prescribed. Serious injuries must be referred to an ophthalmologist immediately.

Penetrating injuries to the eye

Deep, foreign bodies are difficult to identify, produce greater morbidity and yet, initially, may not be as painful as superficial lesions. A good history is essential. There is a high risk of intra-ocular damage in patients with eye pain who have worked with:

- a hammer and chisel;
- glass;
- machinery that emits high-speed fragments;
- high-pressure water jets.

Fragments from grinding wheels rarely cause eye perforation.

The presence of hyphaema or prolapse of intra-ocular contents indicates severe injury, as does distortion of the pupil. Retained ferrous fragments will cause blindness as they are neurotoxic.

> The degree of pain that follows ocular trauma is not a reliable indicator of the severity of the injury.

XR

Fluorescein-aided corneal examination is followed by radiography of the eye. Lateral views with the eye looking up and down are particularly helpful in distinguishing foreign bodies from the unfamiliar but normal bone pattern and from specks on the film.

TX

Immediate specialist referral is essential but acuity should be assessed first and an eye pad applied. Pressure on the eyeball and coughing and straining by the patient must be avoided for fear of dislodging intra-ocular structures.

Severe blunt trauma to the eye

Damage to the globe of the eye most commonly results from sports injuries and assaults. Squash balls are particularly dangerous in this respect as they are small enough to enter the eye socket. Urgent ophthalmic referral is required in all cases. Pressure on the eyeball and coughing and straining by the patient must be avoided for fear of dislodging intra-ocular structures.

Hyphaema

Blood in the anterior chamber is caused by rupture of internal blood vessels (*see Figure 22.1*). The patient is at risk of acute (secondary) glaucoma and requires bed rest and observation. A hyphaema may occasionally be accompanied by iridodialysis – rupture of the insertion of the iris.

Traumatic mydriasis

Fixed dilatation of the pupil is a relatively common observation following blunt injury. The pupil may be distorted. Mydriasis is sometimes permanent. Traumatic miosis (constriction of the pupil) may also occur.

Dislocation of the lens

This is uncommon, although trauma is the most common cause. Cataract may also occur.

Posterior segment injuries

The best sign of this type of trauma is a sudden reduction in visual acuity. Injuries include vitreous haemorrhage and retinal damage such as tears, haemorrhage and detachment. Choroidal rupture and even globe rupture are occasionally seen.

TX

The presence of any of the above conditions is an indication for an urgent ophthalmic opinion. *For blow-out fractures of the floor of the orbit see page 73.*

Subconjunctival haemorrhage

Post-traumatic subconjunctival haemorrhage is common and usually trivial. Fluorescein may be used to reveal any conjunctival lacerations. Failure to visualise the posterior border of the haemorrhage may suggest orbital or retro-orbital trauma.

Spontaneous subconjunctival haemorrhage may follow coughing or straining. It is alarming to the patient but is usually of no consequence. Hypertension should be excluded.

Tx

No specific treatment is required but the patient should be warned that the discoloration may take several weeks to resolve.

The red eye

> **Box 22.3 The Assessment of the Acute Red Eye: Key Observations to Help in Diagnosis**
>
> Is the problem bilateral?
> Is there any associated visual loss?
> Is there a sensation of a foreign body?
> Is the eye uncomfortable and irritating or is it painful?
> Are the eyelids puffy or the conjunctiva oedematous?
> Is there any photophobia?
> Is the pupil irregular, dilated or unreactive?

In the absence of a history of trauma, the cause of a red eye can be difficult to determine. Key observations are shown in *Box 22.3*. Minor trauma is the most common cause of a red eye in the ED; *see previously for information about injuries to the eye.*

> • Topical anaesthetics inhibit epithelial healing and protective ocular reflexes.
> • Topical steroids may exacerbate herpes infections or precipitate glaucoma.

Infective conjunctivitis

This may be caused by several different agents.
• It is often bilateral.
• The eye is red, injected and uncomfortable with a gritty feeling.

Bacteria cause the classical, sticky eye, which is worse on waking.

Viral conjunctivitis results in itchy, watery eyes. There may be a concurrent URTI (upper respiratory tract infection). Injected follicular swelling in the lower fornix is a characteristic finding, as is a preauricular lymph node.

Adenovirus causes a painful, puffy, watery red eye. The condition is slow to resolve and is very infectious.

Tx

As it may be difficult to differentiate between the types of infectious conjunctivitis, it is usual practice to treat them all with a topical antibiotic (e.g. chloramphenicol ointment or gentamicin eye drops).

> Ocular conditions that have not significantly improved after 24 h merit a specialist opinion.

Allergic conjunctivitis

This is caused by exposure to eye-drops, plants or other allergens and is associated with atopy. Chloramphenicol, neomycin and atropine are the most common drug offenders.
• It is the most common cause of a puffy, red eye.
• There is lid swelling and conjunctival oedema (chemosis).
• It is irritating but not painful.

Tx

Remove the offending substance. Eye-drops containing a vasoconstrictor and an antihistamine (e.g. Otrivine-Antistin drops) may be helpful.

Acute conjunctival oedema

Acute conjunctival oedema is sometimes seen without other signs of allergy, especially in children. The conjunctiva may balloon out of the lower fornix in a very alarming way.

Tx

Local application of vasoconstrictor drops may be dramatically effective (*see before*).

Episcleritis

This condition is idiopathic and self-limiting.
- It is uncomfortable and may be painful.
- A discrete area of conjunctiva is injected and swollen.

Tx

Ophthalmological referral is required. NSAIDs can be helpful.

Orbital cellulitis

This is most common in young children and arises from an infection of an adjacent sinus or eyelid. There may be a history of URTI.
- The eye is red and the eyelids are puffy.
- Swelling may be painless at first but within hours there is pain, fever and distress.

Tx

Admission and treatment with IV antibiotics is required. Referral may be made to an ENT surgeon, ophthalmologist or paediatrician, as suggested by the most likely origin of the infection and local policy.

Corneal ulcers

Dendritic ulcers

These are caused by herpes simplex infection of the cornea.
- The eye is red and photophobic.
- There may be a foreign body sensation.
- There is a branching ulcer that stains with fluroscein.

Tx

Referral and therapy with acyclovir is required. Inappropriate steroid therapy can lead to corneal destruction and the need for a graft.

Bacterial corneal ulcers

These may occur in patients with chronic corneal disease or corneal exposure as a result of lid disorders.
- The eye is red and painful.
- There is an intracorneal opacity.

Tx

Referral without antibiotic prescription.

Uveitis (iritis)

This is an idiopathic inflammation of the anterior intra-ocular structures. It is often recurrent and in young adults may be associated with ankylosing spondylitis. There is:
- a red and painful eye with circumcorneal injection;
- tenderness of the eye;
- photophobia;
- adhesions between the pupillary margin and the lens (synechiae), which may cause irregular dilatation of the pupil;
- a haze over the cornea, especially the lower half.

Tx

Local anaesthesia does not relieve symptoms; mydriasis may help. Urgent referral to an ophthalmologist is required.

Glaucoma

Acute angle-closure glaucoma is a disease of the over-40s and especially the elderly. It is associated with severe long-sightedness. Impaired outflow of aqueous humor from the anterior chamber of the eye causes raised intra-ocular pressure. Clinical features include:
- a red, painful eye, which is injected and tender and feels hard on palpation through the lid;
- visual loss, with the appearance of haloes around lights;
- a semidilated, ovoid pupil, which does not react to direct or consensual light stimuli;
- corneal haze caused by oedema;
- malaise, nausea and vomiting.

Tx

Immediate ophthalmic referral is essential. Discuss initial treatment that may include:
• parenteral analgesics and antiemetics;
• pilocarpine eye-drops every 5 min for up to an hour;
• acetazolamide 500 mg orally or by slow IV injection;
• mannitol 20% (up to 500 mL) by slow IV infusion.

Recurrent corneal erosion

There is usually a history of a previous minor corneal injury. The patient describes a sharp discomfort on waking that settles after a few hours and then worsens over a few days. The signs are those of corneal damage.

Tx

Referral and lubricating eye ointment at night for several months.

Marginal keratitis

This is a recurrent condition. There is:
• a red, injected eye;
• photophobia;
• a sensation of a foreign body within the eye;
• small, white patches within the cornea, close to the limbus, which do not stain well with fluorescein. These are sterile inflammatory infiltrates.

Tx

Referral to the next eye clinic.

The eyelids

For injuries to the eyelids see page 74.

Blepharospasm

Spasm of the muscles that close the eye should immediately suggest an underlying problem, such as a corneal abrasion. The application of local anaesthetic drops through the narrow palpebral fissure will usually result in relaxation after a few minutes. The eye can then be examined properly.

Blepharitis

Inflammation of the eyelids should be treated with a topical antibiotic and advice on bathing the eyelids.

Lumps on the eyelids

Small cystic swellings of the eyelid glands are common (Meibomian cysts or chalazia). They may become inflamed. The patient should be given a topical antibiotic ointment and referred to the ophthalmology outpatient clinic.

Sudden loss of vision

Sudden visual loss is distressing for the patient as he or she fears that it will herald permanent blindness.

Retinal detachment

• Visual loss often described as 'like a curtain'.
• Sensation of flashing lights.
• Detached retina appears dark through an ophthalmoscope.
• Associated with severe short-sightedness.

Retinal venous occlusion

• Sudden visual loss of varying degrees.
• Congested, haemorrhagic retina.
• May only involve one tributary of the retinal vein and hence one quadrant of the retina.
• Increasing incidence with age.
• More common than arterial occlusion.

Retinal arterial occlusion

• Acute, unilateral, visual loss.
• Pale, ischaemic retina with a 'cherry-red spot' at the macula and a swollen optic disc.
• May be associated with temporal arteritis (need for urgent ESR) – *see page 232.*

● Pressure on the globe may dislodge the obstruction, which can be thrombus or embolus.
● After about an hour, optic nerve atrophy will result in permanent blindness.

Amaurosis fugax

● Visual loss with the same mechanism and associations as a transient ischaemic attack of other regions of the brain. *See page 235.*
● Often wrongly diagnosed in place of the previously cited conditions.

Vitreous haemorrhage

● Occurs in diabetics with new vessel formation.
● Absent red reflex/retina cannot be visualised.

Macular disease

● Sudden visual reduction with distortion.
● May be related to diabetes or other ocular pathology.
● May need urgent laser photocoagulation.

Cortical blindness

This worrying condition may follow a head injury and may persist for several hours. *See page 46.*

Migraine

This may cause visual distortion or field defects. *See page 232.*

Tx

All patients with acute visual loss require an immediate ophthalmological opinion. Thrombolysis (with streptokinase) may be recommended for central retinal venous or arterial thrombosis.

The ear

For injuries to the pinna see page 73.
For URTI in children see page 341.
For haemotympanum and bleeding from the ear canal see pages 44 and 45.
For barotrauma see page 241.

Earache

Pain in the ear is a distressing condition for both adults and children. Examination of the canal and drum will usually differentiate between otitis media and otitis externa, although the presence of a discharge may make the distinction more difficult. Pain following pressure on the tragus or gentle otoscopy strongly suggests that the canal is inflamed. Pus in the meatus usually comes from the middle ear via a ruptured tympanum, although a boil in the canal may also leak pus.

Tx

Otitis media should be treated with analgesic antipyretics and amoxicillin (or erythromycin). Some patients will require stronger analgesia (e.g. an injectable NSAID). Tympanic rupture should be reviewed after 2 weeks (GP or ENT follow-up). Otitis externa is treated with drops containing both an antibiotic and an anti-inflammatory steroid (e.g. gentamicin and hydrocortisone). Oral flucloxacillin should also be prescribed. The inflamed ear must be kept clean and dry. Patients with debris in the canal should be referred for aural toilet.

Problems with ear-rings

Ear-lobe piercing may introduce infection, including serum hepatitis, but more often it causes problems because of inadequate hygiene in the postoperative period. Not uncommonly, a patient complains of a lost 'butterfly' – the rolled clip used to secure the stud or 'sleeper'. The missing metal can be felt embedded in the inflamed ear-lobe.

Tx

The ear-lobe should be anaesthetised by slowly injecting it with 1–2 mL of lidocaine 2% without adrenaline.

> Do not inject local anaesthetic solutions containing adrenaline into the ear or nose.

The foreign body can then be easily and painlessly removed from behind using splinter forceps. The area should be treated with a local antiseptic.

Foreign bodies in the ear

Patients may present acutely with a missing foreign body or chronically with a discharging ear. In an adult, the lost object is usually the tip of a cotton bud; in a child, more variety can be expected!

Tx

The ear should be examined gently but no attempt made to remove anything but the most superficial objects in a struggling child. Loops can be used as can Hartmann's 'crocodile' forceps and wax hooks. Syringing is another option (*see Box 22.4*). The method used depends on personal experience, although attempts to remove foreign bodies lying close to the ear-drum should be limited to syringing only. If removal is unsuccessful, referral should be arranged to the next ENT clinic. A slight delay before removal is not important but inexpert manipulation, with inadequate instruments, a poor light and a struggling child, can produce major injuries to the tympanic membrane. The chronically discharging ear should also be seen in the ENT clinic.

Insects can crawl or fly into the auditory canal where their movements cause great distress. Before removal, they can be killed by pouring olive oil into the canal.

Sudden hearing loss

Sudden hearing loss is commonly caused by the movement of accumulated wax in the external auditory canal. This causes an obstructive type of deafness. Wax can be removed by syringing, a procedure usually performed at the local health centre. The removal can be eased, and the patient helped, by recommending the purchase of drops to loosen the wax (e.g. Exterol).

Sudden hearing loss of the sensorineural type is an indication for urgent ENT referral. Occasionally, it may be caused by a cerebrovascular accident.

> ### Box 22.4 How to Syringe an Ear
>
> • Ask about possible complications (e.g. known perforation).
> • Warm some sodium chloride 0.9% solution to 38°C. Temperature deviation of any significance may cause profound vertigo.
> • Examine the canal with an auroscope.
> • Drape the patient with towels and position the ear tank. An assistant is usually necessary.
> • Straighten the canal by pulling the pinna upwards and backwards.
> • A manual or, preferably, a pulsed electric ear syringe should be used. Direct the water jet upwards and backwards along the roof of the canal, aiming for the patient's occiput not the eardrum (*Figure 22.2*). A strong jet of water may perforate a scarred drum.
> • Stop immediately if the patient complains of pain or vertigo or if there is any bleeding.
> • During the procedure, re-examine the canal periodically.
> • Mop away excess fluid afterwards.

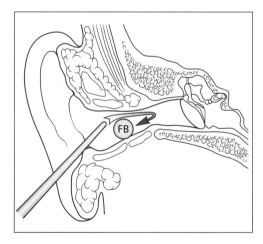

Figure 22.2 Direction of fluid stream to wash out an aural foreign body.

The nose

Nasal foreign bodies

These usually accompany small children and anxious patients. If superficial they can be removed in the ED but often they are deep and surrounded by crusty exudate, having been in place for some days. There may be a purulent discharge.

> Unilateral nasal discharge in a small child is usually caused by a retained foreign body, even if this history is denied.

Tx

Try occluding the unblocked nostril with gentle alar pressure and getting the child to blow with his or her mouth closed. This is often successful. An alternative is to suck the object out with a Yankauer sucker with the side holes taped up. If these measures fail, early specialist referral is recommended. Inexpert probing with forceps or artery clips may push the object further back and cause airway obstruction. Any forceps used for even proximal removal should be of the Tilley's type with a parallel blade, which will not apply a force in a backwards direction.

Epistaxis

Arterial bleeding from Little's area on the anterior wall of the nasal septum is responsible for around 90% of epistaxis in adults. However, in children, nasal bleeding usually comes from the retrocolumellar vein and follows infection or trauma (with a finger). Clotting disorders including drug therapy and telangiectasia must be considered in all patients and there is evidence that epistaxis is associated with regular excessive consumption of alcohol. The blood pressure should be measured.

> Pressure to stop a nose bleed should be applied by firmly squeezing the soft part of the nose between the fingers. The most common reasons for failure are misplaced compression over the nasal bones and lack of constant pressure.

Tx

- Attempt to arrest haemorrhage with alar pressure. A swimmer's nose clip can be used for this purpose.
- Resuscitate if necessary (IV fluids).
- Consider cross-match, full blood count and clotting studies.
- Cauterisation with silver nitrate can be useful for small anterior bleeds.

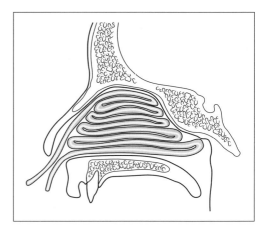

Figure 22.3 Anterior nasal packing.

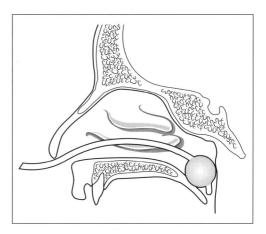

Figure 22.4 Foley catheter in the nasopharynx.

- Anterior bleeding may also be limited by a wet nasal tampon or a pack (*see Figure 22.3*).
- Bleeding from a more posterior site can be controlled by the careful insertion and inflation of a balloon catheter (*see Figure 22.4*).
- Antiseptic cream (e.g. Naseptin) should be prescribed to prevent recurrent bleeding, especially in children.

Urgent ENT referral is required for severe nasal bleeding of any causation. Recurrent epistaxis merits follow-up in the ENT clinic. Patients who have been seen earlier in the ED and who then return with a further episode of epistaxis are also best discussed with an ENT surgeon.

The mouth and throat

For the management of choking see page 205.
For other airway obstruction including foreign bodies see pages 206 and 207.

Small foreign bodies stuck in the throat

Patients commonly complain of a foreign body stuck in the throat, usually after eating fish. Ask about the ability to swallow solids and fluids; this is usually unaffected. *For oesophageal obstruction see below.*

Examination requires a good light and a cooperative patient. An instrument tray for ENT use should be available. Dentures are removed and examined for completeness. The mouth is inspected; the area around the fauces is a common site to find a fish bone. Foreign bodies often lodge in the piriform fossae and are usually radiolucent. A mucosal tear may produce identical symptoms to an impacted foreign body.

XR

A lateral radiograph of the soft-tissues of the neck will occasionally show a radio-opaque foreign body such as a chicken bone. Calcified laryngeal cartilages are a source of confusion.

Tx

Any obvious foreign body should be removed; a topical anaesthetic spray may help with this. Patients with a foreign-body sensation in whom no cause is found should be discussed with an ENT surgeon; they can usually be reviewed in the next clinic. Difficulty swallowing suggests bolus obstruction of the oesophagus – *see below.*

Oesophageal obstruction

A small group of patients have a sudden onset of dysphagia during a meal – often following an attempt to swallow a lump of meat. The blockage is usually localised to the upper chest and, in the most severe cases, the obstruction extends to fluids as well as to solids. If such patients are given a drink of water, regurgitation may be seen within a few seconds. Patients with disorders of oesophageal motility are particularly prone to this problem and devices that reduce palatal sensation (e.g. denture plates) predispose to it.

XR

An oblique radiograph of the chest is the best projection for the detection of radio-opaque material in the oesophagus. Neck films may show an oesophageal fluid level. Surgical emphysema may also be seen.

Tx

The patient must be referred immediately for surgical assessment and oesophagoscopy in theatre. Oesophageal tears may produce mediastinitis, which is often fatal.

Swallowed foreign bodies

This is generally a problem of children and some patients with psychiatric conditions. Rounded objects such as coins are the most frequently swallowed. There may be initial coughing but thereafter the patient is usually symptomless. An oesophageal foreign body is suggested by dysphagia and retrosternal discomfort but this is by no means inevitable. Examination should include the fauces, the upper airway and the lung fields.

The narrowest sites for obstruction are at the cricopharyngeal sphincter, the upper third of the oesophagus at the level of the aortic arch and the cardia. Objects that pass into the stomach will usually traverse the entire gastrointestinal tract within 2–6 days, but may not uncommonly take 2–4 weeks. The two exceptions are:

1 irregularly shaped articles such as open safety pins, which may impact, especially on the pylorus; and
2 very long, straight objects, which may not be able to negotiate the duodenal loop.

415

> Most foreign bodies that cause a problem are lodged in, or have damaged, the oesophagus.

XR

In the case of radio-opaque objects (the majority), X-rays should be obtained of the chest, abdomen and neck (in that order) until the foreign body is located. For a small child this only takes one film. In an anteroposterior view of the neck, a coin in the larynx appears side-on as a bar, whereas a coin in the oesophagus appears as a round disc.

> Thin aluminium objects (e.g. can ring-pulls) and some dental prostheses are not radio-opaque.

TX

For the management of foreign bodies in the airway see page 205.

Patients with foreign bodies in the pharynx or oesophagus should be referred to an ENT surgeon immediately for removal at oesophagoscopy.

Foreign bodies in the stomach or bowel usually pass uneventfully, although this may take several weeks. The parents should be told to bring the child back if abdominal symptoms develop.

Ingested sharp objects require observation and either removal or tracking with frequent radiographs.

Glass may be swallowed, especially by psychiatric patients or those with a personality disorder. It may be seen on X-ray and is usually harmless.

Ingestion of 'button' batteries

Small 'button cell' batteries are sometimes swallowed by children. They may stick and damage the bowel electrically or disintegrate and release toxic contents.

> One in 20 children who have ingested button batteries will have swallowed more than one cell.

There are four main types of button cell:
1 mercury (1.5 V);
2 silver (1.5 V, usually non-toxic);
3 alkaline manganese (1.5 V); and

4 lithium (3 V, but more resistant to corrosion; not usually swallowed as it is used inside watches and replaced by a jeweller).

Mercury batteries are the most dangerous, especially when new. Used cells are less likely to leak or cause tissue injury and, in discharged mercury batteries, the mercuric oxide will be largely converted to elemental mercury, is not absorbed. Late signs of ingestion include:
- fever;
- abdominal pain;
- vomiting;
- blood in the stools.

XR

Obtain radiographs of the chest, neck and abdomen until the exact position of the battery is established. Children with button cells in the stomach need daily abdominal films to show transit and to detect disintegration. Batteries in the bowel should be tracked every 3 or 4 days.

TX

For the management of foreign bodies in the airway see page 205.

> Chemical burns in the mouth suggest that the battery was leaking before ingestion.

- Identify the type of battery involved from the packaging or a matching or similar battery and determine whether it is new or old. Not all button cells are marked with numbers.
- Get more information about the battery contents from:
   1 a poisons information service by phone or modem link;
   2 the battery ingestion guidelines, which are produced by the British Battery Manufacturers' Association and are sent to all UK departments of emergency medicine.
- Oral antacids or milk may help to reduce battery corrosion. Emesis is contraindicated.

For the indications for referral for the removal of button cells see Box 22.5. (Endoscopic or magnetic removal is often possible.)

Box 22.5 Indications for Referral for Removal of Button Cells

Any button cell in the airway.
Any button cell in the oesophagus.
Any button cell remaining in the stomach for more than
    48 h, especially new, undischarged ones.
Any button cell static in the gut for a prolonged period,
    especially new, undischarged ones.
Any button cell where the ingestion is accompanied by
    signs of peritonitis.
Mercury cell in the stomach for more than 24 h.
Mercury cell disintegrating in the stomach.

Batteries in the oesophagus must be removed immediately.

Batteries in the stomach usually pass from the bowel with no problems but all children who have swallowed button batteries should be followed-up after 24 h with a repeat X-ray.

Mercury batteries that are thought to be leaking or have remained in the stomach for more than 24 h must be removed. It is advisable to measure mercury concentrations in the blood and urine when leakage is thought to have occurred.

All children who have swallowed button cell batteries must be admitted or followed-up in clinic.

Sore throat

Pharyngitis, laryngitis and tonsillitis are common and usually result from a viral infection. Some patients will have a bacterial infection but clinical differentiation is almost impossible.

Tx

Symptomatic relief with paracetamol is usually sufficient. Pragmatic treatment is to give antibiotics to patients who are systemically unwell or have severe local symptoms and signs. Penicillin V (phenoxymethylpenicillin), an oral cephalosporin or erythromycin are appropriate.

Amoxicillin or ampicillin may cause a florid rash in patients with glandular fever.

Infectious mononucleosis, cytomegalovirus infection and toxoplasmosis may cause a prolonged sore throat with systemic symptoms.

Diphtheria

Between 1990 and 1999, over 158,000 cases of diphtheria and 4000 deaths were reported in the countries of the former Soviet Union. Diphtheria has re-emerged because of falling levels of immunisation.

Diphtheria is caused by infection with the bacterium *Corynebacterium diphtheriae*, which is droplet spread with an incubation period of 1 to 5 days. Following the introduction of immunisation against diphtheria on a national scale in the United Kingdom in 1940, there was a dramatic fall in the number of notified cases of the disease. From 1986 to 2002, 103 cases of diphtheria were identified and two deaths were reported. The first symptom of diphtheria is usually a mild pharyngitis causing pain with swallowing. Other typical features are:
- low-grade fever (less than 38.5°C);
- headache, nausea and vomiting;
- inflammation of the larynx and nasal passages;
- pharyngeal exudate forming a thick greyish 'pseudomembrane';
- swollen lymph nodes ('bull-neck' appearance);
- pallor and tachycardia;
  Complications include:
- respiratory obstruction;
- pneumonia;
- otitis media and sinusitis;
- myocarditis, peripheral neuritis and nephritis;
- shock and organ failure.

Tx

Patients with suspected diphtheria should be admitted and discussed with a specialist in infectious diseases. Impending respiratory obstruction may require intubation or even tracheostomy. Diphtheria is treated with benzylpenicillin and sometimes with specific antitoxin. It is a notifiable disease – *see pages 383 and 384.*

Epiglottitis

This condition appears to be on the increase in adults. *Haemophilus influenzae* B, beta-haemolytic streptococci or even staphylococci may be responsible. It should be suspected when the degree of hoarseness and dysphagia appear to be disproportionate to the other signs.

Tx

This is the same as in children – *see page 330.*
• Reassure the patient and work calmly. Do not examine the throat.
• Summon skilled anaesthetic and ENT help immediately.
• Position the patient for maximum comfort.
• Administer high-concentration oxygen by mask.
• Consider using nebulised adrenaline (5 mg) by mask to buy time.

IV cefotaxime or chloramphenicol are used to treat *Haemophilus influenzae* epiglottitis.
For stridor in children see page 330.

Swellings in and around the mouth

Dental abscess

Large abscesses arising from dental infections may point externally. There will be a pyrexia and the carous tooth may be tender to the touch. Trismus may limit intra-oral examination.

Swollen salivary glands

Salivary glands may swell because of obstruction, tumour or infection. Obstruction by a stone may cause increased symptoms when the production of saliva is increased (i.e. eating). Mumps must be remembered as a common parotid infection – *see page 420.* Bacterial parotitis may occur in debilitated patients.

Quinsy

Peritonsillar abscess presents as a large, unilateral swelling in an unwell patient with a history of tonsillitis. The oedematous uvula is displaced to the opposite side. Dysphagia, halitosis and trismus are inevitable. The throat pain is often accompanied by earache and the cervical nodes are enlarged and tender. Sometimes the head is flexed to one side.

Retropharyngeal abscess

This condition usually occurs in infants and young children. Infection of the upper respiratory tract leads to a pyogenic adenitis of the retropharyngeal lymph nodes. The resulting abscess is limited to one side of the midline by a median raphe – *see Figure 22.5.* The child is obviously unwell and has:
• a high pyrexia
• dysphagia (dribbling saliva)
• noisy breathing or stridor (not inevitable)
• a smooth unilateral swelling of the posterior pharyngeal wall.

The head may be held flexed to one side.

XR

A lateral soft-tissue view of the neck may show marked soft-tissue expansion in the retropharyngeal space, which pushes the trachea forwards.

Other soft-tissue infections

Cellulitis of the floor of the mouth may cause dangerous swelling (Ludwig's angina). It is most

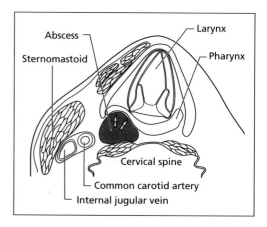

Figure 22.5 Retropharyngeal abscess.

common in young children. There may be associated dental sepsis. Vincent's angina may affect the pharyngeal and tonsillar area.

For diphtheria see page 417.

Tx

Acute swellings with pain or pyrexia are indications for immediate referral to the appropriate specialist. Conditions compromising the airway should be treated in exactly the same way as epiglottitis – *see page 418.*

Other throat and neck symptoms

Several conditions may give misleading symptoms in the throat. In particular, the following should be noted.

Dystonia

Bizarre intermittent problems with speech and swallowing may be the only signs of an acute dystonic reaction – *see page 296.*

Tetanus

Tetanus (which is sometimes called 'lock-jaw') may start with jaw stiffness and trismus – *see page 239.*

Pneumomediastinum

The most common symptoms caused by air in the mediastinum are neck pain and dysphagia – *see page 203.*

Bleeding after tonsillectomy

Patients (usually children) may be brought to an ED with post-tonsillectomy bleeding. This may occur a few hours after the procedure or, if secondary to infection, after a few days. Bleeding may occasionally be severe enough to threaten the airway. The patient should be placed in the recovery position (unless unhappy with this posture) and oxygen administered. Gentle suctioning may

help to clear the airway. FBC and blood grouping should be requested and IV access obtained. Immediate ENT referral is appropriate; an anaesthetic opinion may also be required.

For acquired haemophilia and anticoagulation problems see pages 263 and 264.

Bleeding from a tooth socket after dental extraction

The bleeding must be localised with the aid of a good light and suction. The patient should be:
- sat upright;
- reassured; and
- asked to bite on a gauze pad for 5 min.

If this does not stop the bleeding, an adrenaline pack or a piece of gel foam may be tried. Rarely, the socket may require oversewing. Post-extraction bleeding is more likely to occur in the presence of infection and will itself increase the risk of infection. Antibiotics should be prescribed. Contributory factors such as haemophilia and anticoagulant therapy must be considered – *see pages 263 and 264.*

Toothache

This condition is usually seen in an ED 'out of hours'. The patient is distressed and in pain. The teeth may be generally carous and in need of dental care or show little sign of any problem. The cause of the pain is usually local inflammation – pulpitis or pericoronitis – and gentle tapping of the tooth or gum may exacerbate the pain. Sometimes, a periapical or periodontal abscess may be forming.

Tx

Considerable relief may follow the injection of a NSAID (e.g. tenoxicam 20 mg IM). Antibiotics (amoxicillin or metronidazole) and strong analgesia should also be supplied. The patient must see their own dentist as soon as possible.

For the numbering system that is used to describe teeth see page 72 (Box 5.2).

For dental injuries see pages 72 and 73.

The face

Facial pain

Sinusitis

This can occur in any of the 4 groups of sinuses. There may be facial pain and tenderness in the affected area together with headache and pyrexia. The pain may be periodic. Chemosis, proptosis and other eye signs may be seen. The urgency of referral should depend on the signs. First-line antibiotics for sinusitis are amoxicillin, erythromycin or doxycycline.

Shingles

Herpes zoster infection may cause acute facial pain. Oral acyclovir therapy is effective in limiting prolonged symptoms but is expensive. Shingles of the ophthalmic division of the trigeminal nerve (5a) may damage the cornea and thus requires ophthalmic advice. The usual treatment is with topical acyclovir.

Facial palsy

Bell's palsy is an idiopathic condition causing a unilateral lower motor neuron paralysis of the face. It is associated with discomfort in the vicinity of the mastoid and develops over 48 h. It must be differentiated from a stroke affecting the face. The classical sign used for this purpose is the failure to wrinkle the forehead on the affected side in Bell's palsy. In an upper motor neuron condition this movement is likely to be unaffected as the upper part of the face has bilateral cortical representation.

> Look in the ears of patients with facial palsy. A herpetic infection of the meatus and tympanic membrane may be identified (Ramsay Hunt's syndrome). Severe earache and malaise precedes the development of the palsy by 24–48 h. Vertigo, deafness, loss of taste and vesicles in the fauces may also occur.

Tx

Bell's palsy resolves spontaneously over a few weeks in 90% of patients. To prevent residual problems in the remainder, early prophylactic treatment with steroids has been advocated. Although there is little evidence to support this therapy, many doctors prescribe a short course of high-dose oral prednisolone (40 mg for adults or 1 mg per kg for children daily for 5 days). Patients who have difficulty in closing one eye also need a supply of eye pads to protect the cornea at night.

Suspicion of cerebrovascular disease should prompt medical referral. Patients with facial palsy accompanied by a discharging ear, a cholesteatoma or vesicles should be referred to an ENT specialist.

Mumps

Infection with the mumps virus has a long incubation period (18–21 days or more) and seems to be on the increase. Mumps parotitis causes pyrexia, malaise and progressive tender facial swelling around the angle of the jaw. In 80% of cases, both parotid glands are affected. There may also be cervical adenitis, intra-oral swelling of the orifice of the parotid ducts and occasionally presternal oedema. The illness usually resolves spontaneously within 7–10 days. Complications include meningo-encephalitis, pancreatitis and inflammation of almost any other glandular tissue. Orchitis is seen in about a quarter of postpubertal males with mumps. It is usually unilateral and may lead to testicular atrophy.

For facial swellings originating from the mouth see page 418.

For diphtheria see page 417.

INDEX

Note: Page number in italics refers to figures and tables.